Chronic Illness

Chronic Illness

Impact and Interventions

Sixth Edition

Ilene Morof Lubkin, RN, MS, CGNP
Professor Emeritus
California State University
Hayward, California

and

Pamala D. Larsen, PhD, RN, FNGNA
Professor
Fay W. Whitney School of Nursing
University of Wyoming
Laramie, Wyoming

JONES AND BARTLETT PUBLISHERS
Sudbury, Massachusetts
BOSTON   TORONTO   LONDON   SINGAPORE

World Headquarters
Jones and Bartlett Publishers
40 Tall Pine Drive
Sudbury, MA 01776
978-443-5000
info@jbpub.com
www.jbpub.com

Jones and Bartlett Publishers
Canada
6339 Ormindale Way
Mississauga, Ontario
L5V 1J2
CANADA

Jones and Bartlett Publishers
International
Barb House, Barb Mews
London W6 7PA
UK

Jones and Bartlett's books and products are available through most bookstores and online booksellers. To contact Jones and Bartlett Publishers directly, call 800-832-0034, fax 978-443-8000, or visit our website www.jbpub.com.

Substantial discounts on bulk quantities of Jones and Bartlett's publications are available to corporations, professional associations, and other qualified organizations. For details and specific discount information, contact the special sales department at Jones and Bartlett via the above contact information or send an email to specialsales@jbpub.com.

Production Credits
Acquisitions Editor: Kevin Sullivan
Production Director: Amy Rose
Associate Editor: Amy Sibley
Associate Production Editor: Daniel Stone
Marketing Manager: Emily Ekle
Composition: Auburn Associates, Inc.
Cover Design: Kristin Ohlin
Printing and Malloy, Inc.
Cover Printing: Malloy, Inc.

ISBN-13: 978-0-7637-3594-4
ISBN-10: 0-7637-3594-9

Library of Congress Cataloging-in-Publication Data

Chronic illness : impact and interventions / [edited by] Ilene Morof
Lubkin, Pamala D. Larsen.—6th ed.
       p. ; cm.
   Includes bibliographical references and index.
   ISBN 0-7637-3594-9
   1. Chronic diseases—Psychological aspects.   2. Chronic diseases—
Nursing.   3. Chronically ill—Family relationships.   4. Nurse and patient.
I. Lubkin, Ilene Morof, 1928–   . II. Larsen, Pamala D., 1958–   .
   [DNLM: 1. Chronic Disease—psychology.   2. Professional-Family
Relations.   WT 500 C5577 2006]
RC108.L83 2006
616'.044—dc22
                                         2005025299

6048

Printed in the United States of America
10   09   08   07   06   10 9 8 7 6 5 4 3

CONTENTS

As professional nurses, we are cognizant of our history, the pioneers in our discipline, and those who have made an impact on our profession. Allow me to add Ilene Lubkin to the list of nurses who have made a difference in the nursing discipline. This is the 6th edition of "Ilene's book," but she is not here for its publication because she passed away on April 21, 2005.

In 1986 Ilene published the 1st edition of her book, *Chronic Illness: Impact and Interventions*. At that time I was teaching at another university, and we were developing a master's degree in chronic illness. As we looked for appropriate texts, we found that there were many that discussed chronic disease, but none that addressed what the client and family, were experiencing, until we discovered Ilene's book. Her book discussed the illness experience of the client and family, and interventions that could help these clients. The book talked about the illness experience of the client and *caring* for the *whole* client. Sounds like nursing, doesn't it?

I was privileged to be asked by Ilene to co-edit the 4th edition of her book, the 5th, and now the 6th edition. Although Ilene and I had many phone and email conversations, we never met. What made our relationship work was the passion that we both shared about our clients with chronic illness. Ilene was passionate about everything she did, even in retirement. May you be passionate as you practice nursing, and allow this book to provide a framework for your practice.

Pamala D. Larsen

CONTRIBUTORS

Ilene Morof Lubkin, RN, MS, CGNP
Professor Emeritus
California State University
Hayward, California

and

Pamala D. Larsen, PhD, RN, FNGNA
Professor
Fay W. Whitney School of Nursing
University of Wyoming
Laramie, Wyoming

Susan J. Barnes, RN, PhD
Associate Professor
School of Nursing
Southern Nazarene University
Bethany, Oklahoma

Jill Berg, RN, PhD
Assistant Professor
School of Nursing
University of California, Los Angeles
Los Angeles, California

Sandra Bergquist, RN, PhD
Associate Professor
School of Nursing
University of Kansas Medical Center
Kansas City, Kansas

Diana Luskin Biordi, RN, PhD, FAAN
Professor and Assistant Dean
Research and Graduate Affairs
College of Nursing
Kent State University
Kent, Ohio

Connie Burgess, RN, MS
Managing Partner
Health InterConnexions Inc.
Long Beach, California

Donna Carruthers, RN, PhD
Project Director
School of Nursing
University of Pittsburgh
Pittsburgh, Pennsylvania

Barbara Carson, RN, MSN, CRRN
Assistant Director of Nursing
Johns Hopkins Bayview Care Center
Baltimore, Maryland

Patricia A. Chin , RN, DNSc
Associate Professor
Department of Nursing
California State University, Los Angeles
Los Angeles, California

Jacqueline M. Dunbar-Jacob, RN, PhD, FAAN
Dean, School of Nursing
Professor of Nursing and Epidemiology
Director, Center for Research
  in Chronic Disorders
University of Pittsburgh
Pittsburgh, Pennsylvania

Lienne D. Edwards, RN, PhD
Associate Professor
School of Nursing
University of North Carolina at Charlotte
Charlotte, North Carolina

Judith A. Erlen, RN, PhD, FAAN
Professor and Doctoral Program Coordinator
Associate Director, Center for Research
  in Chronic Disorders
School of Nursing and
Professor, Center for Bioethics and Health Law
University of Pittsburgh
Pittsburgh, Pennslyvania

Lorraine S. Evangelista, RN, PhD
Assistant Professor
School of Nursing
University of California, Los Angeles

Gwendolyn F. Foss, RN, DNSc
Associate Professor
School of Nursing
University of North Carolina at Charlotte
Charlotte, North Carolina

Barbara B. Germino, RN, PhD, FAAN
Professor
School of Nursing
University of North Carolina at Chapel Hill
Chapel Hill, North Carolina

Sonya R. Hardin, RN, PhD
Associate Professor
School of Nursing
University of North Carolina at Charlotte
Charlotte, North Carolina

Faye I. Hummel, RN, CTN, PhD
Professor
School of Nursing
University of Northern Colorado
Greeley, Colorado

Marian Jamison, RN, MBA, PhD
Professor of Nursing
Graceland University
Independence, Missouri

Janet E. Jeffrey, RN, PhD
Associate Professor
School of Nursing
Atkinson Faculty of Liberal and Professional Studies
York University
Toronto, Ontario

Kathryn Jones, MSN, ACNP
Charlotte Cardiology Associates
Charlotte, North Carolina

Gregory P. Knapik, RN, MS
Doctoral Student
Kent State University/University of Akron
Kent, Ohio

Patricia Ryan Lewis, RN, PhD
Director, Rockford Regional Program
College of Nursing
University of Illinois at Chicago
Rockford, Illinois

Rosemary J. Mann, RN, CNM, JD, PhD
Associate Professor
Undergraduate Coordinator
School of Nursing
San Jose State University
San Jose, California

Cheryl P. McCahon, RN, PhD
Undergraduate Program Director
Associate Professor
School of Nursing
College of Education and Human Services
Cleveland State University
Cleveland, Ohio

Sue E. Meiner, EdD, APRN, BC, GNP
Nurse Practitioner – Pain Institute of Nevada
President, Consultant on Health Issues, Inc.
Las Vegas, Nevada

Linda A. Moore, EdD, APRN, BC (ANP, GNP),
  MSCN
Associate Professor
School of Nursing
University of North Carolina at Charlotte
Charlotte, North Carolina

Tama L. Morris, RNC, MSN
Senior Lecturer
School of Nursing
University of North Carolina at Charlotte
Charlotte, North Carolina

Geri B. Neuberger, RN, EdD
Professor
School of Nursing
University of Kansas Medical Center
Kansas City, Kansas

Ann Mabe Newman, APRN, BC, DSN
Associate Professor
School of Nursing
University of North Carolina at Charlotte
Charlotte, North Carolina

Lisa L. Onega, RN, PhD, FNP
Associate Professor of Gerontological Nursing
School of Nursing
Radford University
Radford, Virginia

Judith Papenhausen, RN, PhD
Director, School of Nursing
California State University, San Marcos
San Marcos, California

Margaret M. Patton, RN, MSN, MSEd
Presbyterian School of Nursing
Queens University at Charlotte
Charlotte, North Carolina

Barbara M. Raudonis, APRN, BC, PhD
Associate Professor
Director, Rural Health Outreach Program
School of Nursing
University of Texas at Arlington
Arlington, Texas

Robin E. Remsburg, APRN, BC, FNGNA, PhD
Deputy Director, Division of Health Care Statistics
National Center for Health Care Statistics
Hyattsville, Maryland

Victoria Schirm, RN, PhD
Director of Nursing Outcomes Research
Penn State/Milton S. Hershey Medical Center
Hershey, Pennsylvania

Betty Smith-Campbell, RN, PhD
Associate Professor
School of Nursing
Wichita State University
Wichita, Kansas

Diane L. Stuenkel, RN, EdD
Associate Professor
Curriculum & Professional Development
  Coordinator
San Jose State University
School of Nursing
San Jose, California

Andrea M. Warner, RN, MS
Doctoral Student
Kent State University/University of Akron
Kent, Ohio

Margaret Chamberlain Wilmoth, RN, PhD
Professor
School of Nursing
University of North Carolina at Charlotte
Charlotte, North Carolina

My mother, Ilene Ruth Lubkin, RN, MSN, GNP, died on April 21, 2005, at her home in Walnut Creek, California. In retrospect, at 76, my mom was at the peak of her intellectual and personal life. Physically, she was energetic, vibrant, and always active. Mentally, my mother was an amazing woman who continually impressed her friends, family, and colleagues with her outstanding memory, gentle charm, reassuring perspective, and uncanny wit. She was dedicated to several lifelong passions that included her ongoing education, teaching others, and helping anyone who needed help. She was a humanitarian in the truest sense of the word.

My mother graduated from Wayne State University's Nursing program in 1950. As a student nurse, she developed an interest in helping patients with chronic pain, and the management and prevention of chronic illnesses. She continued this pursuit for decades, staying on the cutting edge of the newest research, attending seminars, and expanding her clinical training. After three decades of clinical nursing, my mother returned to complete her BSN from California State University, Hayward. During that time, she was raising four children and working full time as the Assistant Director of Nursing at John Muir Hospital in Walnut Creek, California. She continued her professional pursuits graduating with a MSN from the University of California, San Francisco. A few years later, she completed the Nurse Practitioner Program at California State University, Long Beach. After receiving her Nurse Practitioner Certificate she was hired as the Medical Director for the VA Hospital in Martinez, California.

During the next few years, she was invited to be a guest lecturer for the Nursing Department at California State University, Hayward. Her reputation as a dynamic lecturer and creative teacher quickly grew and her enthusiasm and excitement about the profession of nursing was contagious. Within two years of her first guest lecture, she was hired as a full time Assistant Professor of Nursing. Her teaching career excelled, like every other aspect of her personal and professional life, and she was quickly promoted to Associate Professor of Nursing. It was during this time that she decided to complete her lifelong "dream" book on the topic of chronic illness. For all of you who are reading this memorial, you are holding her amazing book in your

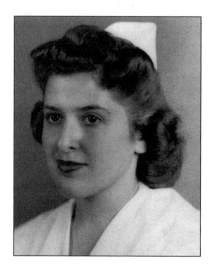

hands. This text is a reflection of my mother's lifelong passion for helping others, and an expression of her amazing dedication to the profession of nursing. This text is a synthesis of over five decades of clinical and academic experiences to better understand the dynamics of chronic illness and how it impacts every facet of a patient's life.

Shortly after the initial publication of this textbook, my mother was promoted to Professor of Nursing. She dedicated the next 15 years of her life to teaching young nurses. She lectured nationwide, and became one of the few nationally recognized experts in the field of chronic illness. When she turned 70, my mother officially retired from teaching. As a retired professor, she worked almost double her previous weekly hours; she had an amazing passion burning in her heart, she was a dedicated advocate for the aged and the ill. For the last five years of her life she served as a Senior Senator, representing Contra Costa County for the California Senior Legislature in Sacramento, researching and advocating legislative bills that supported health care issues and other important legislation for the elderly. Ilene Ruth Lubkin, RN, MSN, GNP, worked every day toward her dreams and goals, up to the day of her death.

Hugh J. Lubkin

To our grandchildren, Ian, Naomi and Kyle Lubkin
and
Cody and Kai Larsen
Jonah and Landon Fanning
and
Abby Larsen

PART I

Impact of the Disease

CHAPTER 1

Chronicity

Pamala D. Larsen

Introduction

Chronic disease is the nation's greatest health care problem. In 2004 it was estimated that there were 133 million individuals living with at least one chronic disease, and it is projected that 50% of the population, roughly 157 million, will have at least one chronic condition by 2020 (Partnership for Solutions, 2004). Perhaps more sobering, however, is data from the 2001 Medical Expenditure Panel Survey (MEPS) which indicates that currently 83% of the nation's medical care costs are associated with treating individuals with chronic conditions (Partnership for Solutions, 2004).

As we examine the range of chronic conditions, one is struck by the wide diversity of services needed to care for such individuals. For example, consider clients with Alzheimer's disease, cerebral palsy, heart disease, AIDS, spinal cord injury, or multiple sclerosis; each of these clients has unique physical needs, and each would need different types of services from a health care system that is currently attuned to delivering acute care.

The first Baby Boomer will turn 65 in 2011, and this anticipated event has brought increased attention to the capabilities of the health care system. This generation, in particular, has been vocal about the inability of the health care system to meet current societal needs, let alone future needs. Additionally, this new group of seniors will be the most ethnically and racially diverse of any previous generation (National Center for Health Statistics, 2004). How will the current system or a future system cope with these diverse seniors and their accompanying chronic conditions?

Multiple factors have produced the increasing number of individuals with chronic disease. Developments in the fields of public health, bacteriology, immunology, and pharmacology have led to a significant drop in mortality from acute disease. Medical success has contributed, in part, to the unprecedented growth of chronic illness by extending life expectancy and by earlier detection of disease in general. Living longer, however, leads to greater vulnerability of people having accidents and disease events that can become chronic in nature. The client who may have died from a myocardial infarction in earlier years now needs continuing health care for heart failure. The cancer survivor has health care needs for the iatrogenic result of life-saving treatment. The adolescent who is a quadriplegic due to an accident may live a relatively long life with our current rehabilitation efforts but needs continuous preventive and maintenance care from the health care system. The child with cystic fibrosis has bene-fited from a lung transplant, but needs continuous care for the rest of their life. Thus, many previously fatal injuries, diseases, and conditions have become chronic in nature.

The current health care system was largely de-signed and shaped in the two decades following World War II (Lynn & Adamson, 2003). It was a sys-tem designed to provide acute, episodic and cura-tive care, and was never intended to address the needs of individuals with chronic conditions. Generally, the system does provide acute care effec-tively and efficiently. However, it is based on a com-ponent style of care in which each component of the system is reimbursed separately, i.e., hospital visit, home care, physician visit. Each component of the health care system views the client from its nar-row window of care. No one entity, practice, insitu-tion, or agency is managing the entire disease, and certainly not managing the illness experience of the client and family. No one is responsible for the over-all care of the individual, just their own indepen-dent component, and with that approach higher costs may occur. As Zitter states "optimizing any component of care separately from other compo-nents often generates higher systemwide costs" (Zitter, 1997, p. 2).

Disease Versus Illness

It is important to distinguish between a *disease* and an *illness,* although the terms are often used in-terchangeably by health care professionals. *Disease* refers to a condition that the practitioner views from a pathophysiological model, such as an alteration in structure and function. *Illness,* on the other hand, is the human experience of symptoms and suffering, and refers to how the disease is perceived, lived with, and responded to by individuals and their families. Although it is important to recognize the pathology of a chronic disease, understanding the illness expe-rience is essential when caring for individuals long term. Thus, the focus of this book is on the *illness* experience of individuals and families, not specific disease processes.

Acute Versus Chronic Disorders

When an individual develops an acute disease, there is typically a sudden onset, with signs and symptoms related to the disease process itself. Acute diseases end in a relatively short time, either with recovery and resumption of prior activities, or with death.

Chronic illness, on the other hand, continues indefinitely. Although a welcome alternative to death, the illness may be seen as a mixed blessing to the individual and to society at large. In addition, the illness often becomes the person's identity. For ex-ample, an individual having any kind of cancer, even in remission, acquires the label of "that person with cancer" (see Chapter 3, on stigma).

Chronic conditions take many forms, and there is no single onset pattern. A chronic disease can ap-pear suddenly or through an insidious process, have episodic flare-ups or exacerbations, or remain in remission with an absence of symptoms for long periods of time. Maintaining wellness or keeping symptoms in remission is a juggling act of balancing treatment regimens while focusing on quality of life.

Historical Perspectives

Throughout history, human beings have recog-nized the presence of illness and attempted to repair or minimize disease. A Sumerian tablet (c. 2158–2008 B.C.) confirms early healing attempts in the form of poultices. This tablet has been considered the oldest medical text, and although it discusses prescriptions and treatments, it does not discuss dis-ease (Majno, 1975). In the 1600s, secondary to tra-ditional interpretation of cause and effect, health authorities ventilated city alleys and legislated the storage of manure in an effort to battle against bad odors and humors, which were thought to be the source of the plague (Cipolla, 1992).

In the nineteenth century, after discoveries in disease causation and process, scientific methodolo-gies began to be applied to health care. Health fields, such as medicine and nursing, now deal with an in-creasing variety of health events that range from acute to chronic, as well as with the iatrogenic effects of successful and wide-ranging interventions.

During the 1940s, the importance of chronic conditions to the health of society became a national concern, and the first National Health Survey was conducted to determine the extent of chronic diseases (Commission on Chronic Illness, 1957). As early as 1977, the Centers for Disease Control (CDC) began to redefine their role to include an emphasis on primary prevention of chronic disease (Benjamin & Newcomer, 1997).

Current health care professionals face the prospect that, in the future, there will be clients with health conditions, chronic and acute as yet unknown, who will require health care by means not yet comprehensible. Health care professionals, scientists and policy makers will need to balance anticipated longer life spans with the economic, societal, and environmental resources needed to maintain those years.

Defining *Chronicity*

Defining *chronicity* is complex. Many individuals have attempted to present an all-encompassing yet clear definition of *chronic illness* (Table 1-1).

Initially, the characteristics of chronic diseases were identified by the Commission on Chronic Illness as all impairments or deviations from normal that included one or more of the following: permanency; residual disability; nonpathological alteration; required rehabilitation; or a long period of supervision, observation, and care (Mayo, 1956). The National Conference on Care of the Long-Term Patient added a time dimension to these characteristics: chronic disease or impairment necessitating acute hospitalization exceeding 30 days, or medical supervision and rehabilitation of three months or longer in another care setting (Roberts, 1954).

Determining a definition for a specific chronic disease is more difficult if one attempts to establish the origin of the condition. Some chronic diseases have multiple factors that take years to accumulate sufficiently to produce symptoms. Do we say that bowel cancer that manifests itself at the age of 50 originated when the first mutant cell divided 30 years earlier? Or is it the result of a particular diet or life-style? Or can we say that it started at the time of biopsy? Like life itself, the time of origin is debatable. For chronic disease, however, origin is highly critical in seeking measures that may prevent or ameliorate the eventual disease.

TABLE 1-1

Definitions of Chronic Illness

Author	Definitions
Commission on Chronic Diseases (1957)	All impairments or deviations from normal which have one or more of the following characteristics: are permanent, leave residual disability, are caused by non-reversible pathological alteration, require special training of the patient for rehabilitation, and may be expected to require a long period of supervision, observation, or care
Feldman (1974)	Ongoing medical condition with spectrum of social, economic, and behavioral complications that require meaningful and continuous personal and professional involvement [summarized]
Cluff (1981)	A condition not cured by medical intervention, requiring periodic monitoring and supportive care to reduce the degree of illness, maximize the person's functioning and responsibility for self-care [summarized]
Curtin & Lubkin (1995)	Chronic illness is the irreversible presence, accumulation, or latency of disease states or impairments that involve the total human environment for supportive care and self-care, maintenance of function, and prevention of further disability

The extent and direction of a chronic disease further complicate attempts to provide a definition. Disability may depend not only on the kind of condition and its severity, but also on the implications it holds for the person. A teen-ager may require greater adjustment to the limitations necessitated by bone cancer than will an individual who is elderly. The degree of disability and altered life style, part of traditional definitions, may relate as much to the client's perception of the disease as to the specific disease.

Long-term and iatrogenic effects of some treatment methods may constitute chronic conditions in their own right, making them eligible to be defined as a chronic illness. For example, this situation is represented by the changes in lifestyle required of clients on hemodialysis for end-stage renal disease (ESRD). Life-saving procedures can create other problems. For instance, abdominal radiation that arrested metastatic intestinal cancer when an individual was age 30 can contribute to a malabsorption problem years later, so that continuous diarrhea results in a now cachectic and exhausted person. Chemotherapy given to a client for an initial bout with cancer may be an influencing factor in the development of leukemia years later.

Chronic illness, by its very nature, is never completely cured or prevented. Biologically, the human body wears out unevenly. Medical advances cause older persons to need a progressively wider variety of specialized services for increasingly complicated conditions. In the words of Emanuel (1982), "Life is the accumulation of chronic illness beneath the load of which we eventually succumb" (p. 502).

From a nursing perspective, the following definition of chronic illness is offered:

> *Chronic illness* is the irreversible presence, accumulation, or latency of disease states or impairments that involve the total human environment for supportive care and self-care, maintenance of function, and prevention of further disability (Curtin & Lubkin, 1995, pp. 6–7).

■ Impact of Chronic Illness

A chronic illness affects all aspects of an individual's life. However, the impact felt by each individual may be different due to the individual's personality traits, beliefs and values, the support systems the individual has in place, and other factors unique to each individual. One 40-year-old woman with primary progressive multiple sclerosis may not have the same illness experience as another individual of the same age with the same diagnosis. Each individual has a unique illness experience.

Growth and Development Factors

The growth and development stage of the individual is a significant factor in the care of the individual with chronic illness. A comprehensive plan for caring for an individual with a chronic illness includes an assessment of the growth and development stage of the individual.

An individual is destined to age. Age and life stages influence the types of problems and consequences that affect the person who has a chronic condition. In spite of illness and/or disability, each individual must accomplish age-specific development tasks that allow psychological and cognitive transition from one stage to the next. Development normally has a centrifugal, or liberating, effect, while illness has a centripetal, or drawing in, effect. An illness diagnosed at a critical period (such as the onset of school for a child) can lead to an incongruity of events and result in ensuing problems (Rolland, 1987).

Chronic illness can have a negative impact on the independence and self-control associated with the individual's developmental level. Increased dependence on others may be necessary: The very young child may be unable to work at self-sufficiency tasks; the school-age child may be unable to stay abreast of school work or participation in after school activities; adolescents and young adults may have obstacles that prevent them from reaching their goals and becoming independent; and the older adult, who may have been independent prior to an illness, is unable to complete the developmental tasks of older age. Managing and complying with a treatment regime at any developmental stage of life provides personal control issues for the individual, may undermine successful disease management, and may negatively affect the illness experience.

Body image is an important component of one's self-concept and is closely tied to the individual's developmental stage. For instance, a child who is becoming aware of his or her own body can be adversely impacted by the onset of a disease that prevents vital body awareness information (e.g., toddlers testing the limits of their bodies). An adolescent going through puberty is similarly affected. An adolescent has a difficult time coping with the normal maturational processes without additional changes to body image due to a chronic disease (see Chapter 8, on body image).

Infancy through Adolescence

It is estimated that approximately 15–18% of children in the United States are living with a chronic illness or disability that requires special health care (Judson, 2004; Perrin, 2004). According to data from the 2001 Medical Expenditure Panel Survey, four conditions are responsible for the majority of the chronic conditions in noninstitutionalized children ages 0–17. These include:

Eye Disorders	6%
Emotional/Behavioral Disorders	15%
Asthma	27%
Respiratory Diseases	35%

Source: Partnership for Solutions, 2004

The percentage of the pediatric population with a chronic condition is increasing as technology, improved treatments, and implementation of public health and preventative measures are instituted. New treatments for chronic conditions, such as cerebral palsy, spina bifida, and cystic fibrosis, have increased these children's life spans. Technological advances have substantially increased the survival of extremely and very-low-birth weight infants (Jackson, 2000). However, the children who survive extreme prematurity may have lifelong chronic health problems. The end result of all of our medical advances is that there are an increasing number of infants, children, and adolescents with long-term health problems. Of importance also is the continuing role that poverty and ethnicity play in the increased incidence and severity of chronic disease in children (National Center for Health Statistics, 2004). Poverty is a common factor that contributes to childhood chronic illness worldwide. Additionally, poverty is often linked with race, social status and education (Judson, 2004).

Because of the unique period of childhood, growth and development needs require sequencing and provision of care different from that of other age groups. Focusing on the child's developmental level rather than the chronological level of the child allows the focus to be on the strengths of the child and not the deficits (Brown-Hellsten, 2005).

Similar to caring for adults with chronic illness, there has been an increasing awareness that a disease-specific approach in caring for children with chronic disorders is perhaps not the best way to work with these children (Schmitke & Schlomann, 2002). In that vein, clinicians have identified six important dimensions of the child with chronic illness that are more appropriate than the specific disease.

■ Nature of the onset
■ Trajectory or progression of the condition
■ Effects on appearance
■ Effects on daily functioning
■ Effects on behavior and ability to relate to others
■ Care required

Source: Schmitke, J. & Schlomann, P. (2002).

Siblings play multiple roles in actively shaping one another's lives and preparing each other for adult life. They experience a gamut of emotional reactions to having a "different" brother or sister; often, their lives reflect the routines made necessary by the affected child's illness or disability. However, there is inconsistency in the literature as to the effect of a sibling having a brother or sister with special needs (Brown-Hellsten, 2005). In fact, there is some evidence in recent years that the effect seems to be decreasing, perhaps due to the fact that there is greater public acceptance of illness and disability (Sharpe & Rossiter, 2002). However, that said, much of the adjustment to a sibling's health problems rests with the parents. Some parents are able to perceive the chronic condition and its effects, and integrate the condition through normalization. Normalization is a management process used by some families of children with chronic illness. The family acknowledges the condition, defines the social effects of the family as minimal, and then engages in activities that demonstrate to others that their family is normal (Knafl & Deatrick, 1986).

The adolescent with a chronic disease may not be able to meet the developmental needs of new levels of independence, but may need to learn to accept a life with limitations. A chronic illness occurring at this time, when there are multiple physical changes, can lead to a feeling that the body is repulsive and can have a damaging effect on interpersonal relationships. A major task confronting an adolescent is growing into a life of "what is and can be" rather than one of "what might have been." Similarly with adolescents as with other age groups, lower socioeconomic status is associated with poorer health status and health outcomes (Newacheck, Hung, Park, Brindis, & Irwin, 2003).

Young to Middle-Aged Adults

The young to middle years of adulthood are typically a time of high activity and productivity. Individuals launch careers and marriages, begin and rear families, experience changes in status, and prepare for retirement. The presence of a chronic condition can complicate the conception and completion of goals and dreams. At a time when creative energy is generally directed outward, the individual may need to utilize most inner resources to cope with the condition.

Older Adults

From the beginning of the 20th century to the end, the concept of aging and dying has changed dramatically. Individuals dying in 1900 tended to die from acute pneumonia, tuberculosis, diarrhea and enteritis and injuries (US Department of Health and Human Services, 2000). Serious illness and/or disability to death was measured in days, weeks or perhaps months, but certainly not years. The family bore the brunt of the medical expenses, and caregiving occurred at home by family members (see Table 1-2).

Leap forward to the 21st century and examine the changes that have occurred. From 1950 to 2000 the proportion of the population 75 and older jumped from 3 to 6%, and by 2050 it is projected that 12% of Americans will be 75 or older (National Center for Health Statistics, 2004). With the greatest proportion of chronic disorders affecting the older population, this increase in population is significant. Also as one ages, diagnoses of chronic disorders frequently multiply. These co-existing conditions are termed *co-morbidities*. In the 21st century, to the older person with chronic illness, longer life expectancy may mean periods of disability, vulnerability to other health problems, financial expense, and increasing care concerns. Lynn and Adamson (2003) categorize chronic illness among the elderly as:

TABLE 1-2

A Century of Change

	1900	2000
Life Expectancy	47 years	75 years
Usual place of death	Home	Hospital
Most medical expenses	Paid for by family	Paid by Medicare
Disability before death	Usually not much	2 years, on average

SOURCE: Reprinted with permission from *Approaching Death: Improving Care at the End of Life.* © 1997 by the National Academy of Sciences, courtesy of the National Academies Press, Washington, DC.

- Nonfatal chronic illness—conditions such as osteoarthritis, hearing or vision problems. Although these conditions contribute to disability and increased health care costs, most individuals can live for many years.
- Serious, eventually fatal chronic conditions—cancers, organ system failures (heart, kidney, liver, respiratory), dementia and strokes
- Frailty—a fatal, chronic condition in which the body has little reserves left, and any disturbance can cause multiple health conditions and costs

The older adult has growth and developmental tasks to complete as well, and the presence of a chronic condition makes it difficult to do so. In general, it is "expected" that the older individual will have one or more chronic diseases and can cope with these conditions as disease comes with age. However, if one uses Erikson's stages of development as a framework for practice, there are tasks to complete at all age stages, including the older adult. The stage of adulthood has the tasks of generativity versus stagnation, and individuals in the stage of "old age" have integrity versus despair. However, society views both the aged and chronically ill negatively (see Chapter 3, on stigma). There is a tendency to look at age and disability in terms of their effect on the national pocketbook. Indeed, persons aged 65 and older account for a significant portion of health care costs. Population projections imply growth in both the amount and percentage of health care dollars for future care of the elderly population (see Chapter 27, on financial impact). Unlike for children, the investment in older adults does not bring a promise of financial return (see Chapters 26 and 24, on politics and policy and long-term care, respectively).

Quality of Life Versus Quantity of Life

Adapting successfully to chronic illness includes the conviction that a meaningful quality of life is worth the struggle. However, the disease is only one of innumerable factors that impact the totality of a person's quality of life. For instance, the same medical condition may be tolerable to one person and overwhelmingly intolerable to another. The characteristics of the disease, age and development of the individual, degree of disability, and extent of medical intervention required to maintain a person with a disease all have implications for the individual, the family, and community (see Chapter 9, on quality of life).

Professional caregivers face changing dilemmas as medical technology creates new methods to preserve and prolong life. The medical community has long been dealing with the question of who receives which life-giving measure and who should finance treatment. With the advent of multiple complex treatment modalities and multiple organ transplants, broad-based planning must establish the guidelines for designating recipients. Most hospitals have ethics committees to decide who of many will receive life-saving measures. Even the process of dying and the moment of death itself can be controlled by machinery that dictates bodily functioning.

The Patient Self-Determination Act of 1990 changed the responsibilities of health care professionals from decision-makers for clients to educators and facilitators. The Act emphasized the active role that clients have in directing their health care and making decisions that could result in their deaths. Two features of the Act that empower patients are a patient's right to refuse treatment and the role of advanced directives in health care (see Chapter 18, on ethics).

Issues of quality versus quantity of life will continue as individuals with chronic conditions become more vocal and participative in their care and treatment. Clients are beginning to see themselves as partners in care as opposed to recipients of care.

Health Disparities

Evidence of racial and ethnic disparities in healthcare is, with few exceptions, consistent across a range of diseases and healthcare services (Smedley, Stith, & Nelson, 2003). These disparities prompted Congress in 1999 to request that the Institute of

Medicine (IOM) assess the level and kinds of disparities. The charges to the IOM included:

■ Assess the extent of racial and ethnic difference in healthcare that are not otherwise attributable to known factors such as access to care

■ Evaluate potential sources of racial and ethnic disparities in health care, including the role of bias, discrimination and stereotyping at the individual, institutional and health system levels; and

■ Provide recommendations regarding interventions to eliminate healthcare disparities.

Source: Smedley et al., 2003, p. 30.

The IOM appointed committee reviewed hundreds of articles and collected data from individuals, data bases and focus groups. Throughout the literature, there were multiple examples of inequities in how healthcare was being provided to ethnic and racial minorities. Some of the strongest and most consistent evidence that demonstrated those health disparities was found in studies of cardiovascular care. The findings and recommendations from this IOM committee are detailed in the book, *Unequal Treatment: Confronting Racial and Ethnic Disparities in Healthcare* (Smedley et al., 2003).

As we look at preventative care of minority populations, similar data exists. From the National Healthcare Disparities Report (NHDR) in 2004, differences exist in the use of evidence-based preventive services for certain populations, particularly people of lower socioeconomic status (SES) and some minorities. For example:

■ People of lower SES and some minorities are less likely to have colorectal and breast cancer screening

■ People of lower SES and Latinos are less likely to have blood pressure and cholesterol screening in addition to counseling and treatment for some cardiac risk factors

■ People of lower SES and African Americans are less likely to have recommended childhood immunizations before the age of four years

■ Children of lower SES and some minority children are less likely to have dental care

■ Lower SES, African American and Latino adults are less likely have recommended immunizations for influenza and pneumococcal disease

Source: Kelley, E. et al. (2004).

Cultural Influences

Illness belief systems form the cultural milieu that defines caregivers' and individuals' attitudes toward illness. Conceptions about the source of disease and required treatment affect the types of therapy the caregiver offers, as well as the outcome the client expects.

The growing diversity of the United States population presents new challenges for health care professionals. How is culturally competent care provided to these clients? The initial question may be, "What is culturally competent care?" In the current health care education system, little time is spent on understanding and learning the culture, beliefs, and values of others. It is often "one size of health care fits all."

Chin (2000) describes three issues in providing culturally competent care in a health care system. These include access to care, utilization, and quality of care. Access to care includes the degree to which services are convenient and obtainable. Part of access is the current health care system's reliance on geographic boundaries for care rather than population-based or community-based boundaries. Another aspect of acess is providing interpreters for non-English-speaking clients, if bilingual care providers are not available. However, there has been controversy over the implementation and cost of interpreter services. In addition, relying on interpreters often entails longer waits for clients, inappropriate translations, and inconvenience in scheduling appointments (Chin, 2000). Additionally, the cost of having interpreters available is not figured into the reimbursement system.

Utilization refers to the availability of services within a system, how frequently the services are used, and whether the use is appropriate. Often immigrants and low-income minority groups lack the enabling services, case management, outreach, transportation, and babysitting services necessary to utilize health services (Chin, 2000).

Although health care professionals typically believe that they are providing quality care, it is from their own perspective that they are viewing quality and not from the client's perspective. An individual from another culture may not view this health care as "quality care" because the health care professional does not consider the individual's religious beliefs, values, and, perhaps, use, for example, of Eastern medicine or Native American medicine. The values and beliefs of the health care provider and the client are often quite divergent, but this aspect is rarely considered when caring for that individual in the current health care system.

Social Influences

The elderly or chronically ill carry a yoke of undesirability. When they become clients in an acute care setting, caring for them is often seen as less rewarding in terms of recovery, reduction of disease states, and economics. It is functionality, not age, that should be used in establishing guidelines for the senior population. Bortz (1988) states that prevention strategies, functional assessment, and rehabilitation therapy should be placed ahead of cure allocations.

To date, society defines *illness* and *debility* largely with a disease-specific focus. This model places chronically ill individuals at a disadvantage. The chronically ill person needs to be considered as "modified" rather than "nonproductive." Such a perspective leads to maximization of well-being, creativity, and productivity.

Nationally recognized individuals have stepped forward to make statements as active persons who, coincidentally, have disabling, chronic, or terminal illnesses. The courage and farsightedness of these persons encourage a more objective and closer appraisal of legislation and funding by lawmakers. Michael J. Fox and Muhammed Ali, with diagnoses of Parkinson's disease; Magic Johnson, with his diagnosis of HIV; and the late Christopher Reeve, as a ventilator-dependent quadriplegic, have each gone public in the hope of decreasing the stigma of chronic disease as well as encouraging lawmakers to change public policy and increase research funding.

Financial Impact of Chronicity

The United States spends more money per capita on health care than any other country in the world (National Center for Health Statistics, 2004). Although the rate of growth in spending was slower in 2003, only 7.7% as compared with 9.3% in 2002, spending amounted to 1.7 trillion dollars (Smith, Cowan, Sensening & Catlin, 2005). For the first time ever, health care spending was greater than 15% of the Gross Domestic Product (GDP), at 15.3% (Smith et al., 2005).

An example of one chronic disease and its financial impact is diabetes. According to the American Diabetes Association, $132 billion dollars were spent in 2002 on costs associated with the disease with $92 billon on direct costs and $40 billion on indirect costs, such as disability, inability to work, premature morbidity, etc. (Kruzikas, Jiang, Remus, Barrett, Coffey & Andrews, 2004). As a result of these costs, the Institute of Medicine has identified diabetes as a priority disease for healthcare quality improvement.

Think about individuals with five or more chronic conditions. These persons have an average of 15 physician visits a year and more than 50 prescriptions/year (Partnership for Solutions, 2004). This translates into multiple health care costs for both the individual as out-of-pocket, for Medicare (typically these individuals are over the age of 65) and any additional health insurance plan that they may have.

One would think that this increased spending on health care would merit confidence from the public in the health care system's ability to manage care. However, just the opposite is true. In a Harris survey of adult Americans, for Johns Hopkins University and the Robert Wood Johnson Foundation (Partnership for Solutions, 2001), it was found that:

- 72 percent of Americans say it is difficult for people living with chronic conditions to get necessary care from their health care providers
- 74 percent say that it is difficult to obtain prescription drug medications
- 89 percent say it is difficult to find adequate health insurance

These increased health care costs bring increased premiums for health insurance. Smaller companies that may have previously paid for insurance coverage of their employees may shift all or part of this expense to employees or simply discontinue it altogether. The average American family has increasingly more difficulty in picking up these costs.

Attitudes of Health Care Professionals

Health care professionals can view chronic illness positively, as a state that can continue to contribute to the potential growth of an individual, a family, or a society, or negatively, as a state of failure to recover completely. Much of this negativity comes from the fact that a majority of health workers participate in a client's care during a crisis or exacerbation of symptoms, because most hospitals provide only episodic care. With this piecemeal exposure, health care professionals often have the perception that a client returns to a prior normal role, even though the client's entire life pattern may actually offer only increasing disability, pain, and deterioration.

Caring for an individual with a chronic condition does not bring the adrenaline rush that comes from saving a life in the emergency room. Educating a client about the long-term effects of their diabetes mellitus diagnosis may not compare with defibrillating a client in cardiac arrest or resuscitating a newborn infant. Unfortunately, there are a number of health care professionals who chose their profession because of the acute care focus, and their attitudes in caring for those with chronic disease are less than positive.

Interventions

One national group that is identifying issues and working on solutions for chronic illness is The Partnership for Solutions. This is a national program funded by the Robert Wood Johnson Foundation and based at Johns Hopkins University. The goal of the program is to improve care and quality of life for the current 133 million Americans with a chronic condition. The Partnership has three major activities: (1) conducting original research and identifying existing research that clarifies the nature of the problem; (2) communicating these findings to policymakers, business leaders, health professionals, and advocates for individuals with chronic disease; and (3) working with these groups to identify solutions to the problems faced by individuals with chronic illness (Partnership for Solutions, 2004). Much of the current literature about chronic illness both for health care professionals and the public can be found in their publications or on their website (http://www.partnershipforsolutions.org).

Professional Education

In addition to models of care that emphasize a chronic, long-term focus for clients, there is a need for "new" models for teaching future health care professionals. If health care education remains static, we will continue to educate our future physicians, nurses, and therapists using an antiquated acute care medical model. Chronic disease has been discussed for several decades now, and it continues to be reiterated that change needs to occur to better care for the chronically ill population. However, little change has occurred in health care professional education.

The Pew Health Professions Commission (1989–1999), funded by The Pew Charitable Trusts, was created to focus on the healthcare workforce. The mission of this commission was to help policy makers and educators better prepare health care professionals to meet the needs of clients in the 21st century. The last report of this Commission was released in December 1998 and contained recommendations for competencies for health care professionals in the twenty-first century (Table 1-3).

With the competencies outlined in Table 1-3, a change in the attitudes of health care professionals is necessary. Health professionals must see caring for individuals with chronic disease as being as impor-

---

TABLE 1-3

Pew Competencies for Health Professionals in the Twenty-First Century

- Embrace a personal ethic of social responsibility and service.
- Exhibit ethical behavior in all professional activities.
- Provide evidence-based, clinically competent care.
- Incorporate the multiple determinants of health in clinical care.
- Apply knowledge of the new sciences.
- Demonstrate critical thinking, reflection, and problem-solving skills.
- Understand the role of primary care.
- Rigorously practice preventive health care.
- Integrate population-based care and services into practice.
- Improve access to health care for those with unmet health needs.
- Practice with communities in health care decisions.
- Provide culturally sensitive care to a diverse society.
- Partner with communities in health care decisions.
- Use communication and information technology effectively and appropriately.
- Work in interdisciplinary teams.
- Ensure care that balances individual, professional, system, and societal needs.
- Practice leadership.
- Take responsibility for quality of care and health outcomes at all levels.
- Contribute to continuous improvement of the health care system.
- Advocate for public policy that promotes and protects the health of the public.
- Continue to learn and help others learn.

SOURCE: Pew Health Professions Commission (1998). Twenty-one competencies for the 21st century. Available on-line at http://www.futurehealth.ucsf.edu/pewcomm/competen.html

---

tant and rewarding as caring for those with acute disease. However, changing attitudes is a slow process. The media are laying a solid foundation of knowledge about the implications of living with chronic illness. Society's lack of empathy and concern, however, may be the result of a lack of interaction with those affected by chronic disease. In the past, because of degree of illness and disability, an unfriendly physical environment, and absence from the workplace, the individual with chronic illness was not integrated into the mainstream of society. At times, still, the individual with chronic illness is identified by their debility rather than their ability.

Another group that has been prominent in making the case for a change in how health professionals are educated is the Institute of Medicine. This group has launched several phases of their quality initiative beginning in 1996. One of their more recent initiatives has recommended changes in health care professional education to better address the healthcare needs of the nation. Briefly, their vision is to have healthcare education address the following:

- Provide patient-centered care
- Work in interdisciplinary teams
- Employ evidence-based practice
- Apply quality improvement
- Utilize informatics

Source: Greiner, A. & Knebel, E. (Eds.) (2003).

Legislation

Changing public policy continues to be a primary intervention in assisting clients and their families with chronic conditions. Institution of national policies and the financing of prevention and health promotion need to occur. Additionally, until health care professionals are able to make a difference in the agency maze and the financing of that maze, clients will continue to have difficulty accessing the chronic long-term care they need. The need for a true continuum of care has never been more apparent.

There has been much discussion about the drug prescription provision of the Medicare Prescription

Drug, Improvement, and Modernization Act of 2003 (MMA). The MMA established a basic out-patient drug benefit as Part D of Medicare and is voluntary for all Medicare beneficiaries. The Congressional Budget Office (CBO) estimates that 87% of Medicare beneficiaries will participate in the prescription drug benefit once it becomes available in 2006 (CBO, 2004). At the present time, there is much talk about how much it is *really* going to cost the government with partisan politics and bureaucrats battling it out. The one thing that is clear is that it is going to cost much more than the original estimates made by the Bush Administration.

However, of note is a component of the MMA that has received relatively little publicity. The MMA includes a provision for a Phase I Voluntary Chronic Care Improvement Program (CMS, 2005). To quote the Centers for Medicare and Medicaid Services (CMS) "this program is the first large-scale chronic care improvement initiative under the Medicare FFS program. CMS will select organizations that will offer self-care guidance and support to chronically ill beneficiaries" (http://www.cms.hss.gov/medicare reform/ccip/). On December 8, 2004, nine awardees were recognized with the first program to be operational by spring 2005.

Phase I awardees and the regions they will serve include:

Humana, Inc.	Central Florida
XLHealth Corporation	Tennessee
Aetna Health Management LLC	Chicago, Illinois
Lifemasters Supported SelfCare, Inc.	Oklahoma
McKesson Health Solutions LLC	Mississippi
CIGNA HealthCare	Georgia
Health Dialog Services Corporation	Pennsylvania
American Healthways, Inc.	Washington DC & Maryland
Visiting Nurse Service of New York	NYC: Queens & Brooklyn
Home Care & United HealthCare Services, Inc.—Evercare	

These programs are poised to serve 150,000 to 300,000 Medicare beneficiaries who are enrolled in traditional fee-for-service Medicare and who have multiple chronic conditions. The agencies were also chosen within geographic areas that have a high prevalence of diabetes and heart failure. CMS data suggest that 14% of Medicare clients have heart failure, but their care accounts for 43% of Medicare spending. Likewise, 18% of Medicare clients have diabetes, and these clients account for 32% of all Medicare spending (CBO, 2004). Participation in the Chronic Care Improvement Program is voluntary, there is no charge to beneficiaries, and it will not affect clients' ability to choose their own physicians.

Providing Culturally Competent Care

The need to provide culturally competent care continues. By the year 2050, the Asian population in the United States is expected to increase from 3 to 8 percent; the African American population from 12.7 to 14.7 percent; and the Hispanic population from 12.6 to 24.4 percent (U.S. Census, 2004). To address the health care needs of this heterogeneous population, new models must be developed that better provide care. Campinha-Bacote's model of cultural competence is one that addresses the needs of a diverse population. This model describes cultural awareness, cultural knowledge, cultural skill, cultural encounters, and cultural desire as constructs of cultural competence (Campinha-Bacote, 1999). The constructs are interdependent—it does not matter where the health care provider enters the process—but all five constructs must be experienced and addressed. It is the intersection of these constructs that depits the true process of cultural competence (Campinha-Bacote, 1999).

The Office of Minority Health of the United States Department of Health and Human Services (DHHS) has developed draft standards for culturally and linguistically appropriate health care services. Table 1-4 depicts these standards as a way to promote equal access to health care.

TABLE 1-4

Recommended Standards for Culturally and Linguistically Appropriate Health Care Services

Culture and language have considerable impact on how patients access and respond to health care services. To ensure equal access to quality health care by diverse populations, health care organizations and providers should:

1. Promote and support the attitudes, behaviors, knowledge, and skills necessary for staff to work respectfully and effectively with patients and each other in a culturally diverse work environment.
2. Have a comprehensive management strategy to address culturally and linguistically appropriate services, including strategic goals, plans, policies, procedures, and designated staff responsible for implementation.
3. Utilize formal mechanisms for community and consumer involvement in the design and execution of service delivery, including planning, policy making, operations, evaluation, training, and, as appropriate, treatment planning.
4. Develop and implement a strategy to recruit, retain, and promote qualified, diverse, and culturally competent administrative, clinical, and support staff that are trained and qualified to address the needs of the racial and ethnic communities being served.
5. Require and arrange for ongoing education and training for administrative, clinical, and support staff in culturally and linguistically competent service delivery.
6. Provide all clients with limited English proficiency (LEP) access to bilingual staff or interpretation services.
7. Provide oral and written notices, including translated signage at key points of contact, to clients in their primary language informing them of their right to receive no-cost interpreter services.
8. Translate and make available signage and commonly-used written patient educational material and other materials for members of the predominant language groups in service areas.
9. Ensure that interpreters and bilingual staff can demonstrate bilingual proficiency and receive training that includes the skills and ethics of interpreting, and knowledge in both languages of the terms and concepts relevant to clinical or non-clinical encounters. Family or friends are not considered adequate substitutes because they usually lack these abilities.
10. Ensure that the clients' primary spoken language and self-identified race/ethnicity are included in the health care organization's management information system as well as any patient records used by provider staff.
11. Use a variety of methods to collect and utilize accurate demographic, cultural, epidemiological, and clinical outcome data for racial and ethnic groups in the service area, and become informed about the ethnic/cultural needs, resources, and assets of the surrounding community.
12. Undertake ongoing organizational self-assessments of cultural and linguistic competence, and integrate measures of access, satisfaction, quality, and outcomes for [culturally and linguistically appropriate services (CLAS)] into other organizational internal audits and performance improvement programs.
13. Develop structures and procedures to address cross-cultural ethical and legal conflicts in health care delivery and complaints or grievances by patients and staff about unfair, culturally insensitive, or discriminatory treatment, or difficulty an accessing services, or denial of services.
14. Prepare an annual progress report documenting the organizations' progress with implementing CLAS standards, including information on programs, staffing, and resources.

SOURCE: Department of Health and Human Services. (1999). Office of Minority Health and Resources for Cross Cultural Health Care. Online: http://www.omhrc.gov/clas/index.htm

Models of Chronic Disease Management

A number of reasons exist why the current health care system cannot address the needs of individuals with chronic illness. Reasons include: (1) inadequate clinical information systems; (2) preventable hospitalizations; (3) insurance coverage; (4) provider payment; and (5) coordination of care (Anderson & Knickman, 2001).

To highlight just one of these areas, inadequate clinical information systems do not allow care providers to share information. An average Medicare beneficiary with one or more chronic conditions is seen by eight physicians during a year. If these care providers do not share information among themselves but rely on the client to share information, how can this work for the client? The Harris Interactive Survey in 2000 indicated that 20 million Americans received contradictory information from different care providers during the year, 18 million received a contradictory diagnosis for the same chronic illness, and 17 million report going to the pharmacist only to be told of a potential drug/drug interaction (Partnership for Solutions, 2001).

Another vulnerable population that suffers from inadequate information systems is the individual who is being transferred or 'transitioned' from care setting to care setting. An example is the frail older adult who lives at home and suffers a hip fracture in a fall. This individual may require treatment and care from a number of individuals and care settings. An exchange of information among all individuals and agencies is critical in achieving successful outcomes with this client (Coleman, 2003).

The current health care system is not designed to provide chronic care. Reimbursement has favored hospitalizations and physicians' visits, and has not been generous in funding long-term care, home health and preventive services (Zitter, 1997, p. 1). In this acute care model, reimbursement is focused on components of care and not the totality of client needs. With that in mind, a concept of care within the health care delivery system has evolved called disease management. *Disease management* programs

are "discrete programs directed at reducing costs and improving outcomes for patients with particular conditions" (Rothman & Wagner, 2003, p. 257).

During the mid to late 1990s many disease management companies were developed, with most having the goal to provide cost-effective care to clients with chronic conditions. By 1999 there were 200 companies nationwide offering disease management services for such conditions as diabetes, asthma and heart failure (Bodenheimer, 2003). Most of those programs did not take place within health care institutions, but were outsourced to separate firms. Today, fewer of those companies exist or are profitable—primarily because their focus was on one specific disease, when typically the older population may have multiple chronic conditions. As an example, fewer than half of the re-hospitalizations among patients initially hospitalized with heart failure are actually attributed to the heart failure. The other hospitalizations are related to conditions that predispose to heart failure, such as coronary artery disease, hypertension, chronic obstructive pulmonary disease and so forth (DeBusk, West, Miller, & Taylor, 1999). These disease management companies offered programs that were just that, programs, and neither a systems approach to the conditions nor an integration of these programs into the health care system. Additionally, a number of these disease management programs are based around physician specialty practice, and not primary practice. However, if we look at our elderly population, they have several chronic conditions that might necessitate their going to several different specialty physicians. Thus, a chronic care program based on specialty practice will be ineffective.

Some commercial health maintenance organizations (HMOs) initiated disease management programs as well. Those programs consisted of providing physicians with clinical practice guidelines, sending client education materials in the mail, and informing physicians if clients were not compliant with their plans of care (Bodenheimer, 2003).

Prevention and maintenance must be a part of a chronic disease management program. Unfortunately, however, admission rates in certain diseases have increased. Between 1994 and 2000, admission rates increased in chronic obstructive pulmonary disease by 20%, hypertension by 13% and bacterial pneumonia by 9% (Kruzikas et al., 2004). Hospitalizations may be prevented by high quality primary and preventive care. If clinicians can diagnose, treat and educate clients, and if clients can then self-manage their care and adopt more healthy lifestyles, hospitalizations may decrease.

So what is the best model for caring for individuals with chronic illness? Much of the work in evaluating programs and developing 'best practice' in this area has come from the work of Edward Wagner, Director of the McColl Institute for Healthcare Innovation at the Group Health Cooperative of Puget Sound, Seattle, Washington. Wagner and his colleagues surveyed 72 chronic disease management programs that were nominated by experts as 'best practice,' innovative and/or effective (Wagner, Davis, Schaefer, VonKorff, & Austin, 2002). To gauge these models, Wagner et al developed a model to determine effectiveness of care (see Figure 1-1). Their model re-

quires an appropriately organized health care system linked with policies and resources from the community. The policies and resources may provide access to supportive or educational services not available in the health care system. Key to their model is the creation of a patient-centered, collaborative care plan, based on timely assessments, that is targeted to each client.

Results of their survey demonstrated that few programs could consistently demonstrate positive results. One-half of the programs could not identify the population of patients they were to serve, and of that number another half reported that they were serving only a minority of the population (Wagner et al., 2002). A clear problem was the lack of organizational strategies to implement the programs and weak linkages to primary care for specialty-based programs (p. 78). Of the 72 programs evaluated, only one had all the elements of an effective chronic illness program according to Wagner's model. Wagner's work suggests that caring for an individual with chronic illness needs a systems approach.

If clients are receiving the majority of their care at a primary care practice, then why not have clients

FIGURE 1-1

A Model for Effective Chronic Illness Care

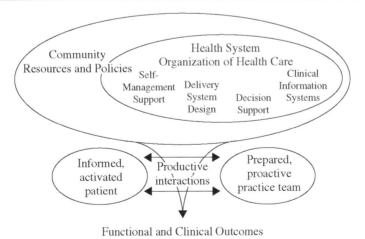

SOURCE: *Key Aspects to Preventing & Managing Chronic Illness.* Funk et al. © Springer Publishing Company, Inc., New York, NY 10036. Used by permission.

receive their chronic illness management there as well, as compared with going to an endocrinologist for diabetes, a cardiologist for heart failure and a rheumatologist for arthritis. If a primary care practice truly practices as such, then continuity, comprehensiveness and coordination, all tenets of primary care, are congruent with the needs of the individual with chronic illness (Rothman & Wagner, 2003, p. 256). But, again, the practice has to meet these expectations in order to be effective in managing chronic illness. In addition, primary care practices often use providers other than physicians, such as nurses, nurse practitioners, and physician assistants. Successful chronic illness interventions and programs include major roles for non-physicians (Rothman & Wagner, 2003).

In addition to the development of their model to evaluate programs, Wagner and associates have developed the Chronic Care Model to be used by organizations to guide services (Bodenheimer, 2003). The Chronic Care Model is an example of how theory grows from practice and then feeds back to improve practice (p. 64). What makes this model different from standard disease management models are the goals. The primary goal of a disease management company is to reduce costs first and then improve chronic care; while the Chronic Care Model's goals are reversed, in that improvement of care is the primary goal followed by reduced costs. The Chronic Care Model utilizes primary care practice as opposed to specialty practice that is often utilized in disease management companies. The Chronic Care Model contains four internal components and two external components (see Table 1-5).

Although the model designed by Wagner and colleagues shows promise, the real test is in its implementation. One concern is whether this model and other similar ones are truly *illness management* models, as opposed to *disease management* models. Clients with a specific chronic disease still must "fit" within a clinical pathway, protocol or map, which is then used to determine interventions. Although Wagner's model of care may be cost effective, it is unclear whether it has the individualism of a true illness management model. Concerns include the issue

---

TABLE 1-5

The Chronic Care Model

*Internal Components
(intrinsic to the provider organization)*

- Self-management support
- Decision support
  - Clinical practice guidelines
  - Clinician education
- Delivery system redesign
  - Planned visits (including group visits)
  - Case management
  - Primary care teams
- Clinical information systems
  - Registries
  - Clinical feedback
  - Reminders

External Components

- Community resources
- Health care organization

SOURCE: Bodenheimer, T. (2003). Interventions to improve chronic illness care: Evaluating their effectiveness. *Disease Management, 6* (2), 63–71.

---

of quality of care versus quantity of care and whether the individual needs of the client will be met.

There will always be unique ways of managing chronic illness. For instance, clients with Multiple Sclerosis (MS) at the Mellen Center for Multiple Sclerosis and nurse case managers have been using email since 1998 to better meet client needs. Client satisfaction continues at a very high level (Cleveland Clinic Foundation, 2005)

Busk and colleagues (1999) sum up what is needed most in caring for clients with chronic illness, "a therapeutic approach that emphasizes treating the patient with disease(s) rather than treating disease(s) in the patient" (p. 2740).

Professional and Community Responsibility

Community professionals must advocate for common sense prevention planning. *Healthy People*

2010 provides a systematic approach to health improvement, including the health of each individual, the health of communities, and the health of the Nation (DHHS, 2000). The objectives of *Healthy People 2010* are based on two overarching goals: (1) Increase the quality and years of healthy life; and (2) eliminate health disparities among subgroups of the population. These goals are being monitored through 467 objectives in 28 focus areas. Many of the objectives focus on interventions designed to reduce or eliminate illness, disability, and premature death among individuals and communities. Other objectives focus on broader areas such as improving access to quality health care, strengthening public health services, and improving the availability and dissemination of health-related information (DHHS, 2000). Additionally, many of the focus areas relate to chronic disease and/or prevention of chronic disease (Table 1-6).

Research

There is a continuing need for research to demonstrate new paradigms of caring for individuals with chronic illness. Although nursing research has made strides in this area, there is a continuing lack of interventional studies. What are the nursing interventions that increase the quality of life of a client with chronic illness?

An example of such an interventional study is examining 'transitional care' in older adults hospitalized with heart failure. In a randomized clinical trial, the experimental group (n = 118) received comprehensive care by an advanced practice nurse (APN) that included individualized care plans; home visits after discharge; and the availability of an APN by phone 24 hours/day-7 days/week. The control group (n = 121) received traditional care with routine discharge instructions. One year after the initial hospitalization, the experimental group had fewer hospital admissions, fewer deaths, fewer hospital days on admission, greater satisfaction with care and their costs were 37.6% less than the con-trol group (Naylor, Brooten, Campbell, Maislin, McCauley, & Schwartz, 2004)

Along with the need for interventional studies is the increased need to measure individual, popu-

---

TABLE 1-6

Focus Areas of *Healthy People 2010*

- Access to Quality Health Services
- Arthritis, Osteoporosis, and Chronic Back Disorders
- Cancer
- Chronic Kidney Disease
- Diabetes
- Disability and Secondary Conditions
- Educational and Community-Based Programs
- Environmental Health
- Family Planning
- Food Safety
- Health Communication
- Heart Disease and Stroke
- HIV
- Immunization and Infectious Diseases
- Injury and Violence Prevention
- Maternal, Infant, and Child Health
- Medical Product Safety
- Mental Health and Mental Disorders
- Nutrition and Overweight
- Occupational Safety and Health
- Oral Health
- Physical Activity and Fitness
- Public Health Infrastructure
- Respiratory Diseases
- Sexually Transmitted Diseases
- Substance Abuse
- Tobacco Use
- Vision and Hearing

SOURCE: Department of Health and Human Services. (2000). *Healthy People 2010*. A systematic approach to health improvement. Available on-line at http://www.health.gov/healthypeople/Document/html/uih/uih_2.htm

---

lation and system outcomes. Some interventional research is, indeed, outcome research; that is, this specific nursing intervention produces this specific client outcome. With health care costs continuing to rise, there is great interest in identifying positive outcomes for the system and the individual. Managed care organizations can describe the population clinical outcomes (i.e., readmission to the acute care setting, medication costs, recidivism, etc.), but there are other outcomes that may be nurse-specific. What are the client outcomes of specific nursing interventions? What difference does that intervention make in the quality of life of an individual?

The interest in outcomes is not new. Florence Nightingale looked at patient outcomes by examining morbidity and mortality rates of soldiers in the Crimean War. The difference now is the mismatch that often occurs between the outcome of the individual client and the outcome of the health care delivery system for a population of clients (Mitchell, Crittenden, Howard, Lawson, Root, & Schaad, 2000).

Within the framework of the health care delivery system, a number of outcomes are monitored. These include service outcomes (i.e., the interval between patient arrival at an emergency room and the beginning of thrombolytic therapy); clinical quality outcomes (i.e., readmission rate); fiscal outcomes (i.e., average length of stay, cost, and readmission rates); and health status (i.e., long-term outcomes) (Brown, 2000). Although these outcomes are salient,

they examine an entire population, and often the individual is lost in the shuffle. It is difficult to measure the quality of life of an individual and family in this manner.

■ Summary and Conclusions

Caring for the client and family with chronic illness is an ongoing challenge in health care. How health care professionals balance quality of care and quantity of care will continue to be an issue. It is essential that the health care system in the United States develop a continuum of care for its population with chronic illness. The acute care system of the past and present, or, as some call it, a "nonsystem", must be redefined to better care for its clients. The increasing elderly population and those with chronic illness do not fit within the current paradigm of care. A new paradigm must emerge to care for individuals with chronic illness.

Study Questions

1. Describe the factors and influences that have led to the increase in chronicity that exists today.
2. In what ways do statistics influence our perspective of chronic illness positively and negatively?
3. Describe the difficulty in defining *chronicity*. What factors should be considered in defining *chronicity*?
4. How does one's developmental stage influence an individual's response to chronic illness?
5. How does our society treat and/or react to someone with chronic illness?
6. What changes in health professional education need to occur to provide better care for the population with chronic illness?

7. What is the relationship between the goals of *Healthy People 2010* and chronic illness?
8. Compare and contrast chronic disease with chronic illness.
9. What changes must occur in the current health care system to better meet the needs of the chronically ill population?
10. How does one's culture affect the chronic illness experience and how health care professionals provide for that individual's care?

References

Anderson, G., & Knickman, J. (2001). Changing the chronic care system to meet people's needs. *Health Affairs, 20* (6), 146–160.

Benjamin, A., & Newcomer, R. (1997). Community level indicators of chronic health conditions. In R. Newcomer & A. Benjamin (Eds.), *Indicators of chronic health conditions*, pp. 1–14. Baltimore: Johns Hopkins University Press.

Bodenheimer, T. (2003). Interventions to improve chronic illness care: Evaluating their effectiveness. *Disease Management 6* (2), 63–71.

Bortz, W. (1988). Geriatrics: Through the looking glass [Commentary]. *Medical Times, 117,* 85–92.

Brown, M. (2000). Stroke management: Beginnings. *Outcomes Management for Nursing Practice, 4* (1), 34–38.

Brown-Hellsten, M. (2005). Chronic illness, disability or end-of-life care for the child and family. In M. Hockenberry (Ed.) *Wong's Essentials of Pediatric Nursing* (7th ed.). (pp. 549–588). St. Louis: Mosby.

Campinha-Bacote, J. (1999). A model and instrument for addressing cultural competence in health care. *Journal of Nursing Education, 38* (5), 203–207.

Centers for Medicare & Medicaid Services (2005). The chronic care improvement program. (http://www.cms.hhs.gov/medicarereform/ccip/) Retrieved 2/20/05.

Chin, J. (2000). Culturally competent health care. *Public Health Reports, 115,* 25–33.

Cipolla, C. (1992). *Miasmas and disease: Public health and the environment in the pre-industrial age.* New Haven, CT: Yale University Press.

Cluff, L. (1981). Chronic disease, function and the quality of care, Editorial. *Journal of Chronic Diseases, 34,* 299–304.

Coleman, E. (2003). Falling through the cracks: Challenges and opportunities for improving transitional care for persons with continuous complex care needs. *Journal of the American Geriatrics Society, 51* (4), 549–555.

Commission on Chronic Illness. (1957) *Chronic illness in the United States, prevention of chronic illness.* Cambridge, MA: Harvard University Press.

Congressional Budget Office. (2004). A detailed description of CBO's cost estimate for the Medicare Prescription Drug Benefit. (http://www.cob/gov/ftpdocs/56xx.doc5668/Report.pdf) Retrieved 10/18/04.

Curtin, M., & Lubkin, I. (1995). What is chronicity? In I. Lubkin (Ed.), *Chronic illness: Impact and interventions* (3rd ed.), (pp. 3–25). Sudbury, MA: Jones & Bartlett.

Debusk, R., West, J., Miller, N., & Taylor, C. (1999). Chronic disease management: treating the patient with disease(s) vs. treating disease(s) in the patient. *Archives of Internal Medicine, 159,* 2739–2742.

Department of Health and Human Services. (2000). *Healthy People 2010. A systematic approach to health improvement.* Available on-line at http://www.health.gov/healthypeople/Document/html/uih/uih_2.htm. Retrieved 2/20/05.

Emanuel, E. (1982). We are all chronic patients. *Journal of Chronic Diseases, 35,* 501–502.

Feldman, D. (1974). Chronic disabling illness: A holistic view. *Journal of Chronic Diseases, 27,* 287–291.

Field, M., & Cassel, C. (1997). *Approaching death: Improving care at the end of life.* Washington, DC: National Academies Press.

Funk et al. (2001). *Key Aspects to Preventing & Managing Chronic Illness.* New York, NY: Springer Publishing, Inc.

Greiner, A., & Knebel, E. (Eds.) (2003). *Health professions education: A bridge to quality.* Washington, DC: National Academies Press.

Healthy People 2010: A systematic approach to health improvement. Available at: http://www.healthpeople.gov/Document/html/uih/uih_2.htm. Retrieved 2/20/05.

Jackson, P. (2000). The primary care provider and children with chronic conditions. In P. Jackson & P. Vessey (Eds.), *Primary care of the child with a chronic condition* (3rd ed.). St. Louis: Mosby.

Judson, L. (2004). Global childhood chronic illness. *Nursing Administration Quarterly, 28* (1), 60–66.

Kelley, E., May, E., Kosiak, B., McNeil, D., et al. (2004). Prevention healthcare quality in America: Findings from the first national healthcare quality and disparities reports. *Preventing Chronic Disease* [serial online] 2004 July. Available at: http://www.cdc.gov/pcd/issues/2004/jul/04_0031.htm.

Knafl, K., & Deatrick J. (1986). How families manage chronic conditions: An analysis of the concept of normalization. *Research in Nursing and Health, 9,* 215–222.

Kruzikas, D., Jiang, H., Remus, D., Barrett, M., et al. (2004). *Preventable hospitalizations: A window into primary and preventive care, 2000.* Agency for

Healthcare Research and Quality, 2004. HCUP Fact book No. 5: AHRQ Publication No. 04-0056.

Lubkin, I. (Ed.). (1995).*Chronic illness: Impact and interventions* (3rd ed.). Sudbury, MA: Jones & Bartlett.

Lynn, J. & Adamson, D. (2003). Living well at the end of life: Adapting health care to serious chronic illness in old age. Available at: http://www.rand.org/publications/WP/WP137/.

Majno, G. (1975). *The healing hand.* Cambridge, MA: Harvard University Press.

Managing chronic illness with technology (2005). *Notable nursing: Revolutionizing nursing practice.* Cleveland, OH: The Cleveland Clinic Foundation.

Mayo, L. (Ed.). (1956). *Guides to action on chronic illness.* Commission on Chronic Illness. New York: National Health Council.

Mitchell, P., Crittenden, R., Howard, E., Lawson, B., et al. (2000). Interdisciplinary clinical education: Evaluating outcomes of an evolving model. *Outcomes Management for Nursing Practice, 4* (1),3–6.

National Center for Health Statistics (2004). *Health, United States, 2004. With Chartbook on Trends in the Health of Americans,* Hyattsville, MD. Washington DC: US Government Printing Office.

Naylor, M., Brooten, D., Campbell, R., Maislin, G., et al. (2004). Transitional care of older adults hospitalized with heart failure: A randomized, controlled trial. *Journal of the American Geriatrics Society, 52*(5), 675–84.

Newacheck, P., Hung, Y., Park, M., Brindis, C., et al. (2004). Disparities in adolescent health and health care: Does socioeconomic status matter? *Health Services Research, 38*(5), 1235–52.

Partnership for Solutions (2001).Available on-line at http://www.partnershipforsolutions.org/statistics/prevalence.htm. A Partnership of Johns Hopkins University and the Robert Wood Johnson Foundation. Retrieved 5/31/01.

Partnership for Solutions. (2004). Available on-line at http://www.partnershipforsolutions.org/statistics/prevalence.htm. Retrieved 2/14/05. A Partnership of Johns Hopkins University and the Robert Wood Johnson Foundation. *Chronic Conditions: Making the Case for Ongoing Care,* September 2004 update.

Perrin, J. (2004). Chronic illness in childhood. In R. Behrman, R. Kleigman & H. Jensen (Eds.) *Nelson textbook of pediatrics* (17th ed.) Philadelphia: Saunders.

Pew Health Professions Commission. (1998). Twenty-one competencies for the 21st century. Available on-line at http://www.futurehealth.ucsf.edu/pewcomm/competen.html.

Powell, S. (2000). *Advanced case management: Outcomes and beyond.* Philadelphia: Lippincott.

Roberts, D. (1954). The overall picture of long-term illness. Address given at a conference on problems of aging, School of Public Health, Harvard University, June 1954. Subsequently published in *Journal of Chronic Diseases,* February 1955, 149–159.

Rolland, J. (1987). Family illness and the life cycle: A conceptual framework. *Family Process, 26,* 203–221.

Rothman, A., & Wagner, E. (2003). Chronic illness management: What is the role of primary care? *Annals of Internal Medicine, 138,* 256–261.

Schmitke, J. & Schlomann, P. (2002). Chronic conditions. In N. Potts & B. Mandleco (Eds.) *Pediatric Nursing: Caring for children and their families.* (pp. 493–515). Clifton Park, NY: Delmar.

Sharpe, D. & Rossiter, L. (2002). Siblings of children with a chronic illness: A meta-analysis. *Journal of Pediatric Psychology, 27,* 699–710.

Smedley, B., Stith, A., & Nelson, A. (Eds.) (2003). *Unequal treatment : Confronting racial and ethnic disparities in healthcare.* Washington, DC: National Academies Press.

Smith, C., Cowan, C., Sensening, A., & Catlin, A. (2005). Health spending growth slows in 2003. *Health Affairs, 24*(1), 185–94.

U.S. Census Bureau (2004). U.S. Interim Projections by Age, Sex, Race, and Hispanic Origin. (http://www.census.gov/ipc/www/usinterimproj/natprojtab01a.pdf). Retrieved 10/18/04.

U.S. Department of Health and Human Services. (1999). *Office of Minority Health and Resources for Cross Cultural Health Care.* Available on-line at http://www.omhrc.gov/clas/index.htm.

U.S. Department of Health and Human Services. (2000). *Healthy People 2010. A systematic approach to health improvement.* Available on-line at http://www.health.gov/healthypeople/Document/html/uih/uih2.htm. Retrieved 6/4/01.

Zitter, M. (1997). A new paradigm in health care delivery: Disease management. In W. Todd & D. Nash (Eds.) *Disease management: A systems approach to improving patient outcomes.* (pp. 1–25). Chicago: American Hospital Publishing.

CHAPTER 2

Illness Behavior and Roles

Pamala D. Larsen ▪ Patricia Ryan Lewis ▪ Ilene Morof Lubkin

Illness is the night-side of life, a more onerous citizen-ship. Everyone who is born holds dual citizenship, in the kingdom of the well and in the kingdom of the sick. Although we all prefer to use only the good passport, sooner or later each of us is obligated, at least for a spell, to identify ourselves as citizens of that other place.
Susan Sontag, *Illness as Metaphor* (1988) p. 3

Introduction

Society establishes both formal and informal guidelines that influence the behavior of its members. The behavior and illness experience of those with a chronic condition are shaped by these societal influences as well. The individual who fully recovers from an illness returns to prior behaviors and roles. However, when there is only partial recovery or continuing illness as with a chronic disease, the individual has to modify or adapt previous roles to accommodate both social expectations and their health status.

Both the presentation of an illness and others' responses to it are determined by socio-cultural factors (Helman, 2001). Cultures have their own *language of distress* which bridges the chasm between the subjective experience and society's acknowledgement of it (p. 85). Each culture decides which symptoms are abnormal, and each shapes the emotional and physical changes into a pattern that defines the illness (Helman, 2001).

Illness Behavior

Disease not only involves the body, but also affects one's relationships, self-image and behavior. The social aspects of disease are related to the pathophysiological changes that are occurring, but may be independent of them as well. The very act of defining something as an illness has consequences far beyond the pathology involved (Conrad, 2005).

> When a veterinarian diagnoses a cow's condition as an illness, he does not merely by diagnosis change the cow's behavior . . . but when a physician diagnoses a human's condition as an illness, he changes the man's behavior by diagnosis: a social state is added to a biophysiological state by assigning the meaning of illness to disease
>
> (Freidson, 1970, p. 223).

Illness behavior refers to the varying ways individuals respond to bodily indications, how they monitor internal states, define and interpret symptoms, make attributions, take remedial actions and utilize various sources of informal and formal care (Mechanic, 1995, p. 1208). The first reference to illness behavior in the literature was by Mechanic in the late 1950s. Although his work was new, the original concept was developed by Talcott Parsons (1951) and an essay by Henry Sigerist in 1929 that described the 'special position of the sick' (Mechanic, 1995). Each individual's interpretation of health status, and thus illness behavior, is influenced by a myriad of factors. Illness behavior, in turn, influences utilization of health care services.

Influences to Illness Behavior and Roles

Social, cultural, economic and demographic factors influence behavior and responses to pathological signs and symptoms. The culture of poverty (Rundall & Wheeler, 1979) influences the development of social and psychological traits among those experiencing it. These traits include dependence, fatalism, inability to delay gratification, and a lower value placed on health (Cockerham, 2001, p. 123). The poor, who have to work to survive, often deny sickness unless it brings functional incapacity (Helman, 2001).

Marital status may influence illness behavior as well. In general, married individuals require fewer services because they are healthier, but utilize other services because they are more attuned to preventive care (Thomas, 2003).

Cultures have distinct concepts of how illness is defined and the behaviors that are valid for themselves or others (Helman, 2001). One's learning, socialization and past experience, as defined by their social and cultural background, mediate illness behavior. Past experiences of observing one's parents being stoic, going to work when they were ill, avoiding medical help, all influence their children's future responses. If children see that 'hard work' and not giving in to illness pays off with rewards, they will assimilate those experiences and mirror them in their own lives.

The Sick Role

Sickness has typically been viewed by sociologists as a form of deviant behavior (Cockerham, 2001, p. 157). This view was corroborated by Talcott Parsons' development of the *sick role*, introduced in his book *The Social System* (1951). Parsons, a proponent of functionalist theory, saw sickness as dysfunctional because it threatened to interfere with the stability of the social system (Cockerham, 2001). From this functionalist viewpoint social systems are linked to systems of personality and culture to form a basis for social order (p. 160). He viewed sickness as a response to social pressure that permitted avoiding social responsibilities. Anyone could take on the role he identified; therefore, the role was achieved through failure to keep well.

There are four major components of the sick role and accompanying behaviors associated with each component (see Table 2-1). Roles are learned, and likewise, the sick role is learned as well. Society is expected to accept the individual in the sick role as long as the individual continues to abide by the four components (Meleis, 1988, p. 366).

Parsons' sick role defines both the patient/client obligations and the physician obligations. Parsons considers the patient-physician relationship as well-defined, stable and predictable. The client is sick and not responsible for his condition; however, he has an obligation to want to get well and seek competent help in the meantime. Thus, the physican enters the relationship as the expert as defined by society and able to help the patient. Although there is mutuality in this patient-physician relationship, the status and power of the individuals is not equal. The physician is in power. Physicians are the ones who create the social possibilities for acting sick because they are society's experts on who is 'really' sick and who define illness (Freidson, 1970, p. 206).

The Impaired Role

The sick role has more applicability to individuals with acute illness and injuries. When it is applied to long-term chronic illness, the role has less

---

TABLE 2-1

Characteristics of the Sick Role

Component of the Role	Associated Expectations and Behaviors
Sick person is exempt from normal social roles	Dependent on the nature and severity of illness. More severe illness allows patient to be exempt from more roles. Requires legitimization (validation) by physician.
Sick person is not responsible for his/her condition	Not responsible for becoming sick, the individual therefore has a right to be cared for. Physical dependency and the right to emotional support are therefore acceptable. Will need a curative process apart from personal willpower or motivation to get well.
Obligation to want to become well	Being ill is seen as undesirable. Because privileges and exemptions of the sick role can become secondary gains, the motivation to recover assumes primary importance.
Obligation to seek and cooperate with technically competent help	The patient needs technical expertise that the physician and other health professionals have. Cooperation with these professionals for the common goal of getting well is mandatory.

SOURCE: Cockerham, W. C. (2001). *Medical Sociology* (8th ed.), (p. 160), Upper Saddle River, NJ: Prentice-Hall.

usefulness. A more appropriate role for those with chronic illness is the 'impaired' role (Gordon, 1966). Although less well known than the sick role, it better addresses the needs of those with chronic illness.

Gordon (1966) identified behaviors, responses and expectations of several socioeconomic groups toward illnesses that differed in both severity and duration. He found, among all groups, that prognosis was the major factor in defining someone as "sick," and that once someone was so defined, behaviors were consistent with Parsons' model. When prognosis worsened, all groups encouraged increased exemption from social responsibility. Socioeconomic groups varied in terms of *who* was defined as sick, with members from lower socioeconomic groups equating sickness with functional incapacity.

Gordon identified two illness role statuses. The first was the *sick role,* as previously defined by Parsons, which was a valid role when the prognosis was grave and uncertain. The second role, which Gordon called the *impaired role,* was considered appropriate for conditions in which the prognosis was known and was not grave. When individuals were seen in the impaired role, 'normal' social expectations and responsibilities were expected (Gordon,

1966). In other words, if society did not consider the individual 'sick', it was expected that the individual return to normal behavior, within the limitations of the condition.

The impaired role assumes the following characteristics:

1. The individual has an impairment that is permanent.
2. The individual does not give up normal role responsibilities but is expected to maintain normal behavior within the limits of the health condition. Modification of life situations may be necessitated by the disability.
3. The individual does not have to "want to get well," but rather is encouraged to make the most of remaining capabilities. The individual must realize potentialities while accepting the existence of the impairment and recognizing limitations and performance commensurate with the disability (Wu, 1973).

Inherent in the impaired role is the attitude that retaining sick role behaviors prevents the individual from managing their own care. However, once the impaired role is accepted, activities that help maintain control of the condition, prevent complications, lead to resumption of role responsibilities, and result in full realization of potentialities are acceptable (Wu, 1973). The impaired role incorporates both rehabilitation and maximization of wellness.

The impaired role, sometimes called the at-risk role, is seen as a transitional state, one in which individuals make changes in a variety of role behaviors that they enacted prior to the illness. This role has some obligations, such as carrying out the medical regimen, but requires much less reduction in other social roles than does the sick role. One important difference between the two roles is that the impaired role has much more uncertainty associated with it than does the sick role. Signs, symptoms, and time boundaries are less clear than those found in the sick role (Meleis, 1988).

■ Issues Related to Illness Behavior and Roles

Criticisms of Parsons' Model

The major deficiency of the sick role model is that it is based on acute episodic illness. It overlooks characteristics of chronic illness, the long-term rather than temporary nature of the illness, the reality that full recovery is not a reasonable expectation, acknowledgment that management is often the responsibility of the client or family, and the individual must adjust to a permanent change. Individuals with chronic illness are often unable to resume prior roles fully and need to focus on retaining (not regaining) optimal role performance, restricted only in relationship to limitations imposed by the disease (Kassenbaum & Baumann, 1965).

Parsons' sick role views patients as victims of illness, and although they take responsibility for their care, the patient must remain the subordinate member of the physician-patient dyad (Meleis, 1988). However, the patient 'role' in 1951 when Parsons

published *The Social System*, and the role of the patient today are quite different. The current healthcare system with increased consumerism and an information laden society with everything available on the internet, have created patients involved with their care and 'in charge' of their health care. Patients today are partners in their care, as opposed to the physician-patient relationship in 1951.

Parsons' sick role has been described as a middle-class pattern of behavior. It emphasizes individual responsibility, striving for normality, and rational problem solving (Cockerham, 2001). It assumes that any effort toward health will result in positive gain. For those in poverty, the sick role is often denied because they have not had the opportunity in the past to enjoy secondary gains from being ill. Additionally, in an environment of poverty, success is the exception to the rule (p. 170).

Exemption from Role Responsibilities

Studies dealing with role responsibilities and performance assume that the person who is willing to consult the doctor is ready to adopt the sick role (Segall, 1976), although the individual's willingness to give up normal work responsibilities or to become dependent on others has not been studied.

Exemption from role responsibilities also requires legitimization, or validation, from others to prevent malingering by those who are not truly ill (Cockerham, 2001). Parsons' model appears to view individuals as helpless victims of illness who have only to seek care and then to cooperate with that care. However, changing health care values have led to the assumption by many Americans that much of the responsibility for health lies with the individual.

Alcoholism and mental illness are both disorders in which obtaining release from role responsibilities is difficult (Segall, 1976). Although alcoholism is now considered a disease needing treatment, most people, including most health professionals, still feel that legitimizing this disorder removes the responsibility that society believes alcoholics should take for their behavior. Consequently, alcoholics are frequently denied the legitimacy that allows them to take on the sick role (Finerman & Bennett, 1994).

Seeking and Cooperating with Competent Help

The four components of the sick role have been studied extensively, especially the component that deals with seeking out and cooperating with technically competent help. Often missing from discussion of this component is the idea that defining oneself as "ill" is a social process, one that involves both subjective experiences of physical or emotional changes and the confirmation of those changes by other people (Helman, 2001). Cultural factors determine which symptoms or signs are perceived as abnormal and the appropriate response that is expected (Buchwald et al., 1994; Mechanic, 1992). Other criticisms concern the oversimplification of behaviors and the model's failure to take into account the personality and orientation of the individual, aspects that influence dependence, knowledge, psychological needs, and so forth (Helman, 2001).

Also missing from this component of the model is a "healthy stage" when individuals may seek contact with the health care system for purposes other than treatment of illness (Hover & Juelsgaard, 1978). Many people are less dependent than Parsons' model would indicate. Mechanic (1961, 1972) takes issue with the assumption that seeking professional care and legitimization is always a condition of assuming the sick role. He demonstrated that individuals can assume a sick role that may or may not include medical treatment.

Who Legitimizes Chronic Illness?

Parsons' model emphasized the physician's role in legitimizing illness; it did not deal with the roles of nurses, social workers, and other health care providers in the process. Legitimizing actions by family and others was also considered less significant. Although the physician may give the final validation with acute illnesses, one must question whether this prerogative applies to situations involving the individual with chronic illness or permanent disability.

Health care management of chronic illnesses occurs primarily in the home, a situation that results in increased dependency on nonprofessional sources for care. Helman (2001) points out that in order for an individual to adopt the rights and benefits of the sick role, the cooperation of his or her social group is required. Once members of the social group deem an individual "sick," they feel obligated to provide care. Honig-Parnass (1981) found that a "more crucial role in their treatment was assigned [by patients] to the lay significant others than to professionals." In other words, care and support by lay caregivers were felt to be more important legitimizing criteria for the chronically ill than was medical care in relation to managing their daily activities.

With some illnesses, especially when symptoms are not well defined, receiving legitimization from the physician or other health care professionals can be difficult and frustrating. Denial of opportunity to move into the sick role leads to "doctor hopping," placing clients in problematic relationships in which they must "work out" solutions alone (Steward & Sullivan, 1982). As a result, symptomatic persons may be left to question the truth of their own perceptions.

As examples, two current chronic conditions often defy diagnosis and are slow to respond to treatment. Chronic fatigue syndrome (CFS) and fibromyalgia are typically seen as diseases of young women. Both diseases are uncertain in regard to etiology, treatment and prognosis. They have been contested illnesses, in that some question their existence (Asbring, 2001). Without legitimatization from physicians or the health care system, these clients get labeled as hypochondriacs or as malingerers. Some of these clients are referred to psychologists or psychiatrists when a physical diagnosis cannot be made and diagnostic tests are normal.

When a diagnosis is finally made, the client frequently shows an initial somewhat joyous response to having a name for the recurrent and troublesome symptoms. This reaction results from the decrease in stress over the unknown. These clients have an enormous stake in how their illnesses are understood. They seek to achieve the legitimacy necessary to elicit sympathy and avoid stigma, and to protect their own self-concept (Mechanic, 1995).

Who Seeks the Sick Role?

Individuals gauge sickness more by the disruption of their ability to function than by organic parameters. Psychological factors such as anxiety and fear play a role. Individuals may have to experience a crisis or realize that symptoms interfere with important activities before they will seek help (Redman, 1993).

Another factor may be previous associations with the sick role. Whitehead and associates (1982) found that individuals who, as children, received rewards (toys, food, and so on) when they were sick tended to move into the sick role more readily, voiced more somatic complaints, made more doctor visits, had more acute and chronic illnesses, and missed a greater number of work days. Further work has also demonstrated that social modeling of illness behavior by parents influences the amount of disability displayed by their children in similar circumstances (Schwartz, Gramling & Mancini, 1994; Whitehead et al., 1994).

Other factors that influence moving into the sick role include economic ability to pay for medical care; a sense of responsibility to one's own health; and personal views of medicine, professionals, surgery, and the body itself (Redman, 1993). As an example, the elderly often see bodily changes as a "natural" part of aging rather than as symptoms, and this attitude adds to their reluctance to seek care, especially when it is coupled with economic concerns.

Mechanic (1972) points out seven important variables that influence an individual's willingness to move into the sick role; some of them tie into an individual's health beliefs:

1. Number and persistence of symptoms
2. Individual's ability to recognize symptoms
3. Perceived seriousness of symptoms
4. Available information and medical knowledge
5. Cultural background of the defining person, group, or agency in terms of emphasis placed on qualities such as tolerance or stoicism
6. Extent of social and physical disability resulting from the symptoms
7. Available sources of help and their social and physical accessibility

Role Changes

Being diagnosed with a chronic disease, either suddenly or gradually, is difficult. Diagnosis influences current roles, and may require the person to incorporate new knowledge, to alter behavior, and to define self in a new social context (Kubisch & Wichowski, 1992). Many believe that our social structure gives confusing messages to those with chronic illness and how they should conduct their roles (Thorne, 1993).

Role Insufficiency

Problems that arise in making role transitions can result in role insufficiency. Disparity in fulfilling role expectations, obligations, or goals as perceived by self or significant others is termed role insufficiency (Meleis, 1988, p. 371). Role insufficiency may be either voluntary or involuntary. Voluntary role insufficiency may be the result of the patient weighing the rewards and costs of a certain role and deciding that the costs are greater than the rewards (Meleis, 1988).

Role Ambiguity

Role insufficiency may also be linked to role ambiguity, which describes a situation in which there is a lack of clarity about the expectations of a role (Hardy & Hardy, 1988). This situation arises when the individual has little information about the behaviors expected in a particular role or when members of an individual's social system do not communicate clear expectations for a particular role.

Role Conflict

Role conflict is a broad term used to describe an individual's experience of conflicting role demands. In *intrarole conflict,* the individual fails to demonstrate role mastery because of conflicting expectations of others for the enactment of a particular role (Nuwayhid, 1991). An example of this type of conflict is a new mother who is trying to adjust to the role of motherhood and is receiving strongly conflicting messages from her own mother and her mother-in-law about how she should care for her child. In interrole conflict, the individual fails to demonstrate appropriate role behaviors as a result of occupying two roles that require behaviors that are incompatible with each other (Hardy & Hardy, 1988). An example of this type of conflict is a woman with a chronic illness who fails to take on the self-care behaviors required for the impaired role because she sees the demands of caring for her children as incompatible with taking the time to care for herself.

Role Strain

When faced with role uncertainty of any kind, the individual may exhibit psychological and physiological signs of role strain. Role strain is the response to feelings that role obligations are difficult or impossible to carry out. Symptoms of role strain may include anxiety, irritation, resentment, hostility, depression, grief, and apathy, as well as typical physiological stress responses (Hardy & Hardy, 1988; Meleis, 1975).

Secondary Gains

The desire to get well is an essential aspect of Parsons' model, but at times clients choose to remain in the sick role; many of their reactions and responses to illness are influenced by premorbid personality, life type, and level of psychosocial competence (Feldman, 1974). Almost everyone, at some point, welcomes illness as a temporary release from stressful situations. Young children quickly discover the manipulative possibilities of sore throats and stomach aches vis-à-vis school, and adults frequently welcome a day in bed with "a touch of the flu" as a sanctioned break from normal pressures.

Adaptation to chronic illness is a lengthy process (Davidhizar, 1994). Patients can be caught between the need to adapt to illness and the urge to return to a higher level of functioning. During this time of fluctuation, the patient may discover secondary gains from certain limitations. These unexpected benefits can make the maintenance or limitations seem attractive.

The uncritical assumption that "everybody wants to be healthy" can blind us to important aspects of health and illness behavior. Few, if any, people want good health at all costs, particularly if the enjoyment of good health seriously curtails all pleasures. Each year millions of Americans smoke, drink, and eat fatty foods in spite of the overwhelming evidence that these behaviors increase the likelihood of illness. Good health competes as a priority with all nonhealth activities, and individual behavior can be understood only in the larger context of life goals.

Life Cycle Differences

Responses to illness differ, depending on people's developmental stages, tasks, and roles. Each age group deals with illness roles, especially the impaired role, differently. Such variations are reflected in the responses of children and the elderly to illnesses.

Children and Chronic Illness

Research demonstrates that the chronically ill child is at significant risk for emotional maladjustment (Pless & Nolan, 1991). Problems include behavioral difficulties, low self-esteem, and poor resolution of developmental tasks. Evidence suggests that a child's risk for development of psychosocial problems is not linked to specific diagnoses or severity of illness (Breslau & Marshall, 1985; Heller et al.,

1985), although children with central nervous system involvement (especially mental retardation) do seem to be at higher risk (Breslau, 1982; Breslau & Marshall, 1985). In addition, the age and developmental stage of a child influence the resources that can be brought to the process of adjustment to chronic illness. Adolescents, already at a tumultuous stage of establishing identity and independence, are at serious risk (Boice, 1998).

Children with a chronic disease use a variety of coping strategies to deal with disease-specific as well as common stressors (Boekaerts & Roder, 1999). Work with diabetic children and adolescents demonstrates that developmental stage influences the way children cope with diabetes (Grey, Camerson & Thurber, 1991). Preadolescents were less depressed and anxious, coped in more positive ways, and were in better metabolic control than were adolescents. Adolescents, already under stress due to development and role changes, demonstrated more avoidance and depression and poorer metabolic control.

The social environment of children with chronic illness, especially the family environment, is very important in their adjustment (Harris, Newcomb & Gewanter, 1991). Chronic illness management is a way of life, and the ability of the family to respond to these demands dictates the quality of the child's and the family's life (McCarthy & Gallo, 1992). A change in the role of one person within the family (the chronically ill child) necessitates changes in the roles of all members of this social system (Meleis, 1975). Christian's (1989) work with families of children with cystic fibrosis suggests that an understanding of the family system is an important framework for explaining the family's adaptation to chronic illness.

It is often difficult, however, to draw conclusions about the direction of the relationship between family problems and maladjustment in chronically ill children. Family dysfunction is often shown to be associated with emotional problems among children with chronic illness (Pless & Nolan, 1991). However, the research has generally focused on families already affected by the stress of chronic illness and does not measure family functioning prior to the onset of the problem.

The Older Adult

The aged, who are involved in many role changes—often in a negative way—also illustrate the interaction of illness and life-cycle roles. Although our society purports to value each individual, many societal actions do not support this contention. Our society values youth, productivity, and independence, and many of these values no longer exist for the elderly as they face more and more role and responsibility losses. The loss of esteemed roles forces the elderly into dependent positions in which they receive little of the positive feedback that allows individuals to consider themselves valued (Kiesel & Beninger, 1979). Being old is sometimes similar to being ill, even for a person who is physically and mentally able (Gilles, 1972). In fact, some social attitudes toward aging and retirement are more appropriate with respect to the soon to be terminally ill than to those who have many long years ahead (Clark & Anderson, 1967).

These role losses affect physical and emotional well-being (Robinson, 1971). Given the greater number of illnesses found among the aged, and given that the sick role is a socially acceptable one, albeit of lower status than others, the aged sometimes find focusing on symptoms easy.

In the elderly, illness can be precipitated by many factors aside from physical and mental deterioration. Limited finances, poor housing and nutrition, social devaluation, and multiple losses all contribute to social isolation and illness (Robinson, 1971). Despite acute onset, most of these illnesses are chronic in nature. Being ill, which allows dependency without obligation, contains many features already present in their lives. For older persons who are alone even when they have families, the onset of symptoms can bring more attention from family members, attention that is unwarranted by the illness but that is considered culturally appropriate behavior (Hyman, 1971). This preferential treatment may become symbolic to the elderly client in two ways: (1) It indicates that some changes in status have occurred, and (2) it reinforces the sense of the sick role. The coupling of a socially acceptable role with the lack of other positive roles for the aged leads to a cycle in which the

The Older Adult and the Sick Role

A.B. had passed most of her adult life without serious health problems. At 68, she was widowed three years after retirement from her job as a candy maker. Her children had long since married and left home, and only one daughter lived in the same community. Her former activities as wife and mother and her involvement with her work had ended. In spite of adequate income to meet her needs and occasional phone contact with her children, A.B. felt lonely and deprived of a meaningful role.

A.B. had some long-standing but mild symptomatology that her physician had evaluated and treated: dysphagia (never diagnosed), mild coronary artery disease, and occasional low back pain. She had also been overweight most of her adult life. Within months of her widowhood, A.B. began making more frequent visits to her physician for evaluation of any symptom, regardless of how minimal. This illness behavior brought forth concerned responses from her family and provided her with a

topic of conversation and a socially acceptable behavior: waiting in the doctor's office. She also enjoyed striking up conversations with others who were waiting, as a change from her daily routine of cleaning house and watching television. No suggestions by her family that she would feel better if she would lose weight and increase her activity were effective. She insisted that the doctor would help her "get well." Visits to the doctor every month or two went on for several years.

By the time A.B. developed a terminal illness, her physician had become insensitive to her ongoing complaints of weakness, pain, fatigue, and so on. At age 74, A.B. consulted another physician, who became concerned by her insistence that she had been growing more fatigued over the last several months. A diagnostic workup revealed acute leukemia, and she entered a true sick role. She died 2 weeks later while undergoing chemotherapy.

SOURCE: From Lubkin (1995).

person adopts the sick role as normal and ongoing, as the case study of A.B. illustrates.

Professional Responses to Illness Behavior and Roles

Health care professionals generally expect those entering the acute hospital setting to conform to sick role behaviors. Most people entering the hospital for the first time are quickly socialized and expect to cooperate with treatment, to recover, and to return to their normal roles. Provider expectations and client responses are in line with social expectations and fit with the traditional medical model of illness as acute

and curable, and discharge is frequently equated with cure. When clients are compliant and cooperative, health providers communicate to them that they are "good patients" (Lorber, 1981). When clients are less cooperative, the staff may consider them problematic.

But the percentage of individuals with chronic illness entering hospitals is increasing. Such admissions occur when symptoms flare or acute illnesses are superimposed. Many of these people have had their chronic illnesses for indefinite periods of time and have had prior hospital experiences. Multiple contacts with the health care system result in loss of the "blind faith" that the individual once had in that system. Chronically ill individuals are seeking a new kind of relationship with health care providers (Thorne & Robinson, 1988). The extent to which a chronically ill patient is included in the formulation of his or her treatment plan will likely influence the assumption of responsibility for it and, ultimately, its success (Weaver & Wilson, 1994).

Being in the impaired role is integral to the daily lives of the chronically ill. Although willing to delegate some responsibility for care to health care personnel, they prefer to retain some control of their regimens when possible. These clients have developed their own competence over time spent dealing with their illnesses, and they have come to expect acknowledgment of that competence in their health care relationships (Thorne & Robinson, 1988).

Thorne's (1990) study of chronically ill individuals and their families found that their relationships with health care professionals evolved from what was termed "naive trust" through "disenchantment" to a final stage of "guarded alliance." She proposed that the "rules" that govern these relationships should be entirely different for acute and chronic illness. While assuming sick role dependency may be adaptive in acute illness, where medical expertise offers hope of a cure, it is not so in chronic illness. Chronically ill individuals are the "experts" on their illnesses and should have the ultimate authority in managing them over time.

When individuals with chronic illness are hospitalized, they view the situation quite differently from the health care providers with whom they interact. Clients with multiple chronic disorders may focus on maintaining stability of quiescent conditions to prevent unnecessary symptomatology, whereas staff are more likely to focus on managing the current acute disorder (Strauss, 1981). In addition, clients who have had multiple prior admissions are more likely to use their hospital savvy to gain what they want or need from the system. During hospitalization, these individuals may demand certain treatment, specific times for treatment, or specific routines. They may keep track of times that various routines occur or complain about or report actions of the staff as a means to an end they consider important. All of these demands increase staff

work and stress, and frequently the client is labeled a "problem patient" (Lorber, 1981).

Health care professionals also receive secondary gains from their work, manifested in a sense of accomplishment and the personal satisfaction that comes from witnessing a client's recovery. The goals of acute care (cure and full restoration of all faculties) provide a subconscious motivation or reward for many nurses, making them feel that they are healers (Wesson, 1965) and generating a sense of omnipotence and self-fulfillment (Table 2-2). The grateful client who recovers makes hospital work worthwhile for those who provide this care.

But cure is not possible for the chronically ill; only stabilization is. Frequent readmissions, often for recurrence of the same problems, can create a sense of frustration for the staff and require repetitive, tiresome care that may become boring. Long-term goals focus on maximizing remaining functional potential and minimizing further deterioration (see Chapter 25, on rehabilitation). These tasks do not provide the dramatic secondary gains that acute care does.

Feelings of frustration and dissatisfaction on the part of the caregiver lead to avoidance of chronically ill patients. Caregiver attitudes may demonstrate a lack of sensitivity to the meaning of illness to the long-term client and to the client's perspective of his or her own best interest. Results of treatment are less predictable, undermining the health care providers' sense of power and efficacy. Power struggles can ensue between clients and providers (Thorne, 1990).

Creating and maintaining satisfactory relationships with health care providers is a major adaptive task for chronically ill individuals. Yet, clearly, this is not a simple task. Thorne (1993) found that chronically ill patients and their families often felt that most health care professionals could not be trusted to understand the requirements of managing a chronic health problem. To some degree, this lack of trust may be adaptive because patients (and families) need to build confidence in their own ability to manage illness. The most productive caregiver–care-recipient relationships described by these subjects were ones in which caregivers were able to

TABLE 2-2

Professional Role: Relationship to the Acute and Chronically Ill

Acute	Chronic
RESPONSIBILITY	
Responsibility for patient health management	Directs care plan but not responsible for it
ACCOUNTABILITY	
Held accountable for care by patient (i.e., lawsuits)	Holds patient accountable for managing own care. Sees patient as problem; easily irritated by patient's use of manipulation or by patient demands
SECONDARY GAINS	
Many for the staff:	Limited for the staff:
1. Patients' gratitude satisfying to staff	1. No available cures; only ability to stabilize condition
2. Feelings of omnipotence when helping to "save" others	2. Repetitive recurrences become tiresome to caregivers
3. Seeing results of efforts through relatively rapid recovery	3. Long-term interactions can lead to valuable relationships

SOURCE: From Lubkin (1995).

recognize limitations in their own expertise and to respect the expertise of patients and their families.

Lack of Role Norms for the Chronically Ill

Chronic illnesses require that a variety of tasks be performed to fulfill the requirements of both medical regimen and personal life style. In spite of residual disability that limits activity, society does not identify the chronically ill as individuals who are experiencing illness. Assuming sick role behaviors is discouraged. These individuals enter and remain in the impaired role, but implicit behaviors for this role are not well defined by society, leading to a situation of role ambiguity. Given this lack of norms, influences on the client include the degree of disability (with different attributes of disability producing different consequences), visibility of the disability (the lower the visibility, the more normal the response), self-acceptance of the disability (resulting in others' reciprocating with acceptance), and societal views of the disabled as either economically dependent or productive (Wu, 1973). Without role definition, whether disability is present or not, individuals are unable to achieve maximum levels of functioning. Individuals

must adapt their definitions of themselves to their limitations, and to what the anticipated future imposes on them by the chronic condition (Watt, 2000).

■ Interventions

The sick role and the impaired role are sociological explanations of behavior responses of individuals; they are states of being, not problems requiring interventions per se. Through knowledge of these roles, though, health care professionals can help their clients cope more effectively with appropriate dependency, elicit a better understanding of the relationship between client and health professional, as well as between those roles and social expectations.

Dealing with Dependency

As noted, dependency is an inherent part of the sick role. But health professionals are not always comfortable about the client's being in this dependent role without making some effort to help him or her move back to independence. Take, for instance, the practice of beginning discharge planning soon after admission, even for the critically ill. Such action is based on several factors: first, the societal expectations that the sick should want to get well; second, wariness of the malingerer or the patient who might want to stay ill for various secondary gains; and third, the pressure created by the economics of our health care system to move clients out of the hospital as quickly as possible. For the client whose disease improves as expected, malingering is generally not a problem, but, at times, individuals, whether suffering from acute or chronic illnesses, remain in dependent states longer than expected.

Severely ill patients are more concerned with physical than psychosocial aspects of care (Hover & Juelsgaard, 1978) and are incapable of making many decisions (Stiggelbout & Kiebert, 1997). Emphasis on the physical aspects of care with these individuals is compatible with Maslow's *hierarchy of needs* model, which emphasizes that meeting physiological and then safety needs precedes the emergence and fulfillment of higher, psychosocial needs. One client noted that during her hospitalization she did not have enough energy to want to survive and was incapable of extending any efforts to improve her condition. Given these factors, the health professional must be able to recognize and accept even total dependency.

Miller (2000) discusses dependency in the chronically ill and links it with the sense of powerlessness that these individuals often confront. Chronic illness is fraught with unpredictable dilemmas. Even when an acute stage is past, the client's energy for recovery may be sapped by the uncertainty about the illness' future course, the effectiveness of medical regimens, and the disruption of usual patterns of living. Awareness of behavioral responses and when they occur can help the professional avoid premature emphasis on independence until the client can collaborate in working toward a return to normal roles (see Chapter 13, on powerlessness).

Miller (2000) recommends several strategies for decreasing clients' feelings of powerlessness as they work toward independence:

1. Modifying the environment to afford clients more means of control
2. Helping clients set realistic goals and expectations

3. Increasing clients' knowledge about their illness and its management
4. Increasing the sensitivity of health professionals and significant others to the powerlessness imposed by chronic illness
5. Encouraging verbalization of feelings

Utilizing knowledge of illness roles in planning interventions allows the health professional to maximize time spent with the client. One such intervention that could benefit from integrating knowledge of illness roles is teaching (see Chapter 15, on client and family education). The client who is still in the highly dependent phase cannot benefit from teaching. As improvement in physical status occurs, emphasis on the desire to return to normal roles creates motivation to learn about the condition and necessary procedures for maximizing health. As the client moves into the impaired role and becomes aware of the necessity to maximize remaining potential, teaching provides a highly successful tool both in the hospital and at home.

Role Supplementation

Role supplementation is the process through which the sick role or the impaired role is clarified by the use of planned interventions (Meleis, 1988). Role supplementation strategies help individuals who are dealing with intrarole conflicts because they are aimed at clarifying roles. Because the individual is dealing with a problem with incompatible role expectations, strategies that clarify alternatives and help the individual to "try them on" may be useful. There are several role supplementation strategies that health professionals can use to help individuals take on new roles successfully.

Role Clarification

Role clarification involves identifying and defining the knowledge, skills, and boundaries of a role (Meleis, 1988). It includes making explicit the expectations of self and others in a new situation through education and the explanation of behaviors expected in the new role. Role clarification is further enhanced when the chronically ill individual successfully rehearses some of the behaviors expected in the new role. For instance, the newly diagnosed diabetic can practice self-injection of insulin.

Role Rehearsal

Role rehearsal enables the individual to anticipate behaviors and feelings associated with a new role (Meleis, 1988). This process can be enhanced if the individual's significant others are identified and included in the rehearsal. Mutually agreed upon roles can then evolve smoothly.

Role Modeling

While information about a role and associated new behaviors may help an individual to clarify ideas about the role, exposure to role models is also an important strategy in helping an individual take on a role. Role modeling occurs when an individual is able to observe a role being enacted and thus learns to understand and emulate the role (Hardy & Hardy, 1988). Health professionals can act as role models themselves or promote contacts with relevant role models. Examples of such contacts might be the Reach to Recovery program for breast cancer patients or Alcoholics Anonymous for the alcoholic.

Role Taking

Role taking focuses on developing an individual's ability to imagine the responses to his or her behavior (Meleis, 1988), to view his or her behavior through the eyes of another, and to adjust his or her performance accordingly (Hurley-Wilson, 1988). Through role taking, behaviors may be rehearsed through fantasies in which patients imagine themselves acting out new roles and also imagine the responses of significant others. Anticipating the responses of others is an important component of taking on a new role, because roles are never enacted in isolation. Patients can then adjust their own role behaviors accordingly (Hurley-Wilson, 1988).

Dealing with Interrole Conflict

An individual experiencing interrole conflict needs help with conflict resolution strategies. Appropriate interventions include teaching relative to the problem-solving process and to time management, teaching significant others, and support provided by the health care professional during the problem-solving process (Nuwayhid, 1991).

Norms for the Impaired Role

Individuals with chronic illness do not have clear role norms to help them define themselves socially, especially because the impaired role, which continues as long as residual pathology or disability does, may limit activity in a variety of ways. For the chronically ill, adaptation requires learning new behaviors, accepting some congruence between old and new behaviors, and being motivated to take on new roles.

But self-definition of roles is not adequate for meeting the challenges of our society. We all need to know the behaviors that society expects and accepts. The political activism of disabled, handicapped, and elderly advocacy groups is creating new norms. These groups are demanding a greater voice in society and more meaningful lives. Their activism has resulted in legislation such as the Americans with Disabilities Act, which took effect in 1992 and assures disabled citizens of access and equal opportunity under the law. Each professional can also help promote the development of norms that lead to greater productivity of a growing segment of the population.

In recent years, the concept of disability as a characteristic of the individual has changed to one that defines *disability* as a lack of fit between the capabilities of individuals and the environment in which they must function (Institute of Medicine, 1991). This broader view suggests that many aspects of the disability process may be issues for social policy and environmental remediation as alternatives to the learning of entirely new roles (Verbrugge & Jette, 1994). In addition, Mechanic (1995) points out that it is possible to design living environments that promote function and allow persons to maintain desired roles.

Norms for the impaired role seem to be shifting. Emphasis on the exploration of the "insider view" of chronic illness has legitimized a role for the patient as an authority about his or her own illness. A focus on "shared decision-making" and "empowerment" casts the patient as a partner in rather than as a recipient of care (Crossley, 1998; Thorne & Paterson, 1998). However, not all patients are comfortable in taking on this more participative role (Stiggelbout & Kiebert, 1997).

Assisting Those in the Impaired Role

Some studies of the relationship among illness response, personality, and stress have found unique responses to specific diseases, as well as variations in affective behavior and cognitive meaning of specific illness (Byrne & Whyte, 1978; Pilowsky & Spence, 1975). These studies, using the same tool, found that individuals who had MIs had different patterns of concerns regarding their bodily functioning, recognition of the gravity of their illness, and responses to stress from those individuals experiencing intractable pain. In fact, patients with MIs initially had difficulty accepting the sick role (Byrne & Whyte, 1978). Such information can be useful in planning care and in devising programs of rehabilitation and prevention. The practicing professional also can consider utilizing such tools to identify characteristics of other chronically ill people in order to plan their short- and long-term care.

Other studies have found commonalities across illnesses in adjustment to the impaired role. Viney and Westbrook (1982) examined psychological reactions of clients who had newly diagnosed chronic illnesses and found that type of illness did not seem to determine client reaction. The best index of patients' emotional reaction to a chronic illness was their perception of how the illness would handicap them. This corresponds closely to work done by Benner and Wrubel (1989) and by Place (1993) that

points out that symptoms are laden with meaning and that getting in touch with this meaning and context of the experience of the illness is essential to caring for clients.

Pollack, Christian, and Sands (1990) established that psychological adaptation did not correspond directly to measures of physiological well-being in chronically ill individuals, regardless of type of illness. Rather, psychological adaptation corresponded to a specific style of handling stress known as the "hardiness characteristic." The personality dispositions of hardiness are specific attitudes of commitment, control, and challenge that mediate the stress response, again indicating individual differences in adjustment to chronic illness (Pollack, 1989).

Not only is ongoing treatment necessary, but individuals in the impaired role are "continually threatened by a decrease in function related to the chronic illness" (Monohan, 1982). This characteristic has led to a modification of the impaired role described as the *at-risk role*, mentioned earlier. Clients who perceive themselves as being at risk of having complications are more highly motivated to greater compliance with regimens (see Chapter 10, on compliance). To encourage movement into this modified role, the health provider needs to persuade the client that compliance is valuable in maximizing health and wellness, when developing symptoms or complications without such adherence is a possibility. The goal should be retaining, not regaining, optimal physical functioning. Helping the client decrease the risks of complications requires that the professional assess the following factors: health beliefs, environmental factors (family setting, role, and composition; medical and social supports; sociocultural factors), and present functioning level and symptoms.

Learning to Deal with Personal Biases

Professionals who have limited awareness of illness roles are often insensitive to these roles, their meaning, and the ways their own responses are affected by and affect the client. The health professional in the hospital setting deals with clients on an episodic basis and often has limited knowledge of the entire situation that these individuals must live with on a daily basis. This limited perspective may hamper efforts to promote recovery or rehabilitation, especially for the chronically ill.

The problem is compounded because chronically ill clients, who are experienced with hospital settings, are not always compliant (Thorne, 1990). Because these individuals are responsible for self-management at home, they may be unwilling to delegate control over all of their care and have acquired ways of continuing aspects of their regimens that they consider important, even though they are in the hospital for other reasons. The chronically ill individual may never fully move into the dependency of the sick role, except during the most acute phases of illness. Health care professionals dealing with such clients often are frustrated because the client is not taking on the expected "sick role." Power struggles may develop between provider and client.

Caring for individuals who have frequent recurrences of the same health problems can lead the provider to feel the same sense of powerlessness over the illness that the chronically ill person feels. Both groups realize that the client will never fully recover. At times, health care providers express their frustration by blaming the client. Such negative feelings about clients inevitably influence interactions with them.

To be helpful, health care professionals must focus on feelings and responses triggered by the client's need to retain autonomy. Only awareness of how these feelings affect care can allow the provider to achieve an objective view of the situation and the realization that chronically ill persons are trying to manage their symptoms and lives and to maximize their remaining potential. Staff members must realize that demands for autonomy indicate that the client is adapting to the illness and its accompanying role while striving to achieve holistic wellness.

Once health care professionals are able to restructure their view, joint goal setting and planning are possible; power becomes shared and a satisfying relationship of reciprocal trust develops between health care provider and client (Thorne & Robinson, 1988). Feeling trusted and respected both fosters satisfaction with the relationship and helps promote and maintain the competence of the chronically ill clients.

Frameworks and Models for Practice

Caring for a client with chronic illness requires a different framework or model for practice than caring for those with acute, episodic disease. The frameworks that follow are examples, and are not intended to be all-inclusive.

These frameworks and models should not be confused with the disease management models discussed in Chapter 1. Disease management models address the physical symptoms of the condition. Some of those models assign an algorithm to the condition where clients receive certain 'care' when their blood work is at an inappropriate level, or their symptoms 'measure' a certain degree of seriousness. These models manage the disease, but not the illness. Illness frameworks and models address the illness experience of the individual and family that occurs as a result of changing health status.

Chronic Illness and Quality of Life

In the early 1960s Anselm Strauss, working with Barney Glaser, a social scientist, and Jeanne Quint Benoliel, a nurse, interviewed dying patients to ascertain what kind of 'care' was needed for those clients (Corbin & Strauss, 1992). As a result of those early interviews, Strauss (1975, 1984) published a rudimentary framework that addressed the issues and concerns of individuals with chronic illness. Although the term 'trajectory' was coined at that time, it did not become fully developed until 20 years later. His framework was simple, but was an early attempt to examine the illness experience of the individual and family as opposed to the disease perspective. If care professionals could better understand the illness experience of clients and families, perhaps more appropriate care would be provided. Basic to this care was understanding the key problems (Table 2-3).

TABLE 2-3

Key Problems

1. The *prevention* of medical crises and their management if they occur
2. *Controlling symptoms*
3. *Carrying out* of prescribed medical regimes
4. Prevention of, or living with, *social isolation*
5. *Adjustment* to changes in the disease
6. Attempts to *normalize* interactions and lifestyle
7. *Funding*—finding the necessary money
8. *Confronting* attendant psychological, marital and familial problems.

SOURCE: Strauss, A. L., et al. (1984). *Chronic illness and the quality of life* (2nd ed.) (p. 16). St. Louis: The C.V. Mosby Company. Used with permission.

After identifying the key problems of the individual and family with chronic illness, what followed were basic strategies, family and organizational arrangements and the consequences of those arrangements (Strauss et al., 1984, p. 17).

The Trajectory Framework

From Strauss and colleagues' work in the 1960s and 1970s, the trajectory framework was further refined in the 1980s. Corbin and Strauss (1992) developed this framework so that nurses could: (1) gain insight into the chronic illness experience of the client, (2) integrate existing literature about chronicity into their practice, and (3) provide direction for building nursing models that guide practice, teaching, research and policy making (p. 10).

A trajectory is defined as the course of an illness over time, plus the actions of clients, families and healthcare professionals to manage that course (Corbin, 1998, p. 3). The illness trajectory is set in motion by pathophysiology and changes in health status, but there are strategies that can be used by clients, families and healthcare professionals that *shape* the course of dying and thus the illness trajectory (Corbin & Strauss, 1992). Even if the disease may be the same, each individual's illness trajectory is different, and takes into account the uniqueness

of each individual (Jablonski, 2004). Shaping does not imply that the ultimate course of the disease will be changed or the disease will be cured, merely that the illness trajectory may be shaped or altered by actions of the individual and family so that the disease course is stable, fewer exacerbations occur and symptoms are better controlled (Corbin & Strauss, 1992).

Within the model, the term 'phase' indicates the different stages of the chronic illness experience for the client. There are nine phases in the trajectory model, and although it could be conceived as a continuum, it is not linear. Clients may move through these phases in a linear way, regress to a former phase, or plateau for an extended period of time. Additionally, having more than one chronic disease influences movement along the trajectory as well (see Table 2-4).

Another term used in the model is biography. A client's biography consists of previous hospital experiences, useful ways of dealing with symptoms, illness beliefs and other life experiences (White & Lubkin, 1998).

The initial phase of the trajectory model is the *pretrajectory phase*, or preventive phase, in which the course of illness has not yet begun; however, there are genetic factors or lifestyle behaviors that place an individual at risk for a chronic condition. An example would be the individual who is overweight, has a family history of cardiac disease and high cholesterol, and does not exercise.

During the *trajectory* phase, signs and symptoms of the disease appear and a diagnostic workup may begin. The individual begins to cope with implications of a diagnosis. In the *stable* phase, the illness symptoms are under control and management of the disease occurs primarily at home. A period of inability to keep symptoms under control occurs in the *unstable* phase. The *acute* phase brings severe and unrelieved symptoms or disease complications. Critical or life-threatening situations requiring emergency treatment occur in the *crisis* phase. The *comeback* phase signals a gradual return to an acceptable way of life within the symptoms that the disease imposes. The *downward phase* is character-

TABLE 2-4		

Trajectory Phases

Phase	Definition	Goal of Management
Pretrajectory	Genetic factors or lifestyle behaviors that place an individual or community at risk for the development of a chronic condition	Prevent onset of chronic illness
Trajectory Onset	Appearance of noticeable symptoms, includes period of diagnostic workup and announcement by biographical limbo as person begins to discover and cope with implications of diagnosis	Form appropriate trajectory projection and scheme
Stable	Illness course and symptoms are under control. Biography and everyday life activities are being managed within limitations of illness. Illness management centers in the home	Maintain stability of illness, biography, and everyday life activities
Unstable	Period of instability to keep symptoms under control or reactivation of illness. Biographical disruption and difficulty in carrying out everyday life activities. Adjustment being made in regimen and care usually taking place at home	Return to stable
Acute	Severe and unrelieved symptoms or the development of illness complications necessitating hospitalization or bedrest to bring illness course under control. Biography and everyday life activities temporarily placed on hold or drastically cut back	Bring illness under control and resume normal biography and everyday life activities
Crisis	Critical or life-threatening situation requiring emergency treatment or care. Biography and everyday life activities suspended until crisis passes.	Remove life threat
Comeback	A gradual return to an acceptable way of life within limits imposed by disability or illness	Set in motion and keep going the trajectory projection and scheme
Downward	Illness course characterized by rapid or gradual physical decline accompanied by increasing disability or difficulty in controlling symptoms	To adapt to increasing disability with each major downward turn
Dying	Final days or weeks before death. Characterized by gradual or rapid shutting down of body processes, biographical disengagement and closure, and relinquishment of everyday life interest and activities	To bring closure, let go, and die peacefully

Source: Corbin, J. (2001). Introduction and overview: Chronic illness and nursing. In R. Hyman & J. Corbin (Eds.) *Chronic illness: Research and theory for nursing practice* (pp. 4–5). © Springer Publishing Company, Inc., New York, NY 10036. Used with permission.

ized by progressive deterioration and an increase in disability or symptoms. The trajectory model ends with the *dying phase* characterized by gradual or rapid shutting down of body processes (Corbin, 2001, p. 4–5).

Shifting Perspectives Model of Chronic Illness

This model resulted from work of Thorne and Paterson (1998) who analyzed 292 qualitative studies pertaining to chronic physical illness that were published from 1980 to 1996. Of these, 158 studies became a part of a metastudy in which client roles in chronic illness were described. Thorne and Paterson's work reflects the 'insider' perspective of chronic illness as opposed to the 'outsider' view, the more traditional view. This change in perspective is a shift from the traditional approach of patient-as-client to one of client-as-partner in care (p. 173). Results from the metastudy also demonstrated a shift away from focusing on loss and burden, and an attempt to view health within illness.

Analysis of these studies led to the development of the Shifting Perspectives Model of Chronic Illness (Paterson, 2001). The model depicts chronic illness as an on-going, continually shifting process where people experience a complex dialectic between the world and themselves (p. 23). Donnelly (1993) first spoke of individuals with chronic illness living in the "dual kingdoms of the well and the sick" (p. 6). Paterson's model considers both the 'illness' and the 'wellness' of the individual (Paterson, 2003). The illness-in-the-foreground perspective focuses on the sickness, loss and burden of the chronic illness. This is a common reaction of those recently diagnosed with a chronic disease. The overwhelming consequences of the condition, learning about their illness, considerations of treatment, and long term effects contribute to putting the illness in the foreground. The disease becomes the individual's identity.

Illness-in-the-foreground could also be a protective response by the individual and be used to conserve energy for other activities. However, it could be used to maintain their identity as a 'sick' person, or because it is congruent with their need to have sickness as their social identity and receive secondary gains (Paterson, 2001).

With wellness-in-the-foreground, the 'self' is the source of identity and not the disease (Paterson, 2001, p. 23). The individual is in control and not the disease. It does not mean, though, that the individual is physically well, cured or even in remission of the disease symptoms. The shift occurs in the individual's thinking that allows the individual to focus

away from the disease. However, any threat that can't be controlled will transition the individual back to the illness-in-the-foreground perspective. Threats could be disease progression, lack of ability to self-manage the disease, stigma or interactions with others. (Paterson, 2001).

Lastly, neither the illness perspective nor the wellness perspective is right or wrong, but each merely reflects the individual's unique needs, health status and focus at the time (Paterson, 2001).

Research

Much of the recent research on the experience of chronic illness has shifted from an 'outsider' perspective, which observes and attempts to draw conclusions about the behavior of groups of patients, to an 'insider' perspective, in which the focus is examination of individual responses to chronic illness. Thorne and Paterson (1998), in a review of this research, note that the insider perspective consistently reveals clients as analysts of their chronic illness experiences and depicts them as active agents in attaining desired outcomes. Health care professionals are seen as limited in their expertise, and there is a shift from the view of chronically ill people as recipients of care to a view of chronically ill people as active partners in their own health care.

This is illustrated in the experiences of many HIV-positive patients. Crossley's (1998) research describes the rejection of the sick role by long-term HIV-positive individuals. This has been, at times, a militant group, skeptical of medical knowledge and expertise. The subjects in her sample demonstrated a need to actively reject the dependency imposed on them by the sick role. Their focus on "empowerment" often involved rejection of medical and societal rules. This raised serious concern because these patients often rejected any obligation to protect others from their disease by reducing their risk behaviors.

Both Crossley (1998) and Thorne and Paterson (1998) note the rise of "self-help" groups as related to this new "active agent" role of the chronically ill client. At the same time, they also note that these more "independent" and "activated" clients are still tied to the health care system for their survival because they need medical care. A static interpretation of this partnership between health care professional and client is not realistic. The evidence demonstrates that the work of managing a chronic illness can sometimes be overwhelming and that many people with chronic illness demonstrate a continuing need to seek and expect help from experts (Cahill, 1996; Stiggelbout & Kiebert, 1997). This research challenges health care providers to develop the clinical expertise to determine when patients want to be in control, when they want to be partners, and when they need to be dependent.

Summary and Conclusions

Illness behavior is influenced by many variables, including the client's health beliefs. At some point along the illness behavior continuum, the acutely ill individual enters the *sick role*, in which it is acceptable to be dependent on others while being relieved of social responsibilities. In exchange, one is obligated to want to become well and to seek and cooperate with technically competent professionals. This role is more applicable to acute, rather than chronic, disorders. According to the *impaired role* model, chronically ill or disabled persons must be responsible for their own health management and can meet normal role expectations within the limits of their health condition. In other words, the impaired role entails adapted wellness.

The sick role's lack of usefulness to chronic illness is a major drawback, especially in light of increasing numbers of individuals with chronic illness. The impaired role is problematic in that society has yet to clearly define role norms that maximize social integration of impaired individuals. The nurse can promote such integration by supporting individualized strategies for each affected individual.

Health care professionals must also come to terms with the differences in behavior of acutely ill and chronically ill clients in the hospital setting by recognizing the internal aspects of their relationships to the clients. Using illness roles as a basis for clinical practice currently has a strong experiential component, because research data are limited. In the meantime, knowledge of illness roles can provide some direction for the health professional.

Society's responses to illness depend on many sociocultural factors, which are not always logical or scientifically based (Helman, 2001). Health care for the individual with chronic illness can be more effectively delivered when health care professionals assist individuals to manage not just their diseases, but also common underlying needs for psychosocial support, coping skills, and a sense of control (Sobel, 1995). Frameworks and models have been developed that allow the health care professional to more appropriately care for those with chronic illness.

Study Questions

1. What is illness behavior, and what factors influence the symptomatic individual to adopt illness behavior?
2. What are the characteristics of the sick role? When do symptomatic individuals take on this role?
3. How does the impaired role differ from the sick role? What are the characteristics of the impaired role?
4. What problems have been identified in relation to the sick role and its characteristics?
5. What role difficulties might an individual encounter when moving into the sick or impaired role?
6. How do children differ in role response to illness? How do the elderly respond?
7. In what ways do professionals' expectations influence their response to clients?

8. In what way does the lack of clarity regarding role norms for the impaired role influence clients' behavior?

9. Consider a client you have cared for in the hospital setting. What criteria could you see in determining whether the individual is in a dependent role? Ready to move toward greater independence?

10. What problems arise from an inadequate societal role for chronically ill or impaired people?

11. Apply both the trajectory framework and the shifting perspectives model to a client with diabetes. What similarities and differences are there between the two models?

References

Asbring, P. (1991). Chronic illness—a disruption in life: Identity transformation among women with chronic fatigue syndrome and fibromyalgia. *Journal of Advanced Nursing, 34* (3), 312–19.

Benner, P., & Wrubel, J. (1989). *The primacy of caring: Stress and coping in health and illness.* Menlo Park, CA: Addison-Wesley.

Boekaerts, M., & Roder, I. (1999). Stress, coping, and adjustment in children with a chronic disease: A review of the literature. *Disability and Rehabilitation, 21* (7), 311–337.

Boice, M. (1998). Chronic illness in adolescence. *Adolescence, 33* (132), 927–939.

Breslau, N. (1982). Psychiatric disorder in children with physical disabilities. *Journal of the American Academy of Child Psychiatry, 24*, 87–94.

Breslau, N., & Marshall, I. A. (1985). Psychological disturbance in children with physical disabilities: Continuity and change in a 5-year follow-up. *Journal of Abnormal Child Psychology, 13*, 199–216.

Buchwald, D., Caralis, P. V., Gany, F., Hardt, E. J., et al. (1994). Caring for patients in a multicultural society. *Patient Care, 26* (11), 105–120.

Cahill, J. (1996). Patient participation: A concept analysis. *Journal of Advanced Nursing, 24*, 561–571.

Christian, B. J. (1989). *Family adaption to chronic illness: Family coping style, family relationships, and family coping status—implications for nursing.* Unpublished doctoral dissertation, University of Texas, Austin.

Clark, M., & Anderson, B. G. (1967). *Culture and aging.* Springfield, IL: Charles C. Thomas.

Cockerham, W. C. (2001). The sick role. In *Medical sociology* (8th ed.) (pp. 156–178). Upper Saddle River, NJ: Prentice-Hall.

Conrad, P. (2005). *The sociology of health and illness: Critical perspectives* (7th ed.) New York: Worth Publishers.

Corbin, J. (1998). The Corbin and Strauss chronic illness trajectory model: An update. *Scholarly Inquiry for Nursing Practice, 12* (1), 33–41.

Corbin, J. (2001). Introduction and overview: Chronic illness and nursing. In R. Hyman and J. Corbin (Eds.) *Chronic illness: Research and theory for nursing practice.* (pp. 1–15). New York, NY: Springer Publishing, Inc.

Corbin, J., & Strauss, A. (1992). A nursing model for chronic illness management based upon the trajectory framework. In P. Woog (Ed.) *The chronic illness trajectory framework: The Corbin and Strauss Nursing Model.* (pp. 9–28). New York: Springer.

Crossley, M. (1998). "Sick role" or "empowerment"? The ambiguities of life with an HIV positive diagnosis. *Sociology of Health and Illness, 20* (4), 507–531.

Davidhizar, R. (1994). The pursuit of illness for secondary gain. *Health Care Supervisor, 13* (3), 49–58.

Donnelly, G. (1993). Chronicity: Concept and reality. *Holistic Nursing Practice, 8*, 1–7.

Feldman D. J. (1974). Chronic disabling illness: A holistic view. *Journal of Chronic Diseases, 27*, 287–291.

Finerman, R., & Bennett, L. A. (1994). Guilt, blame and shame: Responsibility in health and sickness. *Social Science and Medicine, 40* (1), 1–3.

Freidson, E. (1970). *Profession of medicine.* New York: Dodd, Mead.

Gilles, L. (1972). *Human behavior in illness.* London: Faber & Faber.

Gordon, G. (1966). *Role theory and illness: A sociological perspective.* New Haven, CT: College and University Press.

Grey, M., Camerson, M. E., & Thurber, F. W. (1991). Coping and adaptation in children with diabetes. *Nursing Research, 40* (3), 144–149.

Hardy, M. E., & Hardy, W. L. (1988). Role stress and role strain. In M. E. Hardy & M. E. Conway (Eds.), *Role theory: Perspectives for health professionals* (2nd ed.). (pp. 159–240). Norwalk, CT: Appleton & Lange.

Harris, J. A., Newcomb, A. F., & Gewanter, H. L. (1991). Psychosocial effects of juvenile rheumatic disease: The family and peer systems as a context for coping. *Arthritis Care and Research, 4* (3), 123–130.

Heller, A., Rafman, S., Zvagulis, I., & Pless, I. B. (1985). Birth defects and psychosocial adjustment. *American Journal of Diseases of Children, 139,* 257–263.

Helman, C. G. (2001). *Culture, health and illness* (4th ed.). London: Arnold.

Honig-Parnass, T. (1981). Lay concepts of the sick role: An examination of the professional bias in Parsons' model. *Social Science and Medicine, 15A,* 615–623.

Hover, J., & Juelsgaard, N. (1978). The sick role reconceptualized. *Nursing Forum, XVII* (4), 406–415.

Hurley-Wilson, B. A. (1988). Socialization for roles. In M. E. Hardy & M. E. Conway (Eds.), *Role theory: Perspectives for health professionals* (2nd ed.). Norwalk, CT: Appleton & Lange.

Hyman, M. D. (1971). Disability and patient's perceptions of preferential treatment: Some preliminary findings. *Journal of Chronic Diseases, 24,* 329–342.

Institute of Medicine. (1991). *Disability in America: Toward a national agenda for prevention,* Washington, DC: National Academy Press.

Jablonski, A. (2004). The illness trajectory of end-stage renal disease dialysis patients. *Research and Theory for Nursing Practice: An International Journal, 18* (1), 51–72.

Kassenbaum, G. G., & Baumann, B. O. (1965). Dimensions of the sick role in chronic illness. *Journal of Health and Human Behavior, 6* (1), 16–27.

Kiesel, M. Sr., & Beninger, C. (1979). An application of psycho-social role theory to the aging. *Nursing Forum, XVIII* (1), 80–91.

Kubisch, S. M., & Wichowski, H. C. (1992). Identification and validation of a new nursing diagnosis: Sick role conflict. *Nursing Diagnosis, 3* (4), 141–147.

Lorber, J. (1981). Good patients and problem patients: Conformity and deviance in a general hospital. In P. Conrad & R. Kern (Eds.), *The sociology of health and illness: Critical perspectives.* New York: St. Martin's.

Lubkin, I. (Ed.). (1995). *Chronic illness: Impact and interventions* (3rd ed.). Sudbury, MA: Jones & Bartlett.

McCarthy, S. M., & Gallo, A. M. (1992). A case illustration of family management style. *Journal of Pediatric Nursing: Nursing Care of Children and Families, 7* (6), 395–402.

Mechanic, D. (1961). The concept of illness behavior. *Journal of Chronic Diseases, 15,* 189–194.

_____. (1972). *Public expectations and health care.* New York: John Wiley and Sons.

_____. (1992). Health and illness behavior and patient-practitioner relationships. *Social Science and Medicine, 34* (12), 1345–1350.

_____. (1995). Sociological dimensions of illness behavior. *Social Science and Medicine, 41* (9), 1207–1216.

Meleis, A. I. (1975). Role insufficiency and role supplementation: A conceptual framework. *Nursing Research, 24* (4), 264–271.

_____. (1988). The sick role. In M. E. Hardy & M. E. Conway (Eds.), *Role theory: Perspectives for health professionals* (2nd ed.). Norwalk, CT: Appleton & Lange.

Miller, J. F. (2000). *Coping with chronic illness: Overcoming powerlessness* (3rd ed.). Philadelphia: F. A. Davis.

Monohan, R. S. (1982, May). The "at-risk" role. *Nurse Practitioner, 42–44,* 52.

Nuwayhid, K. A. (1991). Role transition, distance and conflict. In C. A. Roy & H. A. Andrews (Eds.), *The Roy Adaptation Model: The definitive statement,* (pp. 363–376). Norwalk, CT: Appleton & Lange.

Parsons, T. (1951). *The social system.* New York: The Free Press.

Paterson, B. (2001). The shifting perspectives model of chronic illness. *Journal of Nursing Scholarship, 33* (1), 21–26.

Paterson, B. (2003). The koala has claws: Applications of the shifting perspectives model in research of chronic illness. *Qualitative Health Research, 13* (7), 987–994.

Pilowsky, I., & Spence, N. D. (1975). Patterns of illness behavior in patients with intractable pain. *Journal of Psychosomatic Research, 19,* 279–287.

Place, B. E. (1993). Understanding the meaning of chronic illness: A prerequisite for caring. In D. A. Gaut (Ed.), *A global agenda for caring* (pp. 281–291). New York: National League for Nursing Press.

Pless, B., & Nolan, T. (1991). Revision, replication, and neglect—Research on maladjustment in chronic illness. *Journal of Child Psychology and Psychiatry, 32* (2), 347–365.

Pollack, S. E. (1989). The hardiness characteristic: A motivating factor in adaption. *Advances in Nursing Science, 11* (2), 53–62.

Pollack, S. E., Christian, B. J., & Sands, D. (1990). Responses to chronic illness: Analysis of psychological and physiological adaptation. *Nursing Research, 39* (5), 300–304.

Redman, B. K. (1993). *The process of patient education.* St. Louis: Mosby.

Robinson, D. (1971). *The process of becoming ill.* London: Routledge and Kegan Paul.

Rundall, T. & Wheeler, J. (1979). Factors associated with utilization of the swine flu vaccination program among senior citizens in Tompkins County. *Medical Care, 17,* p. 191.

Schwartz, S. S., Gramling, S. E., & Mancini, T. (1994). *Journal of Behavior Therapy and Experimental Psychiatry, 25* (2), 135–142.

Segall, A. (1976). The sick role concept: Understanding illness behavior. *Journal of Health and Social Behavior, 17,* 163–170.

Sobel, D. S. (1995). Rethinking medicine: Improving health outcomes with cost-effective psychosocial interventions. *Psychosomatic Medicine, 57,* 234–244.

Sontag, S. (1988). *Illness as metaphor.* Toronto: Collins Publishers.

Steward, D. C., & Sullivan, T. J. (1982). Illness behavior and the sick role in chronic disease: The case of multiple sclerosis. *Social Science and Medicine, 16,* 1397–1404.

Stiggelbout, A. M., & Kiebert, G. M. (1997). A role for the sick role: Patient preferences regarding information and participation in clinical decision-making. *Canadian Medical Association Journal, 157* (4), 383–389.

Strauss, A. (1981). Chronic illness. In P. Conrad & R. Kern (Eds.), *The sociology of health and illness: Critical perspectives.* New York: St. Martin's.

Strauss, A., & Glaser, B. (1975). *Chronic illness and the quality of life.* St. Louis: Mosby.

Strauss, A., Corbin, J., Fagerhaugh, S., Glaser, B., et al. (1984). *Chronic illness and the quality of life* (2nd ed.). St. Louis: Mosby.

Thomas, R. (2003). *Society and health: Sociology for health professionals.* New York: Kluwer.

Thorne, S. E. (1990). Constructive noncompliance in chronic illness. *Holistic Nursing Practice, 5* (1), 62–69.

_____. (1993). *Negotiating health care: The social context of chronic illness.* Newbury Park, CA: Sage.

Thorne, S. E., & Paterson, B. (1998). Shifting images of chronic illness. *Image, 30* (2), 173–178.

Thorne, S. E., & Robinson, C. A. (1988). Reciprocal trust in health care relationships. *Journal of Advanced Nursing, 13,* 782–789.

Verbrugge, L. M. & Jette, A. M. (1994). The disablement process. *Social Science and Medicine, 38* (1), 1–14.

Viney, L. L., & Westbrook, M. T. (1982). Psychological reactions to the onset of chronic illness. *Social Science and Medicine, 16,* 899–905.

Watt, S. (2000). Clinical decision-making in the context of chronic illness. *Health Expectations, 3,* 6–16.

Weaver, S. K. & Wilson, J. F. (1994). Moving toward patient empowerment. *Nursing and Health Care, 15* (9), 380–483.

Wesson, A. F. (1965). Long-term care: The forces that have shaped it and the evidence for needed change. In *Meeting the social needs of long-term patients.* Chicago: American Hospital Association.

White, N., & Lubkin, I. (1998). Illness trajectory. In I. Lubkin & P. Larsen (Eds.) *Chronic illness: Impact and interventions* (4th ed.) (pp. 53–76). Sudbury, MA: Jones & Bartlett.

Whitehead, W. E., Winget, C., Federactivius, A. S., Wooley, S., et al. (1982). Learned illness behavior in patients with irritable bowel syndrome and peptic ulcer. *Digestive Diseases and Sciences, 27* (3), 202–208.

Whitehead, W. E., Crowell, M. D., Heller, B. R., Robinson, J. C., et al. (1994). Modeling and reinforcement of the sick role during childhood predicts adult illness behavior. *Psychosomatic Medicine, 56,* 541–550.

Wu, R. (1973). *Behavior and illness.* Englewood Cliffs, NJ: Prentice-Hall.

CHAPTER 3

Stigma

Rosemary J. Mann ▪ Diane Stuenkel

My car came to a stop at the intersection. I looked around me at all the people in the other cars, but no one there was like me. They were apart from me, distant, different. If they looked at me, they couldn't see my defect. But if they knew, they would turn away. I am separate and different from everybody that I can see in every direction as far as I can see. And it will never be the same again.

Cancer patient

Introduction

This chapter demonstrates how the concept of stigma has evolved and is a significant factor in many chronic diseases and disabilities. It also explores the relationship of stigma with the concepts of prejudice, stereotyping, and labeling. Because stigma is socially constructed, it varies from setting to setting. In addition, individuals and groups react differently to the stigmatizing process. Those reactions must be taken into consideration when planning strategies to improve the quality of life of individuals with chronic disease.

Not all individuals attach a stigma to disease or deformity, even though stigmatizing is common. This chapter does not assume that all who come in contact with those who are disabled or chronically ill devalue them; rather, it insists that each of us examine our values, beliefs and actions carefully.

The *Merriam Webster Dictionary On-Line* (2004) defines *stigma* as a "mark of shame or discredit." The *Merriam Webster Thesaurus On-Line* (2004) lists synonyms such as *blot, slur, spot or stain*. Goffman (1963) traces the historic use of the word *stigma* to the Greeks, who referred to "bodily signs designed to expose something unusual and bad about the moral status of the signifier" (p. 1). These signs were cut or burned into a person's body as an indication of being a slave, a criminal, or a traitor. Notice the moral and judgmental nature of these stigmata. The disgrace and shame of the stigma became more important than the bodily evidence of it.

Stigma, Social Identity, and Labeling Theory

Society teaches its members to categorize persons and defines the attributes and characteristics that are common for persons in those categories (Goffman, 1963). Daily routines establish the usual and the expected. When we meet strangers, certain appearances help us anticipate what Goffman calls "social identity". This identity includes personal attributes, such as competence, as well as structural ones, such as occupation. For example, university students usually tolerate some eccentricities in their professors, but stuttering, physical handicaps, or diseases may bestow a social identity of incompetency. Although this identity is not based on actuality, it may be stigmatizing.

One's social identity may include: (1) physical activities, (2) professional roles, and (3) the concept of self. Anything that changes one of these, such as a disability, changes the individual's identity and therefore potentially creates a stigma (Markowitz, 1998).

Goffman (1963) used the idea of social identity to expand previous work done on stigma. His theory defined stigma as something that disqualifies an individual from full social acceptance. Goffman argued that social identity is a primary force in the development of stigma, because the identity that a person conveys categorizes that person. Social settings and routines tell us which categories to anticipate. Therefore, when individuals fail to meet expectations because of attributes that are different and/or undesirable, they are reduced from accepted people to discounted ones—that is, stigmatized.

During the two decades following Goffman's work in the 1960s, extensive criticism arose concerning the impact and long term consequences of stigma on social identity, particularly in mental health. Antilabeling critics questioned the premise that the impact of stigma and a negative social identity could have profound negative effects on the course of the illness and the nature of social support available to the stigmatized individual. In the area of mental illness, critics resisted the theory that stigma could contribute to the severity and chronicity of mental illness. In a series of studies, Link proposed a modified labeling theory which asserted that labeling, derived from negative social beliefs about behavior, could lead to devaluation and discrimination. Ultimately these feelings of devaluation and discrimination could lead to negative social consequences (Link, 1987; Link et al., 1989; Link et al., 1997).

In 1987, Link compared the expectations of discrimination and devaluation and the severity of de-moralization among clients with newly diagnosed mental illness, repeat clients with mental illness, former clients with mental illness and community residents (Link, 1987). He found that both new and repeat clients with mental illness scored higher on measures of demoralization and discrimination than community residents and former mentally ill clients. Further, he demonstrated that high scores were related to income loss and unemployment.

In 1989, Link and colleagues tested a modified labeling theory on a similar group of clients with newly diagnosed mental illness, repeat clients with mental illness, former clients, untreated clients, and community residents who were well (Link, Cullen, Struening, Shrout, & Dohrenwend, 1989). They found that all groups expected clients to be devalued and discriminated against. Further, they found that, among current clients, the expectation of devaluation and discrimination promoted coping mechanisms of secrecy and withdrawal. Such coping mechanisms have a strong effect on social networks, reducing the size of those networks to persons considered to be safe and trustworthy.

In 1997, Link, Struening, Rahav, Phelan, and Nuttbrock tested modified labeling theory in a longitudinal study that compared the effects of stigma on the well-being of clients who had mental illness and a pattern of substance abuse to determine the strength of the long term negative effects of stigma and whether the effects of treatment have counterbalancing positive effects (Link et al., 1997). They found that perceived devaluation and discrimination as well as actual reports of discrimination continued to have negative effects on clients even though clients were improved and had responded well to treatment. They concluded that health care professionals attempting to improve quality of life for clients with mental illness must contend initially with the effects of stigma in its own right in order to be successful.

Fife and Wright (2000) studied stigma using modified labeling theory as a framework in individuals with HIV/AIDS and cancer. They found that stigma was a significant influence on the lives of persons with HIV/AIDS and with cancer. However, they also found that the nature of the illness had few direct effects on self-perception, whereas the effects on self appeared to directly relate to the perception of stigma. Their findings suggest that stigma has different dimensions which have different effects on self. Rejection and social isolation lead to diminished self-esteem. Social isolation influences body image. A lack of sense of personal control stems from social isolation and financial insecurity. Social isolation appears to be the only dimension of stigma that affects each component of self.

Most recently, Camp, Finlay, and Lyons (2002) questioned the inevitability of the effects of stigma on self based on the hypothesis that, in order for stigma to exert a negative influence on self-concept, the individuals must first be aware of and accept the negative self-perceptions, accept that the identity relates to them, and then apply the negative perceptions to themselves. In a study of women with long-term mental health problems, these women did not accept negative social perceptions as relevant to them. Rather, they attributed the negative perceptions to deficiencies among those who stigmatized them. The researchers found no evidence of the passive acceptance of labels and negative identities. The subjects appeared to avoid social interactions where they anticipated feeling different and being excluded and formed new social networks with groups in which they felt accepted and understood. While they acknowledged the negative consequences of mental illness, there did not appear to be an automatic link between these consequences and negative self-evaluation. Factors that contributed to a positive self-evaluation included membership in a supportive in-group, finding themselves in a more favorable circumstance than others with the same problems, and sharing experiences with others who had knowledge and insight about mental illness.

In summary, stigma, defined as a mark of shame or discredit, arises from widely held social beliefs about personality, behavior and illness and is communicated to individuals through a process of socialization. When individuals display the condition which engenders the mark of discredit, they may experience social devaluation and discrimination. Stigma clearly attaches to individuals with mental illness as well as individuals with infectious and terminal diseases. Stigma may produce changes in perception of body image, social isolation, rejection, and perceived lack of personal control. However, there is some evidence to suggest that stigma does not attach universally to individuals with marked behavior or conditions. Some individuals appear resistant to stigma, identifying flaws in the society conveying the negative beliefs. These individuals share experiences with others who have knowledge of and sensitivity to being stigmatized and benefit from the ability to perceive themselves as equal to or better off than others with the same condition.

Unique Aspects of Stigma

There are special circumstances in which stigma can be perceived with enhanced distinction. Individuals who lack a fully-developed sense of personal identity and who are reliant upon external sources to reinforce their internal sense of worthiness may be uniquely prone to a sense of stigma. Adolescence can be used as an example. There are aspects of society which tend to be highly valued by individuals and when that society communicates stigma, the stigmatizing beliefs are uniquely powerful. Religion and culture are examples as well as issues concerning self-infliction and punishment.

The task of developing a stable, coherent identity is one of the most important tasks of adolescence (Erikson, 1968). To successfully complete this task, the adolescent must be able to utilize formal operational thinking within a context of expanded social experiences to evolve a sense of self that integrates not only the similarities, but also the differences observed between him- or herself and others. Social interactions and messages from the sociocultural environment about what is desirable and what is not desirable guide and direct the adolescent toward an identity that incorporates desired similarities and rejects undesired differences. The influences and preferences of peers become important as the adolescent seeks acceptance of this newly developed sense of identity. The skill of labeling and stigmatizing individuals with intolerable differences is wielded with frightening force and sometimes terrible consequences. The Columbine High School (Colorado) massacre in 1999 is an example:

> Eric and Dylan seemed to relish their roles as outsiders. . . . It wasn't that they were labeled that way. It's what they chose to be. That choice invited taunting by a group of jocks . . . known bullies throughout the school. . . . Some of the jocks and their friends pushed Eric into lockers. They called him 'faggot' . . . Jessica defined Columbine this way. . . . "There's basically two classes of people. There's the low and the high. The low [people] stick together and the high [people] make fun of the low and you just deal with it. (Bartels & Crowder, 1999)

Culture may determine stigma as well. For some conditions, such as traumatic brain injury (Simpson, Mohr, & Redman, 2000), HIV/AIDS (Heckman et al., 2004), and epilepsy (Baker et al., 2000), stigma and social isolation cross cultural boundaries. On the other hand, in a study of attitudes about homelessness in 11 European cities, Brandon et al. (2000) found marked differences in attitudes between countries, with high levels of stigma predominating in former Warsaw Pact countries. A determination of racial and/or cultural inferiority of a minority group by a dominant group may result in racism, discrimination, and stigma (Weston, 2003; Williams, 1999).

Religion may also play a role in stigma. In a study of five large religious groups in London examining attitudes about depression and schizophrenia, it was found that fear of stigma among non-white groups was prevalent, and particularly the fear of being misunderstood by white health care professionals not of the same religious group (Cinnirella & Loewenthal, 1999).

Actual physical or mental disability is not solely responsible for social reaction. The recent incorporation of children with "special needs" (often children with delayed or slowed mental development) into mainstream education has forced the reevaluation of long-held beliefs and stereotypes that have stigmatized these children in the past (Waldman, Swerdloff, & Perlman, 1999). This point is an important one in understanding the concept of stigma. The label produces the negative response from non-labeled people, rather than some aberrant or inadequate behavior producing it. Therefore, the label and associated stigma of a disability or disease exclude individuals from social interaction while their intellectual or physical handicaps alone may or may not (Link et al., 1997). The example of a spoiled identity that leads to stigma effectively removes the individual from the societal interaction that would have otherwise been expected. The social isolation and distress accompanying stigma may then alter the client's health-seeking behavior and result in treatment delays (Baker et al., 2000; Kelly, 1999; Searle, 1999; Williams, 1999).

Most stigmas are considered threatening to others. We stigmatize criminals and social deviants because they create a sense of anxiety by threatening our values and safety. Similarly, encounters with sick and disabled individuals also cause us anxiety and apprehension, but in a different way. The encounter destroys the dream that life is fair. Sick people remind us of our mortality and vulnerability; consequently, physically healthy individuals may make negative value judgments about those who are ill or disabled (Kurzban & Leary, 2001). For example, some sighted individuals may regard those who are blind as being dependent or unwilling to take care of themselves, an assumption that is not based on what the blind person is willing or able to do. Individuals with AIDS are often subjected to moral judgment. Those with psychiatric illness have been stigmatized since medieval times (Keltner, Schwecke, & Bostrom, 2003). As a result, these individuals contend with more than their symptomology; on a daily basis, they contend with those who perceive them as less worthy or valuable: They possess a stigma.

Some individuals are stigmatized because the behavior or difference is considered to be self-inflicted and therefore less worthy of help. Alcoholism, drug-related problems, and mental illness are frequently included in this category (Crisp et al., 2000; Ritson, 1999). Human immunodeficiency virus (HIV), AIDS, and hepatitis B are examples of infectious diseases in which the mode of infection is considered to be self-inflicted as a result of socially unacceptable behavior, and, therefore, affected individuals are stigmatized (Halevy, 2000; Heckman et al., 2004).

In the past, the words *shame* and *guilt* were used to describe a concept similar to stigma—a perceived difference between a behavior or an attribute and an ideal standard. From this perspective, *guilt* is defined as self-criticism, and shame results from the disapproval of others. Guilt is similar to seeing oneself as discredited. Shame is a painful feeling caused by the scorn or contempt of others. For example, a person with alcoholism may feel guilty about drinking and also feel ashamed that others perceive his or her behavior as less than desirable.

Therefore, the concept of *deviance* versus *normality* is a social construct. That is, individuals are devalued because they display attributes that some call deviant (Kurzban & Leary, 2001). At Columbine High School, some teens, labeled *jocks,* stigmatized other teens who were considered as "low" and therefore "expected" to be taunted (Bartels & Crowder, 1999). Indeed, old age, which will one day characterize all of us, is often stigmatized (Ebersole & Hess, 2001). Further, because *stigma* is socially defined, it differs from setting to setting. Use of recreational drugs, for instance, may be normal in one group and taboo in another.

Whenever a stigma is present, the devaluing characteristic is so powerful that it overshadows other traits and becomes the focus of one's personal evaluation (Kurzban & Leary, 2001). This trait, or differentness, is powerful enough to break the claim of all of their other attributes (Goffman, 1963). As an example, the fact that a nurse is a brittle diabetic may cancel her/his remaining identity as a competent health professional. A professor's stutter may overshadow academic competence.

The extent of stigma resulting from any particular condition cannot be predicted. Individuals with a specific disease do not universally feel the same degree of stigma. On the other hand, very different disabilities may possess the same stigma. In writing about individuals with mental illness, Link (1997) describes variations in symptomology among them; however, indivduals without mental illness did not take the variation into account. All those who were disabled were seen as sharing the same stigma— mental illness—regardless of their capabilities or severity of their illness. That is, people responded to the mental illness stereotype rather than to the person's actual physical ability.

Similarly, Herek, Capitanio, and Widaman (2003) reported a study of the stigmatizing effects of the label of HIV/AIDS. They found that those individuals who reported a reduction in the level of stigma attached to HIV/AIDS, generally expressed negative feelings toward people with AIDS and other groups associated with HIV and favored a name-based reporting system.

Types of Stigma

Stigma is a universal phenomenon and every society stigmatizes. Goffman (1963) distinguishes among three types of stigma. The first is the *stigma of physical deformity;* the actual stigma is the deficit between the expected norm of perfect physical condition and the actual physical condition. For example, many chronic conditions create changes in physical appearance or function. These changes frequently create a difference in self- or other-perception (see Chapter 8, on body image). Changes of this kind also occur with aging. The normal aging process creates a body far different from the television commercial "norm" of youth, physical beauty, and leanness, although this norm is changing to include mature and elderly individuals as changes in the demographics of the population occur.

The second type of stigma is that of *character blemishes.* This type may occur in individuals with AIDS, alcoholism, mental illness, or homosexuality.

For example, individuals infected with HIV face considerable stigma because many believe that the infected person could have controlled the behaviors that resulted in the infection (Halevy, 2000; Heckman, 2004; Herek, Capitanio, & Widaman, 2003; Weston, 2003).

Ideals about traits that are considered character blemishes (that is, as undesirable) are culturally derived. For instance, in many African cultures, obesity is considered an expression of beauty and social status. Young women may be placed in a "fattening room" to increase their social status or to treat symptoms such as headaches or weight loss (Brink, 1989).

The third type of stigma is tribal in origin and is known more commonly as *prejudice*. This type originates when one group perceives features of race, religion, or nationality of another group as deficient compared with their own socially constructed norm. Although society is increasingly aware of job discrimination against women and other minority groups, it may be less sensitive to discrimination against individuals with disabilities and former psychiatric illnesses (Katz, 1981).

Most health care professionals agree that prejudice has no place in the health care delivery system. Although some professionals display both subtle and overt intolerance, others strive to treat persons of every age, race, and nationality with sensitivity. However, prejudice against individuals with chronic illnesses exists as surely as racial or religious prejudice.

The three types of stigma may overlap and reinforce each other (Kurzban & Leary, 2001). Individuals who are already socially isolated because of race, age, or poverty will be additionally hurt by the isolation resulting from another stigma. Those who are financially disadvantaged or culturally distinct (that is, stigmatized by the majority of society) will suffer more stigma should they become disabled.

Furthermore, not only is stigma ever-present, but once it occurs it endures (Link et al., 1997). If the cause of stigma is removed, the effects are not easily overcome. An individual's social identity is influenced by a history of the stigmatizing attribute. A person with a history of alcoholism or mental illness continues to carry a stigma in the same way that a former prison inmate does. One's identity is not only spoiled, it is spoiled beyond repair even if there is effective treatment for the stigmatizing condition.

Chronic Disease as Stigma

Individuals with chronic disease present examples of deviations from what many people expect in daily social interchanges. In daily encounters, people do not expect to meet someone in a wheelchair or one with an insulin pump. For example, persons with visible disabilities are not expected to attend social functions.

American values contribute to the perception of chronic disease as a stigmatizing condition. That is, the dominant culture emphasizes qualities of youth, attractiveness, and personal accomplishment. The work ethic and heritage of the western frontier provide heroes who are strong, conventionally productive, and physically healthy. Television and magazines demonstrate, on a daily basis, that physical perfection is the standard against which all are measured, yet these societal values collide with the reality of chronic disease. A discrepancy exists between the realities of a chronic condition, such as arthritis or AIDS, and the social expectation of physical perfection.

A disease characteristic, such as having an unclear etiology, may contribute to the stigma of many chronic diseases. In fact, any disease having an unclear cause or ineffectual treatment is suspect, including Alzheimer's disease (Jolley & Benbow, 2000) and anxiety disorders (Davies, 2000). Diseases that are somewhat mysterious and at the same time feared, such as leprosy, are often felt to be morally contagious.

Stigma can be associated with inequitable treatment, though the relative severity of such inequitable treatment often varies with the degree of severity of the stigmatized condition. For example, public policy about HIV/AIDS has acted both to increase accessibility to treatment and potentially to limit the civil rights of the stigmatized individuals (Herek, Capitanio, & Widaman, 2003). In addition, the shame, guilt, and social isolation of some stigmatized individuals may lead to inequitable treatment for their families. Because of the secrecy associated with being HIV-positive, affected clients and family members may not be able to access needed mental health, substance abuse rehabilitation, or infectious disease therapies (Salisbury, 2000).

So far, this chapter has defined *stigma* as a perceived deficiency between expected and actual characteristics. One is left with imagining the impact of stigma on individuals with chronic illness who have a physical deformity, a shortened life span, reduced energy level, and/or medical and dietary requirements.

All types of stigma share a common tie: In every case, an individual who might have interacted easily in a particular social situation may now be prevented from doing so by the discredited trait. The trait may become the focus of attention and can actually turn others away.

Impact of Stigma

A stigmatizing condition has an impact on both the affected individual and those persons who do not share the particular condition when both confront each other. The stigmatized individual is often unsure about the attitudes of others and therefore may feel a constant need to make a good impression. At the same time, the nonstigmatized individual may worry about whether to acknowledge the stigmatized condition; he or she may be concerned about making unrealistic demands (Goffman, 1963). Individuals with a chronic condition may not be included in groups because others do not know how to act toward them. Responses to stigma vary and will be discussed from the perspective of the stigmatized individual, the nonstigmatized individual, and the professional.

Responses of Stigmatized Individuals to Others

The way an individual deals with the reactions caused by a stigma varies, depending on the length and nature of the condition as well as on the individual's personal characteristics. Dudley (1983, p. 64) eloquently identifies how the stigmatized individual often feels:

> A depreciating remark, cold stare, willful disregard of a person's viewpoint hurts in unimaginable ways. The pain derives not only from each stigma-producing incident, but also from the cumulative effect of numerous previous incidents, with the latest one serving as a further reminder of their inferior status.

In addition to the stigmatized individual, family members, who often acquire a secondary stigma as a result of association (Goffman, 1963), have to deal with their responses to nonstigmatized people. Mothers who are HIV positive expend significant effort to protect their children from the negative effects of disclosure of their HIV status (Sandelowski & Barroso, 2003). Likewise, family members who care for persons with AIDS share the stigma of AIDS and are likewise discredited, resulting in rejection, loss of friends, and harassment (Gewirtz & Gossart-Walker, 2000; Salisbury, 2000). Stigmatized individuals respond to the reactions of others in a variety of ways.

Stigmatized individuals often divide the world into a large group to whom they tell nothing and a small group who are aware of the stigmatizing condition. In the past, medical practitioners have often recommended this type of information management, and this practice continues to some extent today (Goffman, 1963). For example, the diagnosis of leprosy may be listed as Hansen's disease or mycobacterial neurodermatitis. The client then has the option of revealing the alternate name of *leprosy*, with its accompanying historical stigma. Another common example is the abused spouse who provides reasonable explanations for bruises, swelling, and injuries. The practice of "passing" may significantly impair the health-seeking behavior of the abused individual, particularly where sociocultural barriers to disclosure exist (Bauer et al., 2000).

Disregard

A person's first response to a stigmatizing reaction may be *disregard*. In other words, they may choose not to reflect on or discuss the painful incidents. Well-adjusted individuals who feel comfortable with their identity, have dealt with stigma for a long time, and choose not to invest much effort in responding to the reaction of others may disregard it (Dudley, 1983). For example, many proud and confident individuals with chronic conditions choose to disregard demeaning comments directed toward them.

A different example of disregard is provided by wheelchair athletes. They disregard perceptions that their disabilities prohibit them from participating in strenuous, athletic endeavors. Any person who does not have a disability and who has observed these well-conditioned athletes racing their wheelchairs up hills in competitive meets may find it difficult to consider them discounted.

Going public with the diagnosis of AIDS is another example of disregard by acting in the face of negative consequences. One positive aspect of going public is the potential for assertive political action and social change. Former President Gerald Ford's wife, Betty, demonstrated the powerful effect of going public by disclosing her substance abuse problem. Similarly, Muhammed Ali, Earvin (Magic) Johnson, the late Christopher Reeve, Michael J. Fox, and other well-known personalities have captured public attention and acted positively to reduce the stigma attached to their health conditions.

One's perception of stigma may influence the severity that the stigma has on self-identity, and this supports the coping mechanism of disregard. In a study of 206 individuals with HIV/AIDS and cancer, Fife and Wright (2000) found that subjective perceptions of stigma accounted for significant differences in the severity of the impact of the stigma on self-identity. However, the authors also found that the negative impact of stigma (social rejection, in-

ternalized shame, social isolation, and financial insecurity) persisted regardless of illness type.

Isolation

Human beings have a proclivity for separating themselves into small subgroups. This tendency may not necessarily signify prejudice, because staying with one's own group is easier and requires less effort, and, for some individuals, is more congenial. However, this separation into groups tends to emphasize differences rather than similarities (Link, 1989).

Once a group has been set apart, a strategy of *closed interaction* may occur. In this process, the ingroup seldom invites outsiders to participate, and interaction is contained within the group itself. Closed interaction from within enhances one's feelings of normality because the individual is surrounded by others who are similar (Camp, Finlay, & Lyons, 2002). This feeling of normality characterized "The Trenchcoat Mafia" at Columbine High School (Bartels & Crowder, 1999). The process of isolation can occur any time outsiders are seen as threatening or are reminders that the world is different from the ingroup.

Staying with others who are similar is a source of support, but *similar* does not always mean disabled or ill. Some disabled or chronically ill individuals may feel more comfortable when they are surrounded by nondisabled individuals. One young woman, disabled since birth, feels better around nondisabled people because she has always considered herself normal. Her attitude reminds us to use caution when making assumptions about the perceptions of others.

Secondary Gains

Another possible response is to seek *secondary benefits* (Dudley, 1983). For instance, Dudley (1983) describes a docile, dependent individual with mental retardation who behaved in such a way as to gain favors. Health care professionals are familiar with individuals who capitalize on their conditions in order to achieve special favors. They rarely value such behavior, but it is an alternative for a stigmatized individual.

Some secondary gains from a chronic condition may be desirable (Dudley, 1983). For example, supportive work places that accommodate individuals with disabilities may foster social relationships, an important secondary benefit. Furthermore, work places that provide accommodations for disabled individuals promote the economic independence of these individuals and reduce the stigma of having to accept "welfare." Educational institutions that provide accommodations to learning disabled individuals not only promote the education of these individuals, but also help assure eventual employment of such stigmatized students. These examples of secondary gain promote the visibility of stigmatized individuals and may act to reduce the negative stereotypes associated with the stigma.

Resistance

Another response to a stigmatizing situation is *resistance* (Dudley, 1983). Individuals may speak out and challenge rules and protocol if their needs are not met. For many years, individuals using wheelchairs were unable to reach pay telephones. But wheelchair users and others united in voicing their protests of the situation, and now lower pay telephones are a much more common sight, as are ramps on stairs and curbs (curb cuts). Anger often serves as a catalyst for those seeking change. Dudley sees this resistance, at least in the case of individuals who are mentally retarded, as an important step toward autonomy.

Passing

An important potential response is *passing*—pretending to have a less stigmatic identity (Dudley, 1983; Goffman, 1963; Joachim & Acorn, 2000). If the attribute is discreditable (not readily visible), such as being a Type II diabetic or having a positive AIDS antibody test but no symptoms, passing is a viable option. It may begin accidentally and be strongly reinforced. As time goes on, individuals become pro-

ficient at performing activities as though they were normal. Consider, for example, the illiterate individual who buys and carries a newspaper on the bus in order to appear normal (Dudley, 1983) or the person with a hearing impairment who pretends to be daydreaming in order to pass (Goffman, 1963). This process may also include the concealment of any signs of the stigma. Some individuals refuse to use physical equipment, such as hearing aids, because this tells others of their disability.

In addition to visibility, obtrusiveness determines the ability to pass. In other words, how much does the condition interfere with normal functioning? For the individual in a wheelchair, being behind a desk or conference table makes this differentness easier for an observer to ignore (Goffman, 1963). A person with a speech impediment has no visible symbol of stigma, but whenever he or she speaks, others are reminded of the disability.

Learning to pass is one phase of a stigmatized person's career. However, acceptance and self-respect mitigate the need to hide the condition. Voluntary disclosure is a sign of a well-adjusted phase, "a state of grace" (Goffman, 1963).

Occasionally, culture limits the coping choices that are available, particularly in relation to disclosure of mental illness. In a study of West Indian women coping with depression, Schreiber, Stern, and Wilson (2000) found that "being strong" was the culturally sanctioned behavior for depression, rather than disclosure.

Covering

Because of the potential threat and anxiety-provoking nature of disclosure of a stigmatizing difference, most people deemphasize their differentness. This response, called *covering,* is an attempt to make the difference seem smaller or less significant than it really is (Goffman, 1963). Like passing, this process involves understanding the difference between visibility and obtrusiveness; that is, the condition is openly acknowledged, but its consequences are minimized. The object is to reduce tension. For instance, persons with special dietary requirements, in a social situation, may deny the importance of maintaining the restriction, even though they follow it. Minimizing the importance diverts attention from the stigma or defect and creates a more comfortable situation for all.

Another way in which a visible stigma becomes less anxiety producing is the skillful and often light-hearted manner in which the stigmatized individual handles it. The condition is *de-emphasized* by joking about it, thereby reducing the anxiety of others during the encounter. "I make a joke about my wheelchair, and that lets others know it's OK to talk about it" (S. Saylor, personal communication, 1988). The anxiety-producing subject is therefore no longer taboo and can more easily be managed.

Responses of Nonstigmatized People to Stigmatized Individuals

Responses of nonstigmatized individuals to a stigmatized individual vary with the particular stigma and the "nonstigmatized" person's past conditioning. Because society specifies the characteristics that are stigmatized, it also teaches its members how to react to that stigma.

Differences between groups based on nationality and culture have been found in attitudes toward those with disabilities (Brandon et al., 2000; Cinnirella & Loewenthal, 1999). Children learn to interact with others who are culturally different by watching and listening to those around them. In the same way, children learn how to treat chronically ill or disabled individuals by incorporating societal judgments. Unfortunately, these reactions are usually negative, because the stigma usually identifies an individual as discredited.

Devaluing

Nonstigmatized individuals often believe that the person with the stigma is less valuable, less human, or less desired. Unfortunately, many of us practice more than one kind of discrimination and, by so doing, effectively reduce the life chances of the stigmatized in-

dividual (Goffman, 1963). Many may tend to stigmatize persons as inferior or even dangerous and use such words as *cripple* or *moron*. Those who accept the devaluing effect of physical changes see the stigmatized person as having a spoiled social identity.

Stereotyping

Categories simplify our lives. Instead of having to decide what to do in every situation, we can respond to categories of situations. Most of our life's events fall into general categories, and the responses are therefore simplified (Allport, 1954). Church attendance requires appropriate dress. Sometimes, however, the inclination to categorize leads to restricted and inaccurate thinking, such as assuming that disabled people are incompetent.

Stereotypes are a negative type of category. They are a social reaction to ambiguous situations and allow us to react to group expectations rather than to individuals. When nonimpaired individuals meet those with physical impairments, expectations are not clear (Katz, 1981). Nonimpaired people often are at a loss as to how to react, so placing the individual with chronic illness in a stereotyped category reduces the ambiguousness toward him or her and makes the situation more comfortable for those doing the stereotyping. Categories are difficult to change; much less effort is required to sustain a bias than is required to reconsider or alter it.

Using categories and stereotypes to understand individuals decreases our attention to other characteristics (Hynd, 1958). If we are unaware of a person's positive attributes or capabilities, the negative characteristics become the major social identity. When people are put into categories, others not in that category often make quick judgments that are not based on reality. Categorizing tends to make one see the world as a dichotomy. For example, people are categorized as either mentally delayed or not, even though mental capabilities exist on a continuum, with all of us falling somewhere along the line.

Responses such as scapegoating and ostracism to people with AIDS have increased the impact of this disease and delayed treatment (Distabile et al., 1999; Rehm & Franck, 2000; Salisbury, 2000). Indeed, these responses impede appropriate health education aimed at prevention. Regardless of categories, individuals from different groups are similar in some ways and dissimilar in others.

Labeling

The label attached to an individual's condition is crucial and influences the way we think about that individual. For example, the diagnosis of AIDS is a powerful label, resulting in the loss of relationships and jobs not warranted by symptoms or the possibility of infection.

People with learning disabilities sometimes do not mind being called *slow learners,* but may be startled by being called *mentally retarded* (Dudley, 1983). Their response indicates that they see this latter term as a taboo. Individuals who are mentally disabled go to great lengths to explain why they are not retarded when they note that they work, fix their own meals, clean up after themselves, and so on. Their definition of this state is that it is less than human: "Mentally retarded, that's for very low people" (Dudley, 1983, p. 38). That is, the inability to perform certain functions is not as traumatizing to these individuals as the connotations inherent in the negative label.

Professional Responses: Attitudes Toward Stigma

Most health care professionals share the American dream of achievement, attractiveness, and a cohesive, healthy family. These values influence perceptions of individuals who are disabled, chronically ill, or otherwise considered "less than normal."

It is not surprising that society's values and definitions of *stigma* affect professionals' attitudes. These attitudes are also influenced by professional education, because students in health professional schools are enormously affected by their faculty and staff (Cohen et al., 1982). Cohen and associ-

ates describe how faculty influenced medical students in developing attitudes toward clients with cancers. Students assimilated the attitudes they saw around them, so if faculty treated clients with intolerance or a demeaning attitude, the students often adopted that behavior. On the other hand, if humane acceptance of all kinds of clients was observed, that behavior was more likely to be copied.

In addition to the influences of faculty and staff, attitudes were also changed by interactions with clients and chronically ill acquaintances (Sandelowski & Barroso, 2003). Students' confidence in clients' ability to cope with a disease increased with professional experience. In a similar manner, knowing someone with a chronic disease increased positive attitudes.

Another study of medical students' perspectives of illness disclosed a surprising aspect of stigma. Medical students revealed a high level of concern over the perception of social stigma attached to their personal health problems and the resulting professional jeopardy they might encounter upon disclosure (Roberts, Warner & Trumpower, 2000). This perception suggests that, when the health professional feels that she or he has a lot to risk, the fear of being stigmatized is greater and resistance to destigmatizing efforts might be greater.

Health care professionals display all the reactions that any nonstigmatized person has toward those with discrepancies of some sort. Therefore, caregivers need a thorough understanding of potential responses toward stigmatized individuals if they are to overcome the effects of stigmatizing behavior. Understanding the concept of stigma increases one's ability to plan interventions for chronic diseases (Joachim & Acorn, 2000).

Interventions: Dealing with Stigmatized Individuals

A chronic illness or disability imposes various kinds and degrees of constraints on an individual's life. The stigma of that disorder adds additional burdens, often far greater than those caused by the disorder itself (Joachim & Acorn, 2000). Individuals with chronic conditions usually receive medical treatment, but few interventions may be directed at reducing the effects of the associated stigma.

Helping others to manage the effects of stigma is not simple and should be approached with care. At best, change will be slow and uneven. However, consistent and knowledgeable interventions aimed specifically at reducing the impact of stigma are as crucial as those that reduce blood pressure or chronic pain. The following section discusses appropriate strategies for managing stigma.

Responses Toward Self: Changes in Attitudes

Societal norms and values are a major determinant of an individual's sense of self-esteem and self-worth. Children are socialized to adopt the attributes of their particular sociocultural group. Most of our standards of what is normal or expected from our particular society are derived from this socialization. To use Goffman's terms, we expect of ourselves what is expected of those in our particular social category. Specifically, in the United States, achievement and attractiveness are commonly held values.

The person who does not possess the expected attribute is quite aware of this discredit as an equal and desired individual in the society. In addition, individuals with chronic conditions may find that their own deformities or failings decrease their self-respect. That is, not only do stigmatized individuals have to deal with the responses of others, but some experience strong negative feelings about their own self-worth. These internalized perceptions may be more difficult to deal with than the illness or handicap itself.

In contrast, some individuals with chronic conditions can accept deviations from expected norms and feel relatively untouched. They have reordered life's priorities; no longer is the absence of disease or disability their major criterion for self-worth. Rather, an alternative ideology evolves to counter the "standard" ideologies. A strong sense of identity protects them, and they are able to feel acceptable in the face of the stigma (Goffman, 1963). This is also true in groups of culturally distinct individuals, such as Jews or Mennonites, who have pride in the group identity of their members. Similarly, strong extended families and cultural pride provide a strong identity for many members of African American, Hispanic, or other communities.

This identity belief system, also called *cognitive belief patterns,* refers to a person's perspective. It includes one's perceptions, mental attitudes, beliefs, and interpretations of experiences (Link et al., 1997). Individuals who are stigmatized by the major society may believe and perceive that their groups are actually superior or at least preferable. These belief patterns offer protection from the stigmatized reactions of others.

In chronic disease, cognitive belief patterns help individuals achieve identity acceptance and protection in the face of stigmatizing conditions. For example, after mutilating cancer surgery, patients may consciously tell themselves that they are full human beings because the missing part was diseased or useless. The body, although disfigured, is now healthy, whole, and totally acceptable. Similarly, wheelchair athletes take pride in their superb physical condition and competitiveness. That is, one's perception of self-worth influences one's reactions to disease or disability. An individual's question, "Am I worthwhile?" is answered by determining his or her own values and perspective. Therefore, clients' definitions of themselves are crucial factors in self-satisfaction (see Chapter 8, on body image).

In describing studies of clients with cerebral palsy, cancer, facial deformity, arthritis, and multiple sclerosis, Shontz (1977) noted that the personal meaning of the disability to each client was uniformly regarded as crucial. For example, individuals who feel valuable because they are healthy and physically fit usually suffer feelings of worthlessness if they contract a chronic condition. But people with diabetes will never be without a regimen and the necessary paraphernalia; visually impaired individuals will never see normally again. Therefore, the individuals' reactions and ability to accommodate these discrepancies determine their attitudes of worth and value.

Recent social changes have suggested that internalization of stigma based on prevailing social norms may be changing for some health problems. Rehabilitation programs for substance abuse are now commonly covered by health insurance, in part as a result of active consumer demand, evidencing a change of social attitude (Garfinkel & Dorian, 2000). The impact of stigmatizing conditions in women's health, such as abortion and breast cancer with mastectomy, has been reduced (Bennett, 1997). These changes are, perhaps, evidence that visibility and disclosure may have a positive impact on the process of negative stereotyping.

Developing a Support Group of One's Own

Goffman (1963) used the term *the own* for those who share a stigma. Those who share the same stigma can offer the "tricks of the trade," acceptance, and moral support to a stigmatized person. Self-help or support groups are examples of persons who are the own. Alcoholics Anonymous (AA), for instance, provides a community of the own as well as a way of life for its members. Members speak publicly, demonstrating that alcoholics are treatable, not terrible, people. They act as *heroes of adjustment,* to use Goffman's term.

Groups composed of people with similar conditions can be formal or informal and are enormously helpful. First, peer groups can be used to explore all of the potential response options previously discussed, such as resisting and passing. Second, problem-solving sessions in these groups explore possible solutions to common situations (Dudley, 1983). Finally, others who share the stigma provide a source of acceptance and support for both the individuals with the chronic condition and their families.

Again, a word of caution is appropriate. Sometimes stigmatized individuals feel more comfortable with nonstigmatized individuals than with like others as a result of a closer identity with the former. For example, not all women respond positively to Reach to Recovery groups; some may feel more discomfort than support. The "best" solution varies from individual to individual.

Developing Supportive Others

Supportive others are persons (professional and nonprofessional) who do not carry the stigmatizing trait but are knowledgeable and offer sensitive understanding to individuals who do carry it. These people are called *the wise* by Goffman (1963) and are accorded acceptance within the group of stigmatized individuals. The wise see the stigmatized person as normal and do not make affected individuals feel shame. Therefore, they treat such individuals in a normal fashion. One handicapped college student, asked what behaviors she liked from others, indicated a preference for knowledgeable acceptance:

I like to look people in the eye, but that means they need to sit down and come close. I like to be touched. Other students slap each other on the back, why not me? I really feel accepted when they ask to ride with me in my chair up and down the halls. Some people see *me,* not my wheelchair. (S. Saylor, personal communication, 1988)

These desired behaviors are simply the ones two friends or acquaintances would use. The stigmatized person must be seen and treated as a full human being—viewed as more than body changes or orthopedic equipment, seen as a person who is more than a stigmatized condition.

The AIDS epidemic has added to the impetus for the development of groups of supportive others. In many cities, the model of care for those with AIDS depends on volunteer, community-based groups that supply food, transportation, in-home care, acceptance, and support. This community network is an adjunct to hospital care and provides a vivid example of wise others who are essential to the care of these individuals.

The process of becoming wise is not simple; it may mean offering oneself and waiting for validation of acceptance. Health care professionals who encounter individuals with chronic illness cannot prove themselves as wise immediately. Validation requires consistent behavior by the professional that is sensitive, knowledgeable, and accepting.

One way an individual can become wise is by asking straightforward, sensitive questions, such as inquiring about the disabled person's condition. Many disabled individuals would be delighted to have the opportunity to disclose as much or as little as they wish, because that would mean that the disability was no longer taboo. For example, the disabled person may prefer that others ask about a cane or a walker rather than ignore it. This opportunity allows the disabled individual to reply with whatever explanation he or she wishes. Thus, the disability is acknowledged, not ignored. It goes without saying that these questions should be asked after a beginning relationship is established, as opposed to being asked out of idle curiosity.

Wiseness can come from working around individuals with a particular stigma. Health professionals can acquire real-life knowledge about problems, effective strategies, and concerns of a particular illness. This knowledge can enable them to offer the sensitive understanding and practical suggestions of the wise to chronically ill individuals. Nurses who work with AIDS clients, for instance, have the opportunity to find out which behavior is really effective and can learn about outcomes and clients' reactions. This information is extremely valuable to similar clients and their families.

Caring, close friends or relatives are another type of the wise. Siblings, spouses, and parents have the opportunity to be powerfully wise because they can see beneath the disorder to the human being and show that they see ill persons as persons first. However, not all relatives and friends become wise. Many cannot deal with the stigmatizing condition and tend to separate themselves from the ill individual.

Health care professionals are not always wise. Many people who work with the individuals with chronic disease or disability compound the stigma-tization of clients by their lack of acceptance and by their own insensitivity.

Being wise is not a new role for nurses or other caring health professionals. Nurses have traditionally worked in medically underserved areas with discredited persons and are accustomed to treating clients as people, not as conditions. Nurses often assume the predominant role of gatekeepers to the health care delivery system for many devalued individuals. Often, clients with chronic diseases receive effective and efficient care from these nurses and other health professionals, who have great opportunities to perform the role of the wise.

Advocacy

Advocacy is a demonstration of wiseness, because both processes require treating the individual as valuable and worthwhile. Client advocates are persons who support the right of clients to make informed decisions and to determine treatment they will accept. The client advocate supports that right by speaking on behalf of someone in need, combining expertise with a sensitive understanding of an individual or group of individuals (see Chapter 16, on advocacy).

An act of advocacy is obvious when laypersons and professionals speak out against proposed legislation or health policies that unnecessarily deprive those with AIDS or positive HIV antibody tests of their rights. Herek, Capitanio, and Widaman (2003) found a strong linkage between AIDS stigma and negative attitudes toward homosexual men and suggested that strong advocacy by health care professionals would enhance their credibility with key groups affected by HIV.

Stigmatized individuals may engage in advocacy as a means of dispelling the stigma and coping with the problem. A study of mental health consumers in Virginia reported that client-based advocacy was an effective coping mechanism (Wahl, 1999). However, advocacy in the form of protest can have a rebound effect, enhancing rather than suppressing negative stereotypes (Corrigan & Penn, 1999).

Changing Definitions of Disability

As noted earlier, one way to change a stigmatized individual's perception of self-worth is to reassess the criteria by which he or she determines what is normal—to realize that even people with healthy minds and bodies can be crippled by an inability to enjoy happiness (Goffman, 1963). This approach is also applicable for nonstigmatized individuals to use.

Family, friends, and health care providers who interact with the stigmatized person are powerful influences in the self-perception of value and worth (Camp, Finlay, & Lyons, 2002). Being treated as valuable and acceptable by significant persons enhances one's self-esteem. Stigmatized persons may find that this healthy perception of self counteracts the negative reactions of others. Some individuals who are disabled, but have always been treated as if they were valued, do not feel devalued.

Individuals whose self-esteem or identity is dependent on an occupation or hobby may lose these attributes as a result of a chronic condition. Just as a parent whose children are grown may find previously undeveloped personal attributes to fill their lost sense of identity, so many individuals with chronic conditions may find new sources of identity to replace lost functions.

A person should feel intrinsically worthwhile without fulfilling any particular conditions. For instance, a nurse who can no longer work because of a chronic condition may enjoy leisure time with professional friends and former colleagues without suffering a complete loss of self-identity. In the same way, changes in body image may not be catastrophic for those who answer the question, "Who am I?" with intrinsic values rather than physical attributes.

Nonacceptance Versus Nonparticipation

Distinguishing between nonparticipation and nonacceptance is important in caring for stigmatized individuals. *Nonparticipation* is an abstinence from social activities that is based on limitations caused by a handicap or illness. *Nonacceptance,* on the other hand, is a negative attitude—a resistance or reluctance on the part of the nondisabled person to admit the disabled person to various kinds and degrees of social relationships (Ladieu-Leviton, Adler, & Dembo, 1977). A disabled person who chooses not to join a camping trip is a nonparticipant; the physical disability serves as the basis for that person's decision not to participate. Deciding not to invite that person to join the group, whether or not participation is possible, is nonacceptance, preempting the person's choice.

Commonly, non-disabled individuals cannot correctly estimate the limits of potential participation for those with a disease or disability. Usually, the physical limitations imposed by a disability are overestimated. If nondisabled individuals incorrectly assume that a disabled individual is not able to participate, that is a form of nonacceptance. Such nonacceptance is created by the difference between the degree of participation that is actually possible and the degree assumed possible by those who are not disabled. If the difference can be resolved, nonacceptance ceases to be a problem.

The remedy can be simple. Nondisabled individuals can simply indicate that they want the disabled individual to participate, leaving to him or her the decision of whether to become involved. Perhaps the disabled individual would like to participate in a different way. For example, the young adult who has juvenile arthritis may not regret being unable to go fishing if he or she can elect to go along and spend time socializing with friends (Ladieu-Leviton, Adler, & Dembo, 1977).

Professional Attitudes: Cure Versus Care

Traditionally, the goal of health care has been to cure the client. Even today, health care providers tend to measure success in this way. Since chronic disease is now more prevalent than infectious disease or acute illness, this criterion of success may be inappropriate. Cure is neither essential nor necessary in order that the client benefit. Instead, caring, demonstrated by valuing and assisting, should be the criterion. With the increasing number of people who have chronic diseases, providers must learn to accept the characteristics of chronic disease: an indeterminate course of disease, relapses, and multiple treatment modalities. Today cost containment is a central focus in health care delivery. But providers must not lose sight of health policy considerations that include ideas of personhood and equitable health care sensitive to the reality of stigmatizing chronic illness (Gewirtz & Gossart-Walker, 2000; Roskes et al., 1999; Salisbury, 2000).

Selecting an Appropriate Model for Health Care Delivery

The manner in which health care is delivered may increase or decrease the effects of stigma. Encouraging a client's participation in health care decision making is an outward demonstration of respect and regard for that person. Treating a client as a partner in establishing goals demonstrates one's acceptance of the individual as valuable. On the other hand, when health providers make decisions regarding treatment or goals without consulting a client, they reinforce the client's feeling of being discredited. Therefore, any mode of delivery that increases client participation enhances that person's perception of self-worth and therefore reduces the effects of stigma.

All provider-client encounters fall into one of the following three basic health care delivery models (Szasz & Hollander, 1956). For reasons of stigma management, as well as of chronic disease management, it is wise to determine which model of health care delivery is most appropriate for chronic conditions.

Active-Passive The active-passive encounter is not really an interaction, because the client is acted upon and makes no contribution to decision making; the provider is the only active participant. This model is analogous to the relationship between a helpless infant and its parent. In emergency situations, this model may be the most appropriate one, but this form of encounter essentially says that the client is unable to participate in decision making.

Guidance-Cooperation A client seeks help from a provider and is willing to participate in the guidance-cooperation model. In this relationship, the client is expected to respect and obey the health provider; the power is unequal because the client is not expected to question the provider's recommendations. This model of health care delivery makes up the majority of traditional client-provider encounters and is valuable with many acute illnesses. However, it allows little, if any, room for clients' expectations or goals, which may be different from those of the provider.

Mutual Participation Mutual participation divides power evenly between provider and client and leads to a relationship that can be mutually satisfying. In other words, the client should be as satisfied with the recommendations and decisions as the provider is. In addition, each party depends on the other for information culminating in that satisfactory solution. The client needs the provider's experience and expertise; the provider needs not only the client's history and symptoms but his or her priorities, expectations, and goals. Sometimes a choice between treatments with relatively equal mortality rates is necessary—for example, surgery or radiation for cancer treatment. The physician can offer expert knowledge regarding long-term effects of radiation and changes in body image due to surgery. The client must decide the relative value of side effects of the alternative proposed treatments. Because the "right" decision depends on the individual, input from both client and health care provider is necessary to produce a course of action that is mutually acceptable.

An important factor in combating stigma is to allow individuals with limitations the opportunity to become "central participants in the battle" (Dudley, 1983). If the health care professional dominates the interaction, fuller client involvement does not result. The traditional models of client-provider interaction that give power and the right of decision making to the provider must give way to one that allows increased client participation.

When health care professionals become more comfortable with allowing clients a greater range of participation and decision making, the relationship decreases some of the stigmatizing effects of the disability. Wise health professionals create an atmosphere in which individuals with chronic conditions not only are expected to cooperate, but are encouraged to express their concerns, observations, expectations, and limitations.

The mutual participation model is the model of choice in stigmatizing chronic diseases, since it enhances the client's feelings of self-worth. The client is responsible for long-term disease management, and the health care provider is responsible for helping the client help himself or herself (Szasz & Hollander, 1956). Together, they explore alternative strategies and decide on one that is agreeable to both. When a client's priorities and goals are valued and incorporated into the regimen, an increased scnse of acceptance emerges. Therefore, the respect and regard for clients demonstrated by this model provide an effective tool to counteract some stigmatizing effects of illness.

Another benefit of a mutual participation model is increased compliance with a medical regimen. Because, in chronic disease, the client carries out the regimen, compliance becomes a particularly important issue (see Chapter 10, on compliance). Relationships between clients and practitioners that are collegial rather than authoritarian are associated with more compliance. The need for compliance provides further reinforcement for the use of a mutual participation model that increases the client's responsibility for health care. Thus, instead of wondering why the client does not comply with recommendations, providers might consider recommending an acceptable plan.

Inservice Education

Health care professionals' attitudes are representative of general societal views and so can be ex-

pected to include prejudices. Because health professionals have prolonged relationships with chronically ill individuals, the impact of these prejudices can be great. Programs to teach professional staff to identify and correct preconceived and often unconscious notions of categories and stereotypes deserve high priority (Dudley, 1983).

Providing intensive staff education for the purpose of reducing stigma perception by all employees in any particular agency is beneficial. In addition, professional staff are then in a position to practice role model behavior and to give information to help nonprofessional staff treat clients in an accepting manner.

A number of studies point out areas where an inservice program could be helpful. One study of stigma-promoting behaviors provides ideas for health care providers who wish to change their attitudes (Dudley, 1983). In Dudley's study, the most frequent stigma-promoting behaviors included the following: staring, denial of opportunities for clients to present views, inappropriate language in referring to clients, inappropriate restrictions of activities, violation of confidentiality, physical abuse, and ignoring clients.

Another study identifies methods of health communication that were designed to increase public awareness but actually had the opposite effect of increasing public stigma (Wang, 1998). The health communication approaches used conveyed to individuals with obvious disabling characteristics the accompanying message, "Don't be like this." Awareness was heightened at the expense of furthering the stigma of the disabled individual.

One way to increase visibility and heighten awareness about the impact of stigma is to encourage contact between health care professionals and affected individuals (Joachim & Acorn, 2000). This approach should be preceded by group work with a knowledgeable leader who can help identify and work through attitudes and reactions. For example, many nursing students do not like skilled nursing facilities (SNFs) because elderly clients are seen as unappealing. A gerontology nurse specialist spent time with such a group of students before they began working in the SNF. She showed slides of faces etched with character and told stories of interesting experiences these individuals had that helped the students see the elderly as human beings. A group discussion between specialist and students confronted myths and stereotypical thinking regarding the stigma of aging. As a result, these students had a more positive experience at the SNF. Knowledgeable preparation for contact with stigmatized individuals does not solve all problems; it is, however, one way to expose stigmatized reactions such as stereotypes, to examine them, and to provide information to caregivers. The group sessions described here may be appropriate for both nonprofessional and professional caregivers in the community or in agencies.

Community Education Programs

Educational programs that reduce the effects of stigma can be carried to the community at large. Many organizations, such as the American Cancer Society and the American Diabetes Association, provide speakers or literature for the community. Educational programs for young children, who are still being socialized, are effective in preventing the formation of stigma-producing attitudes (Dudley, 1983). Schools, scout troops, and church groups are ideal settings for sensitive introductions of individuals who have many positive values and characteristics but do not meet normal health expectations. For instance, individuals with AIDS have been the focus of group discussions in which children learn to see these people simply as other human beings. Educational programs, such as those that dispel the fears about mental illness, reduce the stigmatizing effects of that disease (Link, 1989).

Much of the stigma attached to chronic conditions still pervades society's attitudes and policies (Herek, Capitanio, & Widaman, 2003), yet, many situations have changed. In the 1970s, an unprecedented and multilayered surge of activism grew among individuals with disabilities and their advocates and resulted in significant social and structural change. Individuals with disabilities began to speak out by publishing magazines, creating movies and

videos, and organizing political action on both the local and national level. Their actions greatly influenced a landmark change, namely, the Americans with Disabilities Act (ADA), which was signed into law in 1990. This legislation requires the government and the private sector to provide disabled individuals opportunities for jobs, education, access to transportation, and access to public buildings.

In addition to formal community education programs, society's attitudes might be changed by increasing contact with disabled individuals. The amount of rewarding, mutual interaction between nondisabled, disabled, and chronically ill individuals can be increased by encouraging service projects, Internet connections, and activities among them.

The media can also be influenced to present a more positive portrayal of people with chronic conditions. Providers and others can write to television networks that show individuals with disabilities functioning well and commend them for these portrayals.

Other points to consider are the issues of "inclusion" and "exclusion" and how they impact stigma. Technology and assistance are significant factors because they underline the fact that "quality of life" is not a static entity. Not many years ago, electric wheelchairs were not available. Now such wheelchairs exist, even in children's sizes, allowing the child with cerebral palsy to "run with the crowd" instead of watch from a corner of the playground. Formerly, a person with paralyzed arms could only type slowly with a stick fastened to a headband; now there are increasingly accurate voice-activated home computers that can type as the person speaks. In the same vein, a person whose speech is unintelligible to most others can press symbols on a display board that produces full sentences spoken in a nonrobotic, smooth human voice.

The opportunity to hire personal assistants is also very important. Having such assistants allows individuals with severe disabilities to have a far richer life than those without such help. Many disability advocates are pressing for public money that is currently spent on nursing homes and other institutions to be redirected to enable individuals who are disabled or chronically ill to live in their own homes (see Chapter 26, on politics and policy, and Chapter 27 on financial impact).

Outcomes

Determining client outcomes, like many of the psychosocial concepts associated with chronic illness, is difficult. Some clients may be stigmatized on a regular basis but have been able to overcome the personal feelings associated with it. Thus, client outcomes of stigma might be the *lack* of other common psychosocial effects of chronic illness. For example:

- The client is *not* socially isolated, but is continuing his or her daily and normal activities without difficulty.
- The client's self-esteem remains high despite the chronic illness and accompanying physical symptoms.
- Healthy relationships continue with family, friends, and supportive others.

The client is not depressed and is interacting with others appropriately.

Summary and Conclusions

Stigma is a concept that historically traces back to the Greeks and attaches an adverse value judgment on another individual who differs in some way. In ancient Greece, stigmata were actually burned into the skin of slaves, criminals, and traitors to permanently mark them as "different." Sociologically, there are three kinds of stigma: actual physical differences, character blemishes, and prejudice. In all cases, stigma is a *perceived* deficiency and is meant to have an adverse impact.

In its present usage, *stigma* continues to signify a mark of discredit. Knowingly or otherwise, all "normals" tend to stigmatize in one way or another so they can socially identify people who are different and thereby minimize their own anxiety while maximizing their own comfort in a social situation. As used here, *normal* refers only to the fact that the person making the judgment does not have the stigmatizing characteristic.

Stigma is often attached to people with chronic illnesses or disabilities. Shortened life span, physical deformities, mobility restrictions, fatigue, medical and dietary requirements, and other limitations are not considered normal. The discrediting and socially isolating effects of stigma transcend any limitations imposed by the actual disease or disability. Devalued characteristics can overshadow other traits and become the focus of evaluation of the person.

Unfortunately, not only do people stigmatize others, but an individual may stigmatize himself or herself—that is, feel a sense of decreased value as a person. In addition, the negative perceptions of society at large are often reflected in the actions and attitudes of professionals who care for those with chronic illness. Professional stigmatization results in inequitable treatment regardless of the severity of the person's condition or ability to function.

A number of actions can be taken to break the cycle of stigmatization. Of major importance is the process of changing attitudes—of society at large, of health care professionals, and of the individual. Criteria by which people value others and themselves need reexamination in relationship to defining a person's worth. The stigmatized individual benefits from the support of like others and from learning to cope with negative responses. Health care providers are encouraged to become "the wise" and to act as knowledgeable and sensitive advocates for individuals bearing the stigma of chronic disease or disability. In addition, a model of health care delivery characterized by a more equitable sharing of power and goals must be developed. Inservice education for professionals and nonprofessionals can increase sensitivity to behaviors that encourage stigma-producing attitudes. Societal education is also necessary to make inroads into underlying causes of stigma.

Case Studies and Discussion Questions

Case Study #1:

Elise Duerr is a 42-year-old, divorced, special education teacher who began experiencing increasing fatigue and ascending muscle weakness approximately four years ago. After a lengthy, and anxiety producing year of testing, she was diagnosed with amyotrophic lateral sclerosis (ALS) three years ago. Her disease course has been progressive, and she is no longer able to work. She is thankful that the union contract with the local school district included long term care insurance benefits. She now is ventilator dependent and requires licensed assistance 24 hours-a-day with all of her activities of daily living and nursing care. Ms. Duerr's insurance has covered 80% of her durable medical equipment needs such as a motorized wheelchair and lift device.

Discussion Questions

1. How might this client be labeled as stigmatized? How would you assess this client's self-perception of stigma?
2. What strategies would you use to reduce the effects of stigma for this client?
3. You are assigned to orient a new respiratory therapist to Ms. Duerr's home health care team. How can health care professionals break down the barriers of stigma among the health care team?
4. What behaviors by Ms. Duerr would suggest that she does not label herself as stigmatized?

Case Study #2:

Domingo Mendez is a 36-year-old married computer software technician with three young sons. He has a history of mild depression that was first diagnosed after the death of his 8-week-old daughter nine months ago. He has been in good physical health, although his blood pressure was "borderline" when he attended an employee health fair event earlier this year. Mr. Mendez particularly is concerned that his employer will "find out" about his depression and has avoided filling the prescription for an anti-depressant medication.

Discussion Questions

1. What suggestions could you give to the health care team to facilitate a culturally appropriate assessment?
2. Are there any specific "labels" that Mr. Mendez may apply to himself? Are there any specific "labels" that the healthcare team may apply thereby creating the barrier of stigma?
3. What stigmatizing situations might arise for Mr. Mendez in the workplace? In the community?
4. What are the benefits and costs of increasing client participation in health care delivery? How does increasing client participation affect the stigma that Mr. Mendez may feel?
5. What strategies might lessen the stigma that Mr. Mendez perceives?

References

Allport, G. (1954). *The nature of prejudice.* Reading, MA: Addison-Wesley.

Baker, G. A., Brooks, J., Buck, D., & Jacoby, A. (2000). The stigma of epilepsy: A European perspective. *Epilepsia, 41* (1), 98–104.

Bartels, L., & Crowder, C. (1999). Fatal friendship. *Denver Rocky Mountain News.* Available on-line at: www.rockymountainnews.com.

Bauer, H., Rodriguez, M., Quiroga, S., & Flores-Ortiz, Y. (2000). Barriers to health care for abused Latina and Asian immigrant women. *Journal of Health Care for the Poor and Underserved, 11* (1), 33–44.

Bennett, T. (1997). Women's health in maternal and child health: Time for a new tradition? *Maternal and Child Health Journal, 1* (3), 253–265.

Brandon, D., Khoo, R., Maglajlie, R., & Abuel-Ealeh, M. (2000). European snapshot homeless survey: Result of questions asked of passers-by in 11 European cities. *International Journal of Nursing Practice, 6* (1), 39–45.

Brink, P. (1989). The fattening room among the Annang of Nigeria. In J. M. Morse (Ed.), *Cross-cultural nursing: Anthropological approaches to nursing research.* Philadelphia: Gordon and Breach Science Publishers.

Camp, D. L., Finlay, W. M. L., & Lyons, E. (2002). Is low self-esteem an inevitable consequence of stigma? An example from women with chronic mental health problems. *Social Science and Medicine, 55* (5), 823–834.

Cinnirella, M., & Loewenthal, K. M. (1999). Religion and ethnic group influences on beliefs about mental illness: a qualitative interview study. *British Journal of Medical Psychology, 72* (4), 505–524.

Cohen, R., Ruckdeschel, J., Blanchard, C., Rohrbaugh, M., et al. (1982). Attitudes toward cancer. *Cancer, 50,* 1218–1223.

Corrigan, P., & Penn, D. (1999). Lessons from social psychology on discrediting psychiatric stigma. *American Psychology, 54* (9), 765–776.

Crisp, A., Gelder, M., Rix, S., Meltzer, H., et al. (2000). Stigmatization of people with mental illness. *British Journal of Psychiatry, 177,* 4–7.

Davies, M. R. (2000). The stigma of anxiety disorders. *International Journal of Clinical Practice, 54* (1), 44–47.

Distabile, P., Dubler, N., Solomon, L., & Klein, R. (1999). Self-reported legal needs of women with or at risk for HIV infection. The HER Study Group. *Journal of Urban Health, 76* (4), 435–447.

Dudley, J. (1983). *Living with stigma: The plight of the people who we label mentally retarded.* Springfield, IL: Charles C. Thomas.

Ebersole, P., & Hess, P. (2001). *Geriatric nursing and healthy aging.* St. Louis: Mosby.

Erikson, E. (1968). *Identity: Youth in crisis.* New York: W. W. Norton.

Fife, B., & Wright, E. (2000). The dimensionality of stigma: A comparison of its impact on the self of persons with HIV/AIDS and cancer. *Journal of Health and Social Behavior, 41* (1), 50–67.

Garfinkel, P. E., & Dorian, B. J. (2000). Psychiatry in the new millennium. *Canadian Journal of Psychiatry, 45* (1), 40–47.

Gewirtz, A., & Gossart-Walker, S. (2000). Home-based treatment for children and families affected by HIV and AIDS. Dealing with stigma, secrecy, disclosure, and loss. *Child and Adolescent Psychiatry Clinics of North America, 9* (2), 313–330.

Goffman, E. (1963). *Stigma: Notes on management of spoiled identity.* Englewood Cliffs, NJ: Prentice-Hall.

Halevy, A. (2000). AIDS, surgery, and the Americans With Disabilities Act. *Archives of Surgery, 135* (1), 51–54.

Heckman, T. G., Anderson, E. S., Sikkema, K. J., Kochman, A., et al. (2004). Emotional distress in nonmetropolitan persons living with HIV disease enrolled in a telephone-delivered, coping improvement group intervention. *Health Psychology, 23* (1), 94–100.

Herek, G. M., Capitanio, J. P., & Widaman, K. F. (2003). Stigma, social risk, and health policy: Public attitudes toward HIV surveillance policies and the social construct of illness. *Health Psychology, 22* (5), 533–540.

Hynd, H. M. (1958). *On shame and the search for identity* (3rd ed.). New York: Harcourt Brace Jovanovich.

Joachim, G. & Acorn, S. (2000). Stigma of visible and invisible chronic conditions. *Journal of Advanced Nursing, 32* (1), 243–248.

Jolley, D. J., & Benbow, S. M. (2000). Stigma and Alzheimer's disease: Causes, consequences, and a constructive approach. *International Journal of Clinical Practice, 54* (2), 117–119.

Katz, I. (1981). *Stigma: A social psychological analysis.* Hillsdale, NJ: Lawrence Erlbaum Associates.

Kelly, P. (1999). Isolation and stigma: The experience of patients with active tuberculosis. *Journal of Community Health Nursing, 16* (4), 233–241.

Keltner, K., Schwecke, L., & Bostrom, C. (2003). *Psychiatric nursing* (4th ed.) St. Louis: Mosby.

Kurzban, R. & Leary, M. R. (2001). Evolutionary origins of stigmatization: The functions of social exclusion. *Psychological Bulletin, 127* (2), 187–208.

Ladieu-Leviton, G., Adler, D., & Dembo, T. (1977). Studies in adjustment to visible injuries: Social acceptance of the injured. In R. Marinelli & A. Dell Orto (Eds.), *The psychological and social impact of the physical disability.* New York: Springer.

Link, B. G. (1987). Understanding labeling effects in the area of mental disorders: An assessment of the effects of expectations of rejection. *American Sociological Review, 52* (1), 96–112.

Link, B. G., Cullen, F. T., Struening, E., Shrout, P. E., et al. (1989). A modified labeling theory approach to mental disorders: An empirical assessment. *American Sociological Review, 54* (3), 400–423.

Link, B. G., Struening, E. L., Rahav, M., Phelan, J. C., et al. (1997). On stigma and its consequences: evidence from a longitudinal study of men with dual diagnoses of mental illness and substance abuse. *Journal of Health and Social Behavior, 38* (2), 177–190.

Markowitz, F. E. (1998). The effects of stigma on the psychological well-being and life satisfaction of persons with mental illness. *Journal of Health and Social Behavior, 39*, 335–347.

Merriam Webster Dictionary and Thesaurus (2004). Available on-line at www.m-w.com.

Rehm, R. S., & Franck, L. S. (2000). Long-term goals and normalization strategies of children and families affected by HIV/AIDS. *Advances in Nursing Science, 23* (1), 69–82.

Ritson, E. B. (1999). Alcohol, drugs, and stigma. *International Journal of Clinical Practice, 53* (7), 549–551.

Roberts, L. W., Warner, T. D., & Trumpower, D. (2000). Medical students' evolving perspectives on their personal health care: Clinical and educational implications of a longitudinal study. *Comprehensive Psychiatry, 41* (4), 303–314.

Roskes, E., Feldman, R., Arrington, S., & Leisher, M. (1999). A model program for the treatment of mentally ill offenders in the community. *Community Mental Health Journal, 35* (5), 461–472.

Salisbury, K. M. (2000). National and state policies influencing the care of children affected by AIDS. *Child and Adolescent Psychiatry Clinics of North America, 9* (2), 425–449.

Sandelowski, M., & Barroso, J. (2003). Motherhood in the context of maternal HIV infection. *Research in Nursing and Health, 26*, 470–482.

Schreiber, R., Stern, P. N., & Wilson, C. (2000). Being strong: How black West-Indian Canadian women manage depression and its stigma. *Journal of Nursing Scholarship, 32* (1), 39–45.

Searle, G. F. (1999). Stigma and depression: A double whammy. *International Journal of Clinical Practice, 53* (6), 473–475.

Shontz, E. (1977). Physical disability and personality: Theory and recent research. In R. Marinelli & A. Dell Orto (Eds.), *The psychological and social impact of physical disability.* New York: Springer.

Simpson, G., Mohr, R., & Redman, A. (2000). Cultural variations in the understanding of traumatic brain injury and brain injury rehabilitation. *Brain Injury, 14* (2), 125–140.

Szasz, T., & Hollander, M. (1956). A contribution to the philosophy of medicine. *American Medical Association Archives of Internal Medicine, 97*, 585–592.

Wahl, O. F. (1999). Mental health consumers' experience of stigma. *Schizophrenia Bulletins, 25* (3), 467–478.

Waldman, H. B., Swerdloff, M., & Perlman, S. P. (1999). Children with mental retardation: Stigma and stereotype images are hard to change. *ASDC Journal of Dentistry for Children, 66* (5), 343–347.

Wang, C. (1998). Portraying stigmatized conditions: Disabling images in public health. *Journal of Health Communication, 3* (2), 149–159.

Weston, H. J. (2003). Public honor, private shame, and HIV: Issues affecting sexual health service delivery in London's South Asian communities. *Health & Place, 9* (2), 109–117.

Williams, D. R. (1999). Race, socioeconomic status, and health. The added effects of racism and discrimination. *Annals of the New York Academy of Science, 896*, 173–188.

CHAPTER 4

Chronic Pain

Janet E. Jeffrey

Introduction

Experiencing pain is a major reason for seeking health care (Clark, 2002; Elliott, Smith, Penny, Smith, & Chambers, 2000; Mantyselkä et al., 2001). "People seek health care for pain not only for diagnostic evaluation and symptom relief, but also because pain interferes with daily activities, causes worry and emotional distress, and undermines confidence in one's health" (Gureje, Von Korff, Simon, & Gater 1998, p. 147).

Melzack (1973) describes pain as "a highly personal experience depending on cultural learning, the meaning of the situation, and other factors that are unique to each individual" (p. 22). The International Association for the Study of Pain defines pain as "an unpleasant sensory and emotional experience associated with actual or potential tissue damage, or described in terms of such damage" (Merksey, 1986, p. S217). In other words, pain is a subjective experience (Turk, 1999; Warfield & Bajwa, 2004), a multidimensional phenomenon that lies at the intersection between biology and culture (Bullington, Nordemar, Nordemar, & Sjöström-Flanagan, 2003) the 'body-self neuromatrix' (Melzack, 1999).

Theories of Pain

Knowledge is limited about the specific mechanism(s) for transmission and perception of pain. However, several theories have been proposed, some of which are briefly noted here. The reader is encouraged to refer to texts, for more detailed information; such as Wall and Melzack (1999—new edition expected in 2005), Turk and Melzack (2001), Warfield and Bajwa (2004), or Weiner (2002).

The specificity theory, one of the oldest theories that serve to explain pain transmission, is based on the concept that there is always a relationship between cause and effect. It proposes that specific pain receptors (nociceptors) project impulses over specific neural pain pathways (A-delta and C fibers) via the spinal cord to the brain.

The *pattern theory* evolved when it was demonstrated that nociceptors respond to stimuli like pressure and temperature and not just to pain. This theory assumes that there are no pain-specific nociceptors and that pain occurs from a combination of stimulus intensity and the central summation pattern of impulses in the dorsal horn of the spinal cord.

The theory used widely in clinical practice today is the *gate control theory* proposed by Melzack and Wall (1965), even though it is not fully supported by incontrovertible experimental evidence. According to this theory, a gating mechanism in the dorsal horn of the spinal cord permits or inhibits the transmission of pain impulses. Peripheral nerve fibers that synapse in the gray matter of the dorsal horn serve as a gate. When the gate is closed, pain impulses are prevented from reaching the brain. Therefore, pain must reach a conscious awareness before it is perceived; if awareness can be prevented, then the perception is decreased or eliminated.

Acute Versus Chronic Pain

Pain can be acute or chronic in nature. Acute pain serves as a protective physiological mechanism that informs us when something is wrong with our bodies (Weiner, 2002) or prevents additional tissue damage by limiting movement in injured parts (Melzack & Wall, 2003). Acute pain presents with autonomic nervous system or behavioral responses and is time limited from minutes to weeks. It subsides when healing occurs and can usually be controlled by medications and other interventions. Even when acute pain is severe, it can often be tolerated because the person experiencing the pain knows that it is temporary.

Pain is chronic when it: (1) persists for a length of time, most commonly lasting more than 3 to 6 months; (2) occurs at intervals for months or years; and/or (3) is associated with chronic pathology (McCaffery & Pasero, 1999; Wall & Melzack, 1999; Warfield & Bajwa, 2004). When an individual has chronic pain, the body's adaptive physiological and autonomic responses are usually absent. Chronic pain can be continuous, intractable, intermittent, or recurrent. Even when mild, it can be so pervasive that it becomes a condition unto itself that requires daily management.

Current terminology differentiates chronic pain as *malignant* (associated with progressive terminal illness), or *nonmalignant* (not associated with terminal illness but unresponsive to treatment). Chronic nonmalignant pain is also known as *chronic benign pain* or *intractable pain*. People with chronic pain often find themselves in a "no-win" situation, because their pain no longer serves the purpose of

acute pain nor does it respond adequately to conventional medical treatment.

Although persons who have chronic health problems can experience either acute and/or chronic pain, it is the ever-present nature of chronic pain that controls much of their lives. This chapter examines some of the problems faced by people with chronic nonmalignant pain and provides general guidelines for interventions. No effort has been made to cover the myriad problems that arise from chronic pain or all of the possible interventions. Many of these interventions can also be used for people with malignant pain. The focus is on information that health care professionals can use to help clients who experience chronic pain.

Problems and Issues

Chronic pain is a common, persistent problem (Elliott et al., 2002). Estimates of the prevalence of chronic pain vary greatly by age, country, and study methods used; for example, 2% to 40% of the general population (Blyth et al., 2001; Elliott et al., 2002; Erikson, et al., 2003; Hasselström, Liu-Palmgren, & Rasjö-Wråak, 2002) to 72% of older adults in the United Kingdom (Thomas et al., 2004). Chronic pain is experienced by many who are disabled and results in secondary economic problems, including lost work productivity and increased health care costs (Blyth, March, Brnabic, & Cousins, 2004; Caudill-Slosberg, Schwartz, & Woloshin, 2004; Maniadakis & Gray, 2000).

Chronic nonmalignant pain can involve any part of the body (Merskey, 1986) and vary in intensity from mild to excruciating (Wall & Melzack, 1999). Chronic pain often results in impaired functional ability (Ljungkvist, 2000), psychological changes (Currie & Wang, 2004; McWilliams, Cox, & Enns, 2003), and changes in family life (Palermo, 2000; Smith & Friedemann, 1999).

Chronic pain is a multidimensional complex phenomenon that can affect every aspect of life for adults (Loeser, 2000; Marcus, 2000; McCaffery & Pasero, 1999) and for children (Palermo 2000; Rapoff & Lindsley, 2000). The *physiological dimension* focuses on the etiology of the pain as well at its location, onset, and duration. The *sensory dimension* focuses on how people describe the intensity, quality, and pattern of their pain. The *affective dimension* is based on clients' feelings about their pain; that is, their mood state, anxiety, fear, and depression (McWilliams, Cox, & Enns, 2003). In fact, affective distress (Turk, 1999) and fear (Crombez et al., 1999) often occur when chronic pain is experienced (Strahl, Kleinknecht, & Dinnel, 2000). The *cognitive dimension* deals with the meaning of pain and other related thought processes (Bullington et al., 2003). The *behavioral dimension* serves to both decrease pain intensity and indicate the presence of pain to others. Finally, the *sociocultural dimension* focuses on the ethnocultural background of the individual—family and social life, work and home responsibilities, recreation and leisure), environmental factors, and social and cultural influences (Davidhizar & Giger, 2004; Riley et al., 2002).

Unrelieved chronic pain affects "all aspects of quality of life . . . [which] has been found to span every age and every type and source of pain" (Katz, 2002, p. S38).

Undertreatment by Professionals

Pain is regularly undertreated by health care professionals. Many health professionals have a poor understanding of pain assessment and pain management. They are often frustrated with clients who do not manifest symptoms of their pain or do not respond well to treatment management. (Green, et al., 2002; Lazarus & Neumann, 2001; McCaffery, Ferrell, & Pasero, 2000; Shvartzman et al., 2003; Weinstein et al., 2000).

Unfortunately, pain relief is not as high a priority among health care professionals as controlling clients' expressions of pain. Tait and Chibnall (2002) concluded that reporting of chronic pain by health care staff was related to displays of discomfort only; whereas clients' pain rating was correlated with displays of discomfort as well with functional independence and depression. In addition, nurses' ratings of pain were predicted by medication administration variables.

Pain intensity is consistently underestimated by health care professionals compared with self-ratings of those experiencing chronic pain (Bergh & Sjostromm, 1999; Tait & Chibnall, 2002). Narcotics are underutilized, even though the need for narcotics is often clearly indicated; there is a "prejudice against use of opioid analgesics" (Weinstein et al., 2000, p. 479). For example, as many as 85% to 90% of clients with acute or prolonged pain from end-stage renal disease could be kept comfortable if narcotics were properly used (McCaffery & Pasero, 1999).

The negative stereotypes of individuals who have chronic pain held by many health care professionals contribute to the discounting of clients' pain complaints. Professionals do not always give credence to pain complaints unless there is identifiable pathology or clients demonstrate autonomic or behavioral responses (Turk, 1999; Weinstein et al., 2000). Professionals often assume that all clients have the same pain perception threshold and, therefore, perceive the same intensity of pain from the same stimuli (Voerman, van Egmond, & Crul, 2000). Many professionals have become desensitized to their clients' pain experience and rate pain as less important than clients do (Shvartzman et al., 2003). Some erroneously assume that the depression that co-exists with chronic pain results in decreased effectiveness of pain relief measures.

Many professionals believe that chronic pain is not as intense as acute pain, especially if there is no evidence of pathology. However, research has demonstrated that the opposite is true. Longstanding pain results in decreased endorphins, which increases the perception of pain from the same stimuli (Takahashi et al., 2000). These misconceptions and others can lead to poor management of chronic pain by physicians who feel ill-prepared to manage their clients' pain (Green et al., 2003).

The pattern of underprescribing analgesics by physicians has been reported for over 30 years (Grossman & Sheidler, 1985; Marks & Sacher, 1973; McCaffery & Ferrell, 1999; Shvartzman et al., 2003). In addition, for the same reasons that medications are underprescribed, they are administered by nurses conservatively by lengthening the interval between doses or giving the low dose in the range prescribed.

Medications are also administered inconsistently, so that relief is neither continuous nor adequate. Some clients further contribute to the inadequate use of narcotics by not taking the recommended medication and/or dose because they share the same misconceptions as health care professionals (Sweeney & Bruera, 2003).

Addiction

Narcotic analgesics are not commonly used to manage chronic pain. Many health professionals are afraid that their clients will become addicted to narcotics (Caracci, 2003; Shalmi, 2004; Sweeney & Bruera, 2003). Their misconceptions about opioid use fuels the controversy about using narcotics to treat chronic pain (Cowan, While, & Griffiths, 2004; McCarberg & Barkin, 2001). They erroneously interpret their clients' behaviors as addiction (Table 4-1). *Addiction* is defined as "a pattern of compulsive drug use characterized by continued craving for an opioid and the need to use the opioid for effects other than pain relief" (McCaffery & Pasero, 1999, p. 36), and does not typically apply to persons who have chronic pain. Addicts do not use drugs to relieve pain; they use them for psychological reasons, compulsively seek drugs, and tend to relapse even after they have undergone physical withdrawal. Table 4-1 describes the common misconceptions about behaviors indicating addiction.

Addiction by clients taking narcotics for pain relief is rare (Laliberte, 2003; Savage, 1999). People in pain who are using narcotics appropriately will stop taking the drug(s) once the pain is relieved. The need to continue drugs indicates that relief from pain has not been obtained and that medications are still necessary. What health care professionals confuse with addiction is usually either physical dependence or drug tolerance.

Physical Dependence

Physical dependence is not a sign of addiction, but is a *physiological response* of the body to repeated doses of a narcotic. If the narcotic is stopped abruptly,

withdrawal symptoms will occur. During the first six to 12 hours after the narcotic is discontinued, clients may manifest anxiety, rhinorrhea, diaphoresis, shaking chills, anorexia, nausea, vomiting, and/or abdominal cramps. By the second to third day, clients may demonstrate excitation, restlessness, insomnia, muscle spasms, low back pain, elevated blood pressure, tachycardia, dehydration, ketosis, and/or leukocytosis. Everyone does not go through demonstrable withdrawal nor do increased doses of narcotics increase the severity of withdrawal. Withdrawal symptoms can be avoided if narcotics are gradually discontinued—a common occurrence as pain subsides (McCaffery & Pasero, 1999). Psychological dependence may be a different matter, but it is rare, with incidence of less than 1% (Goodwin & Bajwa, 2004).

Drug Tolerance

Drug tolerance is an involuntary physiological behavior that occurs when a narcotic begins to lose its effectiveness after repeated administration or when an increasing dose is required to maintain the same effect (McCaffery & Pasero, 1999; Goodwin & Bajwa, 2004). Health care professionals erroneously believe that each narcotic has a maximum dose which results in concern if more medication is needed because of inadequate pain relief. They also fear that increased amounts of narcotics will result in respiratory depression or oversedation. What they need to remember is that a concurrent tolerance to respiratory depression and sedation occurs as tolerance to a narcotic develops (Pasero, Portenoy, & McCaffery, 1999). Individuals with chronic pain require and tolerate higher doses of analgesic medication. They can also use narcotics in addition to other medications to effectively manage their pain.

Effects of Unrelieved Pain

People who have chronic pain may undergo a change from having many roles (e.g., worker, friend, family member) to those who identify only with their pain. Because pain is invisible, clients may feel

TABLE 4-1

Misconceptions: Behaviors Indicating Addiction

Behaviors That Are Often Mistaken as Indicators of Addiction	Correction/Comments—What Else Could It Be?
1. The patient requests analgesics by name, dose, interval between doses, and/or route of administration; e.g., "I'll need two Vicodin every 4 hours." "Morphine, 10 mg IV, works best for my headache."	This is likely to be a well-educated patient who probably has had pain previously or has chronic pain. Patients need to be educated about all their medications, including analgesics. If this patient were a diabetic talking about insulin requirements, it would be welcomed information. This patient is providing helpful information for the pain treatment plan.
2. The patient is "a frequent flyer," frequently visiting several emergency departments (EDs) to obtain opioid analgesics.	This is not desirable behavior, but it may be caused by inadequate pain treatment. If treatment at the ED results in poor pain relief or if staff convey that the patient comes too often, the patient may go to another ED for additional pain relief or to decrease the frequency of visits to a single ED. The patient may have a chronic pain problem that is not well managed by the private physician, so the patient is forced to seek help in the ED. If patients return often to the ED, a plan should be developed and on file to document previous assessments, the effectiveness of treatments, and recommendations for initiating pain relief on subsequent ED visits.
3. The patient obtains opioids from more than one physician.	This is not desirable behavior but, like the aforementioned, may reflect poor pain management. For example, a patient's physician may prescribe an opioid/nonopioid oral analgesic (e.g., Percocet or Tylenol No. 3). The patient may find that one dose in the morning effectively relieves his pain and helps him get moving so that he can work through the day. If the physician refuses to prescribe more than 30 tablets every 3 months and suggests no other methods of pain relief, the patient may seek drugs from another physician. Improved assessment and pain treatment, including use of nonopioids and other modalities, may remedy this situation.
4. The patient requires higher doses of opioids than other patients. "He's hitting his PCA button too much."	There is no set dose of opioid that is safe and effective for all patients. Even a patient who has not received opioids regularly (opioid naive) may require 6 times more opioid than another patient. A patient who is tolerant to opioid analgesia may require 100 times more opioid than the opioid-naive patient. Some conditions, such as sickle cell crisis, are more painful than others. A patient may require much more opioid for a sickle cell crisis than for major abdominal surgery. Frequent use of the PCA button indicates that the pump parameters need to be adjusted.
5. The patient has been taking opioids frequently for a long time.	Length of time on opioids does not appear to increase the likelihood of developing addiction. Many patients with cancer or noncancer pain have taken opioids for months or longer and ceased taking them when the pain subsided. Physical dependence and tolerance may develop with prolonged use, but they are not the same as addiction.

continues

TABLE 4-1
_____

Continued

Behaviors That Are Often Mistaken as Indicators of Addiction	Correction/Comments—What Else Could It Be?
6. The patient is a "clock watcher" and may ask for the analgesic in advance of a specified time. The patient may say, "I'll need my next dose in about 30 minutes."	Sometimes analgesics are prescribed at intervals longer than their duration. When the patient asks for a dose before the interval elapses, the clinician often tells the patient how much time he must wait. For example, "You can't have your next pill for 2 hours." Because the patient must wait in pain for 2 hours, he is likely to note the time and ask for the medication as soon as the 2 hours pass. The patient may then find that it takes the nurse another 30 minutes to deliver the dose. The patient may work with these realities by calculating when the next does can be given and asking for it 30 minutes in advance. This situation strongly suggests that the patient's opioid prescription should be changed to a longer acting opioid or the intervals between doses should be shortened.
7. The patient "prefers the needle to the pill."	When the same dose given parenterally is given orally, the pain relief is likely to be much less. Using an equianalgesic chart often explains the problem. For example, if a patient has been receiving morphine, 10 mg IM or IV q4h, switching the patient to an opioid/nonopioid combination, such as one Tylenol No. 3, provides only one-sixth to one-fifth as much pain relief. The solution may be to use a single entity oral opioid such as morphine. A dose of 30 mg will provide approximately the same pain relief. If pain has decreased by 50%, morphine, 15 mg PO, is indicated.
8. The patient "enjoys his Demerol."	Once pain is relieved, it is natural for the patient to feel happier and engage in more activities, such as talking and ambulating. By contrast, it may look like the patient is "high" or euphoric, but it is simply a return to normal mood, perhaps with some elation at being in less pain.
9. The patient says he is allergic to everything except one particular opioid.	Allergy to opioids is rare, but patients often mistake side effects such as nausea, vomiting, and itching for an allergy. These may have been poorly managed side effects, or the patient may have more severe side effects with some opioids than others. If the patient has more side effects with certain opioids, they should be avoided. If the patient is more convinced of the effectiveness of one opioid over others, it is possible that the patient will try to avoid the others by saying he is allergic to them. Even when an analgesic is not terribly effective, the patient may be afraid to try another analgesic for fear the results will be even worse. If it is not necessary for the patient to change to another opioid, the patient should receive what he prefers. If a change is necessary, perhaps because the opioid preferred by the patient has an active metabolite that is accumulating (a common problem with meperidine), then selection of another opioid will depend on careful assessment to determine whether the patient is allergic or whether he has experienced unmanaged or unmanageable side effects.

May be duplicated for use in clinical practice. From McCaffery M, Pasero C: *Pain: Clinical manual*, pp. 52–53. Copyright © 1999, Mosby, Inc., with permission from Elsevier.

the need to explain or defend the pain in an effort to be believed by health care professionals and others. When faced with skepticism, they may become frustrated, unsupported, and powerless with the health care system (Lane, 2000).

Although many individuals with chronic pain manage to continue with other aspects of their lives, others have limited repertoires for coping with their pain and find the only safe way to respond to symptoms is to call their physicians. Their lives revolve around their pain because the pain "cannot be left behind". Chronic pain is multidimensional and affects many aspects of people's lives.

Depression

A relationship clearly exists between depression and chronic pain, although there is no consensus about the nature of this relationship other than that they coexist (Dersh, Polatin, & Gatchel, 2002; Pincus & Williams, 1999) both in adults and children (Scharff & Turk, 1998). In a review of studies that addressed hypotheses about the causal relationship between depression and chronic pain, Fishbain, Cutler, Rosomoff, and Rosomoff (1997) concluded that the greatest support was for the consequence hypothesis (depression follows the development of chronic pain) and the scar hypothesis (predisposition to depression increases likelihood of depression with chronic pain).

McWilliams et al. (2003) analyzed data from the National Comorbidity Survey (USA) and reported that adults who have chronic pain were more likely to have concurrent depression than those without chronic pain. In a national survey in Canada, adults with chronic low back pain were found to be over three times as likely to also report depression than the general population and "the rate of major depression increased in a linear fashion with greater pain severity" (Currie & Wang, 2004, p. 54). Pain and depression affect ability to complete cognitive tasks and this effect increases with greater pain and depression. Furthermore, the relationship between pain and cognition is mediated by depression, meaning that depression contributes to the impact

of chronic pain on daily life (Brown, Glass, & Park, 2002; Fishbain et al., 1997). Moreover, the success of cognitive-behavioral interventions may be enhanced when depressive symptoms are effectively treated.

There is evidence that depression plays a role in the maintenance of chronic pain because negative thinking contributes to depression, and both affect pain and pain behavior. Spinhoven et al. (2004) reported that cognitive behavioral interventions designed to reduce catastrophizing thoughts about the consequences of pain and promote internal expectations of pain control reduced levels of depression and pain behavior.

However common depression is, it is often unrecognized and consequently, is untreated (Harris, 1999). Given that concurrent chronic pain and depression are associated with greater disability than either pain or depression alone (Currie & Wang, 2004), treating both depression *and* pain is important. In addition, depressive symptoms, in the absence of major depression, should not be ignored. Helping clients manage depression with medications and other interventions can go a long way in reducing the severity and impact of chronic pain. Some pain management programs are designed to address depression and other challenges that coexist with chronic pain, especially those with a cognitive-behavioral component.

Anxiety

Anxiety is experienced by adults who have chronic pain. In recent analysis of national representative samples of adults, McWilliams et al. (2003, 2004) found that the association between pain and anxiety was even greater than the association between chronic pain and depression even when the effect of other variables was controlled. They concluded that anxiety has gone unrecognized in clients with chronic pain.

The high prevalence of anxiety disorders among persons with chronic pain has been clearly documented, with panic disorder and generalized anxiety being the most common (Dersh et al., 2002). Anxiety helps to maintain and/or exacerbate the pain experienced by physiological mechanisms; such as, fear of pain, and fear of movement leading to reducing activities and deconditioning. In addition, cognitive factors may contribute to fear-avoidance behavior (Dersh et al.). One of these factors that has received attention in the past few years is catastrophizing which leads to misinterpretation of sensations associated with pain (Asmundson, Norton, & Norton, 1999; Woby, Watson, Roach, & Urmston, 2004). Some success has been reported in reducing catastrophizing and fear-avoidance beliefs with cognitive-behavior interventions (Woby et al. 2004). More attention needs to be paid to both depression and anxiety experienced by those who have chronic pain.

Worry plays a significant role in the pain experience (Aldrich, Eccleston, & Crombez, 2000). Worry is related to awareness of somatic sensations and can be distracting and intrusive (Eccleston, Crombez, Aldrich, & Stannard, 2001). Worry needs to be addressed for pain management to be effective.

Fatigue and Sleep Disturbance

Fatigue is "a subjective experience of feeling exhausted, tired, weak, or having lack of energy" (Kaasa et al., p. 939) that affects a person's life: work, social activities, and mood (Kaasa et al., 1999). The relationship between chronic pain and fatigue has been recently substantiated by an evidence-based review of the literature; in fact, Fishbain et al. (2003) concluded that there may an etiological relationship between pain and fatigue.

Sleep disturbance is more common in adults who have chronic pain when compared with a healthy control group. The adults with chronic pain had more frequent fragmentation of sleep and longer sleep latency, and resultant poorer quality of sleep (Call-Schmidt & Richardson, 2003). Nicassio, Moxham, Shuman, and Gervitz (2002) found that chronic pain contributed to poor sleep quality which in turn predicted greater fatigue; sleep quality mediated the relationship between chronic pain and fatigue.

Depression and poor sleep quality also contribute to fatigue in adults with fibromyalgia who experience intense pain (Menefee et al., 2000; Nicassio et al., 2002). Not only can depression contribute to poor sleep quality, but the antidepressant medications and sedative/hypnotic commonly used to treat depression and disturbance can also disrupt REM sleep and negatively affect the sleep cycle. Clinicians need to consider the benefits of antidepressants as well as their potential to interfere with sleep and increase fatigue. They also need to consider other interventions to improve sleep and reduce fatigue (see chapter 7, on altered mobility and fatigue).

A negative feedback loop can be created. Sleep disturbance leads to fatigue which leads to less physical activity and contributes to depression, poor concentration and boredom; and all in turn have a negative impact on sleep (Nicassio et al., 2002). Treating the sleep disturbance is as important for children as it is for adults (Lewin & Dahl, 1999).

The disturbed sleep reported by many clients with chronic pain usually indicates either poor pain relief, especially night pain, or psychological disturbance (Smith, Perlis, et al., 2000). Integration of treatment of chronic pain and sleep disturbances can reduce the consequences of fatigue (NIH, 1995).

Life-Cycle Differences

Chronic pain in both children and the elderly is undermanaged even more than in other age groups. It is not uncommon for individuals in these two groups to receive lower than therapeutic doses of medications and less attention in terms of other treatment, which needlessly leaves them in moderate to severe pain.

Children

Pain is a common experience for children. In a cross-sectional population survey of children age 0 to 18 years, 25% of children reported having chronic pain (more than three-month duration) one third of whom reported that pain was very frequent and intense (Perequin et al., 2000).

Inadequate pain control, common in the treatment of very young children, is likely more from a lack of knowledge (including lack of pain assessment) than from lack of concern. Many of the myths that abound about pain in children have no basis in fact such as: (a) very young children, especially neonates and infants, are erroneously believed to feel little if any pain, experience pain to a lesser degree than adults, tolerate pain better than adults, and recover more quickly than adults; (b) the potential side effects of narcotics, including addiction, are believed to make the use of such medication too dangerous with small children; (c) pain is thought not to be life-threatening to young children, and young children do not remember pain (Berde & Masek, 2003; McCaffery & Pasero, 1999; Mitchell & Boss, 2002).

Children of all ages experience pain that can be intense (Perequin et al. 2000). The intensity of chronic pain differs by age in children aged 4 to 7 years who reported less severe pain than younger and older age groups (Perequin et al., 2000). Children demonstrate pain regardless of age; neonates and infants show facial responses to pain and have distinct cries when in pain (Jeans & Johnston, 1985). A recent extensive review of the literature on pain in children concluded that "pain causes stress for babies" and that pain has a long-term effect on neurological development (Whitfield & Grunau, 2000). Once language skills are present, typically, more credence is given to children's expression of pain, even though the pain might not be managed adequately. Children's pain is not innocuous.

In a recent review of the literature on the impact of pain on children and their families, Palermo (2000) concluded that pain has a significant effect on children and their families. Pain interferes with children's sleep, school, play and friendships. There is also widespread interruption of tasks of everyday life for children and their families, as well as parental burden. The same issues of depression and assumption of the sick role are relevant for both children and adults, and the entire "pain puzzle" is as complex for children as it is for adults (Rapoff & Lindsley, 2000).

Depression is associated with chronic pain in children as it is in adults. Williamson, Walters, and Shaffer (2002) reported that depression of mothers predicted depression in their children as did their child's pain. In addition, the relationship between pain and depression in children was ameliorated by the nature of the coping strategies used by their mothers.

Approximately one third of adolescents experience chronic pain (Perequin et al., 2000). A similar relationship between chronic pain and disability, and emotional distress is documented in adolescents as in adults. Depression and anxiety exist concurrently with chronic pain for adolescents (Hunfeld et al., 2001; Kashikar-Zuck et al., 2002; Smith et al., 2003). When compared to adolescents who do not have pain, adolescents with chronic pain report less social acceptance by others, higher fear of failure and poorer quality of life in all domains (Hunfeld et al., 2001; Merlijn et al., 2003). The response of peers and parents to pain has a strong bearing on how adolescents live with their pain; they may hide pain from their peers by staying home because peers do not reward pain behaviors. This reclusive behavior may in turn be rewarded by parents so pain behavior is supported (Merlijn et al., 2003).

Older Adults

As with children, there are misconceptions about pain in the elderly. Myths include: (a) pain is believed to be a natural outcome of growing old and pain increases with age (Gloth, 2004); (b) pain perception and sensitivity decrease with age (Leininger, 2002); (c) the lack of pain behaviors indicates a lack or limited degree of pain (Lansbury, 2000); (d) for the elderly who are depressed and for whom no cause for the pain can be identified, pain will subside when the depression is treated (Scharff & Turk, 1998); and, (e) potential side effects of narcotics make them too dangerous for use with the elderly (McCaffery & Pasero, 1999; McPherson, 2004). However, none of these myths are true (see references noted).

Pain is not inevitable in older adults; in one study, only one third of community-dwelling older adults reported frequent pain (Reyes-Gibby, Aday, &

Cleeland, 2002). As with younger adults and children, pain limits functional ability and should not be considered a normal part of aging. Pain is also associated with fatigue, sleep disturbance, depression and poor quality of life (Jakobsson, Klevsgård, Westergren, & Hallberg, 2003; Roberto & Reynolds, 2002). Therefore, chronic pain needs to be treated.

Failure to diagnose chronic pain and subsequent reluctance to treat the pain and concurrent depression continue to result in "underdiagnosis" and "undertreatment" in the elderly (Gloth, 2004; Scharff & Turk, 1998).

How the elderly differ from younger cohorts, however, is in their presentation of chronic pain which may include fewer pain behaviors in some conditions (Katsma & Souza, 2000; Lansbury, 2000); however, this cannot be generalized to all conditions or all elderly clients with chronic pain. Klinger and Spaulding (1998) concluded that "silence is not golden" and that pain assessment of older persons poses challenges because the older adult may not overtly complain of pain or they have learned to underreport it, given past experiences with health care professionals. Accommodation for the physiological changes that occur with aging is required for both assessment and management of pain whether for medications or other interventions (Gagliese & Melzack, 2003; Miakowski, 2000).

Gender

Gender differences in chronic pain have been documented. A greater proportion of women than men experience chronic pain and their pain is more intense (Keefe et al., 2000; Rustøen et al., 2004; Uhruh, Ritchie, & Merkskey, 1999). Women reported receiving treatment for their pain more often than men, whereas men reported poorer quality of life than women (Rustøen et al., 2004). Edwards, Auguston, and Fillingim (2000) described relationships between pain intensity and anxiety, with greater interference from pain for men than for women. Although there were no gender differences in emotional upset from pain or in the impact of emotional upset, the strategies used to cope with pain were different for men and women (Uhruh et al., 1999).

Given that perceptual ability and other physiological mechanisms explain the gender-related differences in pain intensity and response to treatment, gender is an important factor to consider in pain management (Vallerand & Polomano, 2000). Therefore, clinicians are advised to consider how men and women may respond to chronic pain differently and how different approaches to pain management may be required.

Family Roles

Pain affects the whole family (Ballard & Min, 2002; Smith & Friedemann, 1999). When an individual becomes acutely ill, s/he assumes the sick role (see chapter 2, on illness behavior and roles). This is also true of children (Palermo, 2000).

Family income drops when the individual with chronic pain is no longer employed (Kemler & Furnée, 2002). Redistribution of household tasks that cannot be performed by the individual who is ill to the rest of the family is initially an acceptable alternative because changes in roles and responsibilities are viewed as temporary (Strauss et al., 1984). When pain is chronic in nature, spouses assume increased responsibilities for household management (Kemler & Furnée, 2002). Harris, Morley, and Barton (2003) describe a loss of roles in four domains (friendship, occupation, leisure, and family). Adults from an outpatient pain clinic reported an average loss of 3.4 roles and seven attributes related to these roles. For families who are able to communicate openly, changes necessary for dealing with additional tasks secondary to the illness and pain can be discussed (Strauss et al., 1984), but this is not true for all families.

Smith (2003) explored family relationships of women experiencing chronic nonmalignant pain. Three patterns of family relationships were described: cycle of close involvement of families counterbalanced or compensated with isolation–closeness and separation in a alternating pattern; focus directed toward others as in typical family roles, balanced with feeling guilty about needing help and focusing on themselves; and loss of physical sexual intimacy.

Focusing on chronic pain can contribute to social isolation (McCaffrey, Frock, & Garfuilo, 2003). Whether social isolation is be self-imposed (Zautra, Hamilton, & Burke, 1999), or whether families leave the person who has chronic pain alone, loss of social interaction can lead to further isolation, depression, and poor quality of life.

Spouses are often adversely affected by their partners' chronic pain (Cano et al., 2004). Both are at increased risk for emotional distress or depression (Cano, Weisberg, & Gallagher, 2000), decreased satisfaction with their marriage (Cano et al., 2004), and increased prevalence of health problems (Flor, Turk & Rudy, 1987). In fact, the management of the pain has a greater influence on the coping ability of spouses than either the nature of the illness or the intensity of their partners' pain (Flor et al., 1987).

For adults with chronic pain, marital variables accounted for symptoms of depression and anxiety beyond the contribution of pain variables; "psychological distress in chronic pain is better explained by both pain and marital variables rather than by pain variables alone" (Cano et al., 2004, p. 104). Both clients and spouses may benefit by learning about pain and it management as well as learning to communicate effectively and deal with other marital issues.

There is also a significant impact on children from having siblings who have chronic pain. A meta-analysis indicated that siblings of children with chronic illness were more likely to report depression and anxiety, and less activity with peers when compared to healthy controls. Some of the impact of siblings was a result of the daily treatment regimens required by their sisters/brothers. (Sharpe & Rossiter, 2002)

The family's response to a member who has chronic pain, in turn, affects how that person copes, and vice versa. For example, spouses reinforce pain behaviors by responding to negative cues and attending selectively to their partners' pain and distress. Given the interrelationship among family members, assessment of the entire family should be considered if interventions are to be effective. Interventions that focus only on identified clients may be ineffective if actions/strategies expected of the "patients" are not supported and reinforced by their families. There is new evidence that patients who were in a pain management program that involved spouse-assisted training in pain coping skills were more likely to have improvement in anxiety and depression (Keefe et al., 2004). Families need to be included if interventions for individuals who have pain are to achieve maximum benefit.

Effects of Culture on Pain

Although there is no consensus on how culture influences the perception of pain, there are clear differences in the meaning assigned to pain, how pain is expressed, and how proposed treatment of pain is accepted and/or is perceived to be effective (Beck, 2000; Edwards, Fillingim, & Keefe, 2001; Elliott, Smith, et al., 1999; Galanti, 2004; Green, Baker et al., 2003). Expressions of pain are learned and influenced by the client's environment and social context, primarily by the responses of the family. "Patterned attitudes toward pain behavior exist in every culture, and appropriate and inappropriate expressions of pain are thus culturally prescribed" (Ludwig-Beymer, 2003, p. 407). In some cultures or ethnic groups, pain is not expressed either verbally or nonverbally; these people are stoic. In other cultures, pain is expressed by loud exclamations and/or pain behaviors, such as facial grimacing and hugging the painful body part.

As an example, clients may demonstrate physiological responses that lead the health care provider to inquire about pain (e.g., rapid, shallow breathing; increased heart rate; rigid posture), but there may be no change in facial expression or any verbal expression of pain. In fact, when asked, even by family who translates the question into their clients' language, clients deny experiencing pain and may refuse analgesics when offered. Jorgensen (2000) cautions health care providers to be aware of their paternalistic practice and of clients' concepts of health and their bodies. Body image and how pain is perceived are important for accurate assessment of pain and development of a treatment plan that is acceptable to clients.

Several recent studies have described differences in pain experiences and response to treatment across the world and within North America (Cope, 2000; Green, Baker et al., 2003; McDermott et al, 2000; Soares & Grossi, 1999). Although pain is a universal experience of human existence, pain "acquires specific social and cultural significance" (Davidhizar & Giger, 2004, p. 49). There are differences in characteristics of pain (e.g., pain intensity), and how pain is experienced. Meaning attributed to pain and response to pain are also influenced by culture. For example, pain is reported by Ojibwe elders only when rated above 6 on a 10-point rating scale; and they believe pain is a part of having cancer and that it cannot be relieved (Elliott, Johnson, Elliott, & Day, 1999).

Provision of culturally appropriate care requires health care professionals to understand their own beliefs and attitudes about pain as well as to learn about the beliefs and attitudes of the groups that compose their "client and staff populations." Although there is some truth to the stereotypes of pain responses by cultural groups, the generation of immigration or when clients were dislocated to the health care professionals' practice setting is telling. There are often significant differences across generations. The key point to remember is that individuals' ethnocultural background should be considered when assessing and managing pain. Respect clients as individuals and respect their response to pain to avoid stereotyping an individual on the basis of culture (Ludwig-Beymer, 2002).

Davidhizar and Giger (2004) recommend strategies to promote culturally appropriate assessment and management of pain that take into consideration individuals within the context of their culture. Health care professionals are advised to "appreciate variations in affective response to pain" and to "be sensitive to variations in communication styles" (p. 51). Recognition of the difference in the meaning of pain between cultures and that communica-

tion of pain may not be acceptable within a culture. They advise caution in treatment of pain given the biological differences between racial groups, but also note that there are individual differences within racial groups. "While it is important to understand that both biological and cultural phenomena may be seen in patterns within a culture and thus to increase alertness to them, it is essential to avoid assuming that all persons in the cultural group will behave identically" (p. 53).

Giger and Davidhizar (2004) describe the importance of the way health care professionals communicate with clients about pain, especially the use of touch given what it can mean to clients. The reader is referred to Chapter 4 in Leininger and McFarland (2002) for more specific information about cultural assessment.

Interventions for Dealing with Clients with Chronic Pain

Managing pain requires that both a relationship of trust evolve between health care professionals and that clients experiencing pain take action (Laliberte, 2003). Health care professionals should believe their clients' statements about their pain or at least give their clients the benefit of the doubt. As Katz (1998) noted, clients who have pain are to be respected. Not to believe clients' complaints, in effect, means that clients are being told that they are lying, which is both an unethical and an unprofessional response. In addition, clients who feel that their health care professionals are sincere are more likely to continue to work with them, to follow their recommendations, and continue to seek methods that will help manage their chronic pain.

Problem-Solving Process

The goals for management of nonmalignant pain are to decrease pain intensity, optimize quality of life and to increase functional ability. Problem solving requires that assessment and diagnosis precede the development and implementation of any treatment plan, and that evaluation be performed as a final step to determine the effectiveness of the plan. These steps frequently overlap rather than occur sequentially.

Initial assessment includes history taking, observation, and physical examination. Both objective findings, if present, and subjective factors, such as clients' perceptions and responses to the pain, need to be identified. Care must be taken to consider differences that exist for children, adults, and the elderly. The tool for pain assessment (Figure 4-1) may be practical in any setting, can be easily adapted to clients' needs, and can be useful for any type of pain. Because of the strong influence a family can have on clients, the family system should be included in the assessment as well.

The analysis of collected data allows a diagnosis to be made. Determination of appropriate outcomes and interventions, as well as how they can be attained, should be made jointly by health care professionals and clients.

Interventions for managing nonmalignant pain are greater than the ones presented in this chapter. Those selected for inclusion are useful to the clinical practitioner without requiring additional education or training. The guidelines and general principles are for both pharmacological management and noninvasive measures that diminish, resolve, or prevent the recurrence of the pain state. Information on pain management programs is also included. Much of the included material is drawn from McCaffery and Pasero (1999). When other resources are used, they are so indicated.

Most studies of pain management focus on the individuals who have chronic pain, so little is known about interventions that involve their families. Studies that have examined family involvement in treatment of chronic pain indicate that behavioral methods have promise. The reinforcement of negative pain expressions or behaviors by family members needs to be changed to reinforcement of well-behavior (Keefe et al., 2004; Palermo, 2000; Smith et al., 2003). When well-behavior is reinforced, clients often show improvement in areas such as returning to work, increasing activity levels, and decreased utilization of the health care system. Spouse-assisted pain coping skills resulted in improve coping with pain and psychological disability for the person with chronic pain (Keefe et al., 2004).

Pharmacological Management of Pain[1]

Pharmacological management of pain is the responsibility of the entire health care team, including the individual with chronic pain and his/her family. The goal of management is to attain and maintain the best possible pain control with the fewest side effects. Achieving this goal requires that health care professionals be knowledgeable about the pharmacological parameters of drugs and other strategies/interventions. It is also essential that health care professionals use effective communication skills, and provide research and sources of information to document or support the recommended plan of treatment.

Narcotics are an important class of drugs for pain management. Narcotics work not only by modifying central nervous system perception, but also by interrupting the mechanisms responsible for causing the pain, increasing the pain threshold, blocking peripheral nervous system input, or relieving anxiety or depression. Pain control can sometimes be achieved by nonnarcotics, adjuvant analgesics (antidepressants, anticonvulsants, muscle relaxants, corticosteroids, etc.), antibiotics, and vasodilators. Only general information about narcotics, nonnarcotics, and antidepressants is discussed in this section.

Key Concepts in Administering Narcotics/Nonnarcotics for Pain Control

There are three major concepts to keep in mind when administering pain medication: (1) use a pre-

---

[1]Content on pharmacological and noninvasive methods is drawn from McCaffery, M., & Pasero, C. (1999). *Pain: Clinical manual* (2nd ed.). St. Louis: Mosby. When other sources are used, they are so noted.

FIGURE 4-1

Initial Pain Assessment Tool

INITIAL PAIN ASSESSMENT TOOL   Date_____

Patient's Name_____Age_____Room_____

Diagnosis_____Physician_____

                                        Nurse_____

I. LOCATION: Patient or nurse mark drawing.

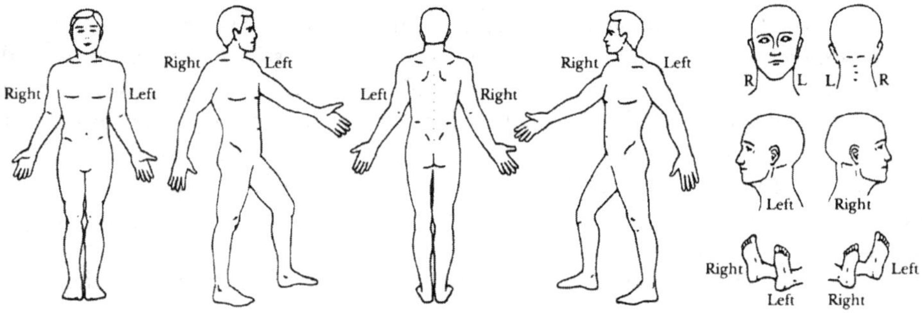

II. INTENSITY: Patient rates the pain. Scale used _____

        Present:_____

        Worst pain gets:_____

        Best pain gets:_____

        Acceptable level of pain:_____

III. QUALITY: (Use patient's own words, e.g., prick, ache, burn, throb, pull, sharp)_____

IV. ONSET, DURATION, VARIATIONS, RHYTHMS:_____

V. MANNER OF EXPRESSING PAIN:_____

VI. WHAT RELIEVES THE PAIN:_____

VII. WHAT CAUSES OR INCREASES THE PAIN?_____

VIII. EFFECTS OF PAIN: (Note decreased function, decreased quality of life)

        Accompanying symptoms (e.g., nausea)_____

        Sleep_____

        Appetite_____

        Physical activity_____

        Relationship with others (e.g., irritability)_____

        Emotions (e.g., anger, suicidal, crying)_____

        Concentration_____

        Other_____

IX. OTHER COMMENTS:_____

X. PLAN:_____

May be duplicated for use in clinical practice. From McCaffery M, Pasero C: *Pain: Clinical manual,* p. 60. Copyright © 1999, Mosby, Inc.

ventive approach, (2) titrate to effect, and (3) give clients as much control as possible. As noted earlier, take into consideration how clients' age and other characteristics that may influence their response to medications and/or dose (McCaffery & Pasero, 1999; Shimp, 1998).

Using a *preventive approach* means giving medication before the onset of or increase in pain. Sticking to an analgesic regimen is recommended (McCaffery, 2000). Prevention may involve administering medication around the clock (ATC) or giving it "as needed" (PRN), that is, as soon as the pain begins so it does not escalate. There are a number of benefits of a preventive approach: pain is experienced for a shorter time; smaller doses of analgesics are required; side effects are reduced; there is less anxiety about the return of pain; and the individual has an increased ability to perform activities. Clients on PRN schedules should be taught to request or self-administer pain medication as soon as the pain occurs and/or before it increases.

Achievement of *titration to effect* requires that the dose of medication given be sufficient to attain the desired pain relief with the fewest side effects. Titrating is performed by tailoring the type of analgesics to clients' needs. It includes: adjusting doses (increasing or decreasing), changing intervals between doses, modifying the route of administration, and/or selecting the drug or drug combination that most effectively achieves the desired results. (McCaffery & Pasero, 1999; Sweeney & Bruera, 2003).

Titrating requires an ongoing evaluation of clients' responses to ensure that safe and effective results are achieved. *Too much medication* is being given if clients are oversedated or have any respiratory depression. *Too little medication* is being given if relief is not achieved and pain recurs too soon. The *wrong medication* should be suspected if relief is not achieved and clients are sedated. *Inadequate frequency* occurs if relief is adequate but does not last long enough.

Giving clients as much control as possible in managing their pain is the third key concept. One method of doing this is to use *patient-controlled analgesia* (PCA), the self-administration of all forms of analgesic by clients. PCA is considered safe and provides clients with control, although it is not an option for everyone (McCaffery & Pasero, 1999). Ideally, all clients should be given the opportunity to make the decision to control their own analgesia. At a minimum, clients should be allowed as much control as they feel they can handle.

Narcotics

As noted earlier, many health care professionals are reluctant to prescribe and provide narcotic analgesics to individuals with chronic pain. The unfortunate consequence is undertreatment and inadequate pain control. Unique responses to medication require tailoring the dose, time interval, route, and choice of drug for each client. Monitoring responses is critical to effective use of analgesics. As tolerance to a medication increases, the dose needs to increase. Fortunately, the concurrent increase in respiratory tolerance eliminates the concern many health care professionals have about the side effect of respiratory depression. (McCaffery & Pasero, 1999; Sweeney & Bruera, 2004)

Several factors contribute to the effectiveness of opioids: (1) client-related factors (e.g., age, gender, psychological distress, prior opioid use); (2) pain-related factors (e.g., usual intensity, breakthrough pain, tempo of pain escalation); and (3) effects of the specific medication (Shalmi, 2004). The use of an equianalgesic chart can guide the amount and route of drugs that are used for pain control (e.g., Lipman & Jackson, 2004, p. 585) as can information about what to consider when prescribing narcotics (e.g., Berde & Masek, 2003 pp. 545–558; Sweeney & Bruera, 2003, pp. 382–385).

Concern about safe administration of medications can be alleviated if a flow sheet is used as a tool for ongoing assessment of medication effectiveness without adverse effects. Flow sheets can be modified, although inclusion of the following factors is recommended: time the assessment is conducted; client's rating of pain intensity; medication name, dose, route, and time of administration; and, client's physiological responses (especially respiratory status).

Health care professionals have no difficulty decreasing medication when necessary, but they typically are not comfortable with increasing doses, especially if greater than usual amounts are needed or if their clients are not getting adequate relief. Professionals may need reeducation to relieve their fear of "addicting" clients; clients do not become addicts as long as medication is being used to control pain. Any decrease in the effectiveness of a given dose requiring greater amounts of medication reflects drug tolerance. A flow sheet provides a quick and easy reference to any increases and decreases in medication that have been given, the client's response, and any supplemental methods that are being used.

Another strategy recommended by Fishman and associates (1999), and based on a review of 90 pain centers, is an opioid contract or written agreement (Canadian Pain Society, 1998; McCaffery & Pasero, 1999; Sweeney & Bruera, 2003). This contract provides health care providers with confidence that the planned opioid administration does not put clients at risk and provides clients with a clear picture of an approach to their pain management, one that they have had a part in negotiating. Although the format of contracts is diverse, the goal is the same—to increase the quality of pain management.

Morphine, the standard narcotic for severe acute pain and chronic cancer pain (American Pain Society, 1987; Gourlay, 1998), is one of four commonly used narcotics (morphine, hydromorphone, levorphanol, and methadone) that are equally capable of relieving pain. Various reasons for selecting one or the other include: prior pain experience, the number and severity of side effects experienced, the concentration or volume of doses available, and the characteristics of the medication (e.g., rate of onset, duration, accumulation).

Although meperidine has been used extensively, primarily because of its rapid onset of action and peak effect for short duration, it is not the narcotic of choice for treatment of chronic pain because of CNS stimulation by its active metabolites (American Pain Society, 1987; McCaffery & Pasero, 1999; Pellegrini, Paice & Faut-Callahan, 1999). In addition, inadequate doses typically prescribed for oral administration are 25% less effective than parenterally administered doses resulting in poor pain control when the oral route is used.

Codeine is not often used in managing chronic pain because of its side effects of constipation and drug tolerance. However, in a study of adults with osteoarthritis, Peloso et al. (2000) found that controlled-released codeine was very effective in long-term treatment of pain.

Newer methods of delivering a narcotic analgesic are being utilized. Fentanyl is one such medication that can be delivered transdermally and is effective for clients whose pain is stable (Sweeney & Bruera, 2003). Methadone has also been evaluated in the treatment of chronic pain (Jamison, Kauffman & Katz, 2000). It has its merits as an alternative medication or for a break from morphine (McCaffery & Pasero, 2000).

Rotation of opioids, both short-acting and long-acting, is recommended to increase control over pain while reducing side effects (McCarberg & Barkin, 2001; Sweeney & Brurea, 2003; Thomsen, Becker, & Eriksen, 1999). The reader is encouraged to refer to guidelines from any of the following sources: the World Health Organization, the Agency for Health Care Policy and Research (AHCPR), the American Pain Society (1987), the American Society of Anesthesiologists, the American Geriatrics Society (1998a, 1998b), and the Canadian Pain Society (1998).

Another strategy recommended to attenuate the need for increased doses of narcotics is concurrent use of *N*-methyl-*D*-asparatate antagonists (NMDA), such as dextromethorphan or ketamine. NMDA, given with reduced doses of morphine, has been reported to control chronic pain (Chevlen, 2000; Katz, 2000; Rabben, Skjelbred & Oye, 1999; Sang, 2000; Weinbroum et al., 2000). Use of NMDA in conjunction with NSAIDS can "improve the balance between analgesia and adverse effects" (Portenoy, 2000, p. S16).

Nonnarcotic Analgesics

Although nonnarcotics, referred to as nonsteroidal anti-inflammatory drugs (NSAIDs), are best known for their anti-inflammatory effect, they can also be used to manage chronic pain (Simon, 2004). Their pain-relieving effects are underestimated. They are underused because both lay people and professionals do not realize how effective these drugs can be as analgesics. These medications work primarily at the level of the peripheral nervous system (please see pharmacology texts for mechanisms of action of NSAIDs or the article by Winzeler & Rosenstein, 1998).

Although NSAIDs have been used effectively to manage a range of musculoskeletal diseases, such as arthritis, they have not been used extensively to treat other malignant or nonmalignant pain. The degree of pain relief varies because some individuals are more responsive to NSAIDs than others or obtain better responses to specific medications (Portenoy, 2000; Simon, 2004).

Selecting the appropriate NSAID depends on individual variations, such as efficacy and side effects (McCaffery, 1998; McCaffery & Gever, 2000). Newer Cox-2 inhibitor NSAIDs have demonstrated promise for effective pain management with reduced gastrointestinal side effects, the primary reason NSAIDs are not well tolerated (Kessenich, 2001; Portenoy, 2000; Simon, 2000). However, older clients are at greater risk of side effects even with Cox-2 inhibitors (Buffum & Buffum, 2000). Equianalgesic tables show that average doses of nonnarcotics can be as effective as low oral doses of narcotics. Please note, acetaminophen (Tylenol), that is available over-the-counter, can be used effectively and safely to provide pain relief on its own or in combination with narcotics and/or non-narcotic medications.

NSAIDs should be used first if pain intensity is in the mild to moderate range. If necessary, they should be given around-the-clock (ATC). If narcotics are needed, NSAIDs should be continued unless side effects contraindicate their concurrent use. Combining narcotics and nonnarcotics is a safe and logical method of pain relief because their pharmacological actions and side effects are different. Nonnarcotics can provide additional pain relief to that of a narcotic. Giving them together poses no more danger than alternating them. The peak effect of nonnarcotics is about two hours after oral administration, about the time that the effectiveness of an intramuscularly administered narcotic tends to decrease. When combined, a lower dose of narcotic may be effective, with the added benefit of a decrease in side effects (Portenoy, 2000).

If oral narcotics do not fully relieve pain, they should be supplemented with ATC doses of nonnarcotics. To obtain the optimal therapeutic doses of each medication in a combination drug, supplement it with an additional amount of the nonnarcotic, because these compounds contain less than optimal doses of the nonnarcotic. For clients receiving parenteral narcotics, who can take oral medications, give an NSAID for ongoing pain or when the narcotic is used for incident pain (McCaffery & Pasero, 1999).

Antidepressants

Antidepressants are being used more frequently in conjunction with narcotic and nonnarcotic analgesics for the management of chronic pain (Jackson & St. Onge, 2003; Macres, Richeimer, & Duran, 2004; Monks & Merskey, 2003). Although the mechanism of action of antidepressants is controversial, they have been found to reduce pain in both depressed and nondepressed clients (Ansari, 2000; Richeimer et al., 1997). Both tricyclic and serotonin reuptake inhibitors can be effective, but results are specific to individuals and the medication used, as is true with most groups of medications (Ansari, 2000). It is also interesting to note that when clients with chronic pain report difficulty sleeping, one of the side effects of many antidepressants, even at low doses, is falling asleep more easily and staying asleep at night. These medications are most effective if they are used in a regimen with analgesics and other strategies to manage pain (Jeffrey, 1996).

Noninvasive Methods of Pain Control

There are many noninvasive, nonpharmacological modalities or methods that can be used to control chronic pain (Laliberte, 2003). Table 4-2 describes misconceptions regarding nondrug approaches to pain. In general, *physical methods* include: counterirritation, vibration, percussion, local application of heat and cold, nerve fatigue from repetitive stimulation, trigger point stimulation, acupuncture, therapeutic touch, physiotherapy, occupational therapy, and neuromodulation. Most of the physical methods involve application of the therapy or modality locally, although a systemic effect may occur (e.g., acupuncture). *Central methods,* which help individuals accept and live with their pain include the doctrines of yoga and transcen-

dental meditation, distraction, and relaxation (progressive muscle relaxation or guided imagery), psychotherapy, operant conditioning, and behavior modification. These methods can be effective, although research is limited. Vessey and Carlson (1996) conclude that such methods can also be useful and effective for children who have chronic pain.

Determining the effectiveness of noninvasive methods for each client requires a trial-and-error approach to determine what works in each unique situation (Table 4-3). Open communication is essential between clients and professionals to identify modalities and to evaluate their effectiveness.

TABLE 4-2

Misconceptions: Nondrug Approaches to Pain

Misconception	Correction
1. Most nondrug methods reduce the intensity of pain for most patients.	Pain reduction is not a predictable outcome of many nondrug techniques for pain management. Most nondrug techniques do, however, have other benefits, such as making pain more bearable, improving mood, reducing distress, giving the patient a sense of control, and sometimes aiding with sleep.
2. The effectiveness of nondrug approaches to pain management has been well established through research.	Research is limited, and results are conflicting and inconclusive. Most nondrug approaches to pain are promoted on the basis of patient testimonials and clinicians' favorable experiences with the techniques.
3. Nondrug measures should be used instead of analgesics or to extend the interval between doses of analgesics.	Nondrug approaches to pain management are never a substitute for appropriate analgesia and anesthesia. They are used in addition to analgesics, after the analgesics have been tailored to the patient's needs.
4. Many nondrug techniques for pain management relieve pain by increasing endorphin levels, the body's natural opioids.	This is mere speculation. No research has been able to show an increase in endorphins as a result of nondrug pain relief measures. Even if endorphin release occurred, it would provide analgesia for only a very short time.
5. Cutaneous stimulation techniques must be used over the site of pain.	Cutaneous stimulation techniques such as heat, cold, and vibration may be effective when used at sites quite distant from the pain (e.g., contralaterally—on the opposite side of the body).
6. The patient who can be distracted from pain does not have very severe pain, or the pain is not as severe as the patient says.	Although distraction may be difficult to use when pain is severe, those who can use it may find that it makes severe pain more bearable or gives them a sense of control. Severe pain cannot be discounted simply because the patient is able to use distraction.

May be duplicated for use in clinical practice. From McCaffery M, Pasero C: *Pain: Clinical manual,* p. 401. Copyright © 1999, Mosby, Inc.

TABLE 4-3

Selection and Use of Nondrug Pain Treatments

1. Clarify the relationship between the use of nondrug pain treatments and the use of analgesics.
   - In most clinical situations (e.g., postoperative pain or cancer pain) nondrug pain treatments should be used in addition to analgesics.
   - Emphasize to the patient that nondrug therapies do not replace analgesics.
2. Assess the patient's attitude toward and experience with nondrug pain treatments.
   - If the patient has used nondrug methods, find out whether they were successful and what, if any, problems were encountered.
   - Find out whether the patient feels that personal attempts at nondrug therapies have been exhausted and that more conventional pain therapies are now appropriate.
   - Find out whether the patient is using nondrug methods to avoid using analgesics. If analgesics are appropriate, discuss the patient's concerns.
3. Ask the patient what, besides taking pain medicine, usually helps with the pain.
   - Try to identify nondrug treatments that are similar to the patient's coping style.
   - Some patients simply want more information about pain or its management, whereas others want to divert their attention away from pain.
   - Many patients naturally use distraction to cope with pain. For these patients, providing a selection of music or videotapes may be helpful.
4. Assess the patient's level of fatigue, cognitive status, and ability to concentrate and follow instructions.
   - Optimal functioning in these areas is desirable to learn and to use a technique such as relaxation imagery but is unnecessary if a cold pack is used.
   - Some patients barely have enough time to perform required activities of daily living. Adding a lengthy relaxation technique may simply increase stress and decrease the patient's sense of control.
5. Ask the patient's family/friends if they wish to be involved in nondrug pain treatments.
   - In home care, the primary caregiver may already be overburdened and have no time or energy to help the patient with a technique such as massage.
   - Some family/friends may welcome a technique like massage that allows them to touch the patient and "do something." However, not all patients or family members are comfortable with techniques that involve touch.
6. Provide the patient and family with adequate support materials.
   - Whenever possible, supply written or audiotaped instructions for even the simplest techniques.
   - Determine whether the appropriate equipment is available. If not, can the patient afford to purchase it? If not, identify less expensive nondrug materials or therapies.

May be duplicated for use in clinical practice. From McCaffery M, Pasero C: *Pain: Clinical manual*, p. 401. Copyright © 1999, Mosby, Inc.

Believing the client is essential. Use of multiple modalities or techniques may be more effective than a single method. Only a few of the myriad methods are reviewed here. For further details, please see McCaffery and Pasero (1999) or any of the other references cited on this topic.

Cutaneous Stimulation

Cutaneous stimulation refers to stimulating the skin for the purpose of relieving pain, especially localized pain. Although the exact mechanism is unknown, the gate control theory suggests that stimulation of the skin may activate the large-diameter fibers that close the gate to pain messages carried by small fibers. Cutaneous stimulation may also work by increasing endorphins and/or decreasing sensitivity to pain.

Cutaneous stimulation is not curative. Although the effects are variable and unpredictable, the intensity of pain is usually reduced during or after stimulation. Some kinds of stimulation work best with acute localized pain; whereas other methods are effective with chronic pain. Many methods of cutaneous stimulation require little participation or action on the part of clients, which makes them appropriate for people who have limited physical or mental energy. Potential benefits include: decreased pain intensity; relief of muscle spasm that is secondary to underlying skeletal or joint pathology, or nerve root irritation; and, increased physical activity (Kubsch, Neveau, & Vandertie, 2000).

Even though cutaneous stimulation covers a number of physical modalities, there is little known about which conditions will respond to what method or how long a method should be used. Beliefs about the use of heat, cold, and other methods are more likely to derive from culture and personal experience than from scientific data.

Selecting the best cutaneous stimulation for a given client can be a challenge. Not only must the most appropriate type of modality be selected, but choices must also be made about the site, duration, frequency of use, and the modifications needed to achieve the greatest relief. The following factors should be considered when selecting a method: potential effectiveness, possible side effects, safety, cost, amount of time required, availability, contraindications, and client acceptability. If possible, clients should be given a choice of available methods.

Some types of cutaneous stimulation, such as electrical transcutaneous stimulation, require special education or training (Gadsby & Flowerdew, 2001), but many do not. Table 4-4 lists some methods that are easy to use in the clinical setting. The "how to" of implementing these methods is not included; the reader is encouraged to seek sources such as McCaffery and Pasero (1999).

Distraction

Distraction from pain is achieved by focusing attention on a stimulus other than the pain sensation. Just as children can be distracted by involving them in other activities, family can provide distraction for either adults or children who have chronic pain (Rapoff & Lindsley, 2000). Reading, singing, listening to music, and humor are some of the methods used for distraction (Mobily, Herr, & Kelley, 1993). Distraction works by relegating the pain to the periphery of awareness, but does not eliminate it.

Distraction is easy to learn and is effective as long as the distracting stimulus is present. Typically, this technique is used for procedural pain when the pain episode lasts for an hour or less, such as with lumbar puncture, bone marrow aspiration, burn or wound debridement, dressing changes, and painful injections. Distraction is not a substitute for medications, but is effective when used as an adjunct prior to and during a painful procedure, or during an acute pain episode.

Even if pain is severe, the pain is less intense if the focus is on another sensory input or on the less bothersome qualities of the pain sensation, such as pressure or warmth. Not only does distraction help to ease pain, but focusing on pleasant things also improves mood, which helps to counteract depression and leads to a sense of control over the painful experience. When pain is greater, the complexity of distraction should increase; with intense pain, simple distraction is more in keeping with clients' level of energy.

Any form of distraction requires clients to understand instructions, have the physical ability and energy to perform the activities, and have the ability to concentrate on the stimulus or stimuli being presented. Although distraction is a useful pain control technique, the time and energy requirements make it inappropriate for long periods of time. In addition, distraction is ineffective for clients who are hypersensitive to stimuli, such as those with migraine headaches. As noted earlier, consideration of clients' abilities and limitations is important to recommending distraction techniques. Individualize distraction techniques by selecting stimuli that have been used previously or are of specific interest to each client. Plan techniques to use before the need arises and provide clients with the opportunity to practice regularly.

Clients with intractable pain do not usually benefit from distraction. However, if they have been

---

TABLE 4-4

Pointers on Selecting a Method of Cutaneous Stimulation

■ Massage	Minimal side effects and contraindications. Backrubs or body massage can be time consuming and may relieve only mild pain, but pain need not be localized and most patients enjoy it. Modest patients may object to touch or disrobing. Massage of feet and hands may be more accessible, acceptable, and even more effective.
■ Pressure, sometimes with massage	Massage/pressure to trigger points or acupuncture points may be very effective but is briefly uncomfortable. Initially it requires time to locate the points. But then patients can learn to work on some trigger points on their own.
■ Vibration	A more vigorous form of massage that may be more effective. Low risk of tissue damage. Check on availability or cost of a vibrator. May be used for trigger points. May be unacceptable due to noise or intensity of stimulation if vibrator is not adjustable. Sometimes this is a less expensive substitute for TENS.
■ Heat and cold	Probably works best for well-localized pain. Both may be done with a minimum of equipment and both should be applied at a comfortable level of intensity. Cold has more advantages than heat. Unwanted side effects (e.g., burns, and contraindications—bleeding and swelling) are more frequent with heating than with cooling. When cold relieves pain, it tends to be more effective than heat. However, patients usually prefer heat to cold, and use of cold often requires some persuasion.
■ Ice application/ massage	A frozen substance applied to the skin is uncomfortable, but only for a few minutes before numbness occurs. Continuous use for ten minutes or less. Pain must be well localized. May relieve severe pain. Simple, low-risk technique for brief, painful procedures. Especially effective in obliterating needle-stick pain. May be used on trigger points. Sometimes this is a very inexpensive substitute for TENS.
■ Menthol	Refers to menthol-containing substances for application to skin. Intensity increases with amount of menthol; may be uncomfortable at higher concentrations. Odor offensive to some people. Use influenced by culture; more restricted use by Americans than other cultures (e.g., Asians). Inexpensive. Once it is applied, it provides continuous stimulation without additional effort. Well suited for nighttime use.
■ TENS	Compared with above methods, much more expensive, less available, and more time needed to teach nurse and patient, but supported by more research and regarded by many as more "scientific."

SOURCE: Reproduced by permission from McCaffery, M., & Beebe, A. (1989). *Pain: Clinical manual for nursing practice.* St. Louis: The C. V. Mosby Company.

deprived of their usual sensory input because of a boring or monotonous environment or an excessive input of meaningless stimuli, simple approaches to normalize daily sensory input may reduce perceived pain intensity. Some clients may be highly motivated to modify their environment. Boredom tends to lead to more boredom, so clients may become passive victims of the very problem that needs to be addressed.

Boring days can be normalized by planning the whole day around activities that are most important or enjoyable to clients. Select activities that clients can perform independently with minimal effort or can be carried out if some help is provided. Written schedules may help to pace activities to avoid overexertion. Clients need to be reminded that developing and carrying out such plans can be a challenge, but one that becomes easier with repeated success. Selected activities should combine as many sensory modalities as possible. For example, a gentle exercise program (kinesthetic) could be done with a friend (possibly verbal), using music (auditory), and written instructions or videotapes (visual). To avoid having the plan itself become boring, the schedule should be changed daily and activities should be varied at regular intervals.

Distraction techniques work best when a combination of sensory modalities is used. For example, focusing visually on a stationary object can be combined with slow rhythmic breathing, comfortable rhythmic massage of part of the body, or singing silently or aloud. Asking the client to describe a picture involves three senses in the distraction (e.g., visual, verbal, and auditory). The volume of recorded music on a cassette or audiotape can be increased when pain increases and decreased when pain decreases.

Interestingly, Cousins (1981) found that laughter lasting for at least 20 minutes created distraction that had a carryover effect—pain was relieved after the laughter stopped. Laughter can be used as an adjunct to relaxation. However, what is thought to be humorous differs from person to person. Although literature dealing with the impact of laughter has focused primarily on clients with cancer, laughter is relevant to all persons who have pain or discomfort. Having the family use laughter as a distraction benefits not only people with pain, but also those living with them.

Clients should be encouraged to combine regulated sensory input with other pain relief methods, such as medications. Combining pain relief measures in this manner allows greater opportunity to be involved in normal activities.

Relaxation

Relaxation should be used as an adjunct to other pain relief methods. It is not a substitute for medications or other methods, because it does not relieve pain directly. The goals of relaxation are to facilitate the reduction of physiological tension (in muscles and other structures) and to provide psy-

chological calming or unwinding. Relaxation breaks the cycle of stress, pain, muscle tension, and anxiety. Ideally, clients achieve the relaxation response: normal blood pressure; decrease in respiratory rate, heart rate, and oxygen consumption; reduction in muscle tension; increase in the brain's alpha waves; and improvement of mood (Laliberte, 2003; McCaffery & Pasero, 1999; Schaffer & Yucha, 2004).

All relaxation methods have been found to be effective for some persons some of the time (Carroll & Seers, 1998). However, to be effective, they must be practiced daily. Just as muscles become weak without daily exercise or use, the effectiveness of these methods are lost without regular practice.

Pain specialists agree that relaxation should be an integral component of a management program for people who have chronic nonmalignant pain given strong evidence of its usefulness (NIH, 1995). Relaxation techniques have been found to lead to a significant reduction in pain and some improvement in the amount of medication required, activity level, and mood. For example, in systematic review of the literature using the steps outlined for the Cochrane Database, Eccleston's et al. (2004) concluded that relaxation is "effective in reducing the severity and frequency of chronic headache in children and adolescents." Clients, whether children or adults, are candidates for relaxation if they: express a need or desire to use one of these techniques to cope with or control their pain; can understand the instructions; and, can focus on and follow directions. As with distraction techniques, health care professionals should provide an array of relaxation strategies from which to choose. Some clients prefer to use one strategy exclusively, while others prefer to use several relaxation methods.

There are many strategies that promote relaxation, including (1) sensory or movement interventions, such as biofeedback, progressive muscle relaxation, music, massage, or therapeutic touch; and (2) cognitive interventions like meditation, guided imagery, and sensory information. Some methods, such as slow rhythmic breathing, are easy to learn. Others, such as yoga, require a training program to build skill. As with distraction, relaxation techniques should be individualized for each client, take into consideration ability, situation, and circumstances. (Laliberte, 2003; McCaffery & Pasero, 1999; Schaffer & Yucha, 2004)

All techniques that can be used for relaxation have four features in common: (1) a mental device (constant stimulus on which to focus, such as slow deep breathing or a word); (2) a passive attitude (involves ignoring distractions while maintaining focus on a mental device); (3) decreased muscle tone; and, (4) a quiet environment (Benson, 1982 cited in Schaffer & Yucha, 2004).

There are various factors to consider in selecting a relaxation technique. Table 4-5 contains practical guidelines to use in matching technique to client. Table 4-6 contains a sample of available relaxation techniques that are easily used in the clinical setting. It is important to remember that some strategies can be independently performed by the person who has chronic pain (such as progressive muscle relaxation or playing music), whereas others require the assistance of another person (such as massage or therapeutic touch).

Clients can be actively involved, or relaxation techniques can be used passively. Active relaxation, especially when used preventively, can: (1) reduce skeletal muscle tension (which, in turn, may reduce strain or pressure on pain-sensitive structures); (2) improve sleep and decrease fatigue (which can increase energy); (3) increase the effectiveness of other pain relief measures; (4) improve mood; decrease distress;

TABLE 4-5

Practical Guidelines for Matching Relaxation Techniques to Patients and Situations

1. Consider the *amount of time* the patient will experience pain vs. the time involved in teaching and using the technique. Usually:
   - Use the less time-consuming techniques for brief episodes of pain (e.g., jaw relaxation or slow rhythmic breathing for procedural or postoperative pain).
   - Be willing to invest more time for patients with chronic pain (e.g., peaceful past experiences or meditative relaxation for cancer pain or recurrent headaches).
   - Beware of introducing time-consuming techniques to patients who are already under considerable stress, even if they have chronic pain, since this may add another stressor.
2. Consider how pain, fatigue, anxiety, and other factors influence the *patient's general ability to learn or engage in an activity.* Usually:
   - Use brief, simple techniques or massage during severe pain, lack of concentration, or along with other pain relief measures (e.g., deep breath/tense, exhale/relax, yawn), when narcotic is given, such as for renal colic.

- Teach more time-consuming techniques when the patient is alert and comfortable (e.g., meditative relaxation when severe back pain is in remission).
- Even if the patient says relaxation is not helpful during pain or the anticipated pain will be too severe for him to use relaxation, suggest he use it before and after pain.
3. Note if the patient has *energy that needs to be dissipated* (e.g., restless, "up-tight," or the "fight or flight" response —meaning that he has generated energy to fight or flee but has nowhere to go). Use a technique that releases energy (e.g., progressive relaxation).
4. For the *patient who misunderstands the purpose of relaxation,* use other terminology and suggest humor, peaceful past experiences, or passive recipient techniques such as a back rub.
5. *Consider whether the focus is inward on the body or outward on peaceful scenes.* An inward focus can increase distress about changes in body image or feelings of failure about physical limitations. Be cautious about using an exclusively inward body focus for patients who are distressed about changes in body appearance or function, severely depressed, or have difficulty maintaining contact with reality.

Source: Reproduced by permission from McCaffery, M., & Beebe, A. (1989). *Pain: Clinical manual for nursing practice.* St. Louis, MO: Mosby.

TABLE 4-6

Characteristics of Specific Relaxation Techniques and Indications for Use

Deep Breath/Tense, Exhale/Relax, Yawn	This takes only a few seconds; is easily learned by patient; is appropriate to introduce when patient is already tense and in pain (e.g., during a procedure) or may be taught prior to brief painful procedures or preoperatively.
Humor	This takes very little of the nurse's time to suggest to patients; patients may spend as much time as they wish using it. It may be appropriate for patients who are elderly; who resist or misunderstand the idea of relaxation; who are depressed or easily lose contact with reality; who have little time or energy for learning the skill of relaxation; or who are from a different culture (assuming a tape from that culture can be obtained). It may be used to relieve boredom of prolonged pain under confining circumstances; also appropriate for brief procedural pain.
Heartbeat Breathing	The nurse may have to teach the patient how to find and count the radial pulse, and some patients may have difficulty with this. If not, it takes very little of the nurse's or patient's time. Heartbeat breathing has an internal focus but is used only briefly. It may relieve a sudden, sharp increase in fear or anxiety and may be used without others noticing. It may be very helpful to patients who are aware of a sudden increase in heart rate during stress.
Jaw Relaxation	This takes very little time for the nurse to teach or for the patient to use. It is considered an abbreviated form of progressive relaxation. Its effectiveness may be due to relaxation of one area of the body, leading to relaxation of the rest of the body. Useful for brief moderate to severe pain (e.g., postoperative pain), especially if taught in the absence of severe pain and tension. Effective with elderly patients.
Slow Rhythmic Breathing	This takes very little of the nurse's time to teach. It is very adaptable; patient can use for 30 to 60 seconds (a few breaths without others noticing) or for up to 20 minutes. It is also a useful technique for initial relaxation prior to engaging in more complex relaxation techniques.
Peaceful Past Experiences	This may prove to be the best of all approaches to relaxation since it relies on what the patient has already found relaxing. It is usually an outward focus (i.e., not focused on the present body state). Recalling a peaceful experience is often a therapeutic process, and this approach may be the most appropriate for patients with chronic pain, particularly those with terminal illness. Remembering certain past experiences may serve many purposes (e.g., releasing or letting go of treasured events or reinforcing the conviction that a valued event will occur again). However, the sharing of a valued past experience may require a trusting relationship between the nurse and patient. This may take a considerable amount of the nurse's time, but not always.
	Give *priority* to this for terminally ill patients, and tape record it.
Meditative Relaxation Script	This usually takes a minimum of three contacts with the patient. The first two take about 15 minutes each. The second usually involves tape recording the script. The third is a follow-up and may take only a minute unless problems occur. The script is highly effective in producing relaxation in English-speaking, middle-class Americans. It is permissive enough that patients can individualize it on their own, and it combines an inward focus (breathing techniques and modified progressive relaxation) with an outward focus (peaceful place). Even when patients say that certain options in the script are not helpful to them, it is seldom necessary to rerecord the tape, since patients usually say they simply ignore what does not help them.

TABLE 4-6	
Continued	
	Give *priority* to this (or peaceful past experiences or progressive relaxation) for patients with prolonged pain. It takes more time than you may have and it is not a miracle, but it often makes a significant difference.
Progressive Relaxation Script	This also usually takes a minimum of three contacts with the patient for a total of 35 minutes or more. The first two contacts take about 15 minutes. The second usually involves tape-recording the technique. The third is a follow-up and may take only a few minutes, unless problems have occurred.
	Its potential advantages are that it involves physical activity that gives a sense of "doing something" (e.g., muscle contraction, dissipates energy), is focused inward without the necessity of keeping the eyes closed, does not rely exclusively on mental activity, and easily gets the patients' attention by asking them to perform specific tasks.
	Give this *priority* for patients with prolonged pain who exhibit signs of moderate to severe anxiety or "fight or flight," especially if they cannot engage in their customary physical exercise. They need to get rid of that muscular energy. Later they may benefit from a more meditative approach.
Simple Touch, Massage, or Warmth	This may be done by the nurse or the patient's family or friends. It need not take much time and is indicated for patients who do not have time or energy to do for themselves whatever would produce relaxation. Loved ones who want to feel useful may benefit themselves and the patient by committing to body rubs of only 3 minutes (e.g., back, feet, hands). Help family and friends identify definite times for performing body rubs. This gives structure for the patient and the loved ones

SOURCE: Reproduced by permission from McCaffery, M., and Beebe, A. (1989). *Pain: Clinical manual for nursing practice*. St. Louis, MO: Mosby.

and, (5) increase confidence along with a sense of control in coping with pain. Previously learned techniques can be integrated into a relaxation program. Ideally, health care professionals can coach their clients through the steps of learning a new technique and then teach the clients' families how to coach if continued external directions are helpful to the clients. Instructions can be tape-recorded and provided to clients and their families to serve as guides and reminders when the professional is not present.

Passive techniques are appropriate for those who: have limited physical or emotional energy; are very young or very old; are confused, agitated, or undergoing sudden distress or pain; or are extremely fatigued or sedated. Family members can learn to use simple touch, massage, or warmth to help achieve relaxation in these clients.

Progressive muscle relaxation is an example of one technique that has proven helpful. It has been practiced for centuries as part of meditation but currently is also used to reduce pain intensity. It can be self-taught, but is usually easier to learn if another person provides verbal direction. Books and videotapes, that can be used when there is no one to read instructions, can be found in the health sections of most large bookstores. Participants are asked to focus on specific muscle groups, to tense or tighten them for 5 seconds, to relax them, and then to focus on the relaxed muscles. This process is repeated in a systematic pattern for the entire body (Laliberte, 2003; Schaffer & Yucha, 2004).

To demonstrate the effectiveness of relaxation, clients can be asked to rate pain intensity or level of calmness before, during, and after practicing the relaxation technique by using a word-scale (improved, the same, or worse) or a ten-point anchored numerical scale (1 indicates no pain and 10 indicates severe pain). Bofeedback, which is not a relaxation technique itself, can also be used to demonstrate reduced heart rate, increased skin temperature, or increased muscle relaxation.

Imagery

Imagery is the interpretation of what humans intentionally visualize and what is experienced in a symbolic manner. Through the use of imagery, clients can learn to modify their outlook, which can be helpful in reducing pain (Burte, 2002; Lewandowski, 2004). The use of imagery for pain relief is based, in part, on two interrelated beliefs. First, it provides partial control over body functions that are not controlled by conscious rational thoughts. Second, the body reacts to images or memories in a manner similar to its functioning or response during the actual event.

Imagery is not a strategy that all clients can use or that all health professionals can teach. When used as a form of distraction from pain, it increases tolerance; when used to produce relaxation, it decreases distress. Imagery can also produce an image of pain relief that decreases the perceived intensity of the pain. *Hypnosis*, which requires additional training on the part of the professional, often uses imagery as a technique (Holroyd, 1996). No form of imagery should be used with resistant clients, regardless of the good intentions of qualified health care professionals.

Like other noninvasive methods, imagery is not a substitute for other methods of pain control but should be considered an adjunctive treatment for pain. When used for pain management, imagery allows one's imagination to develop sensory images that decrease the intensity of pain or change it to a pleasant, more acceptable, or nonpainful substitute, such as numbness or coolness. The use of imagery may lead to greater confidence in the ability to control or heal the painful experience, increase the effectiveness of other pain-relief measures, decrease

pain intensity, reduce related distress, or change the pain sensation to one that is more acceptable.

Imagery may be helpful for those who have pain of clearly defined physical origin because it may alter the physical cause of pain or be beneficial without actually affecting the physiological aspects of pain. An individual can imagine something about the pain that will provide pain relief, rendering this activity therapeutic. Imagery that systematically uses involved techniques for pain relief is often referred to as *therapeutic guided imagery.*

Subtle or conversational imagery, such as routine statements and questions, may already be part of the repertoire of health care professionals. These simpler forms tend to be effective, consume little time, are low risk, and do not require advanced knowledge or skills beyond basic education. There are ways to enhance use of subtle images more naturally and easily. First, when explaining specific pain-relief measures, use words that paint a mental picture of relaxation or have tactile-kinesthetic feelings; such as, *floating, softer healing, lighter, releasing,* and *letting go.* Second, suggest an image of how the pain will subside or be relieved to balance clients' images of what causes the pain. Above all, the professional should use images or descriptors that feel natural to ensure ease and comfort with what is described.

Simple, brief symptom substitution is best when used as an alternative for relieving short-term pain. It allows clients to imagine pain as a more acceptable sensation for a period of time (e.g., pressure instead of aching). Words used should denote greater acceptance and/or less discomfort for clients. Another technique is to guide clients to focus on a substitute sensation (e.g., cold and numbness felt when holding an ice cube) rather than the pain.

More involved forms of imagery, such as meditative imagery, should be taught by professionals who have received specialized training, because there can be adverse effects. Lengthy imagery is *inappropriate* for those who: do not want to try it; have severe emotional problems or a history of psychiatric illness; report hallucinations for any reason, including drug reactions or sensory restriction; have no time or energy for lengthy imagery; or cannot concentrate.

Standardized imagery techniques and *systematically individualized imagery* are more extensive techniques that require a moderate amount of client involvement. Both of these techniques can be used for several minutes or more, and can be practiced regularly and/or used often.

Standardized imagery allows clients to use imagination to visualize and experience positive sensations while they relax to directions such as "see yourself breathing out the pain." Systematically individualized imagery is a personalized image created by clients of what the pain is and how it can be relieved. It is developed in specific detail by each client with guidance from the health care professional.

For any of these techniques, the image used needs to make sense to clients as a means of pain relief. Selected images need not be biologically or medically correct. They can include any variety of things: a sound that gets quieter, a shape that becomes smaller, a vicious animal that becomes friendly, or something of a religious or spiritual nature. Clients should get into a comfortable position and interruptions should be prevented, if possible. Concentrating on the selected image is important and can be performed with the eyes either closed or open. If concentration is difficult, counting with each breath may help. Clients who need to spend more than 20 minutes at a time or more than 1 hour a day may need more pain relief measures. Remember, imagery rarely leads to complete pain relief. Techniques should be used either to prevent regu-

larly recurring pain or to help keep pain from increasing to an intense level, and in conjunction with other pain management strategies.

Cognitive–Behavioral Strategies

The goal of cognitive-behavioral strategies is for clients to question and reappraise thoughts, feelings, and behaviors they have related to their pain. The role of the health care professional is as educator, trainer, and coach. This process is well described by Turk and Okifuji (2003, 2004) and Winterowd, Beck, and Gruener (2003). The five assumptions that form the basis for the cognitive-behavioral perspective are outlined in Table 4-7.

Cognitive therapy is provided by trained professionals, typically psychologists. It is designed to alter the way people think about their pain and illness by modifying their negative thinking patterns (Pilowsky, 1999). This restructuring of cognition is a process to develop positive thoughts (Rapoff & Lindsley, 2000), to increase pain coping strategies (Turk & Okifuji, 2004), and to decrease pain (Wiskin, 1998). The conclusion reached in meta-analyses of randomized control trials that evaluated the effectiveness of cognitive-behavioral interventions is that mood, affect, function, and coping all improved (Eccleston et al., 2002; Morley, Eccleston & Williams, 1999). Walsh and Radcliffe (2002) reported that disability was also reduced. Cognitive-behavioral strategies often form a component of pain management programs.

TABLE 4-7

Assumptions of the Cognitive-Behavioral Perspective

- Individuals are active processors of information and not passive reactors.
- Thoughts (e.g., appraisals, expectations, beliefs) can elicit and influence mood, affect physiological processes, have social consequences, and can also serve as an impetus for behaviour; conversely, mood, physiology, environmental factors, and behaviour can influence the nature and content of thought processes.
- Behaviour is reciprocally determined by *both* the individual and environmental factors.
- Individuals can learn more adaptive ways of thinking, feeling, and behaving.
- Individuals should be active collaborative agents in changing their maladaptive thoughts, feelings, and behaviours.

SOURCE: Turk, D.C., & Okifuji, A. (2003). In R. Melzack, & P.D. Wall. (Eds.). *Handbook of pain management: A clinical companion to Wall and Melzack's textbook of pain,* p. 534. Philadelphia: Churchill Livingstone, with permission from Elsevier.

The effectiveness of cognitive-behavioral programs is not universal, like other interventions for individuals with chronic pain—some interventions work better for some than for others. Cognitive-behavioral strategies work best in combination with other interventions and, as with other noninvasive methods, for persons who are motivated to control their pain. In addition, many clinicians recommend excluding persons with psychiatric problems, including those with clinical depression or significant problems with mood or affect.

Complementary or Alternative Therapies

Although complementary or alternative therapies remain controversial, they are used often used by persons who have chronic pain, typically in conjunction with traditional treatment and on consultation with health care professionals (Haetzman et al., 2003).

Both the lay public and health care professionals have been surprised at the widespread interest and use of a variety of therapies. Although traditional Western medicine recommends caution, it is prudent when considering any form of therapy for the person to weigh the potential benefit and risk (Owens, Taylor, & DeGood, 1999). Health care professionals should talk with their clients about the practices they use to manage their pain to ensure that they complement traditional treatments. For example, some herbal remedies that can be purchased over the counter can potentiate or detract from the effect of prescribed medications.

There is growing scientific evidence that alternative therapies can reduce chronic pain (Berman & Swyers, 1999; Lee, 2000; NIH, 1997). Two of the therapies that have been evaluated are acupuncture and therapeutic touch. Acupuncture, used for centuries in "Eastern medicine," can reduce pain intensity for adults (Ezzo et al., 2000; Leibing et al., 2002; Nabeta & Kawakita, 2002) and for children (Kemper et al., 2000). Therapeutic touch has been shown to decrease both pain and anxiety for older persons who have degenerative arthritis (Lin & Taylor, 1998; Smith et al., 2002).

Health care professionals need to be informed about the most common therapies to understand and support the decisions made by their clients. Maintaining open communication is important so clients feel comfortable talking about all interventions/strategies they are using to manage their pain. These therapies are numerous and beyond the scope of this chapter to describe. The reader is referred to sources such as Laliberte (2003), a book for individuals who have chronic pain, and Caudill (2002).

Involvement of the Family

Families of persons who have chronic pain are often involved in learning how to live with clients' pain because living with someone who has chronic pain is a challenge. Clients and their families need to know what has happened and what to do to manage the pain. Families can learn to play an important role in the pain management program and may benefit from learning how to help the clients manage pain. Some pain management programs include families as participants with clients, other programs use family members to help with the intervention being learned (e.g., Keefe, et al., 2004).

Family members can learn to help with interventions to reduce clients' pain. They can help clients use cutaneous stimulation (e.g., use of heat or cold), distraction, guided relaxation, and cognitive strategies. Families can support clients' behaviors to take their focus off of pain. They also need to learn how to identify and avoid actions or activities that aggravate clients' pain. In other words, any information that benefits clients, benefits their families.

Pain Management Programs

Pain management programs are not new. Aronoff (2004) describes the inception of such programs 30 years ago when there was a shift in focus from traditional medical treatment (e.g., medications, nerve blocks) to treating chronic pain differently than as an extension of acute pain. Growth in the numbers and types of pain management programs is a result of the poor response clients experienced with typical medical treatment for chronic pain.

Pain management programs help clients to better manage their pain and regain some control of their lives. Such programs seek to: decrease pain intensity and pain-related disability; improve mood and decrease depression; decrease use of the health care system and medications; and, increase independence in activities of daily living, involvement with family, and social activities.

Pain management programs are extremely varied. Typically, pain *clinics* are outpatient facilities such as a small unidisciplinary or single-modality clinic (e.g., an anesthesiologist doing nerve blocks). Pain *centers* are facilities that are large multidisciplinary centers, many of which are university based, and have both inpatient and outpatient facilities. Most programs fall somewhere between these two extremes (Aronoff, 2004).

There are now several well designed studies that support the effectiveness of pain programs. Interdisciplinary pain management programs have been found to deliver relief for many of their clients. Pain and disability are reduced, control over pain increase, sleep and physical function improve as does psychological well-being (Becker et al., 2000; Nielson & Jenson, 2004; Wells-Federman, Arnstein, Caudill, 2002; Wilkes, et al., 2003). A recent focus on readiness to self-manage pain can be found in the research literature (Jensen, Nielson, & Kerns, 2003; Jensen et al., 2003, 2004), and in lay publications (Caudill, 2002). This interest reinforces the body-mind alliance in effective pain management (Laliberte, 2003).

One of the key components contributing to the success of pain programs is their multidisciplinary teams. These teams consist of a variety of physicians, nurses, physical therapists, occupational therapists, nurses, psychologists, and other consultants (Coughlin et al., 2000; Jensen et al., 1999). There is an emphasis by all members of the team on diagnosis and assessment of clients' physical, mental, and psychosocial status, so that comprehensive treatment plans can be developed based on the whole person. The client is an important member of the team and participates in all decision making, because s/he carries much of the responsibility for treatment. Many programs also involved the client's family, as much as possible, so they can support the treatment regimen.

Pain programs usually include both physiological and cognitive-behavioral interventions. Medication regimens are reviewed and simplified as much as possible prior to starting such a program. Multiple modalities are used in addition to medication, such as relaxation. Physiological interventions include physical reconditioning (from stretching to strengthening to aerobic fitness and endurance) and activity pacing to enhance pain tolerance. Cognitive-behavioral interventions focus on reappraisal and taking ownership of the pain. Most programs are several weeks in length during which progress is presented to clients, often through graphs or charts that highlight changes over time.

Although initially developed for clients who find that pain has become the central focus of living or do not respond to medical intervention, this comprehensive approach to pain management is indicated for clients who want to learn how to better manage their pain before it manages them. Health care professionals can assist clients in identifying and determining which of these programs best suits their needs. Information about programs can be obtained in literature provided by the programs and in published articles, by visiting a program, or by speaking to others who have attended them. Before making a recommendation, it is important to know about the nature of each pain program; such as, the goals of the program and who sets them (client or program staff), the types of pain that are dealt with, the types of clients treated, and the modalities used and services offered. Additional important information includes the program's accreditation and/or staff credentials, the length of time it has been in existence, and the longevity of the staff.

Outcomes

Pain management is now included as the fifth vital sign by the Joint Commission on Accreditation of Healthcare Organizations (JCAHO) by standards that were implemented January 1, 2001 (Douglas, 1999; Krozek & Scoggins, 2001a, 2001b; JCAHO, 2001). Clients should be asked if they are having pain and if so, to rate its intensity as minimal, moderate, or severe. Moderate or severe pain must be treated.

These "pain standards" appear in several chapters in six of the JCAHO manuals. According to the Rights and Ethics Chapter (JCAHO, 2001), patients have the right "to appropriate assessment and management of pain." This assessment is reinforced in the Assessment of Patients' Function chapter and emphasized in more detail in the Care of Patients' Function chapter and the Education of Patients' Function chapter (www.jcaho.org/standards_frm.html).

Pain control and/or management must be evaluated by the clients. Being without pain may be an achievable outcome in acute pain, but for chronic pain, the level of pain that is determined to be achievable and acceptable may not be a 0 on a 10-point scale. Clients are to be encouraged to set goals with health care providers. For some, this will be low pain intensity, and for others, it may be the ability to be involved in activities of daily living, even with pain present.

Study Questions

1. What are common misconceptions about chronic pain and management of chronic pain for children, adults, and the elderly?
2. Why is it important to consider fatigue, depression, and anxiety for clients who have chronic pain?
3. What factors are to be considered when using analgesics to manage chronic pain? How do these factors influence selection and administration of narcotic and nonnarcotic analgesics to children, adults and the elderly?
4. What aspects of pain assessment are essential for management of chronic pain? Why?
5. Compare the following noninvasive methods of managing pain from the perspective of effectiveness, benefits to client, costs, and ease of implementation:
   a. Cutaneous stimulation
   b. Distraction
   c. Relaxation
   d. Imagery
   e. Cognitive-behavioral strategies
   f. Complementary or alternative therapies
6. How can health professionals assist clients to select an appropriate pain management program?

References

Aldrich, S., Eccleston, C., & Crombez, G. (2000). Worrying about chronic pain: Vigilance to threat and misdirected problem-solving. *Behavior Research and Therapy, 38,* 457–470.

American Geriatrics Society. (1998a). AGS practice guidelines: The management of chronic pain in older persons. *Geriatrics, 53 (Suppl 3),* S6–S7.

_____. (1998b). The management of chronic pain in older persons. AGS Panel on Chronic Pain in Older Persons. *Geriatrics, 53 (Suppl 3),* S8–S24.

American Pain Society. (1987). *Principles of analgesic use in the treatment of acute pain and chronic cancer pain: A concise guide to medical practice.* Washington DC: Author.

Ansari, A. (2000). The efficacy of newer antidepressants in the treatment of chronic pain: A review of current literature. *Harvard Review of Psychiatry, 7,* 257–277.

Aronoff, G. M. (2004). The role of pain clinics. In C. A. Warfield & Z. H. Bajwa. (Eds). *Principles & practice of pain medicine* (2nd ed) (pp. 813–824). New York: McGraw-Hill.

Asmundson, G. J. G., Norton P. J., & Norton, G. R. (1999). Beyond pain: The role of fear and avoidance in chronicity. *Clinical Psychology Review, 19,* 97–119.

Ballard, J. H., & Min, D. (2002). The impact of pain on families. In R.S. Weiner (Ed.). *Pain management a practical guide for clinicians* (6th ed). (pp. 279–284). Boca Raton, FL: CRC Press.

Beck, S. L. (2000). An ethnographic study of factors influencing cancer pain management in South Africa. *Cancer Nursing, 23,* 91–100.

Becker, N., Sjøgren, P., Bech, P., Olsen, A. K., et al. (2000). Treatment outcome or chronic non-malignant pain patients managed in a Danish multidisciplinary pain centre compared to general practice: a randomized controlled trial. *Pain, 84,* 203–211.

Berde, C. G., & Masek, B., (2003). Pain in children. In R. Melzack & P.D. Wall (Eds). (2003). *Handbook of pain management: A clinical companion to Wall and Melzack's textbook of pain. (*pp. 545–558). Philadelphia: Churchill Livingstone.

Bergh, I., & Sjostrom, B. (1999). A comparative study of nurse' and elderly patients' ratings of pain and pain tolerance. *Journal of Gerontological Nursing, 25* (5), 30–37.

Berman, B. M., & Swyers, J.P. (1999). Complementary medicine treatments for fibromyalgia syndrome. *Baillieres Best Practice Research in Clinical Rheumatology, 3,* 487–492.

Blyth, F. M., March, L. M., Brnabic, A. J. M., Jorm, L. R., et al. (2001). Chronic pain in Australia: A prevalence study. *Pain, 89,* 127–134.

Blyth, F. M., March, L. M., Brnabic, A. J. M., & Cousins, M. J. (2004). Chronic pain and frequent use of health care. *Pain, 111,* 51–58.

Brown, S. C., Glass, J. M., & Park, D. C. (2002). The relationship of pain and depression to cognitive function in rheumatoid arthritis patients. *Pain, 96,* 279–284.

Buffum, M., & Buffum, J. C. (2000). Nonsteroidal anti-inflammatory drugs in the elderly. *Pain Management Nursing, 1,* 40–50.

Bullington, J., Nordemar, R., Nordemar, K., & Sjöström-Flanagan, C. (2003), Meaning out of chaos: A way to understand chronic pain, *Scandinavian Journal of Caring Science, 17,* 325–331.

Burte, J. M. (2002). Psychoneuroimmunology. In R.S. Weiner. (Ed.) *Pain management: A practical guide for clinicians* (6th ed). (pp. 807–816). Boca Raton, FL: CRC Press.

Call-Schmidt, T. A., & Richardson, S. J. (2003). Prevalence of sleep disturbance and its relationship to pain in adults with chronic pain. *Pain Management Nursing, 4,* 124–133.

Canadian Pain Society (1998). Use of opioid analgesics for the treatment of chronic pain—A consensus statement and guidelines from the Canadian Pain Society, *Pain Research Management, 3,* 197–208.

Cano, A. Gillis, M., Heinz, W., Geisser, M., et al. (2004). Marital functioning, chronic pain, and psychological distress. *Pain, 107,* 99–106.

Cano, A., Weisberg, J., & Gallagher, M. (2000). Marital satisfaction and pain severity mediate the association between negative spouse responses to pain and depressive symptoms in a chronic pain patient sample. *Pain Medicine, 1,* 35–43.

Caracci, G. (2003). The use of opioid analgesics in the elderly. *Clinical Geriatrics, 11* (11), 18–21.

Carroll, D., & Seers, K. (1998). Relaxation for the relief of chronic pain: A systematic review. *Journal of Advanced Nursing, 27,* 476–487.

Caudill, M. A. (2002). *Managing pain before it manages you.* New York: The Guilford Press.

Caudill-Slosberg, M. A., Schwartz, L. M., & Woloshin, S. (2004). Office visits and analgesic prescriptions for musculoskeletal pain in US: 1980 vs 2000. *Pain, 109,* 514–519.

Chevlen, E. (2000). Morphine with dextromethorphan: Conversion from other opioids analgesics. *Journal of Pain Symptom Management, 19* (Suppl), S42–S49.

Clark, J. D. (2002). Chronic pain prevalence and analgesic prescribing in a general medical population. *Journal of Pain and Symptom Management, 23,* 131–137.

Cope, D. (2000). From research to clinical practice: Cultural and educational issues in pain management Minority cancer patients and their provider: Pain management attitudes and practice. *Clinical Journal of Oncology Nursing, 4,* 237–238.

Coughlin, A. B., Bandura, A. S., Fleischer, T. D., & Guck, T. P. (2000). Multidisciplinary treatment of chronic pain patients: Its efficacy and patient locus of control. *Archives of Physical Medicine and Rehabilitation, 81,* 739–740.

Cousins, N. (1981). *Anatomy of an illness as perceived by the patient.* New York: Bantam.

Cowan, D. T., While, A., Griffiths, P. (2004). Use of strong opioids for non-cancer pain in the community: a case study. *British Journal of Community Nursing, 9* (2), 53–58.

Crombez, G., Eccleston, C., Baeyens, F., van Houdenhove, B., et al. (1999). Attention to chronic pain is dependent upon pain-related fear. *Journal of Psychosomatic Research, 47,* 403–410.

Currie, S. R., & Wang, J. (2004). Chronic back pain and major depression in the general Canadian population. *Pain 107*, 54–60.

Davidhizar, R., & Giger, J. N. (2004). A review of the literature on care of clients in pain who are culturally diverse. *International Nursing Review, 51*, 47–55.

Dersh, J., Polatin, P. B., & Gatchel, R. J. (2002). Chronic pain and psychopathology: Research findings and theoretical considerations. *Psychosomatic Medicine, 64*, 773–786.

Douglas, M. (1999). Pain as the fifth vital sign: Will cultural variations be considered? *Journal of Transcultural Nursing, 10*, 285.

Eccleston, D., Crombez, G., Aldrich, S., & Stannard, C. (2001). Worry and chronic pain patients: A description and analysis of individual differences. *European Journal of Pain, 5*, 309–318.

Eccleston, C., Morley, S., Williams, A., Yorke, L., et al. (2002). Systematic review of randomized controlled trials of psychological therapy for chronic pain in children and adolescents, with a subset meta-analysis of pain relief. *Pain, 99*, 157–165.

Eccleston, C., Yorke, L., Morley S., Williams, A. C., et al. (2004). Psychological therapies for the management of chronic recurrent pain in children and adolescents. *The Cochrane Data Base for Systematic Reviews, Volume 3*. Retrieved October 2004.

Edwards, C. L., Fillingim, R. B., & Keefe, F. (2001). Race, ethnicity and pain. *Pain, 94*, 133–137.

Edwards, R., Auguston, E. M., & Fillingim, R. (2000). Sex-specific effects of pain-related anxiety on adjustment to chronic pain. *The Clinical Journal of Pain, 16*, 46–53.

Elliott, A. M., Smith, B. H., Hannaford, P. C., Smith, W. C., et al. (2002). The course of chronic pain in the community: Results of a 4-year follow-up study. *Pain, 99*, 299–307.

Elliott, A. M., Smith, B., Penny, K., Smith, W., et al. (1999). The epidemiology of chronic pain in the community. *Lancet, 354*, 1248–1252.

Elliott, B. B., Johnson, K. M., Elliott, T. E., & Day, J. J. (1999). Enhancing cancer pain control among American Indians (ECPCAI): A study of the Ojibwe of Minnesota. *Journal of Cancer Education, 14*, 28–33.

Eriksen, J., Jensen, M. K., Sjøgren, P., Ekholm, O., et al. (2003). Epidemiology of chronic non-malignant pain in Denmark. *Pain, 106*, 221–228.

Ezzo, J., Berman, B., Hadhazy, V. A., Jadad, A. R., et al. (2000). Is acupuncture effective for the treatment of chronic pain? A systematic review. *Pain, 86*, 217–225.

Fishbain, D. A., Cole., B., Cutler, R. B., Lewis, J., et al. (2003). Is pain fatiguing? A structured evidence-based review. *Pain Medicine, 4*, 51–62.

Fishbain, D. A., Cutler, R., Rosomoff, H. L., & Rosomoff, R. S. (1997). Chronic pain-associated depression: antecedent or consequence of chronic pain? *Clinical Journal of Pain, 13*, 113–137.

Fishman, S. M., Bandman, T. B., Edwards, A., & Borsook, D. (1999). The opioid contract in the management of chronic pain. *Journal of Pain and Symptom Management, 8*, 27–37.

Flor, H., Turk, D. C., & Rudy, E. T. (1987). Pain and families. II: Assessment and treatment. *Pain, 30*, 29–45.

Gadsby, J. G., & Flowerdew, M. W. (2001). Transcutaneous electrical nerve stimulation and acupuncture-like transcutaneous electrical nerve stimulation for chronic low back pain. Oxford: *The Cochrane Library, 2*.

Gagliese, L., & Melzack, R. (2003). Pain in the elderly. In R. Melzack & P. D. Wall (Eds). *Handbook of pain management: A clinical companion to Wall and Melzack's textbook of pain*. (pp. 559–568). Philadelphia: Churchill Livingstone.

Galanti, G. A. (2004). *Caring for patients from different cultures*. (3rd ed.). Philadelphia: University of Pennsylvania Press.

Gibson, S. J., & Helme, R. D. (2000). Cognitive factors and experience of pain and suffering in older persons. *Pain, 85*, 375–383.

Giger, J. N., & Davidhizar, R. E. (2004). *Transcultural nursing assessment and intervention*. (4th ed.). St. Louis: Mosby.

Goodwin, J., & Bajwa, Z. H. (2004). Understanding the patient with chronic pain. In C. A Warfield, & Z. H. Bajwa (Eds.). *Principles & practice of pain medicine* (2nd ed) (pp. 55–60). New York: McGraw-Hill.

Goth, F. M. (Ed.).(2004). *Handbook for pain relief in older adults: An evidence-based approach*. Totowa, NJ: Humana Press.

Gourlay, G. K. (1998). Sustained relief of chronic pain. Pharmacokinetics of sustained release morphine. *Clinical Pharmacokinetics, 35* (3), 173–190.

Green, C. R., Baker, T. A., Sato, Y., Washington, T. L., et al. (2003). Race and chronic pain: A comparative study of young black and white Americans presenting for management. *The Journal of Pain, 4*, 176–183.

Green, C. R., Wheeler, J. R. C., & LaPorte, F. (2003). Clinical decision making in pain management: Contributions of physician and patient characteristics to variations in practice. *The Journal of Pain, 4*, 29–39.

Green, C. R., Wheeler, J. R. C., LaPorte, F., Marchant, B., et al. (2002). How well is chronic pain managed? Who does it well? *Pain Medicine, 3,* 56–65.

Grossman, S. A., & Sheidler, V. R. (1985). Skills of medical students and house officers in prescribing narcotic medication. *Journal of Medical Education, 60,* 552–557.

Gureje, O., Von Korff, M., Simon, G. E., & Gater, R. (1998). Persistent pain and well-being: A World Health Organization study in primary care. *JAMA, 280,* 147–151.

Haetzman, M., Elliott, A. M., Smith, B. H., Hannaford, P., et al. (2003). Chronic pain and the use of conventional and alternative theory. *Family Practice, 20,* 147–154.

Harris, N. L. (1999). Chronic pain and depression. *Australian Family Physician, 28* (1), 36–39.

Harris, S., Morley, S., & Barton, S. B. (2003). Role loss and emotional adjustment in chronic pain. *Pain, 105,* 363–370.

Hasselström, J., Liu-Palmgren, J., & Rasjö-Wraak, G. (2002). Prevalence of pain in general practice. *European Journal of Pain, 6,* 375–385.

Holroyd, J. (1996). Hypnosis treatment of clinical pain: Understanding why hypnosis is useful. *The International Journal of Clinical and Experimental Hypnosis, 44* (1), 33–51.

Hunfeld, J. A. M., Perquin, C. W., Duivenvoorden, H. J., Hazebroek-Kampschreur, A. A. J. M., et al. (2001). Chronic pain and its impact on quality of life in adolescents and their families. *Journal of Pediatric Psychology, 26,* 145–153.

Jackson, K. C., & St. Onge, E. L. (2003). Antidepressant pharmacotherapy: Considerations for the pain clinician. *Pain Practice, 3,* 135–143.

Jakobsson, J., Klevsgård, R., Westergren, A., & Hallberg, I. R. (2003). Old people in pain: A comparative study. *Journal of Pain and Symptom Management, 26,* 625–636.

Jamison, R. N., Kauffman, J., & Katz, N. P. (2000). Characteristics of methadone maintenance patients with chronic pain. *Journal of Pain and Symptom Management, 19,* 53–62.

Jeans, M. E., & Johnston, C. C. (1985). Pain in children: Assessment and management. In S. Lipton & J. Miles (Eds.), *Persistent pain.* London: Harcourt Brace Jovanovich.

Jeffrey, J. (1996). Role of nursing in the management of soft tissue rheumatic disease. In R. P. Sheon, R. W. Moskowitz, V. W. Goldberg. (Eds). *Soft tissue rheumatic pain: Recognition, management, prevention* (3rd ed). (pp. 329–350). Sudbury, MA: Jones & Bartlett.

Jensen, M. P., Nielson, W. R., & Kerns, R. D. (2003). Toward the development of a motivational model of pain self-management. *The Journal of Pain, 4,* 477–492.

Jensen, M. P., Nielson, W. R., Turner, J. A., Romano, J. M., et al. (2003). Readiness to self-manage pain is associated with coping and with psychological and physical functioning among patients with chronic pain. *Pain, 103,* 529–537.

Jensen, M. P., Nielson, W. R., Turner, J. A., Romano, J. M., et al. (2004). Changes in readiness to self-manage pain are associated with improvement in multidisciplinary pain treatment and pain coping. *Pain, 111,* 84–95.

Jensen, M. P., Romano, J. M., Turner, J. A., Good, A. B., et al. (1999). Patient beliefs predict patient functioning: Further support for a cognitive-behavioral model of chronic pain. *Pain, 81,* 95–104.

Joint Commission on Accreditation of Healthcare Organizations Pain Standards for 2001. (2001). Http://www.jcaho.org/standards_frm.html.

Jorgensen, P. (2000). Concepts of body and health in physiotherapy: The meaning of the social/cultural aspects of life. *Physiotherapy Theory and Practice, 16,* 105–115.

Kaasa, S., Loge, J. H., Knobel, H., Jordhoy, M. S., et al. (1999). Fatigue. Measures and relation to pain. *Acta Anesthesiologica Scandinavica, 43,* 939–947.

Katsma, D. L., & Souza, C. H. (2000). Elderly pain assessment and pain management knowledge of long-term care nurses. *Pain Management Nursing, 1,* 88–95.

Kashikar-Zuck, S., Vaught, M. H., Goldschneider, K. R., Graham, T. B., et al. (2002). Depression, coping, and functional disability in juvenile primary fibromyalgia syndrome. *Journal of Pain, 3,* 412–419.

Katz, N. (2002). The impact of pain management on quality of life. *Journal of Pain and Symptom Management, 24* (1S), S38–S47.

Katz, N. P. (2000). MorphiDex (MS:DM) double-blind, multiple-dose studies in chronic pain patients. *Journal of Pain and Symptom Management, 19* (Suppl), S37–S41.

Katz, W. A. (1998). The needs of a patient in pain. *American Journal of Medicine, 105* (1B), 2S–7S.

Keefe, F., Lefebvre, J. C., Egert, J. R., Affleck, G., et al. (2000). The relationship of gender to pain, pain behavior, and disability in osteoarthritis patients: The role of castastrophizing. *Pain, 87,* 325–334.

Keefe, F. J., Blumenthal, J., Baucom, D., Affleck, G., et al. (2004). Effects of spouse-assisted coping skills training and exercise training in patients with osteoartritic knee pain: A randomized controlled trial. *Pain, 110,* 539–549.

Kemler, M. A, & Furnée, C. A. (2002). The impact of chronic pain in the household. *Journal of Pain and Symptom Management, 23,* 433–441.

Kemper, K. J., LicAc, R. S., Silver-Highfield, E., Xiarhos, E., et al. (2000). On pins and needles? Pediatric pain patients' experience with acupuncture. *Pediatrics, 105* (Suppl), 941–947.

Kessenich, C. R. (2001). Cyclo-oxygenase 1 inhibitors: An important new drug classification. *Pain Management Nursing, 2,* 13–18.

Klinger, L., & Spaulding, S. J. (1998). Chronic pain in the elderly: Is silence really golden? *Physical and Occupational Therapy in Geriatrics, 15* (3), 1–17.

Krozek, C., & Scoggins, A. (2001a). *Patient rights . . . amended to comply with 2000 JCAHO standards.* Glendale, CA: CINAHL Information Systems.

_____. (2001b). *Patient and family education . . . amended to comply with 2000 JCAHO standards.* Glendale, CA: CINAHL Information Systems.

Kubsch, S. M., Neveau, T., & Vandertie, K. (2000). Effect of cutaneous stimulation on pain reduction in emergency department patients. *Complementary Therapies in Nursing and Midwifery, 6* (1), 25–32.

Laliberte, R. (2003). *Doctor's guide to chronic pain: The newest, quickest, and most effective ways to find relief.* Pleasantville, NY: The Reader's Digest Association.

Lane, P. (2000). Adults with chronic low back pain felt frustrated, unsupported, and powerless with healthcare, social, and legal systems. *Evidence Based Nursing, 3* (1), 29.

Lansbury, G. (2000). Chronic pain management: A qualitative study of elderly people's preferred coping strategies and barriers to management. *Disability and Rehabilitation, 22,* 2–14.

Lazarus, H., & Neumann, C. J. (2001). Assessing undertreatment of pain: the patients' perspectives. *Journal of Pharmaceutical Care in Pain and Symptom Control, 9* (4), 5–34.

Lee, T. L. (2000). Acupuncture and chronic pain management. *Annals of Academic Medicine of Singapore, 29* (1), 17–21.

Leibing, E., Leonhardt, U., Köster, G., Goerlitz, A., et al. (2002). Acupuncture treatment of chronic low-back pain—a randomized, blinded, placebo-controlled trial with 9-month follow-up. *Pain, 96,* 189–196.

Leininger, M., & McFarland, M. F. (2002). *Transcultural nursing concepts, theories, research & practice.* (3rd ed.). New York: McGraw-Hill.

Leininger, S. M. (2002). Managing pain in the older adult patient. *Topics in Emergency medicine, 24* (9), 10–18.

Lewandowski, W. A. (2004). Patterning of pain and power with guided imagery. *Nursing Science Quarterly, 17,* 233–241.

Lewin, D. S., & Dahl, R. E. (1999). Importance of sleep in the management of pediatric pain. *Journal of Developmental Behavior in Pediatrics, 20,* 244–252.

Lin, Y., & Taylor, A. G. (1998). Effects of therapeutic touch in reducing pain and anxiety in an elderly population. *Integrative Medicine, 1* (4), 155–162.

Lipman, A. G., & Jackson, K. C. (2004). Opioid pharmacotherapy. In C. A. Warfield , & Z. H. Bajwa. (Eds). *Principles & practice of pain medicine* (2nd ed). (pp. 583–600). New York: McGraw-Hill.

Ljungkvist, I. (2000). Short and long-term effects of a 12-week intensive functional restoration programme in individuals work-disabled by chronic spinal pain. *Scandinavian Journal of Rehabilitation Medicine, 40* (Suppl), 1–14.

Loeser, J. D. (2000). Pain and suffering. *The Clinical Journal of Pain, 16* (Suppl), S2–S6.

Ludwig-Beymer, P. (Ed.) (2003). Transcultural aspects of pain. In M. M. Andrews & J. S. Boyle. *Transcultural concepts in nursing care* (4th ed). (pp. 405–431). Philadelphia: Lippincott.

Macres, S., Bricheimer, S., & Duran, P. (2004). Adjuvant analgesics. In C. A.Warfield & Z. H. Bajwa (Eds). (2004). *Principles & practice of pain medicine* (2nd ed). (pp. 627–638). New York: McGraw-Hill.

Maniadakis, N., & Gray, A. (2000). The economic burden of back pain in the UK. *Pain, 84,* 95–103.

Mäntyselkä, P., Kumpusalo, E., Ahonen, R., Kumpusalo, A., et al. (2001). Pain as a reason to visit the doctor: A study in Finnish primary health care. *Pain, 89,* 175–180.

Marcus, D. A. (2000). Treatment of nonmalignant chronic pain. *American Family Physician, 61,* 1331–1338.

Marks, R. M., & Sacher, E. L. (1973). Undertreatment of medical patients with narcotic analgesics. *Annals of Internal Medicine, 78,* 173–181.

McCaffery, M. (1998). How to make the most out of nonopioid analgesics. *Nursing 1998, 28* (8), 54–55.

_____. (2000). Controlling pain. Helping patients stick to an analgesic regimen. *Nursing 2000, 30* (4), 22.

McCaffery, M., & Beebe, A. (1989). *Pain: Clinical manual for nursing practice.* St. Louis: Mosby.

McCaffery, M., & Ferrell, B. R. (1999). Opioids and pain management: What do nurses know? *Nursing 1999, 29* (3), 48–52.

McCaffery, M., Ferrell, B. R., & Pasero, C. (2000). Nurses' personal opinions about patients' pain and their effect on recorded assessments and titration of opioid doses. *Pain Management Nursing,* 1, 79–87.

McCaffery, M., & Gever, M. P. (2000). Controlling the pain. Heading off adverse reactions from NSAIDS . . . nonsteroidal anti-inflammatory drugs. *Nursing 2000, 30* (4), 14.

McCaffery, M., & Pasero C. (1999). *Pain: Clinical manual for nursing practice* (2nd ed). St. Louis: Mosby.

_____. (2000). Pain control. The merits of methadone. *American Journal of Nursing, 2000* (7), 22–23.

McCaffrey, R., Frock, T. L., & Garguilo, H. (2003). Understanding chronic pain and the mind-body connection. *Holistic Nursing Practice, 17,* 281–189.

McCarberg, B. H., & Barkin, R. L. (2001). Long-acting opioids for chronic pain: Pharmacotherapeutic opportunities to enhance compliance, quality of life, and analgesia. *American Journal of Therapeutics, 8,* 181–186.

McDermott, M. A., Natapoff, J. N., Essoka, C. G., & Rendon, D. (2000). Pain as a mutual experience for patients, nurses and families: International and theoretical perspectives from the four countries. *Journal of Cultural Diversity, 7* (1), 23–31.

McPherson, M. K. (2004). Pharmacotherapy of pain in older adults. In F.M. Goth (Ed.). *Handbook for pain relief in older adults: An evidence-based approach.* (pp. 115–130). Totowa, NJ: Humana Press.

McWilliams, L. A., Cox, B. J., & Enns, M. W. (2003). Mood and anxiety disorders associated with chronic pain: An examination in a nationally representative sample. *Pain, 106,* 127–133.

McWilliams, L. A., Goodwin, R. D., & Cox, B. J. (2004). Depression and anxiety associated with three pain conditions: Results from a nationally representative sample. *Pain, 111,* 77–83.

Melzack, R. (1973). *The puzzle of pain.* New York: Basic Books.

_____. (1999). Pain—An overview. *Acta Anaesthesiologica Scandinavica, 43,* 880–884.

Melzack, R., & Wall, P. D. (1965). Pain mechanisms: A new theory. *Science, 150,* 971–979.

Melzack, R., & Wall, P. D. (2003). *Handbook of pain management: A clinical companion to Wall and Melzack's textbook of pain.* Philadelphia: Churchill Livingstone.

Menefee, L. A., Cohen, M. J. M., Anderson, W. R., Doghramji, K., et al. (2000). Sleep disturbance and nonmalignant chronic pain: A comprehensive review of the literature. *Pain Medicine, 1,* 156–172.

Merlijn, V. P. B. M., Hunfeld, J. A. M., van der Wouden, J.C., Hazebroek-Kampschreur, A. A. J. M., et al. (2003). Psychosocial factors associated with chronic pain in adolescents. *Pain, 101,* 33–43.

Merskey, J. (Ed.). (1986). Classification of chronic pain: Descriptions of chronic pain syndromes and definitions of pain terms. *Pain, Suppl. 3,* S1–S225.

Miaskowski, C. (2000). The impact of age on a patient's perception of pain and ways it can be managed. *Pain Management Nursing, 1,* 2–7.

Mitchell, A., & Boss, B. J. (2002). Adverse effects of pain on the nervous system of newborns and young children: A review of the literature. *Journal of Neuroscience Nursing, 34,* 222–236.

Mobily, P. R., Herr, K. A., & Kelley, L. S. (1993). Cognitive-behavioral techniques to reduce pain: A validation study. *International Journal of Nursing Studies, 30,* 537–548.

Monks, R., & Merskey, H. (2003). Psychotropic drugs. In R. Melzack, & P.D. Wall. *Handbook of pain management: A clinical companion to Wall and Melzack's textbook of pain.* (pp. 353–376). Philadelphia: Churchill Livingstone.

Morley, S., Eccleston, C., & Williams, A. (1999). Systematic review and meta-analysis of randomised trials of cognitive behavior therapy and behavior therapy for chronic pain in adults, excluding headache. *Pain, 80,* 1–13.

Nabeta, T., & Kawakita, K. (2002). Relief of chronic neck and shoulder pain by manual acupuncture to tender points—A sham-controlled randomized trial. *Complementary Therapies in Medicine, 10,* 217–222.

National Institutes of Health. (1995). *Integration of behavioral and relaxation approaches into the treatment of chronic pain and insomnia.* Technology Assessment conference Statement. Bethesda, MD.

_____. (November 3–5, 1997). *Acupuncture. NIH consensus statement: Volume 15(5)*. Rockville, MD: US Department of HHS PUBL Public Health Services.

Nicassio, P. M., Moxham, E. G., Schuman, C. E., & Gevirtz, R. N. (2002). The contribution of pain, reported sleep quality, and depressive symptoms to fatigue in fibromyalgia. *Pain, 100,* 271–279.

Nielson, W. R., & Jensen, M. P. (2004). Relationship between changes in coping and treatment outcome in patients with Fibromyalgia Syndrome. *Pain, 109,* 233–241.

Owens, J. E., Taylor, A. G., & DeGood, D. (1999). Complementary and alternative medicine and psychologic factors: Toward an individual differences model of complementary and alternative medicine use and outcomes. *Journal of Alternative Complementary Therapy, 5,* 529–541.

Palermo, T. M. (2000). Impact of recurrent and chronic pain on child and family daily functioning: A critical review of the literature. *Developmental and Behavioral Pediatrics, 21,* 58–69.

Pasero, C., Portenoy, R. K., & McCaffery, M. (Eds.) (1999). Opioid analgesics. In M. McCaffery, & C. Pasero. *Pain: Clinical manual for nursing practice* (2nd ed). (pp. 161–199). St. Louis: Mosby.

Pellegrini, J. D., Paice, J., & Faut-Callahan, M. (1999). Meperidine utilization and compliance with Agency for Health Care Policy and Research guidelines in a tertiary care hospital. *CRNA, 10* (4), 174–180.

Peloso, P. M., Bellamy, N., Bensen, W., Thomson, G. T. D., et al. (2000). Double blind randomized placebo control trial of controlled release codeine in the treatment of osteoarthritis of the hip or knee. *The Journal of Rheumatology, 27,* 764–771.

Perquin, C. W., Hazebroek-Kampschreur, A. A. J. M., Hunfeld, J. A. M., Bohnen, A. M., et al. (2000). Pain in children and adolescents: a common experience. *Pain, 87,* 51–58.

Pilowsky, I. (1999). Psychiatric approaches to non-cancer pain. *Acta Anaesthesiologica Scandinavica, 43,* 889–892.

Pincus, T., & Williams, A. (1999). Models and measurements of depression in chronic pain. *Journal of Psychosomatic Research, 47,* 211–219.

Portenoy, R. K. (2000). Current pharmacotherapy of chronic pain. *Journal of Pain and Symptom Management, 10* (Suppl), S16–S20.

Rabben, T., Skjelbred, P., & Oye, I. (1999). Prolonged analgesic effect of ketamine, an N-methyl-D-aspartate receptor inhibitor, in patients with chronic pain.

Journal of Pharmacological Experimental Therapy, 289, 1060–1066.

Rapoff, M. A., & Lindsley, C. B. (2000). The pain puzzle: A visual and conceptual metaphor for understanding and treating pain in pediatric rheumatic disease. *Journal of Rheumatology, 27* (Suppl 58), 29–33.

Reyes-Gibby, C. C., Aday, L., & Cleeland, C. (2002). Impact of pain on self-related health in the community-dwelling older adults. *Pain, 95,* 75–82.

Richeimer, S. H., Bajwa, Z. H., Karhamann, S. S., Ransil, B. J., et al. (1997). Utilization patterns of tricyclic antidepressants in a multidisciplinary pain clinic: A survey. *Clinical Journal of Pain, 13,* 324–329.

Riley III, J. L., Wade, J. B., Myers, C. D., Sheffield, D., et al. (2002). Racial/ethnic differences in the experience of chronic pain. *Pain, 100,* 291–298.

Roberto, K. A. & Reynolds, S. G. (2002). Older women's experiences with chronic pain: Daily challenges and self-care practices. *Journal of Women and Aging, 13* (3/4), 5–23.

Rodriquez, C. S. (2001). Pain measurement in the elderly: A review. *Pain Management Nursing, 2,* 38–46.

Rustøen, T., Wahl, A. K., Hanestad, B. R., Lerdal, A., et al. (2004). Gender differences in chronic pain – findings from a population-based study of Norwegian adults. *Pain Management Nursing, 5,* 105–117.

St. Marie, B. (Ed.) (2002). *Core curriculum for pain management for nursing.* Philadelphia: Saunders.

Sang, C. N. (2000). NMDA–receptor antagonists in neuropathic pain: Experimental methods to clinical trials. *Journal of Pain Symptom Management, 19* (Suppl), S21–S25.

Savage, S. R. (1999). Opioid therapy of chronic pain: Assessment of consequences. *Acta Anaesthesiologica Scandinavica, 43,* 909–917.

Schaffer, S. D., & Yucha, C. A. (2004). Relaxation and pain management: The relaxation response can play a role in managing chronic and acute pain. *American Journal of Nursing, 104* (8), 75–82.

Scharff, L., & Turk. D. C. (1998). Chronic pain and depression in the elderly. *Clinical Geriatrics, 6* (9), 30–36.

Shalmi, C. L. (2004). Opioids for nonmalignant pain: Issues and controversy. In C.A. Warfield & Z.H. Bajwa. (Eds). *Principles & practice of pain medicine* (2nd ed). (pp. 601–611). New York: McGraw-Hill.

Sharpe, D., & Rossiter, L. (2002). Siblings of children with a chronic illness: A meta-analysis. *Journal of Pediatric Psychology, 27,* 699–710.

Shimp, L. A. (1998). Safety issues in the pharmacologic management of chronic pain in the elderly. *Pharmacotherapy, 18,* 1313–1322.

Shvartzman, P., Friger, M., Shani, A., Barak, F., et al. (2003). Pain control in ambulatory cancer patients—can we do better? *The Journal of Pain and Symptom Management, 26,* 716–722.

Simon, L. S. (2000). Are the biologic and clinical effects of the COX-2-specific inhibitors more advanced compared with the effects of traditional NSAIDs? *Current Opinions in Rheumatology, 12* (3), 163–170.

Simon, L. S. (2004). Nonsteroidal anti-inflammatory drugs. In C. A. Warfield & Z. H. Bajwa (Eds.). *Principles & practice of pain medicine* (2nd ed). (pp. 616–626). New York: McGraw-Hill.

Smith, A. A. (2003). Intimacy and family relationships of women with chronic pain. *Pain Management Nursing, 4,* 134–142.

Smith, A. & Friedemann, M. (1999). Perceived family dynamics of persons with chronic pain. *Journal of Advanced Nursing, 30,* 543–551.

Smith, D. W., Arnstein, P., Rosa, K. C., & Wells-Federman, C. (2002). Effects of integrating therapeutic touch into a cognitive behavioral pain treatment program: Report of a pilot clinical trial. *Journal of Holistic Nursing, 20,* 367–387.

Smith, M. S., Martin-Herz, S. P., Womack, W. M., & Marsigan, J. L. (2003). Comparative study of anxiety, depression, somatization, functional disability, and illness attribution in adolescents with chronic fatigue or migraine. *Pediatrics, 111,* 376–381.

Smith, M. T., Perlis, M. L., Smith, M. S., Giles, D. E., et al. (2000). Sleep quality and presleep arousal in chronic pain. *Journal of Behavioral Medicine, 23,* 3–13.

Soares, J. J. G., & Grossi, G. (1999). Psychosocial factors, pain parameters, mental health and coping among Turkish and Swedish patients with musculoskeletal pain. *Scandinavian Journal of Occupational Therapy, 6,* 174–183.

Spinhoven, P., ter Kuile, M., Kole-Snijders, A. M. J., Mansfeld, M. H., et al. (2004). Catastrophizing and internal pain control as mediators of outcome in the multidisciplinary treatment of chronic low back pain. *European Journal of Pain, 8,* 211–219.

Strahl, D., Kleinknecht, R. A., & Dinnel, D. L. (2000). The role of pain, anxiety, coping, and pain self-efficacy in rheumatoid arthritis patient functioning. *Behaviour Research and Therapy, 38,* 863–873.

Strauss, A. L., Corbin, J., Fagerhaugh, S., Glaser, B. G., et al. (1984). *Chronic illness and the quality of life.* St. Louis: Mosby.

Sweeney, C., & Bruera, E. (2003). Opioids In R. Melzack & P.D. Wall. *Handbook of pain management: A clinical companion to Wall and Melzack's textbook of pain.* (pp. 377–396). Philadelphia: Churchill Livingstone.

Tait, R. C., & Chibnall, J.T. (2002). Pain in older subacute care patients: Associations with clinical status and treatment. *Pain Medicine, 3,* 231–239.

Takahashi, M., Yoshida, A., Yamanaka, H., Furuyama, Y., et al. (2000). Lower s-endorphin content in peripheral blood mononuclear cells in patients with complex regional pain syndrome. *Journal of Back and Musculoskeletal Rehabilitation, 15,* 31–36.

Thomas, E., Peat, G., Harris, L., Wilkie, R., et al. (2004). The prevalence of pain and pain interference in a general population of older adults: cross-sectional findings from the North Staffordshire Osteoarthritis Project (NorStOP). *Pain, 110,* 361–368.

Thomsen, A. B., Becker, N., & Eriksen, J. (1999). Opioid rotation in chronic non-malignant pain patients. *Acta Anaesthesiologica Scandinavica, 43,* 918–923.

Turk, D. C. (1999). The role of psychological factors in chronic pain. *Acta Anaesthesiologica Scandinavica, 43,* 885–888.

Turk, D. C., & Okifuji, A. (2003). A cognitive-behavioral approach to pain management. In R. Melzack & P. D. Wall (Eds.). *Handbook of pain management: A clinical companion to Wall and Melzack's textbook of pain.* (pp. 533–542). Philadelphia: Churchill Livingstone.

Turk, D. C., & Okifuji, A. (2004). Psychological aspects of pain. In C. A. Warfield & Z. H. Bajwa. (Eds). *Principles & practice of pain medicine* (2nd ed). (pp. 139–147). New York: McGraw-Hill.

Turk, D. C., & Melzack, R. (2001). *Handbook of pain assessment.* (2nd ed.). New York: Guilford Press.

Unruh, A. M., Ritchie, J., & Merskey, H. (1999). Does gender affect appraisal of pain and pain coping strategies? *The Clinical Journal of Pain, 15,* 31–40.

Vallerand, A. H., & Polomano, R. C. (2000). The relationship of gender to pain. *Pain Management Nursing, 1* (Supp 1), 8–15.

Vessey, J. A., & Carlson, K. L. (1996). Nonpharmacological interventions to use with children in pain. *Issues in Comprehensive Pediatric Nursing, 19* (3), 169–182.

Voerman, V. F., van Egmond, J., & Crul, B. J. P. (2000) Elevated detection thresholds for mechanical stimuli in chronic pain patients: Support for a central mechanism. *Archives of Physical Medicine and Rehabilitation, 81,* 430–435.

Wall, P. D., & Melzack, R. (Eds). (1999) *Textbook of pain,* (4th ed). Edinburgh: Churchill Livingstone.

Walsh, D. A., & Radcliffe, J. C. (2002). Pain beliefs and perceived physical disability of patients with chronic low back pain. *Pain, 97,* 23–31.

Warfield, C. A., & Bajwa, Z. H. (Eds). (2004). *Principles & practice of pain medicine* (2nd ed). New York: McGraw-Hill.

Weinbroum, A. A., Rudick, V., Paret, G., & Ben-Abraham, R. (2000). The role of dextromethorphan in pain control. *Canadian Journal of Anesthesia, 47,* 585–596.

Weiner, R. S. (Ed.). *Pain management a practical guide for clinicians* (6th ed). (pp. 279–284). Boca Raton, FL: CRC Press.

Weinstein, S. M., Laux, L. F., Thornby, J. I., Lorimor, R. J., et al. (2000). Physicians' attitudes toward pain and the use of opioid analgesics: Results from a survey from the Texas Cancer Pain Initiative. *Southern Medical Journal, 93,* 479–487.

Wells-Federman, C., Arnstein, P., & Caudill, M. (2002). Nurse-led pain management program: Effect on self-efficacy, pain intensity, pain-related disability, and depressive symptoms in chronic pain patients. *Pain Management Nursing, 3,* 131–140.

Whitfield, M. F., & Grunau, R. E. (2000). Behavior, pain perception, and the extremely low-birth weight subjects. *Clinical Perinatology, 2,* 363–379.

Wilkes, L. M., Castro, M., Mohan S., Sundaraj, S. R., et al. (2003). Health status of patients with chronic pain attending a pain centre. *Pain Management Nursing, 4,* 70–76.

Williamson, G. M., Walters, A. S., & Shaffer, D.R. (2002). Caregiver models of self and others, coping, and depression: Predictors of depression in children with chronic pain. *Health Psychology, 21,* 405–410.

Winterowd, C., Beck, A. T., & Gruener, D. (2003). *Cognitive therapy with chronic pain patients.* New York: Springer.

Winzeler, S., & Rosenstein, B. D. (1998). Non-steroidal anti-inflammatory drugs: A review. *AAOHN Journal, 46,* 253–259.

Wiskin, L. F. (1998). Cognitive-behavioral therapy: A psychoeducational treatment approach for the American worker with rheumatoid arthritis. *Journal of Prevention Assessment and Rehabilitation, 10* (1), 41–48.

Woby, S. R., Watson, P. J., Roach, N. K., & Urmston, M. (2004). Are changes in fear-avoidance beliefs, catastrophizing, and appraisals of control, predictive of changes in chronic low back pain and disability? *European Journal of Pain, 8,* 201–210.

Zautra, A. J., Hamilton, N. A., & Burke, H. M. (1999). Comparison of stress responses in women with two types of chronic pain: Fibromyalgia and Osteoarthritis. *Cognitive Therapy and Research, 23,* 209–230.

CHAPTER 5

Self-Efficacy

Ann Mabe Newman

Introduction

Self-efficacy as a concept has been applied to various domains of psychosocial and physical behaviors spanning more than 30 years, to include phobic disorders (Bandura, Adams, Hardy, & Howells, 1980), depression (Davies & Yates, 1982; Perraud, 2000), achievement behavior (Schunk, 1984; Schunk & Pajares, 2002); addictive behaviors (DiClemente, 1986; DiClemente, Fairhurst, & Pitrowski, 1995); diabetes (Moens, Grypdonck, & vander Bijl, 2002); heart disease (Clark, Janz, Dodge et al., 1997); and arthritis (Lorig et al., 1989; Newman, 2001). This increasing recognition of self-efficacy as a concept is due to its presence in being able to predict health behavior change.

A client's adherence or compliance to a treatment regime is due, in part, to a client's self-efficacy. Behavior change and the maintenance of those changes have great significance for nursing, since as nurses we provide care that maximizes a client's positive interactions with the environment, promotes an optimal level of wellness for the client, and enhances the client's self-actualization.

Many health education programs implicitly enhance self-efficacy. Such programs are designed to help the client feel a sense of accomplishment in performing the tasks required. Self-management or adherence to a medical regime occupies much of the care in working with clients with chronic illness. Thus, a discussion of self-efficacy has the potential to lead nurses to a better understanding of how the client decides to attempt, to continue, or to persist in a health promoting behavior. This knowledge can then be used to design specific interventions and strategies to enhance self-efficacy, and in turn, lead to more effective health practices for individuals with chronic illnesses. Even though the pathology of the illness may not change, the client and the nurse can achieve a therapeutic alliance, with both involved in choosing goals that the client feels personally capable of achieving.

Context of Self-Efficacy

In the text *Social Learning Theory*, Bandura (1977b), stated his attempt to ". . . provide a unified theoretical framework for analyzing human thought and behavior" (p. vi). From this need to distinguish between interventions and applications drawn from social learning theory, Bandura's work on self-efficacy was initiated. A number of social learning approaches had been formulated prior to Bandura's work. The theories of Miller and Dollard (1941) and

Rotter (1954) contributed to the body of knowledge of the relationship between cultural factors and individual adjustment (Rosenthal, 1982). The work of Bandura built upon these earlier theories.

In 1986, Bandura designated the theoretical approach of his work as social cognitive theory. He noted that the previous term, social learning theory, was becoming increasingly inappropriate as psychosocial concepts of the theory became more developed. In social cognitive theory, the social terminology acknowledges the "social origins of much human thought and action. The cognitive portion recognizes the influential causal contribution of thought processes to human motivation, affect, and action" (p. xii). In social cognitive theory, individuals are neither automatically shaped and controlled by external stimuli nor driven by inner forces (Bandura, 1986). Rather, a model of reciprocal determinism explains human functioning in terms of interaction among behavioral, cognitive, other personal factors and the environment (Bandura, 1997). As can be seen in Figure 5-1, the determinants influence each other in a bi-directional way. However, the three factors are not always of equal strength and will exert their influence in different ways under different circumstances.(Bandura, 1997).

FIGURE 5-1

The conditional relationships between efficacy beliefs and outcome expectancies. In given domains of functioning, efficacy beliefs vary in level, strength, and generality. The outcomes that flow from a given course of action can take the form of positive or negative physical, social, and self-evaluation effects. (Bandura, 1997).

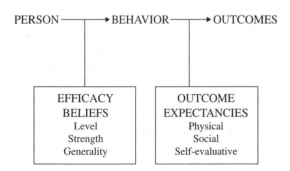

The notion of "reciprocal causation/determinism" is demonstrated in the way individuals manage their chronic illness (see Figure 5-1). Individuals are often able to manage their environments in ways that amaze us, or use cognitive-behavioral techniques to keep going forward day-after-day. Bandura (1997) states that it is through these beliefs of personal efficacy that we exercise control over what we do.

Defining Self-Efficacy

Bandura defined self-efficacy as "the conviction that one can successfully execute the behavior required to produce the outcome" (1977a, p. 193). Self-efficacy is differentiated between "outcome expectancies" and "efficacy expectancies" (self-efficacy), because an individual can believe that a behavior will produce a certain outcome; but if serious doubts exist about whether s/he can perform the necessary tasks to carry out the behavior, the behavior may not be attempted (Bandura, 1977a). It is important to distinguish between outcome expectancies and efficacy expectancies. An "outcome expectancy" is the individual's estimate that a specific behavior will lead to certain outcomes, while an "efficacy expectancy" (self-efficacy) is the conviction that one can successfully execute the outcome" (p. 79). Bandura's belief is that since control is a central concept in our lives, it is these self-beliefs functioning through the mechanism of personal agency that predict our behaviors and actions (see Figure 5-2).

Self-efficacy varies on three dimensions. each with important performance implications. These include *magnitude*, which concerns the level of difficulty; *generality*, some experiences result in mastery while others are generalizable to one's overall increase in self-efficacy; and *strength*, weak expectancies may be extinguished by failure, but persons with strong expectations of mastery will persevere despite failures (Bandura, 1977a).

Human Capabilities in Self-Efficacy

Pajares (2002) notes that "rooted within Bandura's social cognitive theory is the understanding

FIGURE 5-2

The relationships among the three major classes of determinants in triadic reciprocal causation. B represents behavior; P, the internal personal factors in the form of cognitive, affective, and biological events; and E, the external environment. (Bandura, 1986).

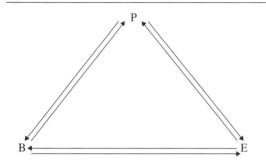

that individuals are imbued with certain capabilities that define what it is to be human." (p. 3). Bandura (1986) defines basic capabilities which influence interactions as:

Symbolizing capability. The capability to use symbols provides individuals with the power to alter and adapt to their environment. Through the use of symbols, individuals store away experiences to be used for future action. Symbols also give continuance to an individual's lived experience. That is not to say, however, that actions based on thoughts are always rational. People may make judgments that are faulty when they don't have the needed information to make a judgment. Thus, thought can be a source of human failing and distress as well as human accomplishment (Bandura, 1986). Because of our ability to symbolize, we are able to model observed behavior.

Forethought Capability. Most behavior is assumed to be purposive and is regulated by forethought rather than by reaction to the immediate environment. Individuals anticipate the likely consequences of their actions based on the stored experiences of the symbolic activity. "Future events cannot serve as determinants of behavior, but their cognitive representations can have a strong causal impact on present actions" (Bandura, 1986, p. 19). Because of forethought capability, we anticipate

what will likely happen and decide to alter our strategies (Pajares, 2002).

Vicarious Capability. Bandura (1986) challenged the notion of psychological theories which assume that learning only occurs by performing responses and experiencing their effects. He maintained that virtually all learned phenomena, which results from direct experience, can occur vicariously; that is, from observing other individuals' behavior and the consequences that occur. Therefore, modeling becomes an indispensable aspect of learning. This phenomenon can be observed through the powerful aspects of the media. If performing the observed behavior meets our values and expectations, we will adopt and repeat the behavior in the future (Pajares, 2002).

Self-Regulatory Capability. The central role of self-regulatory function is a distinctive feature of social cognitive theory (Bandura, 1986). Most behavior is "motivated and regulated by internal standards and self-evaluative reactions to their own actions" (p. 20). Evaluative self-regulation acts as a feedback mechanism after our own personal standards have been set.

Self-Reflective Capacity. The 'distinctly human' (p. 21) capability for reflective self-consciousness enables individuals to analyze their own experiences and think about their own thought processes (Bandura, 1986). Through self-reflection, we monitor our thinking, decide to act on ideas, change them, or judge the adequacy of them. An individual's judgment of their capabilities is a central and pervasive type of thought that affects action. Self-precepts of efficacy are partly responsible for what we choose to do, how much effort we invest in an activity, and how long we will persevere. This product of reflective self-appraisal underlies the exercise of many facets of personal agency (Bandura, 1986).

Concepts Related to Self-Efficacy

Differentiating self-efficacy from similar and related terms may offer further clarification.

Health Locus of Control refers to a generalized expectation about whether one's health is controlled by one's own behavior or by external forces (Wallston

& Wallston, 1984). Within this concept, health is viewed as an outcome, and is differentiated from self-efficacy, which focuses on beliefs about one's capacity to undertake behavior that may or may not lead to desired outcomes (Strecher, DeVellis, Becker, & Rosenstock, 1986). Individuals may believe that they are personally responsible for their health, but if they lack the skill needed to carry out the appropriate health behavior, they would approach the activities with a sense of futility. Self-efficacy, then, is logically differentiated from health locus of control.

Self-esteem refers to respect and liking of one's self that is based on a realistic self-appraisal (Newman, 2003). Self-esteem is concerned with an evaluation of self-worth, while self-efficacy refers to an evaluation of specific capabilities within specific situations (Strecher et al., 1986). Individuals may have high self-efficacy for a task that does not involve self-pride (e.g. tooth-brushing) or low self-efficacy for a task but no loss of self-worth (e.g. being unable to sky-dive) (Bandura, 1977b).

Coping, as conceptualized by Lazarus and Folkman (1984), is a process in which an individual takes into account strategies available, the likelihood of an expected outcome, and whether one can effectively apply the strategy. Coping is not a concept which can be generalized to a person's total concept of self, and in this sense it is closely related to self-efficacy. Thus, when viewed within Lazarus and Folkman's framework, self-efficacy is a component of the coping response.

Learned helplessness results from exposure to uncontrollable events and is mediated through cognitive, affective, and motivational deficits (Strecher et al., 1986). Personal helplessness results when the person feels that s/he cannot control a situation which others might be able to; and a universal helplessness occurs when one feels that s/he lacks any response s/he or others could make (Abramson, Garber, & Seligman, 1980). In terms of self-efficacy, one must feel personally capable before being willing to attempt the behavior. Learned helplessness may be responsible for weak performance expectancies. Within this context, self-efficacy and learned helplessness are related but can be differentiated.

Sources of Self-Efficacy Beliefs

Central to Bandura's theory is that "people's beliefs about their personal efficacy constitutes a major aspect of their self-knowledge" (Bandura, 1997, p. 79). Four principal sources of information allow us to construct our self-efficacy beliefs

- enactive mastery experiences, which give us an indicator of our capabilities;
- vicarious experiences, which may cause us to alter our behavior when we compare ourselves with others;
- verbal persuasion and other social influences that we possess certain capabilities; and
- physiological and affective states that help us judge our capability and vulnerability to dysfunction

Information about judging our personal capabilities is not in-and-of-itself enlightening, whether it is conveyed to us enactively, vicariously, persuasively, or physiologically (Bandura, 1997). Only when information is processed and reflected upon, does it become instructive. Let's explore the four sources of self-efficacy and see how they influence behavior.

Mastery Experience. Performance accomplishments or enactive mastery experiences are the most influential sources of efficacy information because they are based on our own beliefs about whether we have what it takes to succeed (Bandura, 1997). This is personified by the saying that 'nothing succeeds like success itself.' But by like token, failure which comes before success can undermine success. Learning to persevere through failure, then, can help individuals feel more in control of events in their lives. When we become convinced that we have what it takes to succeed, we not only persevere in the face of adversity, we rebound more quickly from setbacks.

The perceived difficulty of a task also influences our personal efficacy judgment of success. When we succeed at an easy task, there is no need for reappraisal of our self-efficacy to try it again. But mastery of difficult tasks brings new efficacy information, which means we must appraise our capabilities again (Bandura, 1997). When we begin a new, complex task, we can not fully know how difficult it will be. This uncertainty and even the ambiguity of the task influences whether we think we will be successful in mastering the task.

Since performance does not occur in a vacuum, many contextual factors may help or hinder increasing an individual's self-efficacy. Contextual factors include help provided by others, the circumstances under which the activity was performed or even whether it is perceived that the right equipment was available and working properly (Bandura, 1997). Even when experience contradicts firmly held self-beliefs, we resist giving up these beliefs about ourselves, if we can find reasons to discount them. For example, if a client believes s/he is unable to measure and give their own insulin, and then is able to do it well with only minimal assistance, the client will not change their efficacy belief about their ability, but rather attribute it to the help provided. In this case, to produce enduring changes in personal efficacy requires powerful, confirming experiences in which the client could successfully manage, under diverse conditions being able to draw up and give his own insulin. According to Bandura (1997), however, as the client gains ability to predict and manage potential threats, s/he will develop increased self-efficacy that will serve in mastering new challenges.

Those who work with individuals with chronic illness know that the road to proficiency is marked by 'spurts and sputters' and that the rate of improvement may vary with the stage of skill acquisition. Often a plateau follows some improvement. Individuals who experience periodic failures but continue to make even small amounts of progress are more likely to experience an increase in their self-efficacy than those who are successful but see their performance leveling off compared with their previous rate of improvement. Clients may think the plateau they have reached means that they have 'maxed out' their capability and are not willing to spend the additional time required to reach a higher level of proficiency. Pajares (2002) summarizes the importance of mastery experience as the most influential source of self-efficacy beliefs by noting "... mastery experiences are only raw data, and

many factors influence how such information is cognitively processed and affects an individual's self-appraisal" (p. 7).

Vicarious Experience. The second most important source of efficacy information is vicarious experience, or observation of the performance of others. In addition to enactive experiences, then, modeling serves as another way of promoting self-efficacy beliefs. When there are no absolute measures of adequacy (such as driving a car, balancing a checkbook, etc), we measure our capabilities with the success of others. Appraisal of our own self-efficacy will vary depending on the talents of those we choose to make comparisons (Bandura, 1997).

There are a number of ways modeling impacts self-efficacy beliefs. When we compare ourselves to those similar to us, we tend to identify with them. Thus, seeing an individual performing successfully will typically cause us to think we have the capability to perform equally as well (Bandura, 1997). We persuade ourselves that if others can do it, so can we! Likewise, however, if the individual we are comparing ourselves with fails, our own efforts may be undermined.

There are other conditions under which vicarious information affects our self-efficacy appraisal. For instance, when we lack knowledge of our own capabilities, we tend to rely more on modeled indicators, and modeling that conveys positive coping can increase our self-efficacy when we have been subjected to countless experiences of personal inefficacy.

Verbal Persuasion. Verbal persuasion, usually from others, is also a major source of efficacy information, although not as strong as performance or vicarious experience. Verbal persuasion, if the positive appraisal is in within realistic bounds, can bolster self-change, even though verbal persuasion alone is limited in terms of creating enduring increases in self-efficacy (Bandura, 1997). When individuals are verbally persuaded that they have the capability to perform a given task, they are more likely to try harder to do what is asked of them. Raising unrealistic beliefs in personal capabilities, however, only discredits the individual using verbal persuasion and further makes the recipient feel that s/he is a failure.

Physiological and Affective States. Emotional and physiological states are the fourth way with which we are provided information about our efficacy beliefs. In health functioning and in coping with stress, somatic indicators of personal efficacy are especially relevant (Bandura, 1997). We often believe that high levels of arousal in stressful situations make us vulnerable to failure; conversely, we believe that we will be more successful when we are not tense or agitated. When we believe that we have no control over the situation, we inadvertently develop increased levels of distress that produce the very dysfunction we fear. Treatments that eliminate emotional reactions through mastery experiences increase beliefs in our self-efficacy to cope, which in turn improves performance (Bandura, 2001). In addition to these autonomic arousal states, other physiological indicators influence self-efficacy information. Individuals judge their fatigue, aches and pains, and even their mood states as indicators of their personal inefficacy. Thus, altering beliefs related to physical status, stress levels, and correcting misinterpretations of bodily states is a major way of enhancing self-efficacy (Bandura, 1991).

Integration of Efficacy Information

The benefits of a strong sense of personal efficacy "do not arise simply from the incantation of capability" (Bandura, 1997, p. 115). Just saying something is so is not the same as believing it is true. Efficacy beliefs are formed through cognitive processing of efficacy information involving performance accomplishments, vicarious experiences, verbal persuasion and emotional arousal. The information which individuals attend to and use to make efficacy judgments has to be weighed and integrated from these four sources of self-efficacy information. As Pajares (2002) states, "....the selection, integration, interpretation, and recollection of information influence judgment of self-efficacy" (p. 8). After one's efficacy beliefs are formed, they contribute to human functioning in many ways through cognitive, motivational, affective and decisional processes (Bandura, 1997).

Self-Efficacy Mediating Processes

Self-efficacy beliefs produce their effects through influencing how we feel, think, and motivate ourselves. Bandura (1997) notes, "A substantial body of literature shows that efficacy beliefs regulate human functioning through four major processes" (p. 116). These different processes, *cognitive, motivational, affective, and selective processes,* operate together rather than in isolation. It is by operating in concert that they influence the regulation of human functioning.

Cognitive Processes

Self-efficacy beliefs affect thought patterns that can help or hinder performance and these cognitive effects take various forms (Bandura, 1987). High self-efficacy beliefs by individuals will cause them to take a futuristic perspective in planning their lives. Purposeful behavior is regulated by forethought in planning goals and is influenced by the self-appraisal of our capabilities. We are more firmly committed to our goals when we have high self-efficacy (Bandura & Wood, 1989; Locke & Latham, 1990)

Most individuals think about an action before initiating it. This act of cognition serves to guide our actions as we develop proficiencies. Beliefs about our efficacy for a task influence how we anticipate and visualize this future action. If we have high self-efficacy we will visualize success but if we have low self-efficacy beliefs, we will visualize failure. High self-efficacy engenders cognitive construction of successful actions and the cognitive thought of success leads to successful courses of action, thereby strengthening self-efficacy beliefs (Bandura, 1997).

A major function of thought is to help us predict what will happen if we take different paths of action and to help us find ways to control the outcome of either path of action. Our problem-solving skills involve judgments about how actions affect outcome. In trying to construct predictive rules, we draw on our pre-existing knowledge in developing options, knowing they will need to be revised when measured against immediate and future options. A strong sense of efficacy is needed to be fully task oriented in the face of causal ambiguities that can have important repercussions. Efficacy beliefs affect the construction and use of problem-solving strategies.

Motivational Processes

Our ability to be self-motivated and carry out purposive action is rooted in cognitive activity (Bandura, 1997). Again, it is this human capacity for *forethought* that allows us to project future activity, although plans for future actions cannot be the cause of current action. Thus, the use of forethought allows individuals to motivate themselves and set goals that guide their actions. Self-efficacy beliefs play a central role in the cognitive process of motivation.

Cognitive motivators are built around three different theories. According to *causal attribution* with the corresponding Attribution Theory of Motivation, retrospective judgments of our performances have motivational effects (Weiner, 1985). When we attribute our success to personal capabilities and our failures to insufficient effort, we will persist in the face of failure to try difficult tasks. Conversely, if we think our failure was due to deficiencies in our ability and success is due to situational factors, we will give up when we encounter difficulties. Bandura (1997) notes that intervention studies which seek to change motivation by changing causal attributions are limited. He further notes that "persuatory attributions can serve as supplementary motivators but not as a primary mode of generating human motivations and accomplishments" (p. 125).

Outcome expectancies based on Expectancy-Value Theory (Ajzen & Fishbein, 1980) support the notion that "people also motivate themselves and guide themselves anticipatorily by the outcomes they expect to flow from given courses of behavior" (Bandura, 1997, p. 125). Bandura notes, however, that regardless of the incentive system, individuals with high self-efficacy and goals, outperform those who doubt their efficacy to meet difficult standards and lower their aspirations accordingly.

Cognized goals and the corresponding Goal Theory (Locke & Latham, 1990) state that the capacity to exercise self-influence by evaluating one's own performance is a major source of motivation and self-directedness. Goals operate more though self-reactive influences than regulating motivation directly. Perceived self-efficacy is one of the important self-influences in creating powerful motivational effects (Bandura, 1997). Further, self-efficacy beliefs influence the level of goal setting, the strength of commitment to them, the amount of effort used in the endeavor, and how efforts are increased when accomplishments fall short.

Affective Processes

Self-efficacy also plays an important role in the regulation of affective states. We can exercise personal control over thought, action, and affect which change the nature and intensity of personal experiences (Bandura, 1997). But when we feel that we cannot influence the events and conditions that will significantly affect our lives, we may experience anxiety and become despondent. Such is the case when living with a chronic illness. When does anxiety and despondency become depression? We experience anxiety when we perceive that we can't manage potentially injurious events. We become saddened and depressed when we perceive that we are unable to gain valued outcomes. Depression results from hopelessness about the future, but because human distress is not neatly packaged, anxiety and despair often accompany perceived inefficacy to alter undesirable life circumstances.

Self-efficacy regulates emotional states in several ways:

1. People who believe they can manage threats are less likely to be distressed by them; those who have low self-efficacy are more likely to magnify risks;
2. People with high self-efficacy can lower their stress and anxiety through acting in ways that make the environment less threatening;

3. People with high self-efficacy have better control over disturbing thoughts;
4. Low self-efficacy can lead to depression.

(adapted by van der Bijl & Shortridge-Baggett, 2002)

Selection Processes

The three self-efficacy activated processes that allow individuals to create helpful environments and have control over them, cognitive processes, motivation, and affective states, set the stage for looking at how individuals shape their environment. By selecting the environment, we help shape what we become. Selection of particular environments can shape our destinies. We avoid activities and environments we believe exceed our capacities, but we will readily undertake activities that we believe we are capable of handling (Bandura, 1997). For example, clients with arthritis with low self-efficacy for arthritis self-management will not attempt difficult tasks such as exercising or practicing relaxation techniques to reduce their pain and depression (Newman, 1993). However, those with high self-efficacy for self-management undertake these challenges as tasks to be mastered.

■ Problems and Issues

Self-management programs based on enhancing self-efficacy are highly successful in reducing symptoms and encouraging behavior change in many chronic illnesses. So why aren't these programs used more? How can these self-management programs be integrated into existing health care? Leaders in the field of self-management in chronic disease cite several conditions that would have to occur for this integration to take place. First, the system needs to identify the population who could benefit from these programs (Lorig, Mazonson, & Holman, 1993; Lorig & Holman, 2003). Secondly, the system needs to identify which evidence-based programs to use. Third, personnel who are dedicated

and trained in self-management skills need to be a part of the health care system (Lorig & Holman, 2003). And last but most importantly, self-management education must be a valued component of the mission of the health care system.

From a cognitive perspective, it is the perceptions and not necessarily the 'true' capabilities that influence behavior (Stretcher et al., 1986). Self-efficacy is task-and-situation-specific, and can not be measured globally. Although related to other concepts such as self-esteem, locus of control, coping and learned helplessness, self-efficacy must be measured within a specific situation (Maibach & Murphy, 1995). In other words, a person may be said to have high or low self-esteem, but stating that a person has high or low self-efficacy would not make sense. For example, a person with diabetes may have high self-efficacy for testing his/her blood-sugar, but low self-efficacy for controlling stress. Thus, measurement issues always become a part of the conversation when self-efficacy is discussed. Instrument development is frequently cited as a challenge in applying the concept to practice.

Self-Efficacy Instrument Development

Tools to measure self-efficacy are somewhat easy to construct. Since self-efficacy is not a global concept, scales to measure self-efficacy are measured in relationship to the specific task you are asking the client to perform. In standard methodology for measurement of self-efficacy, individuals are presented with items describing different tasks and how they rate their belief in their ability to accomplish the tasks. Questions are phrased as *can* do, not *will* do because *can* is a judgment of capability and *will* is a statement of intent.

All instruments use either a 100- or 10-point scale. On a 100-point scale, individuals record the strength of their belief on a 100-point scale, in 10-point intervals from 0 ("Can not do"); to 50 ("Moderately certain can do"); to 100 ("Certain can do"). Individuals are asked to judge their capabilities as of *now*, not what they think they can do in the future. Individuals are asked to rate their perceived efficacy or confidence in their ability to perform a task from 0 to 100 or 0 to 10 for every item in the activity domain. The efficacy strength scores are totaled and divided by the total number of items, which indicate the strength of perceived self-efficacy for that activity domain. A cutoff value is established, and this is "the value below which people judge themselves to be incapable of executing the activities in question" (Bandura, 1987, p. 44).

Since scales must be constructed for the specific tasks relevant to the chronic condition, there can be no single validity coefficient for the self-efficacy scales. Bandura (1997) however, is not apologetic on this point; he notes that the vast body of research reviewed in his text, *Self-Efficacy: The Exercise of Control*, speaks to the validity of the construct.

Kate Lorig is responsible for much of the work in the development of self-efficacy scales to measure chronic illness, the majority of which has been with clients with arthritis. In her early work, Lorig demonstrated that the association between improvement in healthy behaviors and improvement in health status were weak or non-existent in individuals with arthritis who participated in the Arthritis Self-Management Course. (Lorig et al., 1989). In qualitative studies she found that individuals felt the impact of the program was due to their feeling more in control of their illness (Lenker, Lorig, & Gallagher, 1984). Lorig and her colleagues operationalized the concept of control within self-efficacy theory and have developed tools to measure arthritis self-efficacy (Lorig, Ung, Chastain, Shoor, & Holman, 1989).

Other researchers have also developed scales to measure the self-efficacy in chronic illness: macular degeneration (Brody, Williams, Thomas, et al., 1999); heart disease in older adults (Clark, Janz, Dodge et al., 1997); diabetes (Moens et al., 2002). The stem of each question in every scale is the same. . . . 'How confident are you that you can. . . .' You, as the expert clinician, fill in the blank. What is it that you want your client to be able to accomplish?

Interventions

Enhancing Self-Efficacy

The impetus for the development of chronic illness self-management programs is the need to better manage chronic illness (Farrell, Wicks, & Martin, 2004). Since self-management education is focused on client concerns and problems, for each new topic and group of clients, a needs assessment is needed (Lorig & Holman, 2003). For example, Lorig and Holman noted that when working with a group of Latino clients, the clients expressed that they felt neglected or were receiving inferior care when they were assigned to see the nurse practitioner, psychologist, or physical therapist instead of the physician. After discovering this, a section on the training and roles of health care professionals in the U.S. was included in the Spanish version of the self-management course.

Evidence for the Effectiveness of Self-Management

Five programs for individuals with chronic conditions have been developed and evaluated by the Stanford Patient Education Research Center. These include: the Arthritis Self-Management program, the Spanish Arthritis Self-Management Program, the Positive Self-Management Program (for HIV/AIDS), the Back Pain Self-Management Program, and the Chronic Disease Self-Management Program (Lorig, Lubeck, Kraines, Seleznick, & Holman, 1985; Lorig, Sobel, Stewart et al., 1999; VonKorf, Moore, Lorig et al., 1998). The Arthritis Self-Management Course, endorsed by the Arthritis Foundation, has been used by this author to deliver care to more than 100 people with arthritis (Newman, 1993, 1997, 2001). Interventions included self-contracting and goal setting. Participants reported a perceived reduction in pain and other symptoms such as depression.

The Take PRIDE program, developed by Clark and colleagues (1997), used self-management techniques to reduce symptoms and distress for 1 year. In their review of studies of self-management effectiveness, Lorig and Holman (2003) cite the study of Mazzuca and colleagues on diabetes self-management as one which demonstrated positive outcomes (Mazzuca, Mooreman, Wheeler et al., 1986).

Interventions Based on Self-Efficacy

As described earlier, judgments of self-efficacy are based on four sources of information: performance accomplishments enacted through *skills mastery*; vicarious experiences enacted through *modeling;* emotional arousal enacted through *reinterpreting physiologic symptoms;* and verbal persuasion enacted through *social persuasion.* Any program which purports to enhance self-efficacy must contain these four precepts. Lorig and Holman (2003) give examples of how each of these efficacy-enhancing components are used in their Stanford courses.

Interventions using Skills Mastery. Skills mastery or taking action is necessary for behavior change to occur. When people are involved in doing something, it's hard for them to argue that they "can't do it." Action planning requires participants to make a specific plan for the week. Participants can't say, "I'm going to exercise," they have to specify when: "I will walk two blocks Monday and Thursday before lunch." Individuals are then asked how confident they are that they can complete the plan on a scale of 1 (not at all sure) to 10 (very sure). Lorig and Holman (2003) note that if the answer is less than 7 (indicating only moderate confidence in their ability to accomplish what you are asking them to do) then they use problem-solving techniques to adapt or change the plan. The next week, participants report whether they were successful, and if problems were encountered, the problem-solving process is used again.

Nodhturft et al. (2000) taught older adults with arthritis to use self-efficacy techniques by having them first formulate an action plan. Many older people with chronic conditions are so overwhelmed from living with the daily effects of their disease that they have lost their ability to set and accomplish goals. Individuals may need to be taught how to break down goals into small achievable steps: what, when, how much, and how often. Ask clients to contract to try new behaviors every week.

Interventions using Modeling. If an individual sees themselves as very different from the model, their behavior will not be greatly influenced. This idea is especially important when designing programs for modeling behaviors for those with chronic illness. A young man with arthritis would not be the best model for an elderly African American woman with arthritis. Do not pair up individuals who are extremely different for modeling.

Examples of modeling include written and video materials. The materials should 'look like' the participants for whom they were intended. Models should depict different body types, different ages and ethnicity, and both males and females. Focus group participants told Lorig and Holman (2003) that they did not like materials using cartoon figures because they found it demeaning to intimate that chronic illness is funny. Having peers teach the self-management program is a form of modeling as well. Additionally, individuals in a group can act as role models for each other by offering suggestions even before the leader asks. Peer modeling can also be effective by pairing individuals at the same stage of an illness together (Lorig & Holman, 2003). In addition to social comparison, modeling influences our self-efficacy appraisal in other ways. We seek out competent or proficient models who possess the capabilities we desire.

Competent models, through their behavior and ways of thinking, are able to share knowledge and teach those who watch them new skills and ways to manage their lives. Models who exhibit 'undaunted attitudes' are able to influence others to a higher degree by coping with the obstacles thrown at them than by the actual skills they are modeling. By observing the models, the observer may come to believe that the tasks and threats being modeled are more or less difficult than they had imagined. These altered perceptions of task difficulty can change beliefs in our own capabilities.

Depending on the type of information being conveyed, modeling serves different functions. We are exposed to a great deal of modeling in our everyday lives through the media, television, computers, and other visuals. In the past, our only exposure was to models in our own communities. Today, symbolic modeling transcends the globe (Bandura, 1997). Cognitive rehearsal can further enhance the symbolic modeling of self-efficacy beliefs. By visualizing the application of modeled strategies successfully, we strengthen our belief that we can actually do it (Maibach & Flora, 1993).

In complex activities, it is the verbalized thinking skills that guide actions that are more helpful than the modeled skills themselves (Bandura, 1997). In a study almost 30 years ago, Sarason (1975) found that rather than just seeing the modeling of the skills, it is the verbal expression of guiding thoughts, along with the modeling that is most helpful to individuals who do not have problem-solving skills.

Appraisal of personal efficacy is not based on the performance of a single model. We have opportunities in our daily lives to observe the actions of many individuals of similar status. We may discount the success or failure of one individual as an atypical case, but when we see the pattern repeated in many individuals we tend to give more weight to it. Indeed, modeling in which different individuals master difficult tasks produces stronger efficacy beliefs that we, too, can do it, than watching a single model perform the task. Among the various characteristics of models, competency is highly valued by the observer. Model competence can be very influential when the observer perceives him/herself as having a lot to learn and the model as having a lot to offer. This is one time where competence overrides the perceived differences in model and observer. We may seek out models who possess the qualities to which we aspire.

Of the vicarious modes of influencing self-efficacy beliefs, actual modeling, symbolic modeling, videotaped self-modeling or cognitive self-modeling, all are effective in improving performance. "The level to which perceived efficacy is raised is a uniformly good predictor of subsequent performance attainment. The higher the perceived self-efficacy, the greater the performance accomplishment" (Bandura, 1997, p. 95).

Interventions using Verbal Persuasion. Performance feedback is one of the ways verbal persuasion is used to either enhance self-efficacy or undermine it. Evaluative feedback, telling individuals that they have done well in their job, enhances self-efficacy. Conversely, telling individuals that they have the ability and that it was gained by hard work decreases their self-efficacy more than if they were told that they have ability without reference to the effort they had to exert (Bandura, 1997). When social custom frowns on voicing devaluation, the politically correct way of presenting feedback is perceived by the recipient as disingenuous. They are praised excessively for mediocre performances and are generally well-practiced in seeing through these thinly-veiled devaluations, resulting in a lowered judgment of their capabilities. Thus, it is the way in which verbal persuasion and performance feedback are framed that affects the personal appraisal of self-efficacy of individuals.

Some of the support for the effects of framing on perceived self-efficacy comes from the studies of researchers who try to get people to adopt health-promoting behaviors. Bensley et al. (2004) report that health communication emphasizing the Health Behavior Management Model of looking at behavioral intent and persuasive communication to move individuals toward more active stages of change, occurs at the point of stage-specific information. Persuasive health influences framed in terms of threat or loss help individuals with high self-efficacy to strive even harder to make changes, but undermine the efforts of those who feel incapable of exercising control over their behavior (Bandura, 1997).

The effects of verbal framing influences are readily observed in social evaluations of reaching performance goals. We all strive for a certain level of performance, and know that it may occur over time. Social evaluations that focus on achieved progress, to date, emphasize our personal capabilities; while evaluations that focus on our shortfalls from the distant goals emphasize our deficient capabilities. This point of reference can influence the self-evaluation of our capabilities. Feedback framed as 'gains' may increase self-efficacy; whereas, feedback framed in terms of 'shortfalls' is likely to decrease self-efficacy by emphasizing deficiencies. In other words, telling a person how far they have come, rather than how far they have to go is the preferred way to give feedback. All too common in everyday life, good work is taken for granted but shortfalls bring ready criticism (Bandura,1997). Harsh criticism of the performer rather than helpful guidance on how to improve the *performance* undermines people's belief in themselves. Pajares (2002), states ". . . it is usually easier to weaken self-efficacy beliefs through negative appraisals than to strengthen such beliefs through positive encouragement" (p. 8).

As nurses, we are aware that our efforts at verbal persuasion are often unsuccessful in getting individuals with chronic illness to feel capable of making health behavior changes. We serve as role models for our clients and the more believable we are as sources of information, the more likely the client is to develop judgments of personal efficacy that will lead to positive health behaviors. Examples are nurses who smoke, are obese, or suffer from stress-related symptoms themselves. How believable are they as a source of information for a client? Simply telling individuals that they are much more capable than they think they are will not make it so!

Additionally, giving our clients one-time 'pep talks' will do little to change behavior. Verbal persuasion is most effective in increasing self-efficacy when combined with structuring activities in ways that bring success rather than putting them in situations in which they are likely to experience repeated failures. Teach clients to build their success in terms of self-improvement, personal development, rather than in triumphs over others. Health care professionals need to provide efficacy-affirming experiences to clients who spend a lifetime dealing with the consequences of their chronic conditions.

Social Persuasion

A powerful means of enhancing self-efficacy is social persuasion. We are more likely to follow when those around us are, or are not participating in a behavior. Lorig and Holman (2003) cite the example of smoking among teens: when smoking is not the norm, teens are not as likely to begin smoking. If members of a self-management group are participating in exercise and getting positive feedback, other members of the group are more likely to join in. Group support is often the key to self-management education in effecting behavior change. More than pep talks or inspirational talks are involved. Social persuasion works by developing an individual's belief in their capabilities to be successful in overcoming their problem.

Reinterpreting Physiologic Symptoms

Symptomology in chronic illness may have multiple causes. Thus, helping individuals reinterpret or find alternate explanations for their symptoms may also make them willing to try new self-management behaviors (Lorig & Holman, 2003). Providing explanations to the client is important. Fatigue, for example has many causes including disease, poor nutrition, lack of exercise, fear, depression, and medications. When people understand that their fatigue may be due to lack of exercise instead of their disease state, adding exercise to their self-management routine does not seem unreasonable (Lorig & Holman, 2003).

Some individuals dwell on their somatic states and reactions more than others. The less involved we are in activities outside ourselves, the more we focus on our bodies. Physiological reactions are heightened by perceived psychological stress. When one is hyperventilating, sweating, trembling or experiencing a pounding heart or insomnia, it is impossible not to notice the associated agitation and anxiety; however, the attention to it further increases one's internal agitation. High levels of physical activity also produce somatic information on self-efficacy beliefs (Bandura, 1997). When engaging in physical activity, some individuals push themselves to find their limits, to the point of fatigue and pain. Others who are sedentary don't want to know how much their physical capabilities have declined and may cut back on activities to avoid knowing. And finally, physical conditions can draw negative attention to the limitations caused by the physical limitations (Cioffi, 1991). These individuals sometimes become self-monitors of their physical condition and tend to blame other sources, such as sedentariness or fluctuations in their physical state, exclusively for physical impairments (Bandura, 1997). Those who have selective attention to threatening cues judge themselves as inefficacious and are especially prone to misjudging arousal from other sources.

A sense of mastery of previous tasks, validation in comparison with others, and appraisals by knowledgeable others influence the cognitive processing of somatic information when attempting a new task or even in the psychological recovery from physical illness. People who have had a heart attack, for example, are likely to decide how much activity to engage in based on their perception of their cardiac capability (Bandura, 1997). Fatigue, shortness of breath, pain and lack of stamina, which they infer as observable signs of cardiac dysfunction, can also be caused by a sedentary life-style and thus easily misinterpreted. Bandura points out that the difference is in cognitive processing that leads to different perceptions.

In addition to physiological states, mood is an additional source of information for judging self-efficacy beliefs. "People can learn faster if the things they are learning are congruent with the mood they are in and they recall things better if they are in the same mood as when they learned them" (Bandura, 1997, p. 111). This has implications for nurses working with individuals with chronic illness. A positive mood will activate thoughts of past accomplishments and a negative mood will activate thoughts of past failings. So, except for despondency which decreases learning, learning will occur more readily in clients with mood-congruent states. Living with chronic illness can cause despondency, so the nurse can intervene with interventions which increase self-efficacy that, in turn, improve physical and emotional well-being and reduce negative emotional states. By doing so, the nurse sets in motion a process that increases motivation and increases the likelihood of performance accomplishments, which will

increase mood, thereby setting in motion the affirmative reciprocal process (Bandura, 1997).

Outcomes

The most successful self-management programs, using the concept of self-efficacy, have improved outcomes in chronic disease and reduced health care costs by close to 20% (Fries, Koop, Sokolov, Beadle, & Wright, 1998; Lorig et al., 1999). Self-efficacy affects health behavior outcomes in a number of ways. Self-judgments of efficacy can determine which behaviors will be attempted, the amount of effort one will devote to a task, and how long one will persist.

The use of comprehensive self-management programs with individuals who have a chronic disease reveals that those which incorporate self-efficacy have positive effects on health promotion, patient education, clinical practice and patient outcomes (Breslow, 1999; Farrell, Wicks, & Martin, 2004; Fries et al., 1998; Kerse, Flicker, Jolley, Arroll, & Young, 1999; Lorig et al., 1999; Newman, 1993; Nodhturft et al., 2001; Ory & DeFriese, 1998).

The influences of self-efficacy on the pain experience, which is a common symptom in many chronic illnesses, was demonstrated by Dolce and his colleagues (1986). Self-efficacy expectancies were significantly correlated with pain tolerance times and were better predictors of tolerance than pain ratings. Dolce suggested that skills for coping with pain should be taught first if there are deficiencies, and then these skills later reinforced. Again, this supports Bandura's theory that one must believe that one has the skills to perform the behavior before one will attempt the task.

Kaplan, Atkins and Reinch (1984) studied clients with chronic pulmonary obstructive disease and adherence to walking programs. Perceived self-efficacy was a better predictor of participation in the walking program than a locus of control measure.

Helping people find effective, affordable ways to manage "careable"' but not currently "curable" chronic illness presents a formidable task for nurses and all health care professionals. Teaching individuals to cope with the biopsychosocial consequences of chronic illness is an important aspect of care. If we listen, the individual living with a chronic condition tells us how they manage despite the daily hardships they face. We now know that our long held assumption of a sequential progression from intervention to behavior change does not hold true. People report that it is a sense of their ability to effect change that plays an important role in deciding to make behavior change.

Documented successes of self-management programs to reduce pain, increase exercise, improve nutrition, psychological health and differences in hemoglobin Alc should encourage all nurses. We know the programs work, at least partly, because of enhanced self-efficacy. Self-efficacy provides another small piece in the necessary link between knowledge and action in health behavior change and maintenance in chronic illness.

■ Summary and Conclusions

Because chronic disease has become the major cause of disability, research on the relationship between self-efficacy and chronic illness has produced a plethora of studies. Rather than receiving enabling guidance on how to manage their chronic illness, often people are simply given health guidelines which they fail to follow (Bandura, 1987). Issues related to adherence, or their failure to follow these regimens, comes more from lack of belief in their ability to do what is prescribed than from the physical disability, pain or disease activity (Taal, Rasker, Seydel, & Wiegman, 1993). Interventions based on self-efficacy provide hope, because the treatment of chronic illness must focus on a lifetime of self-management.

Study Questions

1. Describe self-efficacy. Differentiate it from coping, health locus of control and self-esteem.
2. Why should we have the goal of self-management of individuals with chronic conditions?
3. What can we as nurses do to enhance self-efficacy in a client with chronic illness?

4. *If you are a circus owner and have to hire a new unicycle rider rather quickly, you would ask the applicants how certain that, given some brief instruction, they could ride a unicycle. You would hire the applicant with the. . . .

*With thanks to Dr. Kate Lorig

References

Abramson, R., Garber, J., & Seligman, M. (1980). Learned helplessness in humans: An attributional analysis. In J. Garber & M. Seligman (Eds.), *Human helplessness: Theory and application.* New York: Academic Press.

Ajzen, J., & Fishbein, M. (1980). *Understanding attitudes and predicting social behavior.* Englewood Cliffs, N.J.: Prentice-Hall.

Bandura, A. (1977a). Self-efficacy: Toward a unifying theory of behavior change. *Psychological Review, 84,* 191–215.

_____. (1977b). *Social learning theory.* Englewood Cliffs, N.J.: Prentice-Hall.

_____. (1986). *Social foundations of thought and actions: A social cognitive theory.* Englewood Cliffs, N.J.: Prentice-Hall.

_____. (1991). Social cognitive theory of self-regulation. *Organizational Behavior and Human Decision Processes, 50,* 248–287.

_____. (Ed.) (1995). *Self-efficacy in changing societies.* New York: Cambridge University Press.

_____. (1997). *Self-efficacy: The exercise of control.* New York: W.H. Freeman and Company.

_____. (2001) Social cognitive theory: An agentive perspective. *Annual Review of Psychology, 52,* 1–26.

Bandura, A., Adams, N., Hardy, A., & Howells, G. (1980). Tests of generality of self-efficacy theory. *Cognitive Therapy and Research, 4,* 39–66.

Bandura, A., & Wood, R. (1989). Effects of controllability and performance standards on self-regulation of complex decision-making. *Journal of Personality and Social Psychology, 56*, 805–814.

Bensley, R. J., Mercer, N., Brusk, J. J., Underhile, R., et al. (2004). The health behavior management model: A stage-based approach to behavior change and management. Preventing Chronic Disease (serial online), retrieved 9/15/2004 from http://www.cdc.gov/pcd/issues/2004/oct/040070.htm.

Breslow, L. (1999). From disease prevention to health promotion, *JAMA, 281*, 1030–1033.

Brody, B., Williams, R., Thomas, R., Kaplan, R., et al. (1999). Age-related macular degeneration: A randomized trial of a self-management interaction. *Annals of Behavioral Medicine, 21* (4), 322–9.

Cioffi, D. (1991). Beyond attentional strategies: A cognitive perceptual model of somatic interpretation. *Psychological Bulletin, 109*, 25–41.

Clark, N., Janz, N., Dodge, J., Sharpe, P. A. et al. (1997). Self-management of heart disease by older adults. *Research on Aging, 19*, 362–382.

Davies, F. & Yates, B. (1982). Self-efficacy expectancies versus outcome expectancies as determinants of performance deficits and depressive affect. *Cognitive Theory and Research, 6*, 23–36.

DiClemente, C. (1986). Self-efficacy and addictive behaviors. *Journal of Clinical and Social Psychology, 4* (3), 302–315.

DiClemente, C., Fairhurst, S., & Piostrowski, N. (1995). Self-efficacy and addictive behavior. In J. E. Maddux (Ed.) *Self-efficacy adaptation and adjustment: Theory, research, and application* (pp. 109–141). New York: Plenum.

Dolce, J., Doleys, D., Raczenski, J., Lossie, J., et al. (1986). The role of self-efficacy expectancies in the prediction of pain tolerance. *Pain, 27*, 261–272.

Farrell, K., Wicks, M. & Martin, J. (2004). Chronic disease self-management improved with enhanced self-efficacy. *Clinical Nursing Research, 13* (4), 289–308.

Fries, J., Koop, C., Sokolov, J., Beadle, C., et al. (1998). Beyond health promotion: Reducing need and demand for medical care. *Health Affairs, 17*, 70–84.

Kaplan, R., Atkins, C., & Reinsch, S. (1984). Specific efficacy expectations mediate exercise compliance in patients with COPD. *Health Psychology, 3*, 223–242.

Kerse, N., Flicker, L., Jolley, D., Arroll, A., et al. (1999). Improving health behavior of elderly people: Randomized controlled trial of a general practice education program. *British Medical Journal, 319*, 683–687.

Lazarus, R. & Folkman. (1984). *Stress, appraisal, and coping.* New York: Springer.

Lenker, S., Lorig, K., & Gallagher, D. (1984). Reasons for the lack of association between changes in health behavior and improved health status: An explanatory study. *Patient Education and Counseling, 6*, 79–72.

Locke, E. & Latham, G. (1990). *A theory of goal setting and task performance.* Englewood Cliffs, N.J.: Prentice-Hall.

Lorig, K. & Holman, H. (2003). Self-management education: History, definition, outcomes, and mechanisms. *Annals of Behavioral Medicine, 26*, 1–7.

Lorig, K., Lubeck, D., Kraines, R., Seleznick M., et al. (1985). Outcomes of self-help education for patients with arthritis. *Arthritis & Rheumatism, 28*, 680–685.

Lorig, K., Mazonson, P., & Holman, H. (1993). Evidence suggesting that health education for self-management in patients with chronic arthritis has sustained health benefits while reducing health care costs. *Arthritis & Rheumatism, 36*, 438–446.

Lorig, K., Seleznick, M., Lubeck, D., Ung, E. et al. (1989). The beneficial outcomes of the arthritis self-management course are not adequately explained by behavior change. *Arthritis & Rheumatism, 32*, 91–95.

Lorig, K., Sobel, D., Stewart, A., et al. (1999). Evidence suggesting that a chronic disease self-management program can improve health status while reducing hospitalization: A randomized trial. *Medical Care, 37*, 5–14.

Lorig, K., Ung, E., Chastain R., Shoor, S., et al. (1989). Development and evaluation of a scale to measure perceived self-efficacy in people with arthritis. *Arthritis & Rheumatism, 32*, 37–44.

Maibach, E. & Flora, J. (1993). Symbolic modeling and cognitive rehearsal. *Communications Research, 20*, 517–545.

Maibach, E. & Murphy, D. (1995). Self-efficacy in health promotion research and practice: Conceptualization and measurement. *Health Education Research, 10*, 37–50.

Mazzuca, S., Moorman, N., Wheeler, M., Norton, J. A. et al. (1986). The diabetes education study: A controlled trial of the effects of diabetes patient education. *Diabetes Care, 9*, 1–10.

Miller, N., & Dollard, J. (1941). *Social learning and imitation.* New Haven, CT: Yale University Press.

Moens, A., Grypdonck, M., & van der Bijl, J. (2002). The development and psychometric testing of an instrument to measure diabetes management self-efficacy in adolescents with type I diabetes. In E. Lentz & L. Shortridge-Baggett (Eds.) *Self-Efficacy in Nursing.* New York: Springer.

Newman, A. (1993). Effects of a self-help program on women with arthritis. In S. Funk, E.Tournquist, M. Champagne, & R. Wiess (Eds.) *Key Aspects of Chronic Pain: Hospital and Home.* New York: Springer.

_____. (1997). Arthritis self-help in minorities: preliminary results. *Arthritis Care and Research, 10* (6), S16.

_____. (2001). Self-management in older African Americans with arthritis. *Geriatric Nursing, 22,* 1–4.

_____. (2003). Self-concept in the nurse client relationship. In F. Arnold & K. Boggs (Eds.), *Interpersonal relationships* (4th ed). St. Louis, MO: Saunders.

Nodhturft, V., Schneider, J., Herbert, P., Bradham, A. D., et al. (2000). Chronic disease management: Improving health outcomes. *Nursing Clinics of North America, 2,* 507–518.

Ory, M., & DeFriese, G. (1998). *Self-care in later life: Research program and policy perspective.* New York: Springer.

Pajares, F. (2002). *Overview of social cognitive theory and of self-efficacy.* Retrieved 10/10/2004 from http://www.emory.edu/EDUCATION/mfp/eff.html.

Perraud, S. (2000). Development of the depression coping self-efficacy scale (DCSES). *Archives of Psychiatric Nursing, 14* (6), 276–284.

Rosenthal, T. L. (1982). Social learning theory. In T. G. Wilson & C. M. Franks (Eds.), *Contemporary behavior therapy* (pp. 339–363). New York: Guilford Press.

Sarason, I. (1975). Test anxiety and the self-disclosing coping model. *Journal of Consulting and Clinical Psychology, 43,* 148–153.

Schunk, D. H. (1984). Self-efficacy perspective on achievement behavior. *Educational Psychologist, 19,* 48–58.

Schunk, D. H., & Pajares, F. (2002). The development of academic self-efficacy. In A. Wigfield & J. Eccles (Eds.) *Development of achievement motivation* (pp. 16–31). San Diego: Academic Press.

Strecher, V., DeVellis, B., Becker, M., & Rosenstock, I. (1986). The role of self-efficacy in achieving health and behavior change. *Health Education Quarterly, 13* (11), 73–91.

Taal, E., Rasker, J., Seydel, E., & Wiegman, O. (1993). Health status, adherence with health recommendations, self-efficacy and social support in patients with rheumatoid arthritis. *Patient Education and Counseling, 20,* 63–76.

Van der Bijl, J. & Shortridge-Baggett, L. (2002). The theory and measurement of the self-efficacy construct. In E. Lentz & L. Shortridge-Baggett (Eds.) *Self-Efficacy in Nursing.* New York: Springer.

Von Korff, M., Moore, J., Lorig, K., Cherkin, D. C., et al. (1998). A randomized trial of a lay person-led self-management group intervention for back pain patients in primary care. *Spine, 23,* 2608–2615.

Wallston, B., & Wallston, K. (1984). Social psychological models of health behaviors: An examination and integration. In A. Brown, S. Taylor, & J. Singer (Eds.), *Handbook of psychology and health: Vol. IV.* Hillsdale, N.J.: Erlbaum.

Weiner, B. (1985). An attributional theory of achievement motivation and emotion. *Psychological Review, 92,* 548–573.

▋ Note

An excellent source of information on self-efficacy can be found at www.emory.edu/EDUCATION/mfp/effpage.html

CHAPTER 6

Social Isolation

Diana Luskin Biordi

Introduction

Most of us actively seek human companionship or relationships. The lives of hermits or cloistered, solitary existences are extraordinary because they so vividly remind us that, usually, life is richer for the human contact we share. As valuable as life may be when we engage in a variety of relationships, time reserved for solitude is also necessary as we seek rest or contemplative opportunity in "our own space." The weaving together of individual possibilities for social engagement or solitude develops a certain uniqueness and texture in personal and community relationships. These distinctive personal configurations of engagement and disengagement have consequences for our work and social lives. It is critical, therefore, that health professionals understand the value of social engagement and solitude.

When Is Isolation a Problem?

Social isolation ranges from the long-term isolate to the voluntary isolate who seeks disengagement from social intercourse for a variety of reasons to those whose isolation is involuntary or imposed by others. Privacy or being alone, if actively chosen, has the potential for enhancing the human psyche. On the other hand, involuntary social isolation occurs when an individual's demand for social contacts or communications exceeds the human or situation capability of others. Involuntary isolation is negatively viewed because the outcomes are the dissolution of social exchanges and the support they provide for the individual or their support system(s). Some persons, such as those with cognitive deficits, may not understand their involuntarily isolation, but their parent, spouse, or other significant person may indeed understand that involuntary social isolation can have a negative and profound impact on caregiver and care recipient.

When social isolation is experienced negatively by an individual or his or her significant other, it becomes a problem that requires management. In fact, according to much of the literature, only physical functional disability ranks with social isolation in its impact on the client and the client's social support network (family, friends, fellow workers, and so forth). Therefore, social isolation is one of the two most important aspects of chronic illness to be managed in the plan of care.

Distinctions of Social Isolation

Social isolation is viewed from the perspective of the number, frequency, and quality of contacts;

the longevity or durability of these contacts; and the negativism attributed to the isolation felt by the individual involved. Social isolation has been the subject of the humanities for hundreds of years. Who has not heard of John Donne's exclamation, "No man is an island," or, conversely, the philosophy of existentialism—that humans are ultimately alone? Yet the concept of social isolation has been systematically researched only during the past 50 years. Unlike some existentialists and social scientists, health care professionals, with their problem-oriented, clinical approach, tend to regard social isolation as negative rather than positive.

The Nature of Isolation

Isolation can occur at four layers of the concept *social*. The outermost layer is *community*, where one feels integrated or isolated from the larger social structure. Next is the layer of *organization* (work, schools, churches), followed by a layer closer to the person, that is, *confidantes* (friends, family, significant others). Finally, the innermost layer is that of the *person*, who has the personality, the intellectual ability, or the senses with which to apprehend and interpret relationships (Lin, 1986).

In the health care literature, the primary focus is on the clinical dyad, so the examination of social isolation tends to be confined to the levels of confidante and person and only extends to the organization and community for single clients, one at a time. For the health care worker, the most likely relationships are bound to expectations of individually centered reciprocity, mutuality, caring, and responsibility. On the other hand, health policy literature tends to focus on the reciprocity of community and organizations to populations of individuals, and so it deals with collective social isolation.

At the level of the clinical dyad, four patterns of social isolation or interaction have been identified; while these were originally formulated with elders in mind, they can be analogized easily to younger persons by making them age relative:

1. Persons who have been integrated into social groups throughout their lifetime

2. The "early isolate," who was isolated as an adult but is relatively active in old age

3. The "recent isolate," who was active in early adulthood but is not in old age

4. The "lifelong isolate," whose life is one of isolation

Feelings That Reflect Isolation

Social isolation can be characterized by feelings of *boredom* and *marginality* or exclusion (Weiss, 1973). Boredom occurs because of the lack of validation of one's work or daily routines; therefore, these tasks become only busy work. Marginality is the sense of being excluded from desired networks or groups.

Description and Characteristics of Social Isolation

The existence of social isolation increases our awareness of the need for humans to associate with each other in an authentic intimate relationship, whether characterized by caring or some other emotion, such as anger. When we speak of social isolation, we think first of the affected person; then we almost immediately consider that individual's relationships. This chapter will demonstrate that, as a process, social isolation may be a feature in a variety of illnesses and disabilities across the life cycle.

As an ill person becomes more aware of the constricting network and declining participation, he or she may feel sadness, anger, despair, or reduced self-esteem. These emotions factor into a changed social and personal identity, but are also separate issues for the person who is chronically ill. Moreover, depending on their own emotional and physical needs, friends and acquaintances may drop out of a person's social support system until only the most loyal remain (Tilden & Weinert, 1987). Families, however, are likely to remain in the social network. As the social network reaches its limitations, it may itself become needful of interventions, such as respite care for the parents of a child who is chronically ill or support groups for the siblings of children with cancer (Heiney et al., 1990).

Social Isolation Versus Similar States of Human Apartness

Social isolation has been treated as a distinct phenomenon, or it has been combined or equated with other states relating to human apartness. The literature is replete with a variety of definitions of *social isolation,* many of which are interrelated, synonymous, or confused with other distinct but related phenomena.

Social Isolation and Alienation

Social isolation and alienation have been linked together or treated as synonymous in much of the health care literature, although they differ from one another. Alienation encompasses powerlessness, normlessness, isolation, self-estrangement, and meaninglessness (Seeman, 1959). *Powerlessness* refers to the belief held by an individual that one's own behaviors cannot elicit the results one desires or seeks. In *normlessness,* the individual has a strong belief that socially unapproved behaviors are necessary to achieve goals. *Isolation* means the inability to value highly held goals or beliefs that others usually value. *Self-estrangement* has come to mean the divorce of one's self from one's work or creative possibilities. Finally, *meaninglessness* is the sense that few significant predictions about the outcomes of behavior can be made. Thus, one can see that isolation is only one psychological state of alienation. However, authors frequently merge the finer points of one or more of the five dimensions of alienation and call the result *isolation.*

Social Isolation and Loneliness

While social isolation is typically viewed today as a deprivation in social contacts, Peplau and Perlman (1986) suggest that it is loneliness, not social isolation, that occurs when an individual perceives her or his social relationships as not containing the desired quantity or quality of social contacts. In an even more subtle distinction, Hoeffer (1987) found that simply the *perception* of relative social isolation was more predictive of loneliness than actual isolation. *Loneliness* has been referred to as an alienation of the self and is sometimes seen as global, generalized, disagreeable, uncomfortable, and more terrible than anxiety (Austin, 1989). Loneliness differs from depression in that in loneliness, one attempts to integrate oneself into new relationships, whereas in depression, there is a surrendering of oneself to the distress (Weiss, 1973).

Nonetheless, loneliness does relate to social isolation. In fact, loneliness is the one concept most invoked when social isolation is considered (Dela Cruz, 1986; Hoeffer, 1987; Mullins & Dugan, 1990; Ryan & Patterson, 1987). However, to use *social isolation* and *loneliness* as interchangeable terms can be confusing. To maintain clarity, loneliness should be considered the *subjective emotional affect* of the individual, while social isolation is *the objective state of deprivation* of social contact and content (Bennet, 1980). Thus, *loneliness* refers to the psychological state of the individual, whereas *social isolation* relates to the sociological status. While it is true that social isolation might lead to loneliness, loneliness is not, in itself, a necessary condition of social isolation. Both conditions can exist apart from each other.

Peplau and Perlman's view of loneliness might be confused with the nursing diagnosis, *Impaired Social Interaction,* defined in almost identical terms (NANDA, 2001). However, this diagnosis refers to a negative state of social exchanges in which the quantity or quality of participation is dysfunctional or ineffective (Gordon, 1982; Tilden & Weinert, 1987). Impaired social interaction and social isolation feed into each other, because they have similar causes and the effects of each diagnosis overlap.

Interestingly, Carpenito (1995) notes that *Risk of Loneliness,* added to the NANDA list in 1994, is a better diagnostic description of the negative state of aloneness. In Carpenito's definition, loneliness is a "subjective state that exists whenever a person says it does and is perceived as imposed by others." Referring to NANDA's lists as response-oriented, she further argues that Social Isolation as a nursing diagnosis is incorrect because it is not a response, but a cause, of apartness, and she recommends that it be dropped as a diagnostic category. However, Carpenito's discussion of loneliness often substitutes social isolation for loneliness, which blurs the distinction she wishes to make. Furthermore, as is demonstrated in this chapter, social isolation becomes cause, process, or response, depending on analysis and circumstances. The complex sets of variables that figure into social isolation lend themselves to a variety of assessments, diagnoses, and interventions: Loneliness is only one aspect of social isolation.

Social Isolation and Aloneness

Tightly linked to social isolation is the need for social support, which is the social context or environment that facilitates the survival of human beings (Lin, 1986) by offering social, emotional, and material support needed and received by an individual, especially one who is chronically ill. While social support literature has focused on the instrumental and material benefits of support, recent literature on social isolation relates isolation more to the negative feeling state of aloneness. This feeling is associated with deficits in social support networks, diminished participation in these networks or in social relationships, or feelings of rejection or withdrawal.

Social Isolation as a Nursing Diagnosis

Social isolation is defined in the nursing literature as "aloneness experienced by the individual and perceived as imposed by others as a negative or threatening state" (NANDA, 2001). That is, despite a need or desire to do so, and because of circumstances imposed on them, individuals are unable to participate fully or meaningfully in social relationships that are important to them (Carpenito, 1995). Note that Carpenito does not include the caveat that the social isolation is imposed by others. It may be that, initially, either the socially isolated withdrew from their social network or that others withdrew from the isolate. Regardless of who initiates it, the isolation frequently becomes reciprocal.

Three critical characteristics were originally described as necessary and sufficient conditions for this diagnosis: (1) absence of supportive significant others, (2) verbalized feeling of aloneness imposed by others, and (3) verbalized feeling of rejection (NANDA, 2001). Other characteristics have since been added to expand these conditions for diagnosis: apathy, seclusion, few contacts with peers, verbalized awareness of isolation, and the lack or absence of contacts with significant others or the community (Gordon, 1989).

At least 20 subjective and objective characteristics of social isolation have now been identified by various nurses, most of which express rejection, alienation, or the absence of critical significant others. An important study of this nursing diagnosis was done in respect to the elderly (Lien-Gieschen, 1993). Eighteen defining characteristics of social isolation were identified, five specific to the elderly. However, the single major identifying characteristic with this population was the absence of supportive significant others. In this study, nurses validated only ages over 75 as characteristic of social isolation.

This single validation study of social isolation as a nursing diagnosis indicates that nurses typically focus on substantive characteristics of social isolation itself (Lien-Gieschen, 1993). As mentioned, the chief characteristic that was validated was lack of supportive others, but several more associated characteristics were identified that fell within broad categories of dull affect, preoccupation with one's own thoughts, loss of meaning or purpose in life, lack of communication, a personal sense or act of apartness, or sensory deficits. As can be seen from the descriptors that have been identified, the nursing view of social isolation is rather holistic and resonates strongly with earlier dimensions of the concepts of alienation and loneliness.

Problems and Issues of Social Isolation

Regardless of how the social isolation occurs, the result is that basic needs for authentic intimacy remain unmet. Typically this is perceived as alienating or unpleasant, and the social isolation that occurs can lead to depression, loneliness, or other social and cognitive impairments that then exacerbate the isolation.

Several predisposing reasons for social isolation have been proposed: status-altering physical disabilities or illnesses; frailties associated with advanced age or developmental delays; personality or neurological disorders; and environmental constraints, which often refer to physical surroundings but are also interpreted by some to include diminished personal or material resources (Tilden & Weinert, 1987).

The Isolation Process

A typical course of isolation that evolves as an illness or disability becomes more apparent is the change in social network relationships. Friends or families begin to withdraw from the isolated individual or the individual from them. This process may be slow or subtle, as with individuals with arthritis, or it may be rapid, as with the person with AIDS. Unfortunately, the process of isolation may not be based on accurate or rational information. For example, one woman with cancer reported that, at a party, she was served her drink in a plastic cup while everyone else had glasses (Spiegel, 1990).

Individuals with serious chronic illnesses come to perceive themselves as different from others and outside the mainstream of ordinary life (Williams & Bury, 1989). This perception of being different may be shared by others, who may then reject them, their disability, and their differentness. Part of this sense of being different can stem from the ongoing demands of the illness. For example, social relationships are interrupted because families and friends cannot adjust the erratic treatment to acceptable social activities. From such real events, or from social perceptions, social isolation can occur, either as a process or as an outcome.

Individuals who are chronically ill often face their own mortality more explicitly than do others. For example, unmarried or younger cancer patients express a loss of meaning in life; suggested to be due to cancer's threat to their lives as they grapple with

the meaning of life; they may withdraw from their networks or the networks may withdraw from them (Noyes et al., 1990; Weisman & Worden, 1977; Woods, Haberman & Packard, 1993).

Even if death does not frighten those who are chronically ill, it frequently frightens those in their social networks, which leads to guilt, and can lead to strained silences and withdrawal. In the case of individuals with cancer (Burnley, 1992; House, Landis & Umberson, 1988; Reynolds & Kaplan, 1990) or heart disease (Kaplan et al., 1988; Orth-Gomer, Unden & Edwards, 1988), social support is significant to their survival. For those who lack this social support, social isolation is not merely a metaphor for death but can hasten it.

Social Isolation and Stigma

Social isolation may occur as one effect of stigma. Many persons will risk anonymity rather than expose themselves to a judgmental audience. Because chronic illnesses can be stigmatizing, the concern about the possibility of revealing a discredited or discreditable self can slow or paralyze social interaction (see Chapter 3, on stigma). In a study examining chronic sorrow in HIV positive patients, stigma created social isolation. Women with children, particularly African American women, were more stigmatized and isolated than gay men because others perceived the women as associated with "dirty sex", contagion, and moral threat (Lichtenstein, Laska, & Clair, 2002). Thus, social roles and the robustness of network support affect social isolation.

The chronically ill or their families grapple with how much information about the diagnosis they should share, with whom, and when (Gallo et al., 1991). If the illness is manageable or reasonably invisible, its presence may be hidden from all but a select few, often for years. Parents of children with chronic illnesses were reported to manage stressful encounters and uncertainty by disguising, withholding, or limiting information to others (Cohen, 1993), an action that may add to limiting their social network. Jessop and Stein (1985) found that invisible illnesses of chronically ill children led to greater difficulty in social interactions because of the uncertainty of ambiguity (disagreement about revealing or passing, or what courses of action to take). For example, parents of a child with cystic fibrosis may tell a teacher that the child is taking pills with meals because of a digestive disease (Cohen, 1993).

As siblings of children with cancer deal with the isolation of their brother or sister, they became vulnerable to being socially isolated themselves (Bendor, 1990). Social isolation not only burdens the chronically ill, it also extends into family dynamics and requires the health professional to consider how the family manages. Nurses must explicitly plan for the isolation in families with children who are chronically ill (Tamlyn & Arklie, 1986). Thus, social isolation is not only a burden for the chronically ill that extends into family dynamics, it requires the health professional to consider how the family manages the illness and the isolation.

Where the stigmatized disability is quite obvious, as in the visibility of burn scars or the odor of colitis, the person who is chronically ill might venture only within small circles of understanding individuals (Gallo et al., 1991). Where employment is possible, it will often be work that does not require many social interactions, such as night work or jobs within protected environments (sheltered workshops, home offices). Regardless of what serves as reminders of the disability, the disability is incorporated into the isolate's sense of self; that is, it becomes part of his or her social and personal identity.

Social Isolation and Social Roles

Any weakening or diminishment of relationships or social roles might produce social isolation for individuals or their significant others. Clients who lose family, friends, and associated position and power are inclined to feelings of rejection, worthlessness, and loss of self-esteem (Ravish, 1985). These feelings become magnified by the client's culture if that culture values community (Siplic & Kadis, 2002; Litwin & Zoabi, 2003). An example of social isolation of both caregiver and care recipient

occurred in a situation of a woman whose husband had Alzheimer's disease. The couple had been confined for more than two years in an apartment in a large city, from which her confused husband frequently wandered. Her comment, "I'm not like a wife and not like a single person either," reflected their dwindling social network and her loss of wifely privileges but not obligations. This ambiguity is common to many whose spouses are incapacitated. Moreover, after a spouse dies, the widow or widower often grieves as much for the loss of the role of a married person as for the loss of the spouse.

The loss of social roles can occur as a result of illness or disability, social changes throughout the life span (e.g., in school groups, with career moves, or in unaccepting communities), marital dissolution (through death or divorce), or secondary to ostracism incurred by membership in a "wrong" group. The loss of social roles and the resultant isolation of the individual have been useful analytical devices in the examination of issues of the aged, the widowed, the physically impaired, or in psychopathology.

The Elderly and Social Isolation

Old age, with its many losses of physical health, social roles, and economic status, contributes to a decreasing social network and increasing isolation (Creecy et al., 1985; Ryan & Patterson, 1987; Trout, 1980; Victor, Scambler, Shah, Cook, Harris, Rink & DeWilde, 2002). The location of the home, access to transportation or buildings, and altered immobility have all been implicated in social isolation for this population.

Strictly speaking, social isolation is not confined to a place. The socially isolated are not necessarily homebound or place-bound, although that is typically the case (Ryan & Patterson, 1987; Stephens & Bernstein, 1984; Watson, 1988). That being said, however, environments that are removed (such as rural locations) or those not conducive to safety (such as high-crime areas) can contribute to social isolation (Glassman-Feibusch, 1981; Kivett, 1979; Krause, 1993; Lyons, 1982, Klinenberg, 2001). Social isolation as a function of location has been demonstrated, particularly for the elderly in urbanized settings, in a number of countries other than the United States. (Klinenberg, 2001; Russell & Schofield, 1999. In these cases, elderly individuals cannot leave their homes for lack of transportation or for fear of assault, so they increasingly isolate themselves from others. This situation is intensified by distrust or by lower levels of education, and it is worse if the elderly have chronic illnesses compounding their constraints.

One objective of planned senior housing is to provide individuals with a ready-made social network within a community (Lawton, Kleban & Carlson, 1973; Lawton, Greenbaum & Liebowitz, 1980; Lawton, Moss & Grimes, 1985), although this objective is not always met. Through such a social network, it is hoped that social isolation would be counteracted among the elderly living in these communities. However, the frail elderly are found to be less interactive with more mobile, healthier elderly, possibly because healthier elderly have few extra resources to expend on others who may have even fewer resources, or they may have better health and networks that are incongruent with, and less likely to cross those of the frail elderly (Heumann, 1988).

Nursing home residents with chronic illness or sensory impairments tend to be more isolated than others. In England, for instance, those in residential care who are ill or disabled are considered socially dead, impoverished by the inactive nature of institutionalization and unable to occupy any positive, valued role in the community (Watson, 1988). Stephens and Bernstein (1984) found that older, sicker residents were more socially isolated than healthier residents. The investigators found that family and longer-standing friendships served as better buffers to social isolation than did other residents.

Social isolation has been linked to confusion, particularly in elderly chronically ill individuals. But when the socially isolated are also immobilized, the combination of isolation and immobilization can lead to greater impairments, such as perceptual and behavioral changes (e.g., noncompliance or time distortions) (Stewart, 1986). Physical barriers (such as physical plant designs) or architectural features (such as too-heavy doors) also contribute to social isolation or homeboundedness (DesRosier, Catanzaro & Piller, 1992). All of these limits contribute to social isolation in ways that motivation alone cannot easily overcome.

Social Isolation and Culture

As globalization increases, with its concurrent absorbing of multiethnic, multilingual, and multireligious individuals into other cultures, there is an overlapping into mainstream health care systems. This is especially true of cultural groups that have not assimilated into the dominant culture. Language differences and traditional living arrangements may impede social adaptations. In addition, many immigrants, especially those who are chronically ill, are less able to engage in support networks, given their long working hours, low-paying jobs, lack of health insurance, and changes in family life-styles and living arrangements. Changes may occur over the second and third generations, but this is less true where the immigrants' home cultures are geographically close, such as Mexican Americans who live along the United States–Mexican border, or have reminders of traditions that are more visible (Jones, Bond & Cason, 1998).

An extensive literature review on health care and its relationship to culture showed two overarching issues: (1) The definitions of culture are conceptually broad and/or indistinct, and (2) mainstream health care struggles to integrate these multicultural groups with varying degrees of success. When one speaks of "culture," many concepts are mixed, even confused (Habayeb, 1995). The dominant White society in the United States and its health care system is secular, individualistic, technology- and science-oriented, and tends to be male dominated (Borman & Biordi, 1992; Smith, 1996). Other European-based cultures have similar situations. Social isolation must be viewed from the client's cultural definition of the numbers, frequency, and quality of contacts, the longevity or durability of these contacts, and the negativism attributed to the isolation felt by the individual involved.

Studies done during the past decade indicate how women, minority groups, the poor, and so forth, have not received the same care as the dominant male Caucasian middle or upper classes (Fiscella et al., 2000). Fortunately, current cultural health care literature indicates a greater awareness of cultural groups and their values. One factor that may be influencing this change is that during the past two decades, other health care providers, including nurses, psychologists, case managers, and a variety of technical support personnel, have made subsequent changes in health care (Biordi, 2000).

Many ethnic and religious groups in the United States value community closeness, family kinship, geographic proximity, and social communication. They seek acknowledgment of their right to mainstream or alternative care (Cheng, 1997; Helton, 1995; Keller & Stevens, 1997; Kim, 1998; Kreps & Kreps, 1997). Attempting to deliver "tailored" culturally competent care to so many groups is overwhelming and lacks an integrating strategy that appeals across all groups. One can now find a large number of articles providing hints, tips, or insights into cultural groups for mainstream health providers.

Social Components of Social Isolation

Mere numbers of people surrounding someone does not cure negative social isolation; an individual can be socially isolated even in a crowd if one's significant social network is lost. This situation is true for such groups as those living or working in sheltered-care workshops, residents in long-term care facilities, or people in prisons. What is critical to social isolation is that, because of situations imposed on them, individuals *perceive* themselves as disconnected from meaningful discourse with people important to them.

Associated with social isolation is reciprocity or mutuality, that is, the amount of give and take that can occur between isolated individuals and their social networks. Throughout the years, much evidence has accumulated to indicate that informal networks

of social support offer significant emotional assistance, information, and material resources for a number of different populations. These support systems appear to foster good health, help maintain appropriate behaviors, and alleviate stress (Cobb, 1979; DiMatteo & Hays, 1981; Stephens & Bernstein, 1984).

Examining reciprocity in the relationships of social networks focuses not only on social roles and the content of the exchange, but also on the level of agreement between the isolated person and his or her "others" in the network (Goodman, 1984; Randers, Mattiasson, & Olson, 2003). The incongruence between respondents in a social network regarding their exchanges can help alert the health care provider to the level of emotional or material need or exhaustion that exists in either respondent. For example, this author observed, during a visit by a nurse, that a homebound elderly woman complained that her children had done very little for her. However, it was discovered that the children visited every day, brought meals, shopped for their mother, and managed her financial affairs. In this case, the elderly mother felt isolated notwithstanding her children's visits and assistance.

Demographics and Social Isolation

Few studies focus directly on demographic variables and social isolation; typically, this topic is embedded in other research questions across a variety of illnesses. Nevertheless, when these disparate studies are taken together, the impact of demographics on social isolation in the chronically ill is evident. Issues of gender, marital status, family position and context, and socioeconomic standing (such as education or employment) have been shown to affect social isolation.

Socioeconomic Factors

Changes in socioeconomic status, such as employment status, have been correlated with social isolation. The lack of employment of both caregiver and care recipient, cited in much of the caregiver literature, can have an adverse effect. A study of caregivers of frail elderly veterans noted that these caregivers are more at risk for physical, emotional, and financial strain than are other populations because disabled elderly veterans receive fewer long-term care services than do other elderly populations (Dorfman, Homes & Berlin, 1996).

Unemployment of the elderly is just one component of the maturational continuum; parents worry about the potential for employment and insurance for their children who have chronic illnesses (Cohen, 1993; Wang & Barnard, 2004). Lower income status, especially when coupled with less education, negatively influences health status and is associated with both a limiting social network and greater loneliness, which, in turn, impacts health status and social isolation (Cox, Spiro & Sullivan, 1988; Williams & Bury, 1989). For instance, almost half of the head-injured clients in one study could not work, which then affected their families' economic status and increased their social isolation (Kinsella, Ford & Moran, 1989).

In addition to problems of employment potential, there are economic and social concerns over the costs incurred by health care, employment discrimination, subsequent inability to secure insurance, and loss of potential friendship networks at work—all of which are factors in increasing social isolation or reducing social interactions. In fact, economics exaggerates the costs of chronic illness. People with disabilities suffer disproportionately in the labor market, which then affects their connections with family and community social networks (Christ, 1987). This is particularly evident in the examination of the mentally ill and their social isolation (Chinman, Weingarten, Stayner, & Davidson, 2001; Melle, Friis, Hauff, & Vaglum, 2000).

General Family Factors

As chronic illness persists, and given tasks that must be managed, relationships are drained, leaving individuals with chronic illness at high risk for social isolation (Berkman, 1983; Tilden & Weinert, 1987). When isolation does occur, it can be a long-term reality for the individual and their family. However, if there is social support and involvement, people with chronic illnesses tend toward psychological well-being. Particularly important is the adequacy, more than the availability, of social relationships (Wright, 1995; Zimmer, 1995).

There is evidence that social isolation does not necessarily occur in every situation. In fact, the negative impact of social isolation on families with children who are chronically ill has been questioned. One study, which used a large community-based, random sample, found that families with children who are chronically ill did not experience a greater degree of social isolation than those with healthy children, nor did they function differently, except for modest increases in maternal dysfunction (Cadman et al., 1991). Cadman and his associates argue that prior studies were subject to biases because the families in those studies were in the clinic populations of the hospital or agency. By definition, such populations were receiving care for illnesses or responses to illnesses and hence were suffering from an unusual aggregation of problems, which is why they were at the clinic or hospital. Therefore, such families were not representative families from those throughout the community.

In another study, classroom teachers evaluated children with cancer or sickle cell disease with a matched sample of controls. The authors found that the children who were chronically ill were remarkably resilient in the classroom setting, although those who survived their brain tumors and could attend regular classes were perceived as more sensitive and isolated (Noll et al., 1992). On the other hand, adolescents with chronic illnesses have been marginalized, which predisposes them to feelings of isolation and low self worth (DiNapoli & Murphy, 2002).

Similarly, some studies of elderly individuals found that isolation did not always occur as they aged (Victor et al., 2002). Although childless elderly individuals tend to be more socially isolated than those with children, when adult children live nearby, older people frequently interact with at least one of them (Mullins & Dugan, 1990). Interestingly, older African American women, even if they lived alone, tended to have more visits from their children than did older African American men; the difference was not explained by needs, resources, or child/gender availability (Spitz & Miner, 1992). It is also interesting to note that older people tend to be less influenced by their children than by contacts with other relatives, friends, and associates (Berkman, 1983; Ryan & Patterson, 1987). One study found no relation between the elders' emotional well-being and the frequency of interaction with their children (Lee & Ellithorpe, 1982).

Findings indicate that in *every* group from 30 to over 70 years of age, it was primarily those with the fewest social and community ties who were nearly three times as likely to die as those with more ties (Berkman, 1983). In other words, maintaining social contacts enhanced longevity. These individuals tended to be widowers or widows and lacked membership in formal groups (Berkman, 1983), thereby limiting their social contacts. In another study, the elderly who lived in senior housing complexes showed little difference in friendship patterns and life satisfaction (Poulin, 1984). Both of these studies found that living alone, being single, or not having family does not necessarily imply social isolation. Rather, if older people have social networks, many developed throughout a lifetime, and if these networks remain available to them, they are provided with support when needed (Berkman, 1983).

Gender and Marital Status

Typically, women have more extensive and varied social networks than do men (Antonucci, 1985). However, if one spouse is chronically ill, married couples spend more time together and less time with networks and activities outside the home (Des-Rosier, Catanzaro & Piller, 1992; Foxall, Eckberg & Griffith, 1986; Smith, 2003). Although gender differences in caregiving occur (Miller, 1990; Tilden & Weinert, 1987), women caregivers indicate greater isolation, increased loneliness, and decreased life satisfaction than do men. Yet both genders show psychological improvement if social contacts, by telephone or in person, increase (Foxall, Eckberg & Griffith, 1986).

While women caregivers may have professional, community, and social networks to aid them in coping with their disabled spouses, over time they reduce their links to these potential supports. Physical work, social costs and barriers, preparation time for care and outings, and other demands of caregiving become so extreme that women curtail access to and use of support networks external to home. As these caregivers narrow their use of social networks, they unwittingly isolate their chronically ill spouse as well. Although women reported needing personal or psychological time alone for relief, the subject of their isolation, the chronically ill person, also became their greatest confidante as the pair struggle in their joint isolation (DesRosier, Catanzaro & Piller, 1992).

Illness Factors and Social Isolation

Chronic illness is multidimensional, and persons who are chronically ill or their networks must assume a variety of tasks: managing treatment regimens, controlling symptoms, preventing and managing crises, reordering time, managing the illness trajectory, dealing with health care professionals, normalizing life, preserving a reasonable self-image, keeping emotional balance, managing social isolation, funding the costs of health care, and preparing for an uncertain future (Strauss et al., 1984) (see Chapter 2, on illness behavior and roles). As people with chronic illnesses struggle to understand their body failure and maintain personal and social identities, they may become fatigued, sicker, or lose hope more readily. Should this happen, they may more easily withdraw from their social networks.

It has been suggested that isolation not only impacts on the individual's social network (Newman et al., 1989), but also can lead to depression and even suicide (Lyons, 1982; Trout, 1980), particularly in the elderly (Frierson, 1991). Women whose illnesses required more physical demands on themselves and greater symptom management reported greater depression but no effect on their relationship with their partner. Women who had concerns about the meaning of their illness reported greater marital distress and lower satisfaction with their family network (Woods, Haberman & Packard, 1993).

Persons with the human immunodeficiency virus (HIV) or acquired immune deficiency syndrome (AIDS) had psychological effects that depended not only on the diagnosis, but also on the age of the person. Older individuals showed significant differences in a number of variables, including social isolation (Catalan, 1998). In addition, HIV-negative men who cared for their partners or friends often lived in social isolation with their care recipients (Mallinson, 1999).

In the case of people with severe head injuries, it was not the chronic physical disability that disrupted family cohesion as much as the resulting social impairment (Kinsella, Ford & Moran, 1989). The greatest burden identified was social isolation brought on by the impaired self-control of the head-injured and their inability to learn from social experience. However, the social isolation was particularly burdensome for the families, because the head injury reduced the client's capacity for recognition of and reflection on the deficiencies in social relationships and precluded formation of new close relationships. Consequently, although friendships and employment possibilities were reduced for the client, the real impact was felt by the constrained family (Kinsella, Ford & Moran, 1989).

Health Care Perspectives

People with chronic illnesses struggle to understand their body failure and its effect on their activities and lives (Corbin & Strauss, 1987). In doing so, they also struggle to maintain their sense of personal and social identity, often in the face of altered self-image and enormous financial, psychological, and social obstacles. If individuals with chronic illness lose hope or become otherwise incapacitated, they may withdraw from their social networks, isolating themselves and others important to them.

Frequently, the daily management of illness means working with health care professionals who often do not recognize the inconspicuous but daily struggles of the person's realities of a "new" body, the issues of care, and the development of a new self-identity (Corbin & Strauss, 1987; Dropkin, 1989; Hopper, 1981).

With the advent of high technology, the aging of the population, and changes in economics, chronic illness has begun to assume major proportions in the United States. Concomitantly, the literature has more articles describing various chronic illnesses, the strategies used to manage them, and issues of social and psychological well-being, including social isolation. More recently, the literature has been extended to consider how chronic illnesses and related technologies are impacted by cultural variety.

The impact of prevailing paradigms of care interventions held by various constituencies is evident. For example, most health care professionals still see clients only episodically, usually using the medical model of "cure" and within the model of the dominant heath care system. But, in the case of children with cancer, the child focuses on the meaning of his or her impairment (which varies by age); the parents focus first on the immediate concern with their child's longevity and cure and later on the impairment and long-term effects; the health professional focuses on client survival; the mental health professional focuses on identifying and minimizing impact, impairments, and social barriers; and the public (third-party payers, employers, schoolmates, partners) focuses on contributions and cost. All of these views center on the interaction and exchange, as well as the specific responsibilities and obligations, incurred by the various networks that touch them. Interactions are intensified by the potential withdrawal of any party from the network (Christ, 1987).

Given the variety of care-versus-cure paradigms, the real, daily micro-impositions of chronic illness on social identity and social networks are often lost. The compassion felt by many health care professionals is evident in the increasing number of articles available and the attempts to present evidence of the isolation felt by clients and their networks. Nevertheless, these articles may not be explicit; therefore, the proposed interventions for the isolate are unclear, irrelevant, or even discouraging. For example, when discussing facial disfigurement, one article noted that the health professional expected evidence of the client's image integration as early as *1 week* postsurgery (Dropkin, 1989). That same article suggested and reiterated that, although the surgery was necessary for removal of the cancer, the resulting *defect* was confined to a relatively small aspect of the anatomy and that the alteration in appearance or function did not change the person (Dropkin, 1989). Both points of emphasis are added. The terminology and the interventions in this article focused on the acute postoperative period and did not take into account what disfigured clients were likely to feel later than 1 week postsurgery or that the word *defect* gives a strong clue to the understanding that the disfiguring surgery is obvious and emotionally charged toward the negative.

For a clearer view of the impact of such surgery as seen by the client, Gamba et al. (1992) asked postsurgical patients, grouped by the extent of their facial disfigurement, questions about their self-image, relationship with their partner and social network, and overall impact of the therapy. Those with extensive disfigurement reported that it was "like putting up with something undesirable" (p. 221), and many patients were unable to touch or look at themselves. Those with extensive disfigurement also reported more social isolation, poor self-image, and/or a worsened sexual relationship with their partner, even though they maintained satisfactory relationships with their children. In another study, reported in the Gamba article, half of the individuals who underwent hemimandibulectomy for head and neck cancers became social recluses, compared with 11 percent of patients who had laryngectomies. As can be seen, in more than one study respondents attached a negative meaning to their disfiguring surgery and its results.

Such findings take into account the client's personal meaning of illness and treatment and their effects on social isolation, demonstrating that the isolating treatment or illness (e.g., disfigurement) often is not associated with objective disability. In fact, others have found that the degree of isolation is *not* directly proportional to the extent of disability (Creed, 1990; Fitzpatrick et al., 1991; Maddox, 1985; Newman et al., 1989). It is important that health professionals not ignore or discount the meaning of illness to the client, regardless of any professional opinion about objective disability or the desirability of treatment.

Interventions: Counteracting Social Isolation

In social isolation, the interventions of choice need to remain at the discretion of the client or caregiver. As can be seen from this chapter, writers focus largely on definitions and correlates of social isolation and relatively less on interventions. When interventions are reported, they often relate to the aggregate, such as the policy-related interventions of community housing. The results of many of these larger scale interventions have been noted in this chapter. Other interventions are mentioned here, although the list is not all-inclusive.

Because the situation of each person with chronic illness is unique, interventions can be expected to vary. Nonetheless, certain useful techniques and strategies can be generalized (Dela Cruz, 1986). Basically, these strategies require that a balance of responsibilities be developed between the health care professional and the client, with the following aims:

1. Increasing the moral autonomy or freedom of choice of the isolate
2. Increasing social interaction at a level acceptable to the client
3. Using repetitive and recognizable strategies that are validated with the client, which correlate to reducing particular isolating behaviors

Another point to remember is that evaluation is a key principle in any problem-solving system, such as the nursing process. Throughout the assessment and intervention phases, the health professional should explicitly consider how effective the intervention is or was. The impact of cultural and social differences should be taken into account. The willingness and flexibility to change an ineffective strategy is the mark of the competent professional.

Assessment of Social Isolation

When social isolation occurs, a systematic assessment can help determine proposed interventions, which the professional must validate with the client before taking action. Guiding people, rather than forcing them to go along with interventions, requires the health care professional to offer a rationale for the proposed interventions. One must ask if one is giving reasonable rationales, assurances, or support. At the same time, the professional should remember that some cultures value the authority and the expertise of other family members over that of the individual. Consequently, the health care professional may have to provide a rationale for suggested interventions to the ranking authority within the support group. Frequently, this is a male figure, often older, who is considered most deserving of any explanation. Other cultures may be matriarchal, so it would be a woman who is the ranking authority.

The key to assessing social isolation is to observe for three distinct features: (1) *negativity,* (2) *involuntary, other-imposed solitude,* and (3) *declining quality and numbers within the isolate's social networks.* Social isolation must be distinguished from other conditions such as loneliness or depression, both often accompanied by anxiety, desperation, self-pity, boredom, and signs of attempts to fill a void, such as overeating, substance abuse, excessive shopping, or kleptomania. In addition, loneliness is often associated with losses, while depression is frequently regarded as anger turned inward. Because

social isolation, loneliness, and depression can all be destructive, the health professional must be resourceful in assessing which issue predominates at any particular point in time.

Properly conducted, an assessment yields its own suggestions for responsive intervention. For instance, the assessment may indicate that the client is a lifelong isolate and that future isolation is a desired and comfortable life-style. In this case, the professional's best intervention is to remain available and observant but noninterfering.

If, on the other hand, the client has become isolated and wants or needs relief, then the intervention should be constructed along lines consistent with his or her current needs and history. In a study designed to be culturally sensitive, Norbeck and associates (1996) applied a standardized intervention using designated individuals for person-to-person and telephone contacts for pregnant African American women who lacked social support networks. Their study showed significantly reduced low-birth-weight infants.

In another example, if the health care professional discovers that a support network is lax in calling or contacting a client, the provider can help the client and support network rebuild bridges to each other. Keep in mind that there are usually support groups to which those in a social network can be referred for aid. As an illustration, if the network is overwhelmed, information can be provided about respite programs. Interventions such as these will help members of the social network maintain energy levels necessary to help their chronically ill relative or friend.

Assessment typically involves the clinical dyad of caregiver and client. It is at this level that assessment is critical to the development of appropriate and effective interventions. Without an adequate and sensitive assessment, interventions are likely to be ineffective or incomplete.

The case study about Will gives some idea about how this client was assessed, his unwanted isolation identified, and, with his knowledge, satisfactory supports contacted that met his needs.

Social Isolation

Will, a 76-year-old childless widower, continued to live alone in his own single-story, urban-area home following the death of his wife, Hazel, three years ago. At the time of her death, he had moderately limited physical mobility from his arthritis, was slightly deaf, and his eyesight, while not severely impaired, was diminishing. Hazel's death had been sudden and unexpected, following complications of treatment for illness. They had been very dependent on each other for material and social support, had lived quietly but interacted to a limited degree with their friends and neighbors, two of whom had lost spouses within the past few years. Although they maintained relationships with family peers about their ages, they interacted with them only rarely. Will described his small social network as follows: "We didn't need for anything and we kept to ourselves."

In the first year following Hazel's death, Will deeply grieved her loss, withdrawing even more from friends and family. During the second year, he was less despairing but began giving away dishes, silverware, and other items, saying, "I won't need these anymore." Over this time span, his physical mobility, vision, and hearing became more limiting, so that he found trips outside the home exhausting and logistically difficult. Consequently, he avoided grocery shopping, going to the barber, worship activities, or any social activities. He used the telephone to contact friends only when he became too lonely, but, for the most part, rarely initiated such contacts.

It was now nearly three years since Hazel's death. Because of his slowly deteriorating health status, he had been referred to the visiting nurse association. In Will's case, the visiting nurse came by twice a month for assessment and treatment of Will's arthritis, deafness, and vision difficulties, as well as his psychological state. He expressed to Ms. B., the visiting nurse, that he sorely missed his wife, rarely saw even the few family members he had, didn't have many friends left, and could not easily leave his home, even to obtain necessities such as food and medicine. Increasingly homebound, Will, a lifelong isolate, had joined the many for whom social isolation becomes problematic or undesirable.

Ms. B., in developing a plan of care, examined the elements of Will's isolation and the levels of identity characterizing Will. She worked with Will to determine the best way to manage the course of his care. In this way, he came to "own" the management of care, that is, the goals of the plan.

First, the nurse *diagnosed* Will as moderately to severely socially isolated, based on his loneliness and unwanted and unpleasant homebound isolation from others in his limited but existing social network. Then Ms. B. acknowledged the *value differentiation* that existed between the two of them. For example, the idea of family was much more important to Ms. B. than to Will. Next, she considered and prioritized relationships and their *meaning* to Will, that is, the relationships that were significant to Will as an individual. The meaning of Will's current situation was defined by him as lonely, unpleasant, confining, and cumbersome.

Moving to the level of *confidante*, she explored his social relationships and their importance to him. In Will's case, the most significant person in his life had been his wife; following in importance were close friends, neighbors, and then some family members. Given that Hazel was no longer part of his social network, the nurse considered which of Will's significant others remained viable alternatives to isolation. Because friends who were also neighbors were available and willing to visit, Ms. B. encouraged Will to accept their overtures of friendship. They then began to visit about every two weeks or telephone every week. Knowing that age mates within the family were also part of Will's limited social network, she helped Will reach out to them. Will later invited a male cousin, who accepted, to come by for a card game about every ten days. Still, none of these individuals could help Will drive to other places, because they themselves were somewhat debilitated or could not help move Will easily in and out of their vehicles.

Ms. B. sought ways of expanding Will's horizons, mentally and spiritually. The local community library rented large-print books and magazines, which were sent to Will on a periodic basis. She also contacted Will's place of worship, and members of his faith made arrangements to visit Will regularly and to transport him to worship services. Gradually, Will was reconnected in some respects to his organizations in addition to his small social network.

Finally, at the level of *community,* Ms. B. considered widening Will's network. To do this, she considered his *physical limitations, needs,* and *barriers.* The nurse not only contacted community social agencies to provide Will with transportation for gro-cery shopping and to get his medications; she also arranged for a neighbor to telephone or look in on Will at least once a day. When the neighbor protested that such a schedule was too demanding, the nurse solicited two other neighbors to develop a rotation scheme so that Will was assured assistance in the event of a fall or some pressing need. In addition, she contacted the postal person to observe for mail or newspapers cluttering the driveway, which would indicate Will was not able to pick them up when he should. Once motivated, Will noted that remote beepers could be used to notify the local hospital or fire department: He made arrangements to obtain such support.

The nurse decided that Will was moving into a *salvaged* identity, although elements of previous identity stages were still present. At no point in the plan was there an attempt to move Will, a lifelong social isolate, into more social activity than he could comfortably manage. Importantly, throughout the development of his diagnosis and plan of care, the nurse and client together validated and negotiated each arrangement. At each new intervention, the nurse evaluated the outcome. For instance: How did Will feel after the visits of the members of his network? Did he go to worship services? Was the nurse hurrying Will into more than he could handle at the time? Ultimately, the desired *outcome* was reached: Will was able to accommodate each step of the plan according to his temperament and resources. This accommodation was verified by Will's ability to articulate whether he felt less isolated than at the beginning of the interventions and whether his social network had, indeed, expanded.

Management of Self: Identity Development

The need for an ongoing identity leads an individual to seek a level where he or she can overcome, avoid, or internalize stigma and, concomitantly, manage resulting social isolation. Social networks can be affected by stigma. Managing various concerns requires people who are chronically ill to develop a new sense of self consistent with their disabilities. This "new" life is intertwined with the lives of members of their social networks, which may now include both health providers and other persons with chronic illnesses. Lessons must be learned to deal with new body demands and associated behaviors. Consequently, the chronically ill must redevelop an identity with norms different from previous ones.

The willingness to change to different and unknown norms is just a first step, one that often takes great courage and time. For instance, one study indicated that clients with pronounced physical, financial, and medical care problems following head and neck surgery exhibited prolonged social isolation 1 year postsurgery (Krouse, Krouse & Fabian, 1989). Although no single study has indicated the time necessary for such identity transformations, anecdotal information suggests that it can last several years, and indeed, for some, it is a lifelong experience.

Identity Transformation

Clarifying how networks form and function is a significant contribution to the management of the struggles of the client who is chronically ill and isolated. The perceptive health care worker should know that much of the management done by the chronically ill and their networks is not seen or well understood by health care professionals today (Corbin & Strauss, 1987). However, we can use Charmaz's findings as guides for assessing the likely identity level of the individual as we try to understand potential withdrawal or actual isolation.

Charmaz (1987), using mostly middle-aged women, has developed a framework of hierarchical identity transformations that is useful in diagnosing a chronically ill individual's proclivity to social networking and in discovering which social network might be most appropriate. This hierarchy of identity takes into account a reconstruction toward a desired future self, based on past and present selves, and reflects the individual's relative difficulty in achieving specific aspirations. Charmaz's analysis progresses toward a "salvaged self" that retains a past identity based on important values or attributes while still acknowledging dependency.

Initially, the individual takes on a *supernormal identity*, which assumes an ability to retain *all* previous success values, social acclamation, struggles, and competition. At this identity level, the individual who is chronically ill attempts to participate more intensely than those in a nonimpaired world despite the limitations of illness. The next identity level that the person moves to is the *restored self*, with the expectation of eventually returning to the previous self, despite the chronic illness or its severity. Health care workers might identify this self with the psychological state of denial, but in terms of identity, the individual has simply assumed that there is no discontinuation with a former self. At the third level, the *contingent personal identity*, one defines oneself in terms of potential risk and failure, indicating the individual still has not come to terms with a future self but has begun to realize that the supernormal identity will no longer be viable. Finally, the level of the *salvaged self* is reached, whereby the individual attempts to define the self as worthwhile, despite recognizing that present circumstances invalidate any previous identity (Charmaz, 1987).

Not only does social isolation relate to stigma; it can develop as an individual loses hope of sustaining aspirations for a normal or supernormal self which are now unrealistic. As persons who are chronically ill act out regret, disappointment, and anger, their significant others and health providers may react in kind, perpetuating a downward spiral of loss, anger, and subsequent greater social isolation. The idea of identity hierarchies thus alerts the caregiver to a process in which shifts in identity are expected.

The reactions, health advice, and the experiences of the chronically ill must be taken into account in managing that particular identity, and also the various factors that help shape it. Both the social network and adapted norms now available play a role at each stage in identity transformation. At the supernormal identity level, individuals who are chronically ill were in only limited contact with health care professionals but presumably in greater contact with healthier individuals who acted as their referents; at the level of the salvaged self, a home health agency typically was used (Charmaz, 1987).

Integrating Culture into Health Care

Isolation, by its very definition, must include a cultural screening through which desired social contacts are defined. When one speaks of social isolation among unique ethnic groups, the number, type, and quality of contact must be sifted through a particularistic screen of that person's culture. Not only the clients, but also the provider's communication patterns, roles, relationships, and traditions are important elements to consider for both assessment and intervention (Barker, 1994; Cheng, 1997; Groce & Zola, 1993; Kim, 1998; Treolar, 1999; Welch, 1998).

Some feel that matching culturally similar providers to clients would be a way to meet needs with effective interventions (Welch, 1998). However, health care educators and service providers recognize the issues of a smaller supply of providers and the greater numbers of clients in a struggling dominant health system coping with multiculturalism. To meet supply and demand issues, as well as cultural needs, the idea of cultural competence is being promoted. Education about cultures is being advanced as the key to effective interventions that intersect the values of two disparate groups of individuals (Davidhizar, Bechtel & Giger, 1998; Jones, Bond & Cason, 1998; McNamara et al., 1997; Smith, 1996). Cultural education not only results in outcomes of culturally relevant compliance (Davidhizar, Bechtel & Giger, 1998) but also helps alleviate the isolation of the chronically ill (Barker, 1994; Hildebrandt, 1997; Treolar, 1999).

For those who find that such culturally-based education is unavailable, and assuming there are more groups and more traditions than can possibly be understood by a single health care provider, a fail-safe strategy remains. This approach requires the provider to approach each person, regardless of their cultural milieu, with respect and dignity, in an explicit good-faith effort to inquire, understand, and be responsive to the client's culture, needs, and person. The provider must set aside prejudices and stereotypes and instead use an authentic sensitive inquiry into the client's beliefs and well-being (Browne, 1997; Treolar, 1999).

By seeking to understand differences, one can find pleasure in the differences and move beyond them to enjoy the similarities of us all. This approach is undergirded by a culture of "caring," and moves toward a model of actively participating groups exchanging concerns of identity, egalitarianism, and needed care (Browne, 1997; Catlin, 1998; Keller & Stevens, 1997; Treolar, 1999). In so doing, social isolation can be managed within the context most comfortable to the client, who is the raison d'etre of the health provider.

Respite

The need for respite has been cited as one of the greatest necessities for the elderly isolated ill and their caregivers, many of whom are themselves elderly (Miller, 1990; Subcommittee on Human Services, 1987). Its purpose is to relieve caregivers for a period of time so that they may engage in activities that help sustain them or their loved ones, the care recipients. Respite involves four elements: (1) purpose, (2) time, (3) activities, and (4) place. The time may be in short blocks or for a longer (but still relatively short-term) period, both of which temporarily relieve the caregiver of responsibility. Activities may be practical, such as grocery shopping; psychological, such as providing time for self-replenishment or recreation; or physical, such as providing time for rest or medical/nursing attention.

Respite may occur in the home or elsewhere, such as senior centers, day care centers, or long-term care facilities. Senior centers usually accommodate persons who are more independent and flexible, often offering social gathering places and events, meals, and health assessment/exercise/maintenance activities. Day care centers typically host individuals with more diminished functioning. Other places, such as long-term care facilities, manage clients with an even greater inability to function.

Finally, respite may be delivered by paid or unpaid persons who may be friends, professionals, family, employees, or neighbors. Although many care recipients welcome relief for their caregiver, some may fear abandonment. The family caregiver and professional must work together to assure the care recipient that he or she will not be abandoned (Biordi, 1993). Therefore, the professional has a great deal of latitude in using the four elements to devise interventions tailored to the flexible needs of an isolated caregiver and care recipient.

Support Groups and Other Mutual Aid

Support groups have been identified for a wide variety of chronic illnesses and conditions, such as breast cancer (Reach to Recovery), bereavement (Widow to Widow), and alcoholism (Alcoholics Anonymous), or for other conditions such as multiple sclerosis or blindness. These groups assist individuals in coping with their illness and the changes in identities and social roles that illnesses may incur for clients. They can help enhance one's self-esteem, provide alternative meanings of the illness, suggest ways to cope, assist in specific interventions that have helped others, or offer services or care for either the isolate or caregiver (Matteson, McConnell & Linton, 1997).

Almost every large city or county has lists of resources that can be accessed: health departments, social work centers, schools, and libraries. Even the telephone book's yellow pages can assist in finding support groups or other resources. The Internet or World Wide Web are also sources of information about support groups and resource listings. Some resources list group entry requirements or qualifications. Because of their variety and number, support groups are not always available in every community, so health professionals may find themselves in the position of developing a group. Therefore, as part of a community assessment, the health profes-

sional should not only note the groups currently available, but also identify someone who might be willing to develop a needed group. The health professional also may have to help find a meeting place, refer clients to the group, assist clients in discussing barriers to their care, and, if necessary, develop structured activities (such as exercise regimens for arthritic individuals). In addition, the use of motivational devices, such as pictures, videos, audio recordings, reminiscence, or games, may be helpful in developing discussion. Demonstrations of specific illness-related regimens, such as exercises, clothing aids, or body mechanics, are also useful to support groups.

Professionals should be alert to problems the isolate may have in integrating into groups, such as resistance to meeting new people, low self-esteem, apprehension over participation in new activities, or the problems of transportation, building access, and inconvenient meeting times (Matteson et al., 1997).

Social activity groups are one way of integrating isolated institutionalized individuals or of reversing hospital-induced confusion; such groups could be recreational therapy groups or those developed particularly to address a special interest (e.g., parents facing the imminent death of a child). Given the limited financial resources typical of most persons who are chronically ill, support groups that are not costly to the chronically ill or their families are more likely to be welcomed.

Spiritual Well-Being

For many, religious or spiritual beliefs offer an important social connection and give great meaning to life. Spiritual well-being typically affirms the unity of the person with his or her environment, often expressed in a oneness with his or her god(s) (Matteson et al., 1997). Consequently, assuring isolates some means of connection to their religious support may help them find newer meaning in life or illness and provide them with other people with whom to share that meaning. The health professional should assess the meaning of religion to the individual, the kind of spiritual meeting place he or she finds most comforting, and the types of religious support available in the community. Religious groups range from formal gatherings to religiously aided social groups.

Frequently, churches or temples have outreach or social groups that will make visits, arrange for social outings, or develop pen pals or other means of human connectedness. The nurse or other health professional may have to initiate contact with these groups to assist in developing the necessary outreach between them and the isolate.

Rebuilding Family Networks

Keeping, or rebuilding, family networks has much to offer. However, families that are disintegrated may have a history of fragile relationships. The health professional must assess these networks carefully to develop truly effective interventions.

The professional must also take into account the client's type of isolation (lifelong versus recent) and the wishes of the isolate: With whom (if anyone) in the family does the isolate wish contact? How often? What members of the family exist or care about the isolate? What is their relationship to the isolate—parent, sibling, child, friend-as-family, other relative? The professional can then make contact with the individuals indicated to be most accommodating to the isolate, explain the situation, make future plans to bring them and the isolate together, and afterward assess the outcome. However, it may not be possible to bring disinterested family members back into the isolate's social network.

For family members who are interested and willing, rebuilding networks means the professional must take into account the location or proximity of family members to the isolate. If they live near each other, and because a "space of one's own" is a critical human need, a balance of territorial and personal needs must be managed if the isolate is to be reintegrated. Should the isolate and family agree to live together, the family's physical environment will require assessment for safety, access, and territorial space. Not only are factors such as sleeping space and heat and ventilation important, but personal space and having one's own possessions are as important to the family members as they are to the ill person. Teaching the family and isolate how to re-

spect each other's privacy (such as by getting permission to enter a room or look through personal belongings, speaking directly to one another, and so forth) is a way to help them bridge their differences.

Understanding Family Relationships

The nature of the relationship between family and isolate must be understood. The family's meanings and actions attached to love, power, and conflict, and observations of the frequency of controlling strategies by various individuals will inform the professional of potential interventions. For example, some clients who live alone were found to be more likely to be satisfied with support when they were feeling depressed, while clients living with others were more satisfied with supporters who cared about them (Foxall et al., 1994). Recalling the earlier example, the elderly woman's use of guilt with an otherwise accommodating family informed the nurse about interventions most likely to succeed.

In some families, love is thought to indicate close togetherness, while, in other families, love is thought to provide members with independence. Love and power can be developed and thought of either as a pyramidal (top-down) set of relationships or as an egalitarian circle. Conflict may be a means of connection or of distance and can be expressed by shouting and insults or by quiet assertion.

Community Resources to Keep Families Together

Using community resources, such as support groups, is a way to help keep a family together. Families draw on each other's experiences as models for coping. For example, families in which there is a child with cancer find ways to help their child cope with the isolation induced by chemotherapy. When necessary, the health professional may wish to refer the isolate and family to psychiatric or specialty nurses, counselors, psychiatrists, or social workers to help them overcome their disintegration. Successful implementation of the wide range of family-related interventions requires sensitive perceptions of the needs not only of the isolate, but also of the various family members with whom that individual must interact.

Two interesting community resources that could help alert families to potential problem situations for isolates are the post office and newspaper delivery services. If these delivery persons observe a build-up of uncollected mail or newspapers, they can call or check the house to see if there is an elderly isolate in distress. Families who are concerned about their isolated family member can provide their post office, regular mail carrier, or news delivery service with information about the isolate that can be used in the event of a problem. Nurses and social workers can also contact mail and news services or help families make these contacts. This intervention can be expanded to include any regular visitor, such as a rental manager, janitor, or neighbor, who might be willing to check on the welfare of the isolate.

In some communities, employees at banks and stores also react to older individuals who may be isolated. Should there be unusual financial activities or changes in shopping patterns, the individual can be contacted to make sure that everything is satisfactory. Although, in some communities, mail and newspaper services and banks and stores are not involved with people in their areas, these resources are valuable and should be expanded throughout the country.

Communication Technologies

Telephones

The telephone is a method used to counteract the effects of place-boundedness. However, findings are equivocal (Kivett, 1979; Praderas & MacDonald, 1986). Still, the telephone is considered almost a necessity in reducing the isolation of a place-bound individual.

Computers

For many persons, including homebound elderly individuals or people with disabilities, computers have helped offset social isolation and loneliness through features such as access to the Internet, which allows the person to reach family and friends or to find new friends, activities, and other common interests. Computers can also be used to provide fun activities, such as computerized games. In the United States, computers are more widely available than elsewhere, and more so among those in higher socioeconomic and educational classes.

Advances in computer technology have created special attachments, such as cameras, breath tubes, or special keyboards, that customize computers to the needs of the isolated or disabled (Imel, 1999; Salem, 1998). In parts of the United States, outreach efforts are increasing, as projects aim to reduce the social isolation of the homebound by providing computers and internet access to caregivers and care receivers.

Font size can be changed, making letters and numbers large enough to aid the visually impaired person in reading or writing letters or documents. Whether connecting with the Internet, using word processing, corresponding via e-mail, taking educational classes, and so on, computers allow isolates to actively fill many hours of otherwise empty time, bringing a measure of relief to tedium while expanding their intellectual and social lives. The caveat, of course, is that the use of the computer, and especially the Internet, could itself be an isolating factor for many individuals. This creates a danger of virtual reality overrunning actual reality, in which case, isolates compound their isolation. That having been said, however, the computer offers many possibilities for overcoming some elements of isolation.

Touch

In cultures where touch is important, families and professionals must learn the use and comfort of touch. American studies indicate that the elderly are the least likely group to be touched, and yet they find touch very comforting. Pets may be useful alternatives to human touch and human interaction; pet therapy is increasingly used as an intervention in families and in group settings such as nursing homes. Feeling loved and having it demonstrated through touch can do much to reduce isolation and its often concomitant lowered self-esteem. Because some individuals find touch uncomfortable, professionals must assess (by simply asking or observing flinching, grimacing, or resignation) the family's or isolate's responsiveness to touch.

Behavior Modification

Behavior modification is a technique that is best used by skilled professionals. It involves the systematic analysis of responses and their antecedent cues and consequences; the use of cognitive therapy to change awareness, perceptions, and behaviors; and the specification of realistic, measurable goals or actual behaviors. Also, reward structures and understanding support persons are necessary in the definition of the problem and its solution. Consistency is needed to develop stable patterns of responses. The time frame of such modification can vary with the problem.

Behavior modification is particularly useful for addressing specific problems, for example, the isolate who is fearful of going outside the house. It is also an important intervention when the environment can be held stable, such as in an institutional setting. Matteson and colleagues (1997) note that where groups are small or the motivation intense, successful behavioral interventions have been instituted for the socially isolated in institutions as well as in the home.

Outcomes

Ideally, the reduction of social isolation and the maintenance of the integrity of the person who is chronically ill and his or her caregiver(s) are preferred outcomes of interventions. However, so many factors can affect social isolation, its assessment, and intervention, that it is difficult to draw simple linear relationships between structure, process, and outcomes. As shown throughout this chapter, a professional must be sensitive to, and prioritize, interventions within the cultural milieu in which the client and support network reside.

Handling the emotionally charged issues surrounding every social isolate requires that professionals recognize in their clients, as well as in themselves, those values that most drive their relationships and build solutions that best deliver culturally and personally competent care toward a better life for their clients.

Summary and Conclusions

Social isolation is not always clearly defined in the literature; it is frequently confused with loneliness, alienation, aloneness, and, at times, impaired social interactions. Social isolation may be either positive, as in the refreshment of the human psyche through solitude, or negative. Where it is involuntary and seen as negative, and where the social network is shrinking in quality or quantity of contacts, it is defined as social isolation.

Where social isolation exists, it becomes a concern for the isolate, his or her social networks, and health care providers. Care should be taken to avoid stereotypical judgments of its existence or intensity. On the other hand, systematic observations of clinical populations argue that social isolation does, in fact, exist and to the detriment of the isolate. This is particularly true in the case of chronic illness. Across various conditions (cancer, heart, or neurological diseases; trauma; and so forth), and across the life span, with its social activities and roles, social isolation contributes to greater risk for mortality and morbidity. Regardless of whether individuals are constrained at the level of the person, his or her confidantes, the organization, or the community, the potential exists for social isolation.

The quality of interactions is the most important variable in reintegrating the isolate. The health professional can help manage the client's situation and its effects on physical and emotional stamina. This requires that the professional recognize the meaning of social isolation to the isolate as well as to the isolate's social network. Furthermore, the professional needs to understand the meaning that chronic illness and isolation has on the identity of the isolate within his or her culture.

Each of these issues needs to be taken into account and considered. Assessments of the client always require validation by the client, and strategies that are agreed on need ongoing evaluation by the health professional. Such action takes the isolated client or social network into an egalitarian relationship that offers full opportunity to exercise moral agency and authority. Because the perception of isolation varies, the health professional must remain vigilant to its symptoms and flexible in attempting interventions.

Wherever possible, the health professional must recognize that the isolate need not exist in a vacuum, but should consider the impact of the person's social network. As social networks deplete their emotional, material, and financial resources, the health professional should consider means to support them.

Finally, social isolation is a model of human disconnectedness. Its systematic examination, therefore, allows the health professional to develop purposeful interventions to reduce the misery of unwanted social isolation.

Study Questions

1. Is loneliness the same thing as social isolation? Why or why not?
2. How might the distance that a manually powered or an electrically powered wheelchair can go relate to social isolation?
3. List six characteristics that might incline a client to social isolation. What criteria did you use to develop these characteristics?
4. Suppose another health professional said about a very new client, "Oh, we must make certain that Mrs. Jones has company. She's a widow, you know." With regard to social isolation, what arguments could you make, pro or con, about this statement?
5. Develop at least five questions you could adapt to assess and validate social isolation in a client. Consider how you might approach identity levels, actual isolation, network assessment, and feelings of the isolate. Add other priorities as you wish, but offer rationales for each of them.
6. Name three community resources you could use to reduce the social isolation of clients.
7. What two principles should guide a health professional when developing any intervention with an isolated client? Why are these important?

8. Suppose a client said to you, "I have had arthritis in my fingers and hands for a long time now. I simply can't do what I used to do. I now have new handles for my kitchen cabinets because the knobs hurt my hands, and new clothes especially made for people like me who can't work buttons. My daughter was shopping and she saw them and told me about them. Now I feel better when I get together with them to see my grandchildren." At what stage of identity might you expect this client to be? Why? Is this person an isolate? Explain your answer.
9. A gay teenager is your client. He has recently "come out" and is now depressed because his schoolmates shun him, his parents are going through a grief reaction to his announcement, and he has few other friends who share his interests or sexual orientation. Is he at risk for social isolation? How would you assess his social network? What interventions, if any, would you recommend? Explain your answers.

References

Antonucci, T. (1985). Social support: Theoretical advances, recent findings and pressing issues. In I. G. Sarason & B. R. Sarason (Eds.), *Social support: Theory, research and application*. Boston: Martinus Nyhoff.

Austin, D. (1989). Becoming immune to loneliness: Helping the elderly fill a void. *Journal of Gerontological Nursing, 15* (9), 25–28.

Barker, J. C. (1994). Recognizing cultural differences: Health care providers and elderly patients. *Gerontology & Geriatric Education, 15* (1), 9–21.

Bendor, S. (1990). Anxiety and isolation in siblings of pediatric cancer patients: The need for prevention. *Social Work in Health Care, 14* (3), 17–35.

Bennet, R. (1980). *Aging, isolation, and resocialization* (chapters 1 and 2). New York: Van Nostrand Reinhold.

Berkman, L. (1983). The assessment of social networks and social support in the elderly. *American Geriatric Society Journal, 31* (12), 743–749.

Biordi, D. (2000). Research agenda: Emerging issues in the management of health and illness. *Seminars for Nurse Managers, 8,* 205–211.

Biordi, D. (primary investigator). (1993). In-home care and respite care as self-care (Grant # NRO20210183). Washington, DC: National Institute of Nursing Research.

Borman, J., & Biordi, D. (1992). Female nurse executives: Finally, at an advantage. *Journal of Nursing Administration, 22* (9), 37–41.

Browne, A. J. (1997). The concept analysis of respect applying the hybrid model in cross-cultural settings. *Western Journal of Nursing Research, 19* (6), 762–780.

Burnley, I. H. (1992). Mortality from selected cancers in NSW and Sydney, Australia. *Social Science and Medicine, 35* (2), 195–208.

Cadman, D., Rosenbaum, P., Boyle, M., & Offord, D. (1991). Children with chronic illness: Family and parent demographic characteristics and psychosocial adjustment. *Pediatrics, 87* (6), 884–889.

Carpenito, L. J. (1995). *Nursing diagnosis: Application to clinical practice* (6th ed.). Philadelphia: Lippincott.

Catalan, J. (1998). Mental health problems in older adults with HIV referred to a psychological medicine unit. *AIDS Care: Psychological and Socio-medical Aspects of AIDS/HIV, 10* (2), 105–112.

Catlin, A. J. (1998). Editor's choice. When cultures clash; comments on a brilliant new book . . . *The Spirit Catches You and You Fall Down*. New York: Farrar, Straus and Giroux.

Charmaz, K. (1987). Struggling for a self: Identity levels of the chronically ill. In J. Roth & P. Conrad (Eds.), *Research in the sociology of health care*. Greenwich, CT: JAI Press.

Cheng, B. K. (1997). Cultural clash between providers of majority culture and patients of Chinese culture. *Journal of Long Term Home Health Care, 16* (2), 39–43.

Chinman, M. J., Weingarten, R., Stayner, D. & Davidson, L. (2001). Chronicity reconsidered: Improving person-environment fit through a consumer-run service. *Community Mental Health Journal, 37* (3), 215–229.

Christ, G. (1987). Social consequences of the cancer experience. *The American Journal of Pediatric Hematology/Oncology, 9* (1), 84–88.

Cobb, S. (1979). Social support and health through the life course. In M. W. Riley (Ed.), *Aging from birth to death*. Boulder, CO: Westview Press.

Cohen, M. (1993). The unknown and the unknowable—Managing sustained uncertainty. *Western Journal of Nursing Research, 15* (1), 77–96.

Corbin, J., & Strauss, A. (1987). Accompaniments of chronic illness: Changes in body, self, biography and biographical time. In J. Roth & P. Conrad (Eds.), *Research in the sociology of health care*. Greenwich, CT: JAI Press.

Cox, C., Spiro, M., & Sullivan, J. (1988). Social risk factors: Impact on elders' perceived health status. *Journal of Community Health Nursing, 5* (1), 59–73.

Creecy, R., Berg, W., & Wright, L. Jr. (1985). Loneliness among the elderly: A causal approach. *Journal of Gerontology, 40* (4), 487–493.

Creed, F. (1990). Psychological disorders in rheumatoid arthritis: A growing consensus? *Annual Rheumatic Disorders, 49,* 808–812.

Davidhizar, R., Bechtel, G. L., & Giger, J. N. (1998). Model helps CMs deliver multicultural care: Addressing cultural issues boosts compliance. *Case Management Advisor, 9* (6), 97–100.

Dela Cruz, L. (1986). On loneliness and the elderly. *Journal of Gerontological Nursing, 12* (11), 22–27.

DesRosier, M., Catanzaro, M., & Piller, J. (1992). Living with chronic illness: Social support and the well spouse perspective. *Rehabilitation Nursing, 17* (2), 87–91.

DiMatteo, M. R., & Hays, R. (1981). Social support and serious illness. In B. H. Gottlieb (Ed.), *Social networks and social support.* Beverly Hills, CA: Sage.

DiNapoli, P., & Murphy, D. (2002). The marginalization of chronically ill adolescents. *The Nursing Clinics of North America, 37* (3), 565–572.

Dorfman, L., Homes, C., & Berlin, K. (1996). Wife caregivers of frail elderly veterans: Correlates of caregiver satisfaction and caregiver strain. *Family Relations, 45,* 46–55.

Dropkin, M. (1989). Coping with disfigurement and dysfunction. *Seminars in Oncology Nursing, 5* (3), 213–219.

Fiscella, K., Franks, M., Gold, M., & Clancy, D. (2000). Social support, disability, and depression: A longitudinal study of rheumatoid arthritis. *Journal of the American Medical Association, 283,* 2579–2584.

Fitzpatrick, R., Newman, R., Archer, R., & Shipley, M. (2000). Inequalities in racial access to health care. *Journal of the American Medical Association,* 25: 284(16), 2053.

Foxall, M., Barron, C., Dollen, K., Shull, K., et al. (1994). Low vision elders: Living arrangements, loneliness, and social support. *Journal of Gerontological Nursing, 20,* 6–14.

Foxall, M., Eckberg, J., & Griffith, N. (1986). Spousal adjustment to chronic illness. *Rehabilitation Nursing, 11,* 13–16.

Frierson, R. L. (1991). Suicide attempts by the old and the very old. *Archives of Internal Medicine, 151* (1), 141–144.

Gallo, A. M., Breitmayer, B. J., Knafl, K. A., & Zoeller, L. H. (1991). Stigma in childhood chronic illness: A well sibling perspective. *Pediatric Nursing, 17* (1), 21–25.

Gamba, A., Romano, M., Grosso, I., Tamburini, M., et al. (1992). Psychosocial adjustment of patients surgically treated for head and neck cancer. *Head and Neck, 14* (3), 218–223.

Glassman-Feibusch, B. (1981). The socially isolated elderly. *Geriatric Nursing, 2* (1), 28–31.

Goodman, C. (1984). Natural helping among older adults. *Gerontologist, 24* (2), 138–143.

Gordon, M. (1982). *Nursing diagnosis: Process and application.* New York: McGraw-Hill.

_____. (1989). Social isolation. *Manual of nursing diagnosis.* St. Louis: Mosby.

Groce, N. E., & Zola, I. (1993). Multiculturalism, chronic illness, and disability. *Pediatrics, 91* (5), 32–39.

Habayeb, G. L. (1995). Cultural diversity: A nursing concept not yet reliably defined. *Nursing Outlook, 43* (5), 224–227.

Heiney, S., Goon-Johnson, K., Ettinger, R., & Ettinger, S. (1990). The effects of group therapy on siblings of pediatric oncology patients. *Journal of Pediatric Oncology Nursing, 7* (3), 95–100.

Helton, L. R. (1995). Intervention with Appalachians: Strategies for a culturally specific practice. *Journal of Cultural Diversity, 2* (1), 20–26.

Heumann, L. (1988). Assisting the frail elderly living in subsidized housing for the independent elderly: A profile of the management and its support priorities. *Gerontologist, 28,* 625–631.

Hoeffer, B. (1987). A causal model of loneliness among older single women. *Archives of Psychiatric Nursing, 1* (5), 366–373.

Hopper, S. (1981). Diabetes as a stigmatized condition: The case of low income clinic patients in the United States. *Social Science and Medicine, 15B,* 11–19.

House, J., Landis, K., & Umberson, D. (1988). Social relationships and health. *Science, 241,* 540–544.

Imel, S. (1999) *Seniors in cyberspace. Trends and issues alerts.* Washington, DC: Office of Educational Research and Improvement (ED). EDD00036.

Jessop, D., & Stein, R. (1985). Uncertainty and its relation to the psychological and social correlates of chronic illness in children. *Social Science and Medicine, 20* (10), 993–999.

Jones, M. D., Bond, M. L., & Cason, C. L. (1998). Where does culture fit in outcomes management? *Journal of Nursing Care Quality, 13* (1), 41–51.

Kaplan, G., Salonen, J., Cohen, R., Brand, R., et al. (1988). Social connections and mortality from all causes and from cardiovascular disease: Prospective evidence from Eastern Finland. *American Journal of Epidemiology, 128* (2), 370–380.

Keller, C. S., & Stevens, K. R. (1997). Cultural considerations in promoting wellness. *Journal of Cardiovascular Nursing, 11* (3), 15–25.

Kim, L. S. (1998). Long term care for the Korean American elderly: An exploration for a better way of services. *Journal of Long Term Home Health Care, 16* (2), 35–38.

Kinsella, G., Ford, B., & Moran, C. (1989). Survival of social relationships following head injury. *International Disability Studies, 11* (1), 9–14.

Kivett, V. (1979). Discriminators of loneliness among the rural elderly: Implications for interventions. *Gerontologist, 19* (1), 108–115.

Klinenberg, E. (2001). Dying alone: The social production of urban isolation. *Ethnography, 2* (4), 501–531

Krause, N. (1993). Neighborhood deterioration and social isolation in later life. *International Journal of Aging and Human Development, 36,* 9–28.

Kreps, G., & Kreps, M. (1997). Amishing "medical care." *Journal of Multicultural Nursing & Health, 3* (2), 44–47.

Krouse, J., Krouse, H., & Fabian, R. (1989). Adaptation to surgery for head and neck cancer. *Laryngoscope, 99,* 789–794.

Lawton, M., Greenbaum, M., & Liebowitz, B. (1980). The lifespan of housing environments for the aging. *Gerontologist, 20,* 56–64.

Lawton, M., Kleban, M., & Carlson, D. (Winter 1973). The inner-city resident: To move or not to move. *Gerontologist,* 443–448.

Lawton, M., Moss, M., & Grimes, M. (1985). The changing service need of older tenants in planned housing. *Gerontologist, 25,* 258–264.

Lee, G. R., & Ellithorpe, E. (1982). Intergenerational exchange and subjective well-being among the elderly. *Journal of Marriage and the Family, 44,* 217–224.

Lichtenstein, B., Laska, M. K., & Clair, J. M. (2002). Chronic sorrow in the HIV-positive patient: Issues of race, gender, and social support. *AIDS patient care and STDs, 16* (1), 27–38.

Lien-Gieschen, T. (1993). Validation of social isolation related to maturational age: Elderly. *Nursing Diagnosis, 4* (1), 37–43.

Lin, N. (1986). Conceptualizing social support. In N. Lin, A. Dean, & W. Ensel (Eds.), *Social support, life events, and depression.* New York: Academic Press.

Litwin, H. & Zoabi, S. (2003). Modernization and Elder Abuse in an Arab-Israeli Context. *Research on Aging, 25* (3), 224–246.

Lyons, M. J. (1982). Psychological concomitants of the environment influencing suicidal behavior in middle and later life. *Dissertation Abstracts International, 43,* 1620B.

Maddox, G. L. (1985). Intervention strategies to enhance well-being in later life: The status and prospect of guided change. *Health Services Research, 19,* 1007–1032.

Mallinson, R. K., (1999). The lived experiences of AIDS-related multiple losses by HIV-negative gay men. *Journal of the Association of Nurses in AIDS Care, 10* (5), 22–31.

Matteson, M. A., & McConnell, E. S. (1988). *Gerontological nursing: Concepts and practice.* Philadelphia: W.B. Saunders.

Matteson, M. A., McConnell, E. S., & Linton, A. (1997). *Gerontological nursing: Concepts and practice* (2nd ed). Philadelphia: WB Saunders.

McNamara, B., Martin, K., Waddel, C., & Yuen, K. (1997). Palliative care in a multicultural society: Perceptions of health care professionals. *Palliative Medicine, 11* (5), 359–367.

Melle, I., Friis, S., Hauff, E., & Vaglum, P. (2000). Social functioning of patients with schizophrenia in high income welfare societies. *Psychiatric Services, 51* (2), 223–228.

Miller, B. (1990). Gender differences in spouse caregiver strain: Socialization and role explanations. *Journal of Marriage and the Family, 52,* 311–322.

Mullins, L., & Dugan, E. (1990). The influence of depression, and family and friendship relations, on residents' loneliness in congregate housing. *Gerontologist, 30* (3), 377–384.

NANDA. (2001). *Nursing diagnoses: Definitions and classification. 2001–2002.* Philadelphia: NANDA.

Newman, S. P., Fitzpatrick, R., Lamb, R., & Shipley, M. (1989). The origins of depressed mood in rheumatoid arthritis. *The Journal of Rheumatology, 16* (6), 740–744.

Noll, R., Ris, M. D., Davies, W. H., Burkowski, W., et al. (1992). Social interactions between children with cancer or sickle cell disease and their peers: Teacher ratings. *Developmental and Behavioral Pediatrics, 13* (3), 187–193.

Norbeck, J., DeJoseph, J., & Smith, R. (1996). A randomized trial of an empirically derived social support intervention to prevent low birthweight among African-American women. *Social Science and Medicine, 43,* 947–954.

Noyes, R., Kathol, R., Debelius-Enemark, P., Williams, J., et al. (1990). Distress associated with cancer as measured by the illness distress scale. *Psychosomatics, 31* (3), 321–330.

Orth-Gomer, K., Unden, A., & Edwards, M. (1988). Social isolation and mortality in ischemic heart disease: A 10-year follow-up study of 150 middle aged men. *Acta Med Scan, 224* (3), 205–215.

Peplau, L. A., & Perlman, D. (Eds.). (1986). *Loneliness: A sourcebook of current theory, research, and therapy.* New York: John Wiley & Sons.

Poulin, J. (1984). Age segregation and the interpersonal involvement and morale of the aged. *Gerontologist, 24* (3), 266–269.

Praderas, K., & MacDonald, M. (1986). Telephone conversational skills training with socially isolated, impaired nursing home residents. *Journal of Applied Behavior Analysis, 19* (4), 337–348.

Randers, I., Mattiasson A., & Olson T. H. (2003). The "social self": the 11th category of integrity—implications for enhancing geriatric nursing care. *Journal of Applied Gerontology, 22* (2), 289–309.

Ravish, T. (1985). Prevent isolation before it starts. *Journal of Gerontological Nursing, 11* (10), 10–13.

Reynolds, P., & Kaplan, G. (1990). Social connections and risk for cancer: Prospective evidence from the Alameda County study. *Behavioral Medicine, 16* (3), 101–110.

Russell, C., & Schofield, T. (1999). Social Isolation in Old Age: A qualitative exploration of service providers' perceptions. *Ageing and Society, 19* (1), 69-91

Ryan, M., & Patterson, J. (1987). Loneliness in the elderly. *Journal of Gerontological Nursing, 13* (5), 6–12.

Salem, P. (1998). Paradoxical impacts of electronic communication technologies. Paper presented at the International Communication Association/National Communication Association Conference, Rome, Italy, July 15–17, 1998.

Seeman, M. (1959). On the meaning of alienation. *American Sociological Review, 24,* 783–791.

Siplic F., & Kadis, D. (2002). The psychosocial aspect of aging. *Socialno Delo, 41* (5), 295–300.

Smith, A. (2003). Intimacy and family relationships of women with chronic pain. *Pain Management Nursing, 4* (3), 134–142

Smith, J. W. (1996). Cultural and spiritual issues in palliative care. *Journal of Cancer Care, 5* (4), 173–178.

Spiegel, D. (1990). Facilitating emotional coping during treatment. *Cancer, 66,* 1422–1426.

Spitz, G., & Miner, S. (1992). Gender differences in adult child contact among black elderly parents. *Gerontologist, 43,* 213–218.

Stephens, M., & Bernstein, M. (1984). Social support and well-being among residents of planned housing. *Gerontologist, 24,* 144–148.

Stewart, N. (1986). Perceptual and behavioral effects of immobility and social isolation in hospitalized orthopedic patients. *Nursing Papers/Perspectives in Nursing, 18* (3), 59–74.

Strauss, A., Corbin, J., Fagerhaugh, S., Glaser, B., et al. (1984). *Chronic illness and the quality of life* (2nd ed.). St. Louis: Mosby.

Subcommittee on Human Services of the Select Committee on Aging: U.S. House of Representatives (1987). *Exploding the myths: Caregiving in America* (Committee Print # 99–611). Washington, DC: US Government Printing Office.

Tamlyn, D., & Arklie, M. (1986). A theoretical framework for standard care plans: A nursing approach for working with chronically ill children and their families. *Issues in Comprehensive Pediatric Nursing, 9,* 39–45.

Tilden, V., & Weinert, C. (1987). Social support and the chronically ill individual. *Nursing Clinics of North America, 22* (3), 613–620.

Treolar, L. L. (1999). People with disabilities—the same, but different: Implications for health care practice. *Journal of Transcultural Nursing, 10* (4), 358–364.

Trout, D. (1980). The role of social isolation in suicide. *Suicide and Life Threatening Behavior, 10,* 10–22.

Victor, C., Scambler, S.J., Shah, S., Cook D.G., et al. (2002). Has loneliness amongst older people increased? An investigation into Variations among Cohorts. *Ageing and Society, 22* (5), 585–597.

Watson, E. (1988). Dead to the world. *Nursing Times, 84* (21), 52–54.

Weeks, J. R., & Cuellar, J. P. (1981). The role of family members in the helping networks of older people. *Gerontologist, 21,* 388–394.

Weisman, A. D., & Worden, J. W. (1976–1977). The existential plight in cancer: Significance of the first 100 days. *International Journal of Psychiatry in Medicine, 7,* 1–15.

Weiss, R. S. (1973). *Loneliness: The experience of emotional and social isolation.* Cambridge, MA: Massachusetts Institute of Technology Press.

Welch, C. M. (1998). The adult health and development program: Bridging the racial gap. *International Electronic Journal of Health Education, 1* (3), 178–181.

Williams, S., & Bury, M. (1989). Impairment, disability, and handicap in chronic respiratory illness. *Social Science and Medicine, 29* (5), 609–616.

Wright, L. (1995). Human development in the context of aging and chronic illness: The role of attachment in Alzheimer's disease and stroke. *International Journal of Aging and Human Development, 44,* 133–150.

Woods, N., Haberman, M., & Packard, N. (1993). Demands of illness and individual, dyadic, and family adaption in chronic illness. *Western Journal of Nursing Research, 15* (1), 10–30.

Zimmer, M. (1995). Activity participation and well being among older people with arthritis. *Gerontologist, 351,* 463–471.

CHAPTER 7

Altered Mobility and Fatigue

Sandra Bergquist ▪ Geri B. Neuberger ▪ Marian Jamison

Mobility and motion are integral to health and well-being across the life span. Being active in daily life involves coming and going at will, walking, running, playing, driving, working away from home or at home, and interacting with other people. Young children learn about their environment through movement. As one ages, the capacity for activity and sustained motion becomes increasingly crucial to maintaining independence.

Health problems, psychosocial factors, increasing age, and disuse can interfere with a daily life of motion by altering mobility and inducing fatigue. Altered mobility and fatigue can, in turn, exacerbate preexisting health care problems, compromise a number of organ systems, and perpetuate further losses in mobility and increased fatigue. This chapter focuses on the problems and issues associated with altered mobility and fatigue and discusses interventions to prevent or ameliorate their effects.

Altered Mobility

Introduction

Impaired physical mobility is defined as a state in which the individual experiences limitation of movement (Carpenito-Moyet, 2004). The individual may be unable to move one or more body parts, be unable to freely move within the environment, or both. An estimated 18.6 million people in the United States have some mobility impairment; and approximately 5.6 million of these people have major mobility problems (Iezzoni, McCarthy, Davis, & Siebens, 2000).

Problems and Issues with Altered Mobility

Causes of Altered Mobility

The causes of altered mobility are numerous and often multifactorial. Musculoskeletal and neurological disorders are among the most common causes of altered mobility, but lifestyle, cardiovascular disease, diabetes, sensory deficits, iatrogenic factors, pain, and environmental factors may contribute to the problem. The population of people with altered mobility has changed over the past few decades (Ostchega, Harris, Hirsch, Parsons, & Kington, 2000). Factors that may account for these changes include (1) advances in medical science and assistive technology which have decreased mortality rates at birth, increased survival from traumatic injuries, and decreased mortality rates for a variety of disabling illnesses and injuries; and (2) an aging population.

Advances in Neonatal Medicine

Improvements in neonatal medicine and advanced technologies have reduced the mortality rate among low-birth-weight (LBW < 2,500 g) and very-low-birth-weight infants (VLBW < 1,500 g) (Hamvas, 2000). More LBW and VLBW infants are surviving into childhood and young adulthood. VLBW has been shown to be associated with a diagnosis of developmental delay and disability before three years of age (Thompson, Edwards, & Ross, 2003). A corresponding rise in cerebral palsy has also been noted among industrialized countries, and the increased prevalence of this condition has been linked to the increased survival rate of LBW infants (Hack & Fanaroff, 1999). As cerebral palsy is often manifested by contractures, hemiplegia, and quadriplegia, the number of young children with impaired mobility may increase.

Trauma

The mortality rate from serious injury has decreased over the past several decades with im-

provements in trauma medicine and advanced technologies. In a study of 87 survivors of multiple trauma one year after discharge from the intensive care unit, Dimopoulou et al. (2004) found that 59% experienced moderate to severe disability and 64% reported problems related to physical mobility.

Brain injury often occurs during a trauma event. The Centers for Disease Control and Prevention (CDC) estimate that 1.5 million Americans sustain traumatic brain injuries (TBIs) annually (Thurman, Alverson, Dunn, Guerrero, & Sniezek, 1999). Of these, approximately 80,000 to 90,000 experience long-term disability (Thurman et al., 1999). The more severe the TBI, the greater the functional limitations (Dikmen, Machamer, Powell, & Temkin, 2003; Dimopoulou et al., 2004). The estimated prevalence of Americans now living with disabilities resulting from TBIs is 5.3 million (Thurman et al., 1999). Similarly, more people are surviving traumatic spinal cord injury and living longer with paraplegia and quadriplegia.

Age

Some decline in physical ability is an inevitable result of the normal aging process. The number of muscle fibers, for example, decreases with age, ultimately reducing muscle strength and endurance (Carlson, Ostir, Black, Markides, Rudkin & Goodwin, 1999). The proliferative capacity of bone and cartilage also changes with increasing age, and the ability of these cells to perform their specialized functions diminishes (Buckwalter & DiNubile, 1997). In cartilage, declining chondrocyte function reduces the cells' ability to repair cartilage matrix, and cartilage surfaces deteriorate (Dieppe & Tobias, 1998). Collagen fibers increase in diameter and cross-linking, resulting in increased tissue stiffness, decreased strength, and decreased joint mobility (Dieppe & Tobias, 1998). Gradual calcium loss from bone begins in the fourth decade of life and accelerates in women following menopause. Bone strength declines from loss of bone mass that occurs when bone reabsorption exceeds bone formation.

In the past, few people lived past age 65, whereas, today, the average male adult lives 74.7 years, and the average female adult lives 79.9 years (Kochanek & Smith, 2004). This increased life expectancy has led to an unprecedented growth in the 65+ and 85+ population (Desai, Zhang & Hennessy, 1999) and has been accompanied by a relative and absolute decline in long term care institutionalization (Manton & Gu, 2001). The impact of aging on mobility is expected to peak when the Baby Boom cohort reaches age 85+. By the mid twenty-first century, a significant portion of the community-dwelling U.S. population is expected to have impaired functional abilities. Interestingly, rates of chronic disability in long term care have declined from 26.2% in 1982 to 19.7% in 1999 (Manton & Gu, 2001).

Neurological

Stroke is a leading cause of death in the United States and an important cause of altered mobility among older adults. Over the past several decades, stroke mortality rates have declined, falling from 66.3 deaths per 100,000 in 1970 to 25.1 deaths per 100,000 by 1998 (NSA, 2000). Medical advances in the treatment of hypertension, heart disease, and diabetes mellitus have been credited for the reduction in stroke mortality rates. Unfortunately, the decline in stroke mortality has not been matched by a corresponding decrease in stroke incidence. Every year, approximately 730,000 Americans have a new or recurrent stroke and, two-thirds of these strokes occur in people over age 65 (NSA, 2000). The increased number of stroke survivors suggests an increased number of individuals with residual altered mobility. This same trend has been noted for persons with Parkinson's disease and dementia.

Musculoskeletal

Joint disease, musculoskeletal deformities, osteoporosis, and fractures are common conditions that alter mobility. Podiatric problems such as bunions and calluses can cause pain and reluctance or inability to walk (Kane, Ouslander & Abrass,

1999). The prevalence of self-reported arthritis or chronic joint symptoms is estimated to be 33%, or one in three adults in the United States (CDC, 2002a). The high prevalence of arthritis in combination with an increasing older population produces a high incidence of altered mobility.

An estimated 323,000 hip fractures resulted in hospitalization in 1999 (Popovic, 2001). Often associated with osteoporosis, hip fractures are most common among women over 50 years of age. Evidence suggests that the number of hip fractures will increase concomitant to an increase in the number of older adults (Stevens et al., 1999).

Lifestyle

Lifestyle refers to a typical way of life for an individual, group, or culture and generally encompasses such things as diet, exercise, smoking, and alcohol consumption. These behaviors are known to have an impact on general health and well-being, and may have an impact on long-term functional ability.

Using data from the 1999–2001 National Health Interview Survey conducted by the Centers for Disease Control and Prevention, Schoenborn and colleagues (2004) found that almost 40% of adults were physically inactive during their leisure time (Schoenborn, Adams, Barnes, Vickerie, & Schiller, 2004). With aging and with retirement, individuals frequently develop a more sedentary life-style. The reduction in normal activities can lead to muscle atrophy, loss of flexibility, and diminished endurance (Carlson et al., 1999). This disuse disability perpetuates further reduction of activity and sets up a vicious cycle of disuse and declining function.

Smoking, obesity, and excessive alcohol consumption have been linked to a number of disorders associated with disability. In 1999-2001, 23.1% of adults in the U.S. were current smokers, almost 60% of adults were overweight (body mass index ≥ 25), and 5% of adults were classified as heavy drinkers (Schoenborn et al., 2004). These behaviors have been found to affect mobility in middle-aged and older adults. In a large study of 12,652 Americans aged 50 to 61 years and 8,124 community-dwelling older persons aged 70 years and older; smoking, obesity, alcohol consumption, and exercise predicted impaired mobility and recovery of lost mobility (Ostbye, Taylor, Krause, & Van Scoyoc, 2002). In another study among 1,526 women and 1,391 men aged 70 and older, a high percentage of body fat and high body mass index were associated with greater functional limitations (Davidson, Ford, Cogswell, & Dietz, 2002).

Cardiovascular Disease

Coronary artery disease with frequent angina, myocardial infarction with progression to congestive heart failure, and peripheral vascular disease with frequent claudication compromises strength and endurance and eventually affects activity levels. Continued advances in medical science have decreased cardiovascular disease mortality rates. Individuals with chronic cardiovascular conditions are now managing the disease for a longer period of time and may be facing more years of altered mobility.

Diabetes

Over six percent of the population in the United States is estimated to have diabetes (CDC, 2003). Diabetes is associated with a wide range of disabilities. Diabetes, for example, is a common cause of foot deformity and lower extremity amputation, which often lead to significant mobility alterations (Sinacore, 1998). Diabetes is also a common cause of vision loss in adults. The vision loss associated with diabetic retinopathy frequently leads to restrictions in mobility (Lamoureux, Hassell, & Keeffe, 2004). Some evidence suggests that the relationship between diabetes and disability may be partially independent of the vascular comorbidities and risks (Maty et al., 2004).

Because Type II diabetes is strongly associated with age, the number of persons with impaired mobility from this disease is expected to rise. Type II diabetes also has increased among adolescents at the same time obesity has increased in this same age

group (Bobo et al., 2004). Changes in the population of those with Type II diabetes imply more individuals with more years of altered mobility.

Sensory Impairment

Visual and hearing loss can dramatically impact freedom of movement within an individual's environment. Impaired vision diminishes the individual's awareness of obstacles, hazards, and other sources of danger and increases the risk for accidents and falls. Accidents and falls that do occur may subsequently leave the individual immobilized. Individuals who are fearful of falling or encountering danger may self-restrict activity levels. In institutional settings, clients with impaired vision may be inappropriately restricted to bed or chair. Individuals who have hearing loss may be also vulnerable to injury, because they are unable to hear warning signals.

Iatrogenic Factors

Prescribed medications and their accompanying side effects may affect mobility. Narcotics, sedatives, and hypnotics can cause drowsiness and ataxia. Psychiatric medications may have adverse effects on muscle function and diminish mobility.

Pain

Pain is a common symptom experienced by individuals of all age groups. Although federal guidelines on the clinical management of pain have been published, research continues to document inadequate relief for persons experiencing pain (Ducharme, 2000). Pain in infants and children also remains undertreated (American Medical Association, 2003).

Chronic pain can make the simplest task difficult or even impossible and depletes energy. Individuals experiencing pain may be reluctant to mobilize or engage in activities of daily living, especially when such activities produce pain. Chronic pain can evoke an ever-intensifying cycle of pain, anxiety, and immobilization until the cycle is broken (see Chapter 4, on chronic pain).

Environmental Factors

Environmental factors that restrict mobility include such conditions as slick floors and pathway obstructions. A lack of mobility aids (e.g., canes, walkers, and appropriately placed railings) reduces mobility in institutional and home settings. Architectural barriers to mobility include lengthy stairways and narrow corridors and doorways. In the public setting, high steps and curbs, steep ramps, and limited bathroom space discourage mobility. Disabled older adults ($\geq$ 70 years), for example, reported greater avoidance of environmental challenges to mobility than nondisabled older adults (Shumway-Cook et al., 2003).

Effects of Immobility

Altered mobility, regardless of etiology, can adversely affect physical and psychosocial health. The most profound effects of immobility occur when individuals are placed on bedrest (Table 7-1), but negative consequences are manifest with even mild alterations in mobility, especially when the individual is already physiologically compromised.

Cardiovascular

Cardiovascular deconditioning is a significant adverse effect of immobility. Cardiac muscle atrophies and maximal work capacity decreases rapidly with bedrest (Convertino, 1997; Levine, Zuckerman & Pawelczyk, 1997). Resting heart rate increases, and heart rate with exercise is higher during bedrest than pre-bedrest rates (Convertino, 1997).

Immobility also reduces skeletal muscle pumping action on peripheral veins. Venous stasis and pooling of blood in the lower extremities may lead to the development of venous thrombosis. Individuals on bedrest for 4 days or longer are at risk for thrombosis (Anderson & Spencer, 2003). A deep venous thrombus can dislodge or fragment and travel to the lungs, causing pulmonary embolism.

TABLE 7-1

Effects of Bedrest

Cardiovascular	Metabolism
1. Increased workload on the heart	1. Decreased metabolic rate
2. Hypotension	2. Impaired glucose tolerance
3. Thrombus formation	3. Negative nitrogen balance
Pulmonary	Gastrointestinal
1. Limited chest expansion	1. Constipation
2. Poor ventilation and gas exchange	
3. Increased and pooled secretions	Genitourinary
	1. Urinary infection
Musculoskeletal	2. Urinary calculi
1. Loss of muscle tone and mass	
2. Decreased range of motion	Psychological
3. Contractures	1. Decreased social interaction
4. Osteoporosis	2. Altered mentation
	3. Sensory deprivation
Skin	4. Sleep pattern disturbance
1. Pressure ulcers	5. Role change

SOURCE: Summarized from Olson et al. (1967).

The combination of deconditioned cardiovascular reflexes and diminished plasma volume can lead to postural hypotension (Kane, Ouslander & Abrass, 1999). After 4 days on bedrest, plasma vasopressin decreases, producing plasma volume loss (Sigaudo et al., 1996). Impaired baroreflex function and changes in autonomic balance also begin after 4 days of bedrest (Pavy-Le Traon et al., 1997). These responses in combination with reduced skeletal muscle pumping action on peripheral veins may produce postural hypotension. Postural effects related to immobilization are slow to reverse.

Respiratory

Respiratory function is compromised with immobility. In the supine position, the diaphragm is displaced cephalad, and functional residual capacity is decreased. The work of breathing increases, and there are fewer deep breaths or sighs. Hypoventilation results in atelectasis and a decline in PO2. Coughing is less effective in the supine position, and secretions pool in small airways, predisposing the individual to the development of pneumonia. Immobility was identified as a significant risk factor for lower respiratory tract infections in elderly long-term patients (Loeb et al., 1999).

Musculoskeletal

Joint stiffness increases and range of motion progressively decreases after short periods of immobility. With immobilization muscle fibers begin to shorten, limiting full range of motion of the attendant joint (Singer, Dunne, Singer, & Allison, 2002). Measurable changes in joint range of motion are noted in animal models after just two weeks of immobility (Trudel, Uhthoff & Brown, 1999).

Decreased mobility also produces loss of skeletal muscle mass (atrophy). Skeletal muscle atrophies rapidly within the first 7 days of decreased weight bearing (Bloomfield, 1997). Muscle mass declines by 7% to 14% after four weeks of immobilization and is accompanied by loss of strength and endurance (Berg, Dudley, Haggmark, Ohlsen, & Tesch, 1991).

Although strength and muscle mass can be regained after bedrest, at least one week of rehabilitation is required for each week of immobilization (Berg et al., 1991). Recovery takes twice as long in the elderly client (Brummel-Smith, 1996).

Bone

Altered mobility adversely effects bone integrity. Diminished weight bearing increases osteoclastic (bone reabsorbing) activity above oseoblastic (bone building) activity. Bone loss begins within seven days of immobilization (Bloomfield, 1997; LeBlanc et al., 1995). Scheld et al. (2001) found that renal calcium excretion was elevated after two weeks of bedrest and renal excretion of N-telopeptide (a bone resorption marker) were highest after weeks 10 and 14 of bedrest.

For the older individual, bone loss resulting from prolonged bedrest compounds bone loss resulting from aging and menopause. Pluijm and colleagues (1999) found that an immobile period of longer than four weeks was a strong predictor of hip and other fractures. Although bone mineral may be gradually restored after bedrest, the rate of restoration is much slower than the rate of loss (Bloomfield, 1997). Residual deficits may persist following remobilization (Jorgenson et al., 2000).

Skin

Pressure ulcer development is a serious and costly consequence of immobility. When unable to change or control body position or a body part, soft tissue between a bony prominence and an external surface, such as the bed mattress or chair seat, is compressed. Capillary blood flow may be obstructed, causing tissue ischemia and hypoxia. Exposure to prolonged and intense pressure or pressure of low intensity and long durations will produce cell death and pressure ulcer development (Husain, 1953; Kosiak, 1961). Age-related skin changes, poor nutritional states, and diminished central or peripheral sensory perception can also interact with immobility and pressure to produce ulcer development.

Metabolic Effects

Immobility markedly reduces the energy requirements of cells and their metabolic processes. Impaired glucose tolerance can develop after only three days of bedrest (Yanagibori et al., 1994). A negative nitrogen balance may develop within seven days of immobilization due to muscle mass loss (Ferrando et al., 1996) but is highest after 14 days of bedrest (Scheld et al., 2001).

Gastrointestinal

Impaired mobility affects the gastrointestinal system by altering one or more of its three functions: ingestion, digestion, and elimination (Olson et al., 1967). Immobility decreases colonic motility. Muscle weakness and the inability to use gravity to aid in defecation worsen constipation and increase the risk for fecal impaction. Decreased colonic activity as well as lowered metabolic rates reduce appetite. An inadequate supply of nutrients eventually interferes with digestion and cellular metabolism.

Genitourinary

Immobility alters physiological urinary flow and increases the risk for urinary tract infections and calculi formation. Urine drains from the renal pelvis by gravity. With bedrest, drainage of urine from the renal calyces is impaired, and bladder emptying may be incomplete. Urine stasis in the kidney and bladder allows for bacterial growth and increases the time for precipitation and aggregation of the calcium crystalloids that have been excreted as a result of mobilization of calcium from the skeletal system (Ruml et al., 1995).

Neurological–Psychological and Social Effects

Altered mobility and impaired activity may decrease social interaction and reduce sensory stimulation. Anxiety, hostility, depression, auditory and visual alterations, time and spatial distortions, neu-

rosis and sleep disturbances also have been noted (Ishizaki et al., 1994; Monk et al., 1997; Ryback et al., 1971, Stewart, 1986). These factors may, in turn, further reduce mobility, reduce social interactions, and increase isolation. Bates-Jensen et al. (2004) found that nursing home residents observed in bed during the daytime experienced increased daytime sleeping and less social engagement. Social status, employment, familiar life-style, and personal goals that are altered by impaired mobility may lower self-esteem.

Impaired mobility frequently increases dependency on family or other caregivers to perform activities of daily living. The client and caregiver(s) may be faced with functional and role changes. Loss of independence and control may increase psychological stress and initiate the grieving process. Psychological stress can exacerbate disease activity or associated pain and further affect mobility. Grief over impaired mobility may persist, particularly with continued decline in mobility.

Patterns of Mobility Alteration

In many chronic diseases, levels of activity and altered mobility are seldom static. Individuals with chronic illnesses often exhibit patterns of activity and altered mobility, which, in some cases, are a defining characteristic of the disease state. These patterns can be classified as intermittent changes in mobility, progressive changes in mobility, and permanent changes in mobility. Although each of these patterns is described within this chapter as if it were a separate entity, individuals may fluctuate between patterns, depending on the activity of the disease.

Intermittent Changes in Mobility

Individuals with a chronic illness may experience intermittent acute exacerbations of the disease. Levels of activity and mobility may temporarily decline in response to the acute episode (Figure 7-1). For example, the client with congestive heart failure (CHF) may experience increased shortness of breath and be less active while being treated for the CHF.

FIGURE 7-1

Pattern of Intermittent Change in Mobility

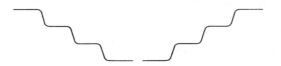

Once symptoms have abated and the client feels better, energy, activity, and mobility improve. Exacerbations of a chronic disease may be rare or frequent but often occur unpredictably. This unpredictability creates difficulty for the client and family in planning activities of any kind because of the ambiguity of what will happen in the future.

Progressive Changes in Mobility

Progressive changes continue over time in a given steplike direction (Figure 7-2). A negative progression has continuous downward steps; a positive direction demonstrates some kind of improvement. The level of altered mobility may stabilize or plateau for a period of time during the process.

In some disease states, progressive immobility may occur with physical or functional decline, increasing pain, or fatigue. An individual with multiple sclerosis (MS), for example, may experience a sudden decline in physical and functional abilities, which may be stabilized with an adjustment to the medical regimen. However, these individuals show steplike deterioration in mobility over time. Coping with a downward trajectory of mobility is often difficult for a client and family. Stabilization at a plateau provides opportunities to adjust before another change occurs. Expectations for continued improvement can exceed the client's potential or ability, and the client and family may be greatly disappointed when their hopes are not realized.

Permanent Changes in Mobility

Permanence refers to mobility loss that is irreversible, even when appropriate rehabilitative care has been provided (Figure 7-3). Permanent change can occur after a period of intermittent or progressive change but frequently results from sudden trauma or injury, as with spinal cord injuries or cerebrovascular accidents. Permanent changes in mobility may place a heavy burden of financial, emotional, and psychosocial demands on the client and significant others. The family unit must adjust to the disability in order to function in a reasonably stable manner.

FIGURE 7-2

Pattern of Progressive Change in Mobility

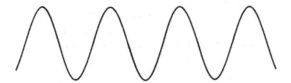

FIGURE 7-3

Pattern of Permanent Change in Mobility

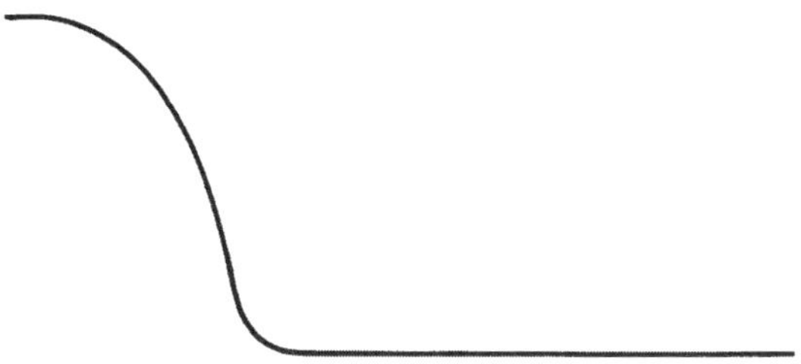

Interventions for the Client with Altered Mobility

A major goal of the health care professional is to help the client gain optimum health and mobility. This requires a detailed assessment of the physiological, psychosocial, and environmental factors limiting mobility as well as the complications encountered from the impaired mobility. Interventions for clients with altered mobility should address the causative factors and focus on preventing or ameliorating complications, providing psychological support, and reducing environmental barriers.

Preventative Health Care

Clients with chronic illness may not be receiving adequate preventative health care to promote optimal wellness and prevent comorbid conditions. The reduction in preventative care may be a result of the focus of care on the chronic illness, overshadowing the need for preventative health care. Shabas and Weinreb (2000) surveyed 220 women with multiple sclerosis and found that 85% had never taken a bone density test, 50% were not taking supplemental calcium, and 71% were not taking vitamin D, despite their increased risk for premature osteoporosis. They reported that 50% of the women did not receive regular preventative examinations, 25% did not receive regular pelvic examinations, and 11% had not had a pap smear in three to five years.

Researchers have found disparities in preventative services based on mobility. Among women aged 18 to 75 years who had not had their uterus removed, Iezzoni and colleagues (2000) found that those with major mobility problems were less likely than those without mobility problems to have received a Papanicolaou test within the previous three years (63.3% compared to 81.4%). Among women who were older than 50 years, they found that those with major mobility problems were less likely than those without mobility problems to have had a mammogram within the previous two years (45.3% compared to 63.5%). Iezzoni et al. also noted that persons with major mobility problems were less likely than persons without mobility problems to be asked about their use of tobacco, alcohol, and drugs; and to receive a tetanus shot.

Physical impairments present a barrier to some of these preventative health care services. For example, clients with mobility impairments generally require greater assistance and longer appointment times than clients who do not have impaired mobility (Iezzoni et al., 2000) Wheelchair access to health care offices and clinics can be a problem. Equipment may not be user-friendly for clients with mobility problems. For example, most equipment for mammography requires women to stand for the procedure, and most examining tables are high and non-adjustable, making it difficult for wheelchair-bound clients to get onto them.

Physical Activity

Physical activity can prevent, minimize, or reverse many of the adverse consequences of altered mobility. Specifically, physical activity enhances musculoskeletal strength and functioning to facilitate functional capacity and self-sufficiency and improves circulation, appetite, digestion, elimination, respiration, mood, sleep, and self-concept. Habitual exercise also plays an important role in the prevention and treatment of many disabling chronic diseases, such as cardiovascular disease, stroke, osteoporosis, and diabetes. Among older persons with impaired mobility, physical activity may be associ-

Altered Mobility—Case Study

Gracy Williams is a 78-year-old widow who, until recently, lived with her dog, an Irish Setter, in a two-bedroom single story house with a fenced-in yard. She has one daughter who lives nearby and a close circle of friends. She is overweight and has a history of hypertension, hypothyroidism, and osteoarthritis, with pain in her low back which made it more difficult to take her dog for walks.

A year ago Ms. Williams fell in the back yard after her dog bumped up against her. Her hip was fractured in the area of the femoral neck and she was hospitalized. Treatment consisted of surgery to insert a hip joint prosthesis. Inpatient rehabilitation began the day after surgery and included bed level and chair level exercises, which consisted of range of motion, strengthening, and conditioning exercises. Nurses administered pain mediation 45 minutes before physical therapy sessions to help keep the pain under control during physical therapy sessions. By the fourth post-operative day, Ms. Williams was practicing standing pivot transfers from bed to chair, wheelchair skills, pre-gait and gait activities, bathroom skills, and training for activities of daily living. By the eighth post-operative day, Ms. Williams was practicing advanced skills in transfer, mobility, and activities of daily living. The therapists encouraged Ms. Williams' daughter to be present during

therapy so that she could help with strengthening and conditioning exercises, and could learn to use equipment that would be needed after discharge.

Because Ms. Williams' progress was slower than expected, she was transfered to a rehabilitation unit on the tenth postoperative day where she received comprehensive rehabilitation. Plans were made during this time to discharge Ms. Williams to her daughter's home. With the help of the home health nurse and the physical therapist, Ms. Williams' daughter purchased grab bars, a chair, and non-slip mats for the shower; new light fixtures, and a raised toilet seat. Throw rugs and electrical cords that might present a safety hazard were removed. After 4 weeks on the rehabilitation unit, Ms. Williams was discharged to her daughter's home where she continued to receive home health physical therapy for 8 weeks after discharge. Periodically, Ms. Williams' home health nurse reviewed her medications for potential side effects and interaction that might increase her risk for another fall.

One year later, Ms. Williams continues to ambulate with a cane and tries to maintain a program of regular exercise. Although she no longer drives or takes the dog for a walk, she goes to church and family events with family and friends.

---

ated with a reduced risk of disability and mortality (Hirvensalo, Rantanen, & Heikkinen, 2000).

Increasing Activity in the Client Who Is Bedridden

Bedrest is sometimes required to decrease functional demands on the body. When bedrest is im-

posed, it should be kept to a minimum. Individuals placed on bedrest should turn, cough, and deep breathe every two hours. A 30-degree side-lying position is recommended because a 90-degree lateral position places excessive pressure on tissue over the trochanter bone. Turning the client from a 30-degree or 40-degree side-lying position to the same position on the opposite side will help mobilize secretions. The combination of turning, coughing, and deep breathing also provides stimulus to the cardiovascular reflexes, alters intravascular pressure, relieves pressure on tissue over bony prominences, and prevents urinary stasis. When repositioning, clients should be placed in proper body alignment to maximize respiratory function and avoid contracture formation.

As important as turning the client from side to side is changing the client's position from horizontal to vertical. Simply helping the client stand on her or his feet for a few minutes each day may prevent bedrest-related bone loss (Mahoney, 1998) and orthostatic hypotension as well as maximize respiratory, gastrointestinal, and genitourinary mechanics. When standing is not possible, the client who is immobile should sit upright for multiple times each day for short intervals. Frequency is key to maintaining physical ability and reducing the negative sequelae of immobility for clients who may have little energy or tolerance for activity.

Health care professionals should encourage clients to dress, bathe, and use the toilet, with assistance if needed. The performance of activities of daily living provides joint exercise, maintains task-specific muscle training, and fosters independence within a person's limitations (Carlson et al., 1999; Mahoney, 1998).

Exercise

Although physical activity may reduce many of the adverse effects of immobility, added exercise is necessary to maintain and improve physiological and psychological health. Exercise can be classified as flexibility training, resistance or strength training, endurance or aerobic training, and balance training.

Flexibility Training Flexibility training maintains or improves joint motion, muscle strength and muscle mass (Mahoney, 1998). During flexibility exercises, each joint is moved through its range of motion in all planes and muscles associated with each joint are lengthened and flexed. Range-of-motion exercises and muscle stretching should be slow and of even cadence. Several repetitions should be performed multiple times per day. Special em-

phasis should be paid to hip extension, knee extension, ankle dorsiflexion, and shoulder flexion, because joint motion is more likely to become restricted in these directions (Mahoney, 1998). For those on bedrest, exercises should be performed in a seated position whenever possible to maximize respiratory, gastrointestinal, and genitourinary mechanisms and place a greater load on the spine.

Flexibility exercises also help prevent venous thrombus formation. The exercise activity causes contraction of the skeletal muscles, which exerts pressure on the veins, promotes venous return, and reduces venous stasis.

Resistance or Strength Training Strength training is a form of active exercise in which muscular contraction is resisted by an outside force. Strength training maintains or improves muscle strength and muscle fiber area and can increase functional performance and capability (Hurley & Roth, 2000).

Resistance exercises can be carried out isometrically, isokinetically, and isotonically. Isometric exercise is a static form of exercise during which muscles contract but do not shorten. No joint movement occurs because muscle length does not change. When performed, each voluntary contraction should be held from six to ten seconds. Ten sets of five repetitions are commonly recommended. Welsh and Rutherford (1996) demonstrated that strength training using isometric contractions maintained or modestly increased muscle strength.

Isokinetic exercise is a form of dynamic exercise during which muscle movement occurs at a constant speed that is controlled by a mechanical device. Resistance to movement is applied, but the amount of resistance accommodates to the tension-producing capabilities of the muscle throughout the range of motion (Kisner & Colby, 1996). Clients undergoing knee surgery may have the affected leg placed in this type of device. Range of motion is performed automatically at a prescribed degree, level of resistance, and length of time. Isokinetic systems are also available for training other extremity or trunk musculature. Isokinetic exercise has been shown to be an effective means of increasing muscle strength and endurance.

During isotonic exercises, muscles shorten or lengthen against a constant or variable load. Having the client close a fist and squeeze tightly is an example of an isotonic exercise that can be done while resting in bed. More strenuous isotonic exercises that can be conducted in bed include performing active range-of-motion exercises against resistance, adding weights to the extremities during range-of-motion activities, and performing bed chin-ups by pulling the body directly upward toward an overhead trapeze. Examples of isotonic exercises for ambulatory clients include lifting hand-held weights, walking in a swimming pool, and use of weight machines. Frequent sets of one to three repetitions throughout the day are preferable to fewer sets of more repetitions for clients who have little endurance (Mahoney, 1998).

Research has suggested that isotonic exercises may forestall or reverse age-related declines in muscle strength among the elderly (Hurley & Roth, 2000). In a study that examined the effects of a strength-training program in older men, participants showed significant improvement in knee extension strength and contraction velocity after 12 weeks (Trappe et al., 2000). Nursing home residents who performed progressive resistance training of the hip and knee extensors for 45-minute sessions three days a week showed significant improvement in muscle strength tests, gait speed, stair-climbing, power, and ambulatory competence (Fiatarone et al., 1994). Benefits of strength training have even been noted in the oldest old (Schulte & Yarasheski, 2001).

Resistance exercise programs have been used effectively in clients with a variety of chronic illnesses. Aquatic exercise programs, for example, have been found to reduce postural sway in women with lower extremity rheumatoid or osteoarthritis (Koceja, 2000) and improve gait and flexibility in older individuals with arthritis (Alexander, Butcher, & MacDonald, 2001).

Resistance training may be an important adjunct to aerobic exercise for clients with heart failure. The addition of weight training may improve functional adaptations in the neuromuscular system, prevent muscle atrophy and deconditioning, and increase muscle strength and endurance (King, 2001).

Clients with amyotrophic lateral sclerosis (ALS) may benefit from an exercise program designed to increase muscle endurance. In a prospective study of 25 patients with ALS, 15-minute periods of exercise performed twice daily had a mild and temporary positive effect on motor deficit and disability (Drory, Goltsman, Rexnik, Mosek, & Korczyn, 2001).

The effectiveness of an eight-week home-based resistance exercise program for adults with multiple sclerosis was examined by DeBolt and McCubbin (2004). The exercises included chair raises, forward lunges, step-ups, heel-toe raises, and leg curls. The exercise program increased leg extensor power and did not cause injury or exacerbate the symptoms of multiple sclerosis. Four participants stopped using their canes.

Endurance or Aerobic Training Aerobic capacity or endurance is determined by the body's capacity to take up oxygen, deliver oxygen to muscle cells, and efficiently extract it for cellular metabolism during exercise. Aerobic exercises maintain or enhance the body's capacity to effectively perform these processes. Walking, dancing, treadmill exercises, bicycling, running, swimming, hiking, cross-country skiing, and rope-skipping are all types of aerobic exercises.

For clients on bedrest, aerobic exercises such as air punches and supine cycling may be of benefit. Liu et al. (2003) found that one hour of supine cycling per day was beneficial for preventing bone loss in adults during bedrest. While seated, clients may perform light exercises such as circling or scissor-like crossing of the arms, leg kicks, and stepping feet alternately onto a low step or cushion placed approximately 18 inches in front of the chair (Eliopoulos, 1997; Mahoney, 1998).

Weight-bearing activity such as walking prevents bone loss in the lumbar spine and lower extremities (Kelley, 1998). Moderate intensity aerobic exercises increase ventilatory volume, improve cardiovascular performance, and decrease blood pressure, body fat, weight, serum triglycerides, and insulin resistance when performed 3 to 5 days per week (NIH Consensus Panel, 1995). Aerobic exercise also enhances muscle protein synthesis and improves maximal oxygen consumption and leg blood flow in older adults (Beere, Russel, Morey, Kitzman, & Higginbotham, 1999; Short, Vittone, Bigelow, Proctor, & Nair, 2004). When aerobic exercises cannot be performed for 30 minutes or more, some health benefits may be gained over time when aerobic activity is performed daily in several short 10-minute sessions (Surgeon General, 1996). A moderate amount of occupational physical activity also has been shown to protect against subsequent impaired physical mobility (Gregory, Gallo, & Armenian, 2001).

Balance Training   Balance is the ability to control upright posture under a variety of conditions and is prerequisite to physical activity. Forty minutes of balance training program performed two to three times weekly for 12 weeks improved static balance function among Japanese frail elderly (Uchiyama & Kakurai, 2003). Dynamic balance exercise in the form of tai chi is the only *individual* intervention that demonstrates a significant reduction in the risk of falls (Wolf et al., 1996). Balance training otherwise does not increase range of motion, muscle strength, or endurance (Province et al., 1995). Otherwise, balance training combined with other forms of exercise appears to be more effective in increasing stability and lessening falls (Carlson et al., 1999).

Exercise Prescription

Flexibility, strength, endurance, and balance are each important in preventing and ameliorating the causes and consequences of altered mobility. The different types of exercise are best done in combination to achieve desired outcomes. For example, a nine-week exercise and education program held twice weekly that included stretching, strengthening, endurance, and balance was shown to improve physical performance and mental health among older adults (mean age 73 ± 6.4 years) with moderate to severe osteoarthritis or rheumatoid arthritis (Gunther, Taylor, Karuza, & Calkins, 2003).

Encouragement to exercise by health care professionals has been shown to increase the chances that individuals will increase their level of physical activity. In one study, older men and women (aged 65 to 84 years) who remembered receiving advice to exercise by a health care professional initiated supervised exercise classes five to six times more frequently than similar men and women who did not recall having received such advice (Hirvensalo, Heikkinen, Lintunen, & Rantanen, 2003). Structured exercise activities are essential for clients with spinal cord injury and many other health care problems to reduce the risk of complications related to a sedentary lifestyle and immobility and to increase physical capacity (Jacobs & Nash, 2004).

Interdisciplinary collaboration is important in developing an effective exercise plan that carries a low risk of injury. Nurses, physicians, and physical and occupational therapists should develop an individualized exercise program that is based on the client's past medical history, functional limitations and motivation. Together, they can monitor client tolerance to the prescribed exercises.

Clients, families, and caregivers must be taught the importance of physical activity in preventing and minimizing alterations in mobility. They should be instructed on the elements of the exercise prescription, possible adverse events and subsequent action. Family and caregivers play a crucial role in encouraging clients to perform range-of-motion exercises, sit up in a chair, and ambulate as much as possible. They can also encourage or assist the client to perform prescribed exercise routines.

Adequate Nutrition

Proper nutrition is essential for the maintenance of body structure and function and requisite for activity and motion. Adequate amounts of protein and carbohydrates are needed to reduce a negative nitrogen balance, maintain normal tissue repair, and support exercise performance (Volek, 2003). Nutritional interventions to correct individual deficiencies should also focus on supplementing needed micronutrients, vitamins and minerals. Calcium intake in recommended amounts prevent bone absorption and maintains bone mass. Adequate fluid intake also is necessary to prevent dehydration, decrease urinary stasis, maintaining electrolyte balance, blood viscosity, and the viscosity of pulmonary secretions in immobile individuals.

Pain Control

Pain control is necessary to prevent or minimize alterations in mobility and break the pain, anxiety, and immobility cycle. Nonnarcotic analgesics, such as acetaminophen and nonsteroidal antiinflammatory drugs (NSAIDs) may be prescribed to control mild to moderate pain and reduce the inflammation associated with musculoskeletal disorders. Narcotic preparations such as morphine, codeine, and fentanyl are usually used for more severe pain. Relief from joint pain may also require the injection of steroids into the affected joint.

Comfort measures may facilitate reduction of pain. Specific comfort techniques such as relaxation therapy, massage, biofeedback, acupuncture, and imagery may provide pain relief. Vibration and the application of heat and cold may also relieve acute and chronic pain.

The health care professional must learn to listen actively to the client's description of the type and quality of experienced pain in order to take effective individualized action (McCaffery & Pasero, 1999). Careful assessment of pain is especially important in children and the elderly and should be performed with tools that are age appropriate. Pain management also should include monitoring for the side effects of prescribed medications.

Aids for Sensory Impairment

Professionals should be knowledgeable about the services and assistive technologies available to those with sensory impairment. They should ask clients how the sensory impairment affects their participation in activities of daily living. Referrals for low-vision rehabilitation services may help these individuals increase their mobility and participation in essential and meaningful activities (Lamoureux et al., 2004). For individuals with partial vision, improved lighting, especially floor lighting, helps reduce falls or other home accidents. Steps with edges in colors, vibrant contrasting colors to mark changes in height or location, or enlarged lettering can alert the person to surroundings and enhance mobility. The removal of bifocals when descending stairs may improve visual reception sufficiently to maintain balance.

Tactile or auditory interventions generally are useful. Tactile aids include raised lettering or Braille to designate doorways, business location, elevator floors, and so on. Books on tape and enlarged-print products are readily available. An array of auditory cues such as bells and alarms also can be used to present information to the visually impaired.

Effective interventions to compensate for hearing loss include the use of visual cues (blinking lights and hand and facial gestures) or tactile cues (touching the individual to gain attention or creating vibratory contact such as pounding on a table or floor). General measures include facing the auditorially impaired person to allow him or her to focus on the speaker's face and gestures. Telecommunication devices for the deaf (TDD) enhance telephone communication for persons with hearing impairments.

Psychosocial Interventions

Health care professionals should encourage clients to assume responsibility for maintaining mobility and preventing further losses to mobility. Knowledge and perceived control may enhance feelings of self-efficacy and improve mood and depression. Clients also may need to be referred for counseling and psychological treatment to help them work through changes to self, loss, and grief.

Prior roles may no longer be possible or may be significantly altered. Changes in employment, occupation, home responsibilities, and daily routines may be necessary. Clients may need encouragement to be socially active and require support from rehabilitative services to establish a different life-style.

The client's social network also may require support. A realistic understanding of the client's limits, abilities, and goals assists these individuals in working together cohesively. Respite time may be needed to provide caregivers time away from responsibilities. Referral for financial, emotional and spiritual support may facilitate psychological and social adjustment for involved members.

Management of Equipment

Assistive devices and equipment are sometimes necessary to maximize mobility. An overbed trapeze will enable some individuals to reposition themselves independently and perform chin-ups. Additional devices for mobility include walkers, wheelchairs, canes, transfer devices for lifting, and orthotics. Care should be taken to ensure that the mobility aid is the correct device, appropriately sized and in good repair. Devices for hygiene include bathtub benches and seats for washing and showering. Raised toilet seats reduce the difficulties associated with rising to a standing position and reduce stress on the hip and knee (Alexander, Koester & Grunawalt, 1996). Devices for furnishing and adaptation of homes include special tables, handrails, elevators, stair-lifts, and ramps. The client should be instructed in the correct use of the mobility aid.

Reducing Environmental Barriers

Health care professionals need to be aware of the environmental barriers that affect mobility. Clients should be encouraged to wear clothing that facilitates unencumbered movement. Footwear should be carefully fitted, with low heels and non-skid soles. It is also important to anchor loose rugs and reduce the hazards of wet, waxed, or slick floor surfaces. Pathways should be kept free of obstacles and clutter to encourage ambulation and prevent falls. Restrictions to mobility that are imposed by treatments such as intravenous tubing and foley catheters. may be remedied by using feasible alternatives, such as intravenous locks and leg bags.

Education of individuals, groups, and federal, state, and local agencies about the importance of removing environmental barriers to mobility is important. The passage of the Americans with Disabilities Act (ADA) in 1990 provided a legal means to assure equality of opportunity, full participation, independent living, and economic self-efficiency for persons with disabilities. Federal and state laws now require physical and vocational access to private as well as federally funded businesses and vocational and educational institutions for those with disabilities.

Health care professionals can become advocates by encouraging agencies to move toward greater accessibility and by finding creative alternatives for the client and other involved individuals. Jones and Sanford (1996) suggested that a reduction in the slope of access ramps may be needed, as may the design of signage, alarm systems, and door and window hardware to accommodate an aging America. Requirements for accessibility also may need to accommodate personal assistants and better account for assistive technology. Currently, architectural drawings of barrier-free homes feature bathrooms that accommodate both the wheelchair-bound individual and a caregiver (Blaney, 2000).

Cultural Influences

Social norms and expectations may influence the level of mobility. Individuals who interact with others at higher levels of mobility may strive to achieve a similar level of functional ability, while individuals who interact with individuals with more impairment may be willing to accept less mobile states (Mobily & Kelley, 1991). Similarly, individuals may strive for higher levels of mobility when high levels of mobility are expected or, conversely, accept lower levels of mobility when personal, family, or cultural expectations foster dependency. Decreased opportunities for socialization with other individuals may foster inactivity, altered mobility, and social isolation. Differences in the prevalence of physical activity vary by race and ethnicity. In data collected in 1999–2001, White adults (63.5%) and Asian adults (61.9%) were more likely than Black adults (49.3%) to engage in some type of physical activity during their leisure time; and adults of Hispanic or Latino origin (45.0%) were less likely than non-Hispanic adults (63.4%) to engage in physical activity during their leisure time (Schoenborn et al., 2004).

Differences in the incidence of smoking, alcohol use, and body weight also varied by race and ethnicity. In 1999–2001, Asian adults, for example, exhibited healthier behaviors in terms of smoking, alcohol use, and body weight than other racial groups examined. Black women had higher rates of obesity than White and Asian women. Non-Hispanic women had much higher rates of smoking compared to Hispanic women (Schoenborn et al., 2004). Not all cultures view these behaviors the same. For example, some may view an obese woman as strong and healthy, whereas another may view an obese woman as weak and in poor health.

Among 77,000 non-institutionalized adults who responded to the 1994 National Health Interview Survey, more Black adults than White or Hispanic adults reported problems related to mobility (Iezzoni et al., 2000). After adjusting for age and gender, the percentages of adults who reported mobility problems were 15.7% for Blacks, 11.1% for Hispanics, and 10.0% for Whites.

The prevalence of chronic diseases that contribute to altered mobility also differs by cultural or ethnic group. In the United States, for example, Black adults have a higher incidence of hypertension and stroke than do White or Hispanic adults. The incidence of diabetes is higher among Hispanics and Native Americans.

Life-expectancy rates vary by cultural group. Life expectancy is lowest in Third World countries. In the United States, the life expectancy for the White population is greater than the average life expectancy for all races (Kochanek & Smith, 2004), suggesting that some groups may live longer with alterations in mobility.

Biological variations between cultural groups may attenuate or potentiate the effects of altered mobility. For example, bone density is highest among the Black population, as is muscle mass of select muscle groups. The long, thin bones of older White women leave them at greater risk for osteoporosis and bone loss and thus increased risk for immobility.

Cultural influences may modify interventions for altered mobility. For example, it may be considered inappropriate in some cultures for women to be involved in certain types of physical activity. Alternately, cultural activities may be a method of increasing physical activity for select individuals. In some cultures, family members may be reluctant to stop doing everything for a family member with impaired mobility. Such behaviors may interfere with active participation of the client in a rehabilitation program.

Some clients may have specific beliefs regarding the types of foods or food preparation techniques that promote health. Two nutritional deficiencies that are seen with greater frequency in some racial groups include lactose intolerance and glucose-6-phosphate dehydrogenase (G-6-PD) (Giger & Davidhizer, 2004). Thus, some persons may be unwilling or physically unable to eat certain Western foods. These factors should be incorporated into the plan of care.

Written educational materials, such as pamphlets and brochures, for clients with problems related to impaired mobility should be developed with careful consideration of the age, reading level and culture of intended readers. Patients who have problems related to impaired mobility are frequently elderly, and the elderly generally have a lower reading ability compared to other age groups. In an examination of ten pamphlets and brochures designed to provide information to clients on how to care for their skin and pressure ulcers, Wilson and Williams (2003) found that the average readability level was tenth grade and none of the educational materials addressed cultural needs of clients or the experience of having a pressure ulcer from a cultural point of view.

Specific information on the perception and management of immobility across cultural groups is lacking in the literature, suggesting that research in this area is needed. DiCicco-Bloom and Cohen (2003) found that nurses who provided home care for culturally diverse clients frequently did not recognize cultural differences. For those nurses who did recognize cultural differences, the differences were often viewed in terms of the nurses' cultural norms. In other cases nurses appreciated cultural differences and requested help from their supervisors to meet identified needs, however, the supervisors rejected their recommendations. DiCicco-Bloom and Cohen suggested that nurses learn to recognize and accept cultural differences and develop strategies for integrating cultural practices and beliefs into the care of clients.

Outcomes

A variety of client outcomes can be identified to determine the effectiveness of interventions for altered mobility.

- The client demonstrates muscular strength and endurance, joint flexibility, skeletal strength and alignment, balance, bone mass and density, and functional capacity
- The client demonstrates cardiac muscle conditioning, circulation, and cardiovascular reflexes within normal limits
- The client demonstrates pulmonary functioning, including vital capacity, gas exchange, removal of secretions, and absence of infection

- The client demonstrates nutritional adequacy and colonic activity
- The client demonstrates glucose tolerance, serum calcium levels, nitrogen balance, and body weight within normal limits
- The client demonstrates normal voiding patterns and absence of infection and renal calculi
- The client demonstrates proper use of assistive devices
- The environment is barrier-free
- The client verbalizes relief of pain
- The client demonstrates increased independence
- The client reports well-being

Fatigue

Introduction

Fatigue is a nonspecific symptom that is common in individuals with chronic diseases or conditions (McPhee & Schroeder, 1999). For many of these diseases, fatigue is present every day to some degree and often worsens with increased disease activity. Fatigue affects every aspect of a client's life and may interfere with his or her ability to carry out activities of daily living related to self-care as well as the ability to perform family and societal roles.

The goal in caring for the individual with fatigue is to find ways to reduce fatigue or assist the client in managing its effects. Care of the individual with a chronic disease involves the active participation of the client, who is in charge of managing the illness on a daily basis.

Significance of Fatigue

Initial research on fatigue was done by industry (Grandjean, 1968, 1969, 1970; Kashiwagi, 1971) and by aerospace researchers (Burton, 1980; Schreuder, 1966). Both groups were interested in the relationship between fatigue and the productivity and safety of their workers. Early health research in fatigue conducted by nurses included studies of clients with cancer (McCorkle & Young, 1978; Haylock & Hart, 1979) and multiple sclerosis (Freel & Hart, 1977; Hart, 1978).

Fatigue commonly occurs with illnesses that induce pain, fever, infection, diarrhea, bedrest, extreme stress, disturbed sleep, and anxiety or depression. Common disease states that induce fatigue are hypothyroidism, chronic renal failure, malignancies, congestive heart failure, anemia, nutritional disorders, chronic lung diseases (McPhee & Schroeder, 1999; Oh, Kim, Lee, & Kim, 2004), AIDS (Barroso, 2001; Bormann, Shiverly, Smith, & Gifford, 2001; Phillips et al., 2004), Parkinson's disease (Shulman, Taback, Bean, & Weiner, 2001), and multiple sclerosis (Colombo et al., 2000; Stuifbergen, Seraphine & Roberts, 2001). Fatigue is a side-effect of cancer treatment (Meek et al., 2000; Stone, Hardy, Huddart, A'Hern & Richards, 2000; Stone, Richards, A'Hern, & Hardy, 2001). It has also been associated with postpolio syndrome, although clients with this syndrome frequently have other concurrent medical conditions that contribute to the experience of fatigue (Schanke

& Stanghelle, 2001), Chen (1986) analyzed fatigue from data collected in a large probability sample (n = 2,362) of adults ages 25 to 74. In men, fatigue was associated with the four chronic conditions—arthritis, asthma, emphysema, and anemia—and in women, it occurred with arthritis and anemia. In both sexes, subjects who were physically inactive were more than twice at risk for being fatigued compared with those who were active. Reduced physical activity can lead to fatigue, but, conversely, fatigue can lead to reduced physical activity.

Defining Fatigue

Multiple factors contribute to the experience of fatigue, and the pattern of onset, duration, and the progression of fatigue may vary with specific disorders (Piper, 1997). With multiple factors involved, defining fatigue has been a challenge. Fatigue has been described from different perspectives (Aaronson et al., 1999). At the cellular level, studies have been conducted with muscle fatigue—a condition in which recovery can occur after rest (MacLaren et al., 1989). From a neurological perspective, fatigue has been described as central (malfunction of the central nervous system) and peripheral (impaired neuromuscular transmission). From a psychological perspective, fatigue has been described as a product of boredom or reduced motivation (Lee, Hicks & Nino-Murcia, 1991). Clients often experience difficulty describing their fatigue, relying on metaphors to describe their experience (Potter, 2004). Further complicating definitions of *fatigue* is the fact that the exact mechanism that causes fatigue in many chronic diseases is unknown. Fatigue can be documented subjectively and objectively, but little is known about the pathophysiology involved.

Fatigue has been defined "as an unpleasant sensation of tiredness, weakness, or lack of energy" (Stone, Richards, A'Hern, & Hardy, 2001, p. 1007). Everyone experiences this type of fatigue after a long, busy day. Piper (1989) differentiates this normal "acute fatigue" from chronic fatigue. She describes chronic fatigue as having an unknown

purpose or function, as primarily affecting ill clinical populations, and as having multiple additive or unknown causes, and often unrelated to activity or exertion. Piper's integrated model of fatigue identifies six general dimensions that define fatigue:

1. Temporal
2. Sensory
3. Cognitive/mental
4. Affective/emotional
5. Behavioral
6. Physiological

The model also identifies 13 risk factors that contribute to the occurrence of fatigue (Table 7-2).

In integrating the physical and mental aspects of fatigue, Carpenito-Moyet (2004) defined fatigue as "the self-recognized state in which a person experiences an overwhelming, sustained sense of exhaustion and decreased capacity for physical and mental work that is not relieved by rest" (p. 309). Although multiple factors may contribute to fatigue, it is the client's perception of fatigue as a symptom of generalized tiredness or lack of energy that is the concern of both the client and the health care provider.

TABLE 7-3

Risk Factors Contributing to Fatigue

- Life event patterns
- Social patterns
- Environmental patterns
- Changes in regulation/transmission patterns
- Oxygenation patterns
- Psychological patterns
- Symptom patterns
- Innate host factors
- Accumulation of metabolites
- Changes in energy and energy substrate patterns
- Activity/rest patterns
- Sleep/wake patterns
- Treatment patterns

SOURCE: Data from Piper et al. (1989).

Problems and Issues with Fatigue

Fatigue is an all consuming symptom that disrupts normality in the following ways:

- *Affecting physical functioning:* Fatigue can interfere with performance of self-care activities of daily living such as dressing, bathing, and eating. The client may seek help from others or avoid doing these activities with regularity. If fatigue interferes with the preparation or eating of food, malnutrition and weight loss can occur, which can increase fatigue. Withdrawal from an active life-style of many forms of physical activity may hasten problems of immobility, such as constipation, decreased muscle strength, and overall endurance.

- *Changing roles/relationships:* Fatigue has profound psychological and cognitive effects on the client. One's self-esteem, mood, self-motivation, memory, ability to concentrate, and relationships with others are often negatively affected. Fatigue interferes with one's ability to perform the roles of cook, parent, housekeeper, friend, wife, or breadwinner, and clients may disengage partially or totally from some of these roles (Dzurec, 2000; Potter, 2004).

- *Causing social isolation:* The fatigued client may avoid contact with others, feeling that it takes too much energy to communicate effectively or participate in group activities. This normal reaction may remove the client from those who could be most supportive. Invitations to social events may diminish or cease completely if the ill person consistently declines such invitations. This leaves the person isolated, with a sense of loss, and may initiate the grief process. Grief can manifest itself in many forms, such as denial, pain, depression, loss of appetite, disturbed sleep, and/or guilt.

- *Affecting sexual functioning:* Fatigue also may affect a very personal aspect of the life of the client. Results of a study of sexual satisfaction in 130 subjects with arthritis indicated that fatigue, joint pain, and joint stiffness disturbed sexual adjustment of the rheumatoid arthritis (RA) subjects more than these factors affected matched control group subjects without RA (Blake et al., 1987).

- *Affecting spirituality:* Fatigue may have an impact on spirituality, especially if the fatigue occurs in the context of terminal illness. Results of a study of the fatigue experience in clients with advanced cancer revealed that clients used fatigue as an indicator of where they were in process of their illness (Potter, 2004). Potter suggested that the meaning of fatigue may be integrated into the process of coping with a terminal illness and impending death, and may determine reactions to fatigue.

- *Affecting quality of life:* Fatigue may have an impact on quality of life. Fatigue has been negatively associated with global quality of life in clients with prostate cancer receiving hormone therapy (Stone, Hardy, Huddart, A'Hern, & Richards, 2000), and with different aspects of the quality of life in patients with ankylosing spondylitis (van Tubergen et al., 2002). The different domains of quality of life were explained by different dimensions of fatigue.

Measurement of Fatigue

Measurement of fatigue is important for clinicians and researchers particularly, because they determine whether interventions have been effective in decreasing fatigue levels in their clients. There are a number of instruments that have been developed to measure fatigue. Instruments include the Fatigue Severity Scale (Krupp et al., 1989), the Visual Analog Scale for Fatigue (Lee, Hicks & Nino-Murcia, 1991), the Multidimensional Assessment of Fatigue (Tack, 1991), the Profile of Mood States short form fatigue subscale (McNair, Lorr, & Droppleman, 1992), the Short Form-36 Vitality Subscale of the Short Form Health Survey, and the Fatigue Questionnaire (Chalder et al., 1993). A discussion of these instruments is beyond the scope of this chapter, but Neuberger (2003) provides a thorough description and brief critique of many of them. An instrument designed to measure fatigue in pediatric clients is the Pediatric Quality of Life Inventory Multidimensional Fatigue Scale. It was designed for use in children and adolescents age 2 to 18 years and has demonstrated reliability and validity with this population (Varni, Burwinkle, Katz, Meeske, & Dickinson, 2002).

A decision must be made about which aspect of fatigue one is interested in measuring: Severity? The distress it causes? Activities with which it interferes? Another decision must focus on the population to be assessed: Clients with cancer? Clients with rheumatoid arthritis? Clients of a particular age group? Asking these questions helps the health care professional decide which instrument is appropriate to use. For example, the Fatigue Severity Scale (Krupp et al., 1989) may be a better measure of fatigue-related severity, symptomatology and functional disability for persons with Chronic Fatigue Syndrome (Taylor, Jason, & Torres, 2000). Meek et al. (2000) compared the psychometric properties of several fatigue instruments in adults with cancer. The Profile of Mood States short form received their highest recommendation for the assessment of cancer-related fatigue and the evaluation of the impact of cancer treatment on fatigue.

Fatigue in Chronic Disease

Two chronic diseases, rheumatoid arthritis (RA) and cancer, typify the effects, predictors, and related factors associated with fatigue.

Rheumatoid Arthritis

Individuals with RA report fatigue as one of the three most problematic aspects of having the disease (Jump, Fifield, Tennen, Reisine, & Giulliano, 2004; Tack, 1990). Clients described fatigue as an overall sense of tiredness and heaviness that was associated with the desire to sleep. Conditions under which the onset of fatigue occurred were joint pain, disturbed sleep, dealing with environmental barriers, emotional stress, certain household tasks, and working long hours. Effects of fatigue included increased feelings of irritability, frustration, helplessness, pain, and hopelessness.

Another study found that 40% of 133 persons with RA reported that fatigue occurred every day. Analyses of data showed that pain, sleep quality, physical activity level, comorbid conditions, functional status, and duration of disease affected levels of fatigue (Tack, 1991).

Crosby (1991) studied factors related to fatigue in clients with RA and found disease activity, disturbed sleep, and increased physical effort associated with increased fatigue. In another study, Huyser and colleagues (1998) found that best predictors of fatigue were higher levels of pain, more depressive symptoms, and being female. In addition, longer duration of RA and less perceived adequacy of social support were associated with greater fatigue.

Neuberger and colleagues (1997) conducted a study of 25 persons with RA who participated in an exercise intervention program. The purpose of the study was to determine factors that correlated with fatigue and to determine the effects of a 12-week low-impact exercise class on the experience of fatigue. Data analyses supported significant positive relationships among fatigue and depression, sleep disturbance, anger, and tension. Subjects who attended more exercise classes significantly decreased their fatigue without increasing measures of disease activity. All subjects, on average, showed increased aerobic fitness, increased right- and left-hand grip strength, decreased pain, and decreased time to walk 50 feet. Evidence of the benefits of aerobic and strengthening exercises for persons with RA has increased (Stenstrom & Minor, 2003). However, there is little research on the effects of exercise on RA symptoms such as fatigue, pain and quality of life (Stenstrom & Minor).

Cancer

Irvine et al. (1991) reviewed 24 research articles exploring the experience of fatigue in individuals with cancer. These authors found that fatigue is a prevalent problem among individuals with cancer who are receiving chemotherapy and radiation therapy. Their review found that fatigue occurred in 80% to 96% of individuals receiving chemotherapy. Fatigue was positively associated with pain, negative mood, and cumulative dose of interferon therapy. In clients receiving radiation therapy, the prevalence of fatigue increased over the course of therapy and gradually diminished after treatment. However, a small percentage of clients had continuing fatigue up to three months post-treatment. In the studies reviewed on radiation therapy, fatigue was related to weight loss, negative mood, pain, and length of treatment (Irvine et al., 1991).

In a subsequent prospective study conducted by Irvine and colleagues (1994), fatigue was measured in clients receiving radiation or chemotherapy compared with a healthy control group. Individuals with cancer experienced a significant increase in fatigue over a 5- to 6-week course of radiotherapy or 14 days after treatment with chemotherapy. As weight decreased in the treatment groups, fatigue increased. Symptom distress, mood disturbance (anxiety, confusion, depression, anger), and alteration in one's usual functional activities were all significantly and positively correlated to fatigue.

More recent evidence supports the association between fatigue and cancer therapy. In clients with prostate cancer, fatigue severity increased after three months of hormonal therapy (Stone et al., 2000). Modest increases in fatigue were noted among clients with cancers of the breast or prostate who were receiving radical radiotherapy (Stone et al., 2001).

Few conceptual frameworks are available that explain cancer-related fatigue. In a study of 103 women in remission from breast cancer following treatment, researchers used the stress-process theory developed by Herbert and Cohen to conceptualize fatigue as a consequence of prolonged stress (Géninas & Fillion, 2004). The results indicated that participants' perception of cancer stressors and coping strategies were related to persistent fatigue. "The more a woman perceived cancer stressors the more fatigued she was. . . . the more she used active coping, the less fatigue she reported" (p. 275). The research supported the stress-process theory in explaining cancer-related fatigue. Berger and Walker (2001) tested a conceptual model to determine variables that influence fatigue in women receiving adjuvant breast cancer chemotherapy. Predictors of fatigue differed at treatment time.

Fatigue and Other Symptoms

Fatigue does not occur in isolation from other symptoms of chronic illness, and other symptoms may affect the experience of fatigue (Dodd, Miaskowski, & Paul, 2001; Gift, Stommel, Jablonski, & Given, 2003). Symptoms such as anorexia and/or cachexia, leading to weight loss, can affect the energy available for daily activities. Other symptoms such as breathlessness or dypspnea (Oh et al., 2004; Potter, 2004), negative mood states such as anxiety or depression (Oh et al.; Phillips et al., 2004), and poor sleep quality (Phillips et al., 2004) can increase the severity of fatigue. An holistic approach is necessary to assess all of the factors that may be contributing to the fatigue experience of each client.

Research with clients with RA (Belza, 1993; Huyser et al., 1998; Neuberger, et al., 1997, Stone et al., 2001) and HIV disease (Phillips et al., 2004) supports the belief that depression is positively correlated with or can predict increased fatigue levels. A history of an affective disorder has been found to be associated with higher levels of fatigue in patients with RA, even if the depressive episode was experienced years ago (Jump et al., 2004). Jump and colleagues found that self-efficacy to perform self-management behaviors may mediate the relationship between history of affective disorder and higher levels of fatigue. In other words, a history of affective disorder influenced the experience of fatigue in RA both directly and indirectly through confidence in the ability to manage the arthritis. The relationship between fatigue and depression has also been found among persons with HIV disease (Phillips et al., 2004).

Depressed persons lack energy and motivation for activity or social interaction. Being fatigued and without energy for a day planned with numerous activities can lead to depression; however, being depressed may also lead to fatigue.

Coping with pain takes both physical and mental energy. Research supports a positive relationship between pain and fatigue in clients with RA (Belza, 1993; Huyser et al., 1998; Neuberger, 1997) and in clients with ankylosing spondylitis (van Tubergen et al., 2002). For many chronic conditions, such as arthritis, complaints of pain do not always match

Fatigue

Bonica Anderson is a 35-year-old single mother of 3 school aged children who was diagnosed with systemic lupus erythematosus five years ago. Her children are active in sports and are able to participate in sports after school. Ms. Anderson was unfamiliar with the disease at the time of diagnosis and has attempted to learn all she can about the disease through written materials provided through her physician, the internet, and a support group that she attends intermittently. She works full-time as a mail clerk in a large organization, and is able to get a fair amount of exercise at work delivering mail to the various departments.

Her most annoying problems include fatigue, painful hand joints, and an occasional discoid rash. Ms. Anderson takes nonsteroidal anti-inflammatory drugs to treat the cutaneous lesions and for the symptoms of arthritis, plaquenil, and topical steroids. Recently she experienced an extremely severe flare and was treated with intravenous methylprednisolone sodium succinate for three days followed by low-maintenance prednisone. Ms. Anderson was unable to work during this time and found it difficult to maintain her usual household activities.

Once the flare was resolved, she was able to return to work but had little energy for anything else. Ms. Anderson's nurse taught her how to conserve her energy through careful planning. Ms. Anderson learned to make easy-to-prepare meals that were healthy and enlist the help of her children in meal preparation. She learned to slide objects across the kitchen counter or floor rather than lift them, and she purchased a cart with wheels for transporting laundry and other items from room to room. She found she had to prioritize and give up activities that were less important. For her, that meant not making her bed every morning, allowing the children to pick up after themselves, and vacuuming less often. Although she missed many of her children's practices, she made a point to attend their games. On low energy days at work she was able to trade with coworkers her mail delivery activities for other more sedentary activities. By pacing herself and delegating more responsibility to her children, she was able to continue to work and maintain her household.

observable signs of disease activity such as joint swelling or sedimentation rate (Dworkin, Van Korff & Le Resche, 1992). The influence of psychosocial factors on the pain experience is supported by studies of pain in persons with RA (Bradley, 1989; Cavalieri, Salaffi & Ferraccioli, 1991).

Cultural Influences

The cultural background of the client can affect her or his perception of fatigue and the willingness to seek treatment. Specific information on how culture may affect the perception of fatigue and its management is currently not found in the literature, indicating that research is needed in this area.

The prevalence of chronic diseases that have fatigue as a common symptom varies by race and culture. For example, in Latino elders, major health concerns include diabetes, cardiovascular disease, cerebrovascular disease, and cancer, all of which can have fatigue as a symptom (Brangman, 1997). AIDS disproportionately affects Black and Hispanic communities (CDC, 2002b).

Biological differences among racial groups may influence the ability to detect factors that can contribute to fatigue. Dark skin color, for example, may influence the ability to detect the presence of pallor, jaundice, cyanosis, and rashes. When assessing clients with darker skin, nurses should use adequate lighting, and should focus on skin surfaces that have the least amount of pigmentation, such as the palms of the hands, soles of the feet, the abdomen, and buttocks. The nurse should also examine the mouth, conjunctivae and nail beds for color.

Cultures have different activity orientations, which refers to the group's perception of themselves as "doing" or "being." People from "doing"-oriented cultures value achievement, whereas, persons from "being"-oriented cultures value inherent existence (Giger & Davidhizer, 2004). Compared to persons from a being-oriented culture, a person from a doing-oriented culture may have a more difficult time coping with fatigue and may find it more difficult to set personal limits on activities.

Clients may use a variety of approaches to help reduce or limit the effects of fatigue. A variety of alternative and complementary therapies are available and attractive to such persons. Examples of such therapies include acupuncture, biofeedback, meditation, diet-based therapies, homeopathic treatments, folk medicine, massage, hypnosis, therapeutic touch, aromatic therapy, and guided imagery. According to the National Center for Complementary and Alternative Medicine (2004), approximately 36% of adults are using some form of complementary and alternative medicine in the United States, and the percentage increases to 62% when megavitamin therapy and prayer specific for health reasons are added. In addition, many people consult the *Old Farmer's Almanac* or the Zodiac to determine the best time to perform activities or receive health-related procedures; others may depend on dreams as a reliable source of guidance (Giger & Davidhizer, 2004). By the time some clients with fatigue seek conventional medicine, the nurse might correctly assume that every home remedy known to the client, as well as a variety of alternative and complementary therapies, has been tried.

Nurses and other health care professionals should assess remedies the patients have used to reduce the level of fatigue, and try to determine if the client's current practices are harmful, neutral, or beneficial. To determine whether a current practice is harmful, Giger and Davidhizer (2004) suggest that nurses ask the client if the practice has worked. If the client answers "no," the nurse may suggest that a different approach be tried. If the client believes that the harmful practice is beneficial the nurse must provide education on the potential consequences of the harmful practice (Giger & Davidhizer).

Interventions

Assessment of Fatigue

The health care professional needs to assess the client for the presence of fatigue and then plan with the client possible approaches to reduce the fatigue. As mentioned previously, there are several quantitative measurement tools available to measure fatigue. However, much data can be obtained from interviewing the client. Potential interview questions about fatigue include the following (Dzurec, 2000):

- In your own words, how would you describe your experience with fatigue?
- How long have you been bothered with fatigue?
- Has fatigue had any effect on your relationships with other people, especially with family or significant others?
- What time of day does your fatigue occur?
- What activities increase your fatigue?
- Has anything helped your fatigue?

Encourage the client to keep a diary for one week of their daily activities and times when fatigue occurs. These data can assist the health care provider and the client in planning appropriate interventions. At follow-up in a busy clinical setting, nurses may simply ask clients to rate their level of fatigue on a scale of 0 to 10. Recording these verbal assessments at each client visit or contact will aid the nurse in assessing whether interventions are helpful in reducing fatigue.

Support Groups

Lack of support may prevent a client from seeking care. Research strongly supports the belief that social support is a moderator of health behavior and physical and mental health status (Hubbard, Muhlenkamp & Brown, 1984; Langlie, 1977). Many studies have identified that it is the support the client *perceives* to be available that is more consistently related to outcome measures rather than the actual support received (Cohen & Wills, 1985; Kessler & McLeod, 1984; Wethington & Kessler, 1986).

Health care providers need to assess clients' perceptions of their social support. Clients can be encouraged to create or help expand support groups that are accessible at different locations in the community. Support groups can give clients a place to discuss problems and solutions with others with similar health problems. With modern computer technology, there are now support group mechanisms available on the Internet, enabling clients who are confined to home to interact with supportive others. An example of this appeared in a recent article in *Computers in Nursing*, entitled "Cyber Solace," which reported on Internet support groups for persons with cancer (Klemm et al., 1999).

Managing Fatigue

Nursing interventions for the client with fatigue focus on educating the client on the following interrelated energy-conservation and exercise strategies: setting priorities, delegating, planning, acting during times of peak energy, and pacing (Whitmer, Tinari, & Barsevick, 2004). *Setting priorities* involves making a list of daily activities for each day and identifying which are essential, desirable, transferable, and optional. At first, clients may overestimate the number of tasks that can be achieved in a day, but eventually they will learn to be more realistic.

Delegating activities may be difficult; clients may need counseling to determine which activities should be delegated and how to request help from others (Whitmer et al., 2004). Sometimes, roles within the family can be modified or shared. When a particular task is bothersome for the client, it needs to be reassigned to another family member. For example, vacuuming is a strenuous task for a person with arthritis affecting the wrists and small joints of the

fingers. If the client lives alone, a cleaning service may be the answer, or trading vacuuming for another more manageable task with a neighbor or friend.

Planning refers to the process of anticipating needed resources and determining the easiest way to carry out the most important activities (Whitmer et al., 2004). It involves rearranging home and work environments to minimize obstacles in performing tasks and to consolidate similar tasks. One example is arranging items in home or office work areas to have items used frequently closer to the workspace. Occupational therapists have special expertise in these areas and should be consulted when indicated (Mahowald & Dykstra, 1997). *Acting during times of peak energy* involves planning to complete high-priority tasks when energy is at its peak.

Pacing involves planning for periods of rest and exercise, breaking up big tasks into smaller more manageable ones, and spreading out the smaller activities over the week. *Resting* involves planning for short rest periods so that the fatigue produced by overactivity is prevented. An example of pacing is to teach the client to lie down for 20 to 30 minutes after arriving home from work in the late afternoon, before starting to prepare dinner for the family. Rest periods can involve reading or listening to music; naps should be limited to avoid a dysfunctional diurnal rhythm (Whitmer et al., 2004). Regular exercise at low or moderate intensity can increase endurance and decrease fatigue (Burnham & Wilcox, 2002). Increasing physical activity has been recommended by the National Arthritis Action Plan (1999) as one strategy to preserve function and independence among people with arthritis.

Maintaining one's role as a spouse or significant other, including sexual intimacy, is important for both the client and partner. Open discussion, negotiation, and compromise between sexual partners as to time, place, and alternate positions for sexual intercourse are necessary to preserve this important aspect of a couple's life together.

Knowledge of the results of research studies of fatigue in specific populations of clients can help the nurse assess those factors that may be modified to help reduce or manage fatigue. For example, among patients with multiple sclerosis, heat has been found to exacerbate fatigue. Cooling therapies may be beneficial for those clients (Ward & Winters, 2003).

Bormann et al. (2001) found a negative relationship between fatigue and self-efficacy to manage fatigue among adults who were HIV-positive. Thus, the HIV-positive individuals with greater confidence to manage fatigue reported less fatigue. Conversely, those individuals with less confidence to manage fatigue reported greater fatigue. Thus, teaching strategies that promote self-efficacy may help some clients cope with fatigue.

In another example, Potter (2004) found that the energy conservation strategies described previously were of little to no benefit among fatigued individuals with advanced cancer. Clients with advanced cancer reported that the most helpful strategies for them were talking about their experiences with a health care professional and receiving explanations regarding their symptoms. Other strategies that helped them to cope with fatigue included using relaxation techniques and having troublesome symptoms controlled.

The nurse or health care professional can educate clients with newly diagnosed cancer to anticipate that fatigue may occur and what measures they can take to alleviate its effects. The nurse can teach the client that pain can increase fatigue and that it is important that pain is adequately controlled. Remind clients to be assertive in asking for help if their pain is not under control. It also may be helpful to suggest that clients allow extra rest periods on treatment days but continue to do some light exercise such as walking on nontreatment days to help maintain muscle strength and endurance. Explore with clients activities that elevate their mood, such as music, reading, or visiting an art museum, and encourage them to schedule these activities to help elevate their mood and remain positive. Remind clients to report problems with nausea and to eat healthy, nutritious meals to avoid weight loss, which can increase fatigue. Eating small snacks more frequently may be better tolerated by clients than eating three large meals.

The National Comprehensive Cancer Network (NCCN) and the American Cancer Society (ACS) recently released new guidelines for the treatment of cancer-related fatigue and anemia. The guidelines were designed to help both patients and health care providers make informed decisions about cancer treatments. Nurses can refer clients who are at risk for cancer-related fatigue to the website, which can be found at www.nccn.org.

It is important that clients understand the mechanisms that medications and/or other treatments provide in decreasing fatigue. Clients may tend to reduce the number of medications taken as their fatigue and other symptoms improve. Some clients may do this to save money or because they are reluctant to take medications on a regular basis. Thus, it is important to teach clients how other treatments help lessen fatigue.

Insomnia or disrupted sleep secondary to pain or other discomfort may contribute to fatigue. Validate with the client that he or she is taking pain medication properly. If pain is unrelieved, obtain an order for new or additional medications. Teach the client adjuvant pain-relief methods such as music, visual imagery, relaxation technique, massage, and/or application of heat or cold when appropriate. Teach the client sleep hygiene methods such as avoiding caffeine, use of their bed only for sleeping or napping and not for reading or doing work, and establishing a regular time for sleep and awakening. If these measures are not effective, the client may need an antidepressant or nonaddictive sedative to promote sleep.

When fatigue is present, clients tend to reduce physical activity and increase rest periods to eliminate the feeling of fatigue. Such inactivity contributes to increased fatigue levels. Teach the client to increase performance of appropriate *aerobic exercises* that will increase muscle strength and endurance (Mahowald & Dykstra, 1997). Consultation with a physical therapist may be indicated when specific therapeutic exercises are indicated (e.g., for clients who have had a stroke or have multiple sclerosis).

Regardless of the type of chronic illness causing fatigue, a healthy nutritious diet is vital. Being underweight or overweight can contribute to fatigue.

Therefore, it is important to teach the client the effect of nutrition on fatigue. Consultation with a dietician may be indicated.

Fatigue management programs may be beneficial for some clients. Ward and Winters (2003), for example, found evidence that a fatigue management program designed for clients with multiple sclerosis was effective in reducing the impact of fatigue on clients' lives, and increased performance and satisfaction in everyday living. The program focused on energy conservation techniques and provided opportunities for patients with multiple sclerosis to interact with one another, socialize, and share personal experiences with fatigue.

Outcomes

Although each disease process is different, the outcomes that should be expected from managing fatigue are the same.

- The client's fatigue lessens or occurs later in the day.
- The client/family is able to describe how to prioritize daily activities to avoid or decrease fatigue.
- The client has more restful sleep.
- The client maintains normal body weight.
- The client increases muscle strength and cardiopulmonary endurance.
- The client displays positive affect and denies feelings of depression.

Summary and Conclusions

Activity and motion are a part of everyday life. Health problems, psychosocial factors, and increasing age can alter mobility and induce fatigue. Physical activity, activity management, improving nutritional status, and relieving pain prevent or minimize the physiological and many of the psychological consequences of altered mobility and fatigue. Early intervention is crucial, as complications develop rapidly and recovery of preexisting physiological states is prolonged.

Individuals with mobility alterations and fatigue face many psychological and sociological adjustments. Psychologically, the individuals must handle loss and face changes in self-image. Sociologically, they may experience role and life-style changes. Health care professionals need to be sensitive to and facilitate needed psychosocial adjustments created by the loss of mobility and ongoing fatigue.

Study Questions

1. How have advances in medical science and assistive technologies increased the number of young persons with altered mobility?
2. What age-related disorders affect mobility? For each of these disorders, how have advances in medical science and assistive technologies increased the number of persons with altered mobility?
3. What psychosocial factors impact mobility?
4. What physiological systems are affected by altered mobility? Describe these effects.
5. How does altered mobility affect psychological health?
6. How does altered mobility affect the individual's social environment?
7. How would you describe the patterns that characterize mobility alterations? Select a chronic medical condition. How would this condition "fit" within these patterns?
8. What normal physical activity interventions can be conducted for the individual on bedrest?
9. What normal physical activity interventions should be promoted for individuals who are more mobile?
10. What flexibility, resistance, and aerobic exercises can be done with the individual on bedrest?

What flexibility, resistance, aerobic, and balance exercises can be done with the individual who has fewer alterations in mobility?

11. What does the individual who is engaging in exercise need to know about performing exercise?

12. How is sensory impairment a barrier to mobility? What interventions can reduce this barrier?

13. How does pain affect mobility? What interventions help manage pain?

14. What are the environmental barriers to mobility? What interventions can help reduce these barriers and enhance mobility?

15. What common disease or illness states and alterations in health induce fatigue?

16. What psychosocial factors are associated with fatigue?

17. Differentiate between acute fatigue and chronic fatigue.

18. How is fatigue assessed?

19. What produces fatigue among patients with rheumatoid arthritis? What factors are associated with fatigue in cancer patients?

20. What interventions can be used to relieve fatigue?

References

Aaronson, L. C., Teel, C. S., Cassmeyer, V., Neuberger, G. B., et al. (1999). Defining and measuring fatigue. *Image, 31* (1), 45–50.

Alexander, M. J. L., Butcher, J. E., & MacDonald, P. B. (2001). Effect of water exercise program on walking gait, flexibility, strength, self-reported disability and other psycho-social measures of older individuals with arthritis. *Physiotherapy Canada, Summer 2001,* 203–211.

Alexander, N. B., Koester, D. J., & Grunawalt, J. A. (1996). Chair design affects how older adults rise from a chair. *Journal of the American Geriatric Society, 44,* 356–362.

American Medical Association. (2003). Pain management: Pediatric pain management. http: www.ama_cme online.com/pain_mgmt/module06/index.htm

Anderson, F. A., & Spencer, F. A. (2003). Risk factors for thromboembolism. Circulation, *107* (23 Suppl. 1), 19–16.

Barroso, J. (2001). "Just worn out": A qualitative study of HIV related-fatigue. In S. G. Funk, E. M. Tournquist, J. Leeman, M. S. Miles, & J. S. Harrell (Eds.), *Key aspects of preventing and managing chronic illness* (pp. 183–186). New York: Springer.

Bates-Jensen, B. M., Schnelle, J.F., Alessi, C. A., A-Samarrai, N. R., et al. (2004). The effects of staffing on in-bed times of nursing home residents. *Journal of the American Geriatrics Society, 52* (6), 931–938.

Beere, P. A., Russel, S. D., Morey, M. C., Kitzman, D. W., et al. (1999). Aerobic exercise training can reverse age-related peripheral circulatory changes in healthy older men. *Circulation, 100,* 1085–1094.

Belza, B. L., Henke, C. J., Yelin, E. H., Epstein, W. V., et al. (1993). Correlates of fatigue in older adults with rheumatoid arthritis. *Nursing Research, 42* (2), 93–99.

Berg, H. E., Dudley, G. A., Haggmark, T., Ohlsen, H., et al. (1991). Effects of lower limb unloading on skeletal muscle mass and function in human. *Journal of Applied Physiology, 99,* 137–143.

Berger, A. M., & Walker, S. N. (2001). An explanatory model of fatigue in women receiving adjuvant breast cancer chemotherapy. *Nursing Research, 50* (1), 42–52.

Blake, D., Maisiak, R., Alarcon, G., Holley, H., et al. (1987). Sexual quality of life of patients with arthritis compared to arthritis free controls. *Journal of Rheumatology, 14,* 570–576.

Blaney, B. (2000). Home, barrier-free home. *Arthritis Today, 14* (6), 68–72.

Bloomfield, S. A. (1997). Changes in musculoskeletal structure and function with prolonged bed rest. *Medicine and Science in Sports and Exercise, 29,* 197–206.

Bobo, N., Evert, A., Gallivan, J., Imperatore, G., et al. (2004). An update on type 2 diabetes in youth from the National Diabetes Education Program. *Pediatrics, 114* (1), 259–263.

Bormann, J., Shively, M., Smith, T. L., & Gifford, A. L. (2001). Measurement of fatigue in HIV positive adults: Reliability and validity of the Global Fatigue Index. *Journal of the Association of Nurses in AIDS Care, 12* (3), 75–83.

Bradley, L. A. (1989). Psychosocial factors and disease outcomes in rheumatoid arthritis: Old problems, new solutions, and a future agenda. *Arthritis and Rheumatism, 32,* 1611–1614.

Brangman, S. A. (1997). Minorities. In R. J. Ham & P. D. Sloane (Eds.) *Primary care geriatrics: A care based approach* (pp. 82–93). St. Louis: Mosby.

Brummel-Smith, K. (1996). Rehabilitation. In R. J. Ham & P. D. Sloane (Eds.), *Primary care geriatrics: A case-based approach* (3rd ed.) (pp. 139–152.) St. Louis, MO: Mosby.

Buckwalter, J. A., & DiNubile, N. A. (1997). Decreased mobility in the elderly. *The Physician and Sports Medicine, 25* (9), 127–133.

Burnham, T. R., & Wilcox, A. (2002). Effects of exercise on physiological and psychological variables in cancer survivors. *Medicine and Science in Sports and Exercise, 34* (12), 1863–1867.

Burton, R. R. (1980). Human responses to repeated high G simulated aerial combat maneuvers. *Aviation, Space & Environmental Medicine, 51,* 1185–1192.

Carlson, J. E., Ostir, G. V., Black, S. A., Markides, K. S., et al. (1999). Disability in older adults 2: Physical activity as prevention. *Behavioral Medicine, 24,* 157–168.

Carpenito-Moyet, L. J. (2004). *Nursing diagnosis: Application to clinical practice* (10th ed.). Philadelphia: Lippincott Williams & Wilkins.

Cavalieri, F., Salaffi, F., & Ferraccioli, G. F. (1991). Relationship between physical impairment, psychological variables, and pain in rheumatoid disability: An analysis of their relative impact. *Clinical and Experimental Rheumatology, 9,* 47–50.

Centers for Disease Control and Prevention (2002a). Prevalence of Self-Reported Arthritis or Chronic Joint Symptoms Among Adults – United States, 2001. *Morbidity & Mortality Weekly Report, 51* (42), 948–950.

Centers for Disease Control and Prevention (2002b). HIV/AIDS Surveillance Report 2002, *14,* 1–48.

Centers for Disease Control and Prevention (2003). National diabetes fact sheet: General information and national estimates on diabetes in the United States, 2002. Atlanta, GA: U. S. Department of Health and Human Services, Centers for Disease Control and Prevention.

Chalder, T., Berelowitz, G., Pawlikowska, T., Watts, L., et al. (1993). Development of a fatigue scale. *Journal Psychosomatic Research, 37,* 147–153.

Chen, M. K. (1986). The epidemiology of self-perceived fatigue among adults. *Preventive Medicine, 15,* 74–81.

Cohen, S., & Wills, T. A. (1985). Stress, social support, and the buffering hypothesis. *Psychological Bulletin, 98,* 310–357.

Colombo, B., Boneschi, F. M., Rossi, P., Rovaris, M., et al. (2000). MRI and motor evoked potential findings in nondisabled multiple sclerosis patients with and without symptoms of fatigue. *Journal of Neurology, 247,* 506–509.

Convertino, V. A. (1997). Cardiovascular consequences of bed rest: Effect on maximal oxygen uptake. *Medicine and Science in Sports and Exercise, 29* (2), 191–196.

Crosby, L. A. (1991). Factors which contribute to fatigue associated with rheumatoid arthritis. *Journal of Advanced Nursing, 16,* 974–981.

Davidson, K. K., Ford, E. S., Cogswell, M. E., & Dietz, W. H. (2002). Percentage of body fat and body mass index are associated with mobility limitations in people aged 70 and older from NHANES III. *Journal of American Geriatrics Society, 50,* 1802–1809.

DeBolt, L. S., & McCubbin, J. A. (2004). The effects of home-based resistance exercise on balance, power, and mobility in adults with multiple sclerosis. *Archives of Physical Medicine and Rehabilitation, 85,* 290–297.

Desai, M. M., Zhang, P., & Hennessy, C. H. (1999). Surveillance for morbidity and mortality among older adults—United States, 1995–1996. *Morbidity and Mortality Weekly Report, 48* (SS8), 7–26.

DiCicco-Bloom, B., & Cohen, D. (2003). Home care nurses: A study of the occurrence of culturally competent care. *Journal of Transcultural Nursing, 14* (1), 25–31.

Dieppe, P., & Tobias, J. (1998). Bone and joint aging. In R. Talles, H. Fillet, & J. C. Brocklehurst (Eds.), *Geriatric medicine and gerontology* (pp. 1131–1136). Edinburgh, United Kingdom: Churchill Livingstone.

Dikmen, S. S., Machamer, J. E., Powell, J. M., & Temkin, N. R. (2003). Outcome 3 to 5 years after moderate to severe traumatic brain injury. *Archives of Physical Medicine and Rehabilitation, 84,* 1449–1457.

Dimopoulou, I., Anthi, A., Mastora, Z., Theodorakopoulou, M., et al. (2004). Health-related quality of life and disability in survivors of multiple trauma one year after intensive care unit discharge. *American Journal of Physical Medicine and Rehabilitation, 83,* 171–176.

Dodd, M. J., Miaskowski, C., & Paul, S. M. (2001). Symptom clusters and their effect on the functional status of patients with cancer. *Oncology Nursing Forum, 28* (3), 465–470.

Drory, V. E., Goltsman, E., Rexnik, J. G., Mosek, A., et al. (2001). The value of muscle exercise in patients with amyotrophic lateral sclerosis. *Journal of Neurological Sciences, 191*, 133–137.

Ducharme, J. (2000). Acute pain and pain control: State of the art. *Annals of Emergency Medicine, 35*, 592–603.

Dworkin, S. F., Von Korff, M. R., & LeResche, L. (1992). Epidemiologic studies of chronic pain: A dynamic-ecologic perspective. *Internal Medicine, 14* (1), 3–11.

Dzurec, L. C. (2000). Fatigue and relatedness experience of inordinately tired women. *Image, 32*, 339–345.

Eliopoulos, C. (1997). *Gerontological nursing* (4th ed.). Philadelphia: Lippincott.

Ferrando, A. A., Lane, H. W., Stuart, C. A., Davis-Street, J., et al. (1996). Prolonged bedrest decreased skeletal muscle and whole body protein synthesis. *The American Journal of Physiology, 270*, E627–633.

Fiatarone, M. A., O'Neil, E. F., Ryan, N. D., Clements, K. M., et al. (1994). Exercise training and nutritional supplementation for physical frailty in very elderly people. *New England Journal of Medicine, 330*, 1769–1775.

Freel, M. I., & Hart, L. K. (1977). Study of fatigue phenomena of multiple sclerosis patients. (Grant No. 5R02-NU-00524-2), Division of Nursing, USDHEW.

Géninas, C., & Fillion, L. (2004). Factors related to persistent fatigue following completion of breast cancer treatment. *Oncology Nursing Forum, 31*, 269–278.

Gift, A. G., Stommel, M., Jablonski, A., & Given, W. (2003). A cluster of symptoms over time in patients with lung cancer. *Nursing Research, 52* (6), 393–400.

Giger, J. N., & Davidhizar, R. E. (2004). *Transcultural nursing: Assessment and intervention* (4th ed.). St. Louis, MO: Mosby.

Grandjean, E. P. (1968). Fatigue: Its physiological and psychological significance. *Ergonomics, 11*, 427–436.

_____. (1969). *Fitting the task to the man—An Ergonomic Approach.* London: Taylor & Francis.

_____. (1970). Fatigue: Yant memorial lecture. *American Industrial Hygiene Association Journal, 31*, 401–411.

Gregory, P. C., Gallo, J. J., & Armenian, H. (2001). Occupational physical activity and the development of impaired mobility: The 12-year follow-up of the Baltimore Epidemiologic Catchment Area Sample. *American Journal of Physical Medicine & Rehabilitation, 80*, 270–275.

Gunther, J. S., Taylor, M. J., Karuza, J., & Calkins, E. (2003). Physical therapist-based group exercise/education program to improve functional health in older health maintenance organization members with arthritis. *Journal of Geriatric Physical Therapy, 26* (1), 12–20.

Hack, M., & Fanaroff, A. A. (1999). Outcomes of children of extremely low birthweight and gestational age in the 1990's. *Early Human Development, 53* (3), 193–218.

Hamvas, A. (2000). Disparate outcomes for very low birth weight infants: Genetics, environment or both? *The Journal of Pediatrics, 136*, 427–428.

Hart, L. K. (1978). Fatigue in the patient with multiple sclerosis. *Research in Nursing and Health, 1*, 147–157.

Haylock, P. J., & Hart, L. K. (1979). Fatigue in patients receiving localized radiation. *Cancer Nursing, 2*, 461–467.

Hirvensalo, M., Heikkinen, E., Lintunen, T., & Rantanen, T. (2003). The effect of advice by health care professionals on increasing physical activity in older people. *Scandinavian Journal of Medicine Science Sports, 13*, 231–236.

Hirvensalo, M., Rantanen, T., & Heikkinen, E. (2000). Mobility difficulties and physical activity as predictors of mortality and loss of independence in the community-living older population. *Journal of American Geriatrics Society, 48* (5), 493–498.

Hubbard, P., Muhlenkamp, A. F., & Brown, N. (1984). The relationship between social support and self-care practices. *Nursing Research, 33*, 266–270.

Hurley, B. F., & Roth, S. M. (2000). Strength training in the elderly: Effects on risk factors for age-related diseases. *Sports Medicine, 30* (4), 249–268.

Husain, T. (1953). An experimental study of some pressure effects on tissues with reference to the bed-sore problem. *Journal of Pathology and Bacteriology, 66* (2), 347–358.

Huyser, B. A., Parker, J. C., Thoreson, R., Smarr, K. L., et al. (1998). Predictors of subjective fatigue among individuals with rheumatoid arthritis. *Arthritis & Rheumatism, 41*, 2230–2237.

Iezzoni, L. I., McCarthy, E. P., Davis, R. B., & Siebens, H. (2000). Mobility impairments and use of screening and preventative services. *American Journal of Public Health, 90*, 955–961.

Irvine, D. M., Vincent, L., Bubela, N., Thomson, L., et al. (1991). A critical appraisal of the research literature investigating fatigue in the individual with cancer. *Cancer Nursing, 14* (4), 188–199.

Irvine, D. M., Vincent., L., Graydon, J. E., Bubela, N., et al. (1994). The prevalence and correlates of fatigue in patients receiving treatment with chemotherapy and radiotherapy. *Cancer Nursing, 17* (5), 367–378.

Ishizaki, Y., Fukuoka, H., Katsura, T., Katsura, T., et al. (1994). Psychological effects of bed rest in young healthy subjects. *Acta Physiologica Scandinavia, 150* (Suppl 616), 83–87.

Jacobs, P. L., & Nash, M. S. (2004). Exercise recommendations for individuals with spinal cord injury. *Sports Medicine, 34*, 727–751.

Jones, J. L., & Sanford, J. A. (1996). People with mobility impairments in the United States today and in 2010. *Assistive Technology, 8* (1), 43–53.

Jorgensen, L., Jacobsen, B. K., Wilsgaard, T., & Magnus, J. H. (2000). Walking after stroke: Does it matter? Changes in bone mineral density within the first 12 months after stroke. A longitudinal study. *Osteoporosis International, 11* (5), 381–387.

Jump, R. L., Fifield, J., Tennen, H. Reisine, S., et al. (2004). History of affective disorder and the experience of fatigue in rheumatoid arthritis. *Arthritis Care and Research, 51* (2), 239–245.

Kane, R. L., Ouslander, J. G., & Abrass, I. B. (1999). *Essentials of clinical geriatrics* (4th ed.). New York: McGraw-Hill.

Kashiwagi, S. (1971). Psychological ratings of human fatigue. *Ergonomics, 14*, 17–21.

Kelley, G. (1998). Aerobic exercise and lumbar spine bone mineral density in postmenopausal women: A meta-analysis. *Journal of the American Geriatric Society, 46*, 143–152.

Kessler, R. C., & McLeod, J. D. (1984). Sex differences in vulnerability to undesirable life events. *American Sociological Review, 49*, 620–631.

King, L. (2001). The effects of resistance exercise on skeletal muscle abnormalities in patients with advanced heart failure. *Progress in Cardiovascular Nursing, 16*, 142–151.

Kisner, C., & Colby, L. A. (1996). *Therapeutic exercise: Foundations and techniques* (3rd ed.) (pp. 1–142). Philadelphia: F. A. Davis Company.

Klemm, P., Hurst, M., Dearholt, S. L., & Trone, S. R. (1999). Cyber solace: Gender differences on Internet cancer support groups. *Computers in Nursing, 17* (2), 65–72.

Koceja, S. R. (2000). Postural sway characteristics in women with lower extremity arthritis before and after exercise intervention. *Archives of Physical Medicine and Rehabilitation, 81* (6), 780–785.

Kochanek, K. D., & Smith, B. L. (2004). Deaths: Preliminary Data for 2002. *National Vital Statistics Reports, 52* (13), 1–48.

Kosiak, M. (1961). Etiology of decubitus ulcer. *Archives of Physical Medicine and Rehabilitation, 42* (1), 19–29.

Krupp, L. B., LaRocca, N. G., Muir-Nash, J., & Steinberg, A. D. (1989). The fatigue severity scale: Application to patients with chronic fatigue syndrome. *Archives of Neurology, 46*, 1121–1123.

Lamoureux, E. L., Hassell, J. B., & Keeffe, J. E. (2004). The impact of diabetic retinopathy on participation in daily living. *Archives of Ophthalmology, 122*, 84–88.

Langlie, J. K. (1977). Social networks, health beliefs and preventive health behavior. *Journal of Health and Social Behavior, 18*, 244–260.

LeBlanc, A., Schneider, V., Spector, E., Evans, H., et al. (1995). *Bone, 16*, 301S–304S.

Lee, K. A., Hicks, G., & Nino-Murcia, G. (1991). Validity and reliability of a scale to assess fatigue. *Psychiatry Research, 36*, 291–298.

Levine, B. D., Zuckerman, J. H., & Pawelczyk, J. A. (1997). Cardiac atrophy after bed-rest deconditioning: A nonneural mechanism for orthostatic intolerance. *Circulation, 96*, 517–525.

Liu, Y. S., Huang, W. F., Li, L. P., Zong, C. F., et al. (2003). Preventive effects of exercise training on bone loss during 21 day—6 degrees head down bed rest. *Space Medicine and Medical Engineering, 16* (2), 96–99.

Loeb, M., McGeer, A., McArthur, M., Walter, S., et al. (1999). Risk factors for pneumonia and other lower respiratory tract infections in elderly residents of long-term care facilities. *Archives of Internal Medicine, 159*, 2058–2064.

MacLaren, D. P. M., Gibson, H., Parry-Billings, M., & Edwards, R. H. T. (1989). A review of metabolic and physiological factors in fatigue. *Exercise and Sport Science Review, 17*, 29–66.

Mahoney, J. E. (1998). Immobility and falls. *Clinics in Geriatric Medicine, 14* (4), 699–726.

Mahowald, M. D., & Dykstra, D. (1997). Rehabilitation of patients with rheumatic diseases. In J. H. Klippel, C. M. Weyland, & R. L. Wortmann (Eds.), *Primer on the rheumatic diseases* (pp. 407–412). Atlanta: Arthritis Foundation.

Manton, K. G., & Gu, X. (2001). Changes in the prevalence of chronic disability in the United States black and nonblack population above age 65 from 1982 to 1999 [Electronic version]. *Proceedings of the National Academy of Sciences U.S.A. 98* (11), 6354–6359.

Maty, S. C., Fried, L. P., Volpato, S., Williamson, J., et al. (2004). Patterns of disability related to diabetes mellitus in older women. *Journal of Gerontology, 59A*, 148–153.

McCaffery, M., & Pasero, C. (1999). *Pain: Clinical manual* (2nd ed.). St. Louis, MO: Mosby.

McCorkle, R., & Young, K. (1978). Development of a symptom distress scale. *Cancer Nursing*, 373–378.

McNair, D. M., Lorr, M., & Droppleman, L. F. (1992). Profile of mood states manual (2nd ed.). San Diego, CA: Educational & Industrial Testing Service.

McPhee, S. J., & Schroeder, S. A. (1999). General approach to the patient: Health maintainence and disease prevention and common symptoms. In L. M. Tierney, S. J. McPhee, & M. A. Papadakis (Eds.), *Current medical diagnosis and treatment* (pp. 1–32). Stanford, CT: Appleton and Lange.

Meek, P. M., Nail, L. M., Barsevick, A., Schwartz, A. L., et al. (2000). Psychometric testing of fatigue instruments for use in cancer patients. *Nursing Research, 49* (4), 181–190.

Mobily, P. R., & Kelley, L. S. (1991). Iatrogenesis in the elderly. *Journal of Gerontological Nursing, 17* (9), 5–10.

Monk, T. H., Buysse, D. J., Billy, B. D., Kennedy, K. S., et al. (1997). The effects on human sleep and circadian rhythms of 17 days of continuous bedrest in the absence of daylight. *Sleep, 20* (10), 858–864.

National arthritis action plan: A public health strategy (1999). Retrieved November 1, 2004 from http://www.cdc.gov/nccdphp/naap.pdf.

National Center for Complementary and Alternative Medicine (2004). Retrieved October 7, 2004 from http://nccam.nih.gov/news/camsurvey_fs1.htm

National Institute of Health Consensus Panel. (December 18–20, 1995). Physical activity and cardiovascular health. *NIH Consensus Statement, 13* (3), 1–33.

National Stroke Association. (2000). Stroke mortality. Available on-line at http://www.stroke.org.

Neuberger, G. B. (2003). Measures of fatigue. *Arthritis Care and Research, 49* (5S), S175-S183.

Neuberger, G. B., Press, A. N., Lindsley, H. B., Hinton, R., et al. (1997). Effects of exercise on fatigue, aerobic fitness, and disease activity measures in persons with rheumatoid arthritis. *Research in Nursing and Health, 20*, 195–204.

Oh, E., Kim, C., Lee, W., & Kim, S. (2004). Correlates of fatigue in Koreans with chronic lung disease. *Heart & Lung, 33* (1), 13–20.

Ostbye, T., Taylor, D. H., Krause, K. M., & Van Scoyoc, L. (2002). The role of smoking and other modifiable lifestyle risk factors in maintaining and restoring lower body mobility in middle-aged and older Americans: Results from the HRS and AHEAD. *Journal of the American Geriatric Society, 50*, 691–699.

Ostchega, Y., Harris, T. B., Hirsch, R., Parsons, V. L., et al. (2000). The prevalence of functional limitations and disability in older person in the US: Data from the National Health and Nutrition Examination Survey III. *Journal of the American Geriatrics Society, 48*, 1132–1135.

Pavy-Le Traon, A., Sigaudo, D., Vasseur, P., Fortrat, J. O., et al. (1997). Orthostatic tests after a 4-day confinement or simulated weightlessness. *Clinical Physiology, 17*, 41–55.

Phillips, K. D., Sowell, R. L., Rojas, M., Tavakoli, A., et al. (2004). Physiological and psychological correlates of fatigue in HIV Disease. *Biological Research for Nursing, 6* (1), 59–74.

Piper, B. F. (1989). Fatigue: Current basis for practice. In S. G. Funk, E. M. Tornquist, M. T. Champagne, L. Copp, & R. A. Wiese (Eds.), *Key aspects of comfort* (pp. 187–198). New York: Springer.

_____. (1997). Measuring fatigue. In M. Frank-Stromberg & S. J. Olsen (Eds.), *Instruments for clinical healthcare research* (pp. 482–496). Sudbury, MA: Jones & Bartlett.

Piper, B. F., Lindsey, A. M., Dodd, M. J., Ferketich, S., et al. (1989). The development of an instrument to measure the subjective dimension of fatigue. In S. G. Funk, E. M. Tornquist, M. T. Champagne, L. A. Copp, & R. Wiese (Eds.), *Key aspects of comfort* (pp. 199–208). New York: Springer.

Pluijm, S., Graafmans, W., Bouter, L., & Lips, P. (1999). Ultrasound measurements for the prediction of osteoporotic fractures in elderly people. *Osteoporosis International, 9*, 550–556.

Popovic, J. R. (2001). 1999 National Hospital Discharge Survey: Annual summary with detailed diagnosis and procedure data. *Vital Health Statistics, 13* (151), 1–206.

Potter, J. (2004). Fatigue experience in advanced cancer: A phenomenological approach. *International Journal of Palliative Nursing, 10* (1), 15–23.

Province, M. A., Hadley, E. C., Hornbrook, M. C., Lipsitz, L. A., et al. (1995). The effects of exercise on falls in elderly patients: A preplanned meta-analysis of the FICSIT trials. *Journal of the American Medical Association, 273*, 1341–1347.

Ruml, L. A., Dubois, S. K., Roberts, M. L., & Pak, C. Y. (1995). Prevention of hypercalciuria and stone-forming propensity during prolonged bedrest by alendronate. *Journal of Bone and Mineral Research, 10* (4), 655–662.

Ryback, R. S., Trimble, R. W., Lewis, O. F., & Jennings, C. L. (1971). Psychobiological effects of prolonged weight-lessness (bed rest) in young health volunteers. *Aerospace Medicine, 42*, 408–415.

Schanke, A., K., & Stanghelle, J. K. (2001). Fatigue in polio survivors. *Spinal Cord, 39,* 243–251.

Scheld, K., Zitterman, A., Heer, M., Herzog, B., et al. (2001). Nitrogen metabolism and bone metabolism markers in healthy adults during 16 weeks of bedrest. *Clinical Chemistry, 47* (9), 1688–1695.

Schoenborn, C. A., Adams, P. F., Barnes, P. M., Vickerie, J. L., et al. (2004). Health behaviors of adults: United States, 1999–2001. *Vital and Health Statistic, Series 10* (219), 1–89.

Schreuder, O. P. (1966). Medical aspects of aircraft pilot fatigues with special reference to the commercial jet pilot. *Aerospace Medicine, 37,* 1–44.

Schulte, J. N., & Yarasheski, K. E. (2001). Effects of resistance training on the rate of muscle protein sythesis in frail elderly people. *International Journal of Sport Nutrition and Exercise Metabolism, 11* (Suppl.), S111–118.

Shabas, D., & Weinreb, H. (2000). Preventative healthcare in women with multiple sclerosis. *Journal of Women's Health & Gender-based Medicine, 9* (4), 389–395.

Short, K. R., Vittone, J. L., Bigelow, M. L., Proctor, D. N., et al. (2004). Age and aerobic exercise training effects in whole body and muscle protein metabolism. *American Journal of Physiology—Endocrinology and Metabolism, 286* (1), E92–101.

Shulman, L. M., Taback, R. L., Bean, J., & Weiner, W. J. (2001). Comorbidity of the nonmotor symptoms of Parkinson's disease. *Movement Disorders, 16* (3), 507–510.

Shumway-Cook, A., Patla, A., Stewart, A., Ferrucci, L., et al. (2003). Environmental components of mobility disability in community-living older persons. *Journal of the American Geriatrics Society, 51,* 393–398.

Sigaudo, D., Fortrate, J. O., Maillet, A., Allevard, A. M., et al. (1996). Comparison of a 4-day confinement and head-down tilt on endocrine response and cardiovascular variability in humans. *European Journal of Applied Physiology, 73,* 28–37.

Sinacore, D. R. (1998). Acute charcot arthropathy in patients with diabetes. *Journal of Diabetes and Its Complications, 12,* 287–293.

Singer, B., Dunne, J., Singer, K. P., & Allison, G. T. (2002). Evaluation of triceps surae muscle length and resistance to passive lengthening in patients with acquired brain injury. *Clinical Biomechanics, 17* (2), 152–161.

Stenstrom, C. H., & Minor, M. A. (2003). Evidence for the benefit of aerobic and strengthening exercise in rheumatoid arthritis. *Arthritis and Rheumatism, 49,* 428–434.

Stevens, J. A., Hasbrouck, L. M., Durant, T. M., Dellinger, A. N., et al. (1999). Surveillance for injuries and violence among older adults. *Morbidity and Mortality Weekly Report, 48* (SS8), 27–50.

Stewart, N. (1986). Perceptual and behavioural effects of immobility and social isolation in hospitalized orthopedic patients. *Nursing Papers, 18* (3), 59–74.

Stone, P., Hardy, J., Huddart, R., A'Hern, R., et al. (2000). Fatigue in patients with prostate cancer receiving hormone therapy. *European Journal of Cancer, 36,* 1134–1141.

Stone, P., Richards, M., A'Hern, R., & Hardy, J. (2001). Fatigue in patients with cancers of the breast or prostate undergoing radical radiotherapy. *Journal of Pain and Symptom Management, 22* (6), 1007–1015.

Stuifbergen, A. K., Seraphine, A., & Roberts, G. (2001). Maximizing health for those with multiple sclerosis. In S. G. Funk, E. M. Tournquist, J. L. Leeman, M. S. Miles, & J. S. Harrell (Eds.), *Key aspects of preventing and managing chronic illness,* (pp. 195–206). New York: Springer.

Surgeon General. (1996). *Surgeon General's report on physical activity and health.* (S/N 017-023-00196-5). U. S. Department of Health and Human Services, Centers for Disease Control and Prevention, National Center for Chronic Disease Prevention and Health Promotion, The President's Council on Physical Fitness and Sports; Washington, DC: Government Printing Office.

Tack, B. (1990). Self-reported fatigue in rheumatoid arthritis: A pilot study. *Arthritis Care and Research, 3* (3), 154–157.

_____. (1991). Dimensions and correlates of fatigue in older adults with rheumatoid arthritis. Unpublished doctoral dissertation. University of California, San Francisco.

Taylor, R. R., Jason, L. A., & Torres, A. (2000). Fatigue rating scales: An empirical comparison. *Psychological Medicine 30,* 849–856.

Thompson, J. R., Edwards, A. R., & Ross, N. L., (2003). A population-based study of the effects of birth weight on early developmental delay or disability in children. *American Journal of Perinatology, 20* (6), 321–332.

Thurman, D. J., Alverson, C., Dunn, K. A., Guerrero, J., et al. (1999). Traumatic brain injury in the United States: A public health perspective. *Journal of Head Trauma Rehabilitation, 14,* 602–615.

Trappe, S., Williamson, D., Godard, M., Porter, D., et al. (2000). Effect of resistance training on single muscle fiber contractile function in older men. *Journal of Applied Physiology, 89* (1), 143–152.

Trudel, G., Uhthoff, H. K., & Brown, M. (1999). Extent and direction of joint motion limitation after prolonged immobility: An experimental study in the rat. *Archives of Physical Medicine and Rehabilitation, 80,* 1542–1547.

Uchiyama, Y., & Kakurai, S. (2003). Specific effects of balance and gait exercises on physical function among the frail elderly. *Clinical Rehabilitation, 17,* 472–479.

Varni, J. W., Burwinkle, T. M., Katz, E. R., Meeske, K., et al. (2002). The PedsQL in pediatric cancer: Reliability and validity of the Pediatric Quality of Life Inventory Generic Core Scales, Multidimensional Fatigue Scale, and Cancer Module. *Cancer, 94,* 2090–2106.

Volek, J. S. (2003). Strength nutrition. *Current Sports Medicine Reports, 2* (4), 189–193.

Ward, N., & Winters, S. (2003). Results of a fatigue management programme in multiple sclerosis. *British Journal of Nursing, 12,* 1075–1080.

Welsh, L., & Rutherford, O. M. (1996). Effects of isometric strength training on quadriceps muscle properties in over 55 year olds. *European Journal of Applied Physiology and Occupational Physiology, 72,* 219–223.

Wethington, E., & Kessler, R. C. (1986). Perceived support, received support, and adjustment to stressful life events. *Journal of Health and Social Behavior, 27,* 78–89.

Whitmer, K., Tinari, M. A., & Barsevick, A. (2004). How do we manage fatigue in cancer patients? *Rehabilitation Nursing, 29,* 112–113.

Wilson, F. L., & Williams, B. N. (2003). Assessing the readability of skin care and pressure ulcer patient education materials. *Journal of Wound Ostomy Continence Nurses, 30* (4), 224–230.

Wolf, S. L., Barnhart, H. X., Kutner, G. G., McNeely, E., et al. (1996). Reducing frailty and falls in older persons: An investigation of *Tai Chi* and computerized balance training. *Journal of the American Geriatrics Society, 44,* 489–497.

Yanagibori, R., Suzuki, Y., Kawakubo, K., Makita, Y., et al. (1994). Carbohydrate and lipid metabolism after 20 days of bed rest. *Acta Physiologica Scandinavica, 150* (Suppl 616), 51–57.

CHAPTER 8

Body Image

Diana Luskin Biordi ▪ Andrea M. Warner ▪ Gregory P. Knapik

Introduction

Body image serves as a standard or frame of reference people use when relating to themselves. Body image, or one's view of one's body, changes over time, depending on life tasks such as learning one's gender role, performing a job or sport, creating a family, or aging. Body image is both a modifier of, and is modified by, chronic illness. Chronic illness, in its capacity to change the body, typically necessitates revisitations of one's body image. These revisitations are modified by the psychology of the individual, whether to *persevere* in meeting an ideal, *reformulate or readjust* the ideal to conform to one's own attributes, or *reject* the ideal of one's own body.

Significant research in body image has occurred only recently, despite being the subject of the literature since the late 1800s. In nursing, there appears to be a large gap from an initial spate of studies in the 1970s to those of the 1990s, with a substantial increase in research over the last decade. Most of the literature examining the theories of body image is found in psychology, chronic illness (particularly examining cancer), and gender studies; applied disciplines such as nursing, bioengineering, and vocational counseling typically contribute to examination of interventions.

Definitions of Body Image

Body image is the mental image of one's physical self, including attitudes and perceptions of one's physical appearance, state of health, skills, and sexuality. Body image is how one perceives one's own body, including its attractiveness, and how that body image influences interactions and others' reactions. Consequently, body image is a major delimiter of social interactions, and as such has a profound effect on physical health, social interaction, psychological development, and interpersonal relationships. Moreover, because body image is conceptual, even if it is expressed inferentially, as in anorexia nervosa, most of the literature describes body image from information taken from cognitively intact, communicative human beings. Issues of profoundly retarded individuals and their body images, for example, are more likely examined from the perspective of deviance from norms and societal reactions.

The literature on body image refers to body image in two ways. First, body image is conceptualized as a final product or end state, a state of being, e.g., "Charles's body image is that of a muscular young man." Second, body image is also portrayed as a process, in a continuous examination by its incumbent, whereby one's body is defined and redefined. In both of these conceptualizations, there are a number of factors that influence body image. Furthermore, the attitudes and perceptions about one's body guide evaluation and investment in body image which affects physical and psychosocial functioning. Attitudes about body image are related to one's self esteem, interpersonal functioning, eating and exercise patterns, self-care activities, and sexual behaviors (Cash & Fleming, 2002).

Historical Foundations of Body Image

Although body image has been discussed in the literature since the 1880s, not until Schilder first presented his work in 1935 did a new understanding of this concept arise. In his book, *The Image and Appearance of the Human Body,* Schilder (1950) explored the dimensions of body image and stated, "The image of the human body means the picture of our own body which we form in our mind, that is to say the way in which the body appears to ourselves" (p. 11). He believed that the perception of one's body is based on a three-dimensional image that comprises physiological, psychological, and social experiences.

Schilder's work affected several subsequent researchers, even into the twenty-first century. Critiquing Schilder's broad and complex theory, Cash and Pruzinsky (1990) claim that Schilder's chief contribution was not just the idea of body image, but that the idea that body image has "central pertinence not only for the pathological but also everyday events of life" (p. 9). Subsequently, Cash and Pruzinsky (2002) claim that Schilder also "single handedly moved the study of body image beyond the exclusive domain of neuropathology" (p. 4).

Most current discussions now view body image as having a perceptual component, a psychological component, and a social component (Cash & Fleming, 2002; Thompson & Gardner, 2002; Thompson & Van Den Berg, 2002). For example, with regard to eating and weight disorders, the perceptual component is the accuracy of the person's body size estimation, the psychological component is the person's

attitudes or feelings toward their own body, and the social component might be the cultural context in which body image is assessed.

Like others, Thompson & Fleming argue that body image is not a simple perceptual phenomenon, but is highly influenced by cognitive, affective, attitudinal, and other variables. Recent research builds on these studies by recognizing that the already complex physical and psychological development of body image can vary by the complexity of different social situations (White, 2000). Moreover, a cultural overlay, whether from the larger societal culture or the more immediate culture of ethnicity or family, affects body image.

Of particular importance to health care professionals in chronic illness is the empirically derived idea that the perceptual elements of body image are complex. Fisher (1986) found that people not only compartmentalized their body image, but also differed in how they did so: Some localized their body image, while others had a more global view of their body. For instance, people with serious body defects might approach their bodies as separate regions, specifically isolating the defective region so that it will not influence their overall evaluation of self. Fisher believed that this ability suggests "important defensive and maturational significance in how differentiated one's approach to one's body is" (p. 635). He also argued that the rubric of body image itself is vague, representing a number of dimensions of the same and different constructs.

Defining Body Image

Definitions of body image, though varied, share similarities. Common to many of the definitions is the belief that body image develops in response to multiple sensory inputs (visual, tactile, proprioceptive, and kinesthetic). The body is experienced as a reflection of the self. Body image is the way people perceive themselves and, equally important, the way they think others see them. Body image is brought into immediate focus of the individual by pain, physical or psychological illness, age, or weight (Krueger, 2002)

Yet body image is more than a personal view of one's physical appearance, although physicality is included in one's image, body image is very subjective and dynamic (Cash, 2002; Pruzinsky, 2004). Kinesthetic perceptions of function, sensation, and mobility are also part of our image. Children without sensation of body parts (e.g., spina bifida) often do not include in their art those body parts where they lack sensation. Body image also includes feelings and thoughts. How one thinks and feels about one's body will influence social relationships and other psychological characteristics. Furthermore, how we feel and think about our bodies influences the way we perceive the world (Cash & Fleming, 2002).

Body image also takes into account one's perception of attractiveness. Part of this perception is based on the social actions and attitudes of others. In a study of body image and social interaction, Nezlek (1999) found that three factors were included in the definition of body image. These included body attractiveness, social attractiveness (how attractive people believed others found them to be), and general attractiveness. For both men and women, self-perceptions of body attractiveness and social attractiveness were positively related to intimacy. Because body attractiveness is an important function of body image, this concept frequently is confused with body image itself, but body image encompasses more than attractiveness.

Many definitions of body image today involve the notions of the real and the ideal. Theorists would argue that the ideal image of oneself and the real image must be compatible, or dissonance results. A discrepancy between the real and the ideal body image may lead to conflicts that adversely affect personality, interactions, and health. For example, "normative discontent" refers to the pervasive negative feelings women and girls experience when they negatively distort their appearance, experience body image dissatisfaction, or overevaluate the appearance in defining a sense of self (Striegel-Moore & Franko, 2002).

For the health professional, definitions of body image indicate the complexity of the concept, but more importantly, emphasize how significantly the client's cultural, social, historical, and biological factors affect body image. Perhaps even more important to health care professionals and their professionally derived norms is that body image and the factors affecting it are not merely cosmetic. A client's perceptions and attitudes about his or her body can affect health, social adjustment, interpersonal relationships, and general well-being. These perceptions are profoundly affected by chronic illness, as can be seen in this and other chapters.

Perhaps because body image is so vital to issues of ordinary health as well as chronic illness, it has come to be associated with, or even confused with, several other terms. The terms *body image, self-concept,* and *self-esteem* are frequently used interchangeably. Body image is not the same as body attractiveness but is related to both attractiveness and to self-esteem. Body image is a mental image of one's physical self, moderated by one's psychology and the social environment. Body image, thus, is an integral component of self-concept. Self-concept is the total perception an individual holds of self—who one believes one is, how one believes one looks, and how one feels about one's self (Mock, 1993). Research extends self-concept to include not only ongoing perceptions of one's self, but also the idea that self concept so mediates and regulates behavior that it is one of the most significant regulators of behavior (Markus & Wurf, 1987). Finally, self-esteem is related to "the evaluative component of an individual's self-concept" (Corwyn, 2000, p. 357).

Factors Influencing Adjustment to Body Image

Meaning and Significance

As critical as each influence may be to the individual's adaptation, it is most important that the *meaning of the event* to the individual be ascertained. Knowing that clients may compartmentalize both the meaning and the body part, the health care professional must recognize and accept how each client assesses the changes occurring, their importance, and the way that client chooses to incorporate (or not) change and image into their body image.

Treatment of chronic illness, body image, external changes, functionality, or appearance cannot be far removed from the meaning attributed to such by the client or significant other. In most cultures, body parts carry emotional attribution quite aside from functionality. The hands, for instance, are critical portrayals of metaphysics of religions, whether shown invitingly open, in clasped position, or thumbs and forefingers together. While the mind is connected with the brain, with all the significance attached to that in a knowledge society, the heart is universally seen as a major font of emotions. The heart is, to many, the symbol of love, courage, and life, and the seat of joy, hate, and sorrow. Indeed, in some cultures, the heart is seen as the location of the soul. Consider the emotional significance, then, that damage to the heart would engender in the body image of the affected client. Most nurses have been taught about clients who, after sustaining a myocardial infarction, are so anxious that they become a "cardiac cripple" due to their fear of death from exercise or normal activity. Clearly, the self-image of such clients has sustained a serious insult. To counter the insult, giving a reasonable sense of hope for future improvement may sustain a more positive body image. Building false hope, of course, can lead to false trust and, perhaps, a dire consequence. Thus, the health care professional must find ways to encourage the client to move toward a more robust body image, while recognizing that, for the client, losing trust may be nearly as catastrophic as losing hope.

Body image and the functionality insults of chronic illness cannot be isolated from the meaning and significance the client gives to them. Furthermore, the meaning and significance to family members or significant others can also play an important role in the client's response. These are crucial factors to consider in offering and performing effective and sensitive care. Of all the aspects of body image in chronic illness, the appreciation and understanding of the meaning and significance to the client are the areas to which nursing can most contribute. The client's

meaning and significance placed on the change in body image must not be overlooked or downplayed. Nursing's empathic and holistic approach can be of great value in this arena of healthcare.

The cause of the person's chronic illness and associated body image insult can be an important coping factor. If it is due to an accident, healthcare mismanagement, or personal negligence, the person may harbor unresolved anger, blame, and shame. The person may also be guarded about sharing and discussing such matters, which confounds and makes more difficult, recovery. On the other hand, if the cause is due to recommended or life-saving interventions, the person perceives body image insult as an unavoidable consequence and a relatively small price to pay (Rybarczyk & Behel, 2002).

Another important factor the nurse must not forget is the "fifth vital sign" or pain. If pain is associated with the cause of the body image change, the meaning and significance of the altered body image can be negatively influenced. Pain may also nourish a persisting and even worsening negative body image and also impair recovery in functionability (Rybarczyk & Behel, 2002). Hence, it is essential to assess the person for pain and discomfort.

Influence of Time

The length of time during which body changes occur may influence one's body image and subsequent psychological adjustment (White, 2002). Changes in body image may occur slowly, over a lifetime, or quickly, within hours or days. Although some might argue that more time gives individuals greater opportunity to reformulate a body image, the fact remains that some individuals will never adapt to their body image. A person experiencing Type II diabetes may have a slow progression of changes and ample time for denial and grief resolution, whereas trauma and sudden illness, such as a stroke, and certain surgeries may lead to abrupt changes in the body and in body image. Individuals who experience sudden traumatic illnesses have no warning, and thus little opportunity to adjust to the changes (Bello & McIntire, 1995). A classic example is the lag time between perceived body image and the phantom pain experienced in limb amputations. To adjust to rapid change, the client must grieve the loss as well as physically adjust to the changes. Otherwise, the client who cannot cope with the dysfunction is at a higher risk for infection, noncompliance with therapeutic care, depression, social isolation, and obsession with or denial of the changes in body image (Dropkin, 1989).

The permanence of the change in appearance also affects adjustment to changes in body image. A person may better cope with changes in appearance that are temporary (i.e., temporary ileostomy) more so than those that are permanent (i.e., limb amputation). However, adjusting to body image changes depends partly on the meaning the individual ascribes to the changes and, in some cases, more so than the length of time during which the change occurs (White, 2002).

Social Influences

Each sociocultural group establishes its own norms governing the acceptable, especially in terms of physical appearance and personality attributes (Jackson, 2002). Societies can hold a persistent, pervasive view using standards dictating ideal physical appearance and role performance. These standards, although some with caveats, serve all members of that social group, including those who have chronic illness and those who do not.

Groups target their social influence and affect the self-images of individuals. Family relationships are often important to the person with a chronic illness and their initial perception of their own body image. Negative family reactions about appearance, behavior, performance, and body image have been linked with recurrent poor body image consequences (Byely et al., 1999; Kearney-Cooke, 2002). Peer relationships are important mediating groups, particularly for those who are uncertain how to structure their life-styles (e.g., adolescents). On one hand, peers can help shape conformance to a model. An example is the currently popular view of the muscle-bound, minimal-body-fat male model that is popular among young people (Olivardia, Pope & Hudson, 2000). On the other hand, peer groups can call into question the appropriateness of such modeling for their own age group (e.g., seniors' perception of the aforementioned male model).

Persons with disfigurements are often forced to deal with their body image and the prevailing societal view with little choice in the matter. Depending on the visibility of the disfigurement and the coping of the disfigured person, sanctions such as staring, whispering, or shunning can negatively affect body image and personal value (Pruzinsky, 2002; Rumsey, 2002).

Untoward issues of body image often begin early in individuals. There is evidence now that in the United States, both girls and boys as young as 6 years old are overly conscious of their body weight and begin dieting in an attempt to meet social norms of idealized thin and handsome young men and women. The body image issues begun in early years often persist through adolescence and into adulthood (Striegel-Moore & Franko, 2002).

The effect of the society and environment on body image is reciprocal. Just as societal reactions can affect body image, the individual is not entirely passive, and so can react to such standards. Nevertheless, societal influences weigh heavily on behavior and body image, frequently leading to stereotypical assignments that affect individual body image adjustments. For example, persons with cranial-facial disfigurement or those who are chronically obese have been subjected to societal reactions and expectations of ideal beauty throughout their lives. Over the years, having been constantly compared with the "ideal" beautiful or thin person, the individual with chronic illness has had to manage their own responses as well as those of others in the obvious discrepancy between an ideal body and their own real bodies.

Cultural Influences

Many aspects of culture affect body image. A cultural map has been suggested by Helman (1995) in which a view of the body is shared by the members growing up within a particular cultural or social group. This cultural map tells individuals how their body is structured and how it functions, includes ideal body definitions, and identifies "private" and "public" body parts as well as differentiating between a "healthy" and an "unhealthy" body (Helman, 1995).

The perceptions of health and illness and their effects on body image vary from culture to culture. In Altabe's study (1998) on ideal physical traits and body image, ethnic groups were similar in their identification of ideal body traits but different in assigning values to the body traits (e.g., valuing skin color or breast size). Findings indicated that African Americans had the most positive self-view and body image, while Asian Americans placed the least importance on physical appearance. Some non-Caucasians had a more positive body image than did Caucasians.

African Americans view health as a feeling of well-being, the ability to fulfill role expectations, and the experiencing an environment free of pain and excessive stress. In the United States, the Hispanic culture perceives health as being and looking clean, feeling happy, getting adequate rest, and being able to function in expected roles. An imbalance in the emotional, physical, and social arenas may produce illness. Hispanic individuals often do not seek health care until they are very sick, and those with chronic illness may view themselves as victims of malevolent forces, attributed to God or punishment (Rhode Island Department of Health, 1998).

Native Americans view health as a balancing of mind, body, spirit, and nature. The practice of medicine is viewed as cooperative and offers choice and individual involvement in the pursuit of health. The Southeast Asian culture's health beliefs focus on the concept of Yin and Yang (balance) and maintaining this balance to achieve wellness. Obesity is viewed as a sign of contentment and socioeconomic status (Rhode Island Department of Health, 1998).

Influence of Health Care Team Members

The care given to persons with a chronic disease or disability has a direct influence on their ability to adapt to societal pressures. Members of the health care team, while subject to the norms of the larger society, also have perceptions of illness and certain disabilities shaped by such professional norms as objectivity, compassion, or moral judgment. When caring for an individual with chronic illness, reactions from the health care team are important in the clients' adjustment and acceptance of body image.

Health care team members must understand that they are often the first person to see the changes engendered by the chronic illness or treatment. Their reactions often set the stage for body image expectations of clients. Seeing their caregiver's reactions may reinforce a body image for clients that continues for a long period of time, whether that image is positive or negative. Health care team members, therefore, must learn to manage their demeanor, voice, tone, and body reactions, avoiding any obvious rejections or trivialization of clients with chronic illness. One of the goals of the health care team should be to assist clients in having and/or maintaining a positive image and acceptance of self. For example, the client who has recently undergone breast reconstructive surgery following a mastectomy may have problematic issues of body image. The support and guidance by health team members in helping the client with information about surgery, pain relief, self-care, positive reinforcement, family relationships, and emotional support are important to positive body image building (Van Deusen, 1993). Assessing concerns related to appearance and allowing clients to express fears, beliefs, thoughts, and life experiences also contributes to adjustment to body image changes (White, 2002).

Age

Erik Erikson's classic developmental theory is useful in examining phases of psychosocial development, particularly as this theory examines various stages throughout the life span which encourage or inhibit body image and personal feelings of value (Erikson, 1963). In younger age groups, conflicts about industry versus inferiority are changed into feelings of worth and competence (Cash & Pruzinsky, 1990). If there were negative effects during early developmental stages, altered or poor body image may result.

It is thought that younger children may be able to adapt more easily to changing body images because they have not fully come to recognize or appreciate their body image, unlike an adolescent or adult. Because their bodies are constantly changing, and because they are attending to their peers, adolescents can have an especially difficult time adapting to body image changes brought on by chronic illness. Juvenile diabetics or adolescents with visible physical disfigurements, such as skin or neural diseases, frequently act out their frustrations via risky behaviors, depression, or withdrawal.

Body image in an adult has likely been well established and serves as an identity base. Adaptation to changes in body image can be more difficult to accept in an older group of individuals because illness challenges their fundamental identity. The older adults' acceptance of body image changes tends to be related more to ability to be useful in society, loss of independence and health status, and, possibly, attractiveness to others (Krauss-Whitbourne & Skultety, 2002). Elderly persons may still feel young at heart but as their bodies age, they are subject to changes in skin, hair, posture, strength, or speed of action, which are compounded by various chronic illnesses such as cardiac, respiratory, orthopedic, visual, or hearing problems. They may feel young, but their outer appearances demonstrate their age and associated conditions in a culture that values the young. The elderly often want to maintain an accepted social body image, so it is important to consider these issues when possible body image disturbances arise.

Gender

The gender of a person may influence his or her response to a change in body image. Although both genders are subject to norms of beauty, women with burns, for example, generally have a more negative body image than do men with burns, although the effect of burns on body image depends on locus of the burn and the percentage of body surface in-volved (Orr, Reznikoff & Smith, 1989). It is important to note, however, that females tend to have negative body image perceptions more often than males across age and cultures, therefore, women may experience more disturbances in body images than males when faced with chronic illnesses (Striegel-Moore & Franko, 2002).

Typically, the male gender is associated with a "masculine, strong" appearance, and the female gender is associated with a "feminine, softer" appearance. Role behaviors are less strictly segregated now than in the decades of the 1950s, 1960s, and 1970s, yet, many older clients were socialized to gender roles during those years and have strong expectations of clear role behaviors: Men are expected to be strong, active, rational, and silent, while women are expected to be indirect, passive, capable, and emotional. These views have an impact on their self-image and the differences engendered by chronic illness. Older chronically ill men or widowers who need assistance in learning to cook, or women learning to be more assertive even as their bodies are less conducive to these activities, often must change their body image. Often they do so gracefully, as we hear in the admonition, "Growing old is not for sissies." However, it behooves health care professionals, many of whom were not born in the times generating the social norms governing the body images of the elderly, to learn about the histories of the elderly whose chronic illnesses they treat. In that way, the health professional can become more empathetic and understand the possible sources of body images of their clients. This is particularly important for the chronically ill diabetic woman, whose diet is strictly managed but who yet needs to be a good cook to accommodate her self-image as a competent woman. Another example is the hypertensive man whose medication limits his libido or sexual performance.

Prior Experience and Coping Mechanisms

Body image is thought to be individually developed through each person's concept of his or her "ideal" perception and based on his or her previous experiences within society as well (Cash & Pruzinsky, 2002). Because past experiences, positive or negative, can substantially affect present circumstances, understanding how a client is likely to perceive an event, and cope with it, is one of the more important assessments performed by the health care professional. This awareness is particularly beneficial to the individual who has not had much exposure to the health care system and may require advocacy by the health professional.

Coping mechanisms already developed by the individual through support from family, the health care team, or the client's social group, are helpful in promoting adaptation to changes in body image during chronic illness. Understanding the individual's perception of body image before and during a diagnosis of chronic illness can be helpful to the health care professional in easing the client's adjustment to body image changes. Knowing that body image is an inferential diagnosis, it is helpful for the health care professional to estimate which stage of body image is most likely to reflect the client's situation, whether persevering, reformulating, or rejecting one's body image.

Most clients have an exacerbation of their typical coping mechanisms during illness. Therefore, under the stress of chronic illness and depending on its familiarity to the client, the health care professional is most likely to initially observe an exaggerated coping style, however inadequate it may be. Using that information as a first step in assessing a client, and moving from there to infer body image changes on the continuum presented in this chapter, is a good beginning for the health care professional and client.

Assessment of Body Image

Assessing the behaviors of individuals who have experienced an alteration in function or change leading to a disruption in body image is vital in planning appropriate interventions. This assessment leads to a determination of perceptions and meanings associated with the change that is unique to the client, and allows recognition of barriers to health.

This assessment is done by observing and interviewing the client to determine the nature and meaning of the threat. Only after such an assessment and validation of its correctness may the health care professional provide interventions.

A key to a successful assessment is a therapeutic relationship with the client. Trust, sensitivity to the client's thoughts and feelings, and provision of accurate and realistic support all help to build and strengthen the therapeutic relationship between the client and provider (Hayslip et al., 1997).

A complete assessment of a client's experience and meaning of change is facilitated by asking questions related to the client's perception of the experience, knowledge of the illness and its effects, and others' perceptions of the client's illness. Accounting for these in the assessment process creates a client-centered knowledge base for choosing appropriate interventions. Additionally, assessing the client's psychosocial history and support systems allows the provider to elicit greater support for the client in areas already known to the client.

Assessing a client's unique influencing factors is essential in planning interventions. Knowing how much value is placed on the appearance or functioning of the body helps the health care professional to determine the impact of the image disruption. Assessing self-esteem and the client's perceived attitudes of others is also important in discovering the meaning and impact of the disruption to the client. Ascertaining the phase of recovery of the client is essential, and is particularly important in planning specific client-centered interventions. Knowing *when* to implement educational, supportive, or rehabilitative interventions makes them most useful.

In some instances, it may be necessary to use a standardized assessment tool to measure body disturbances and number and types of support systems. Many tools are available for this use (Cash & Pruzinsky, 2002). Tools about body disturbances generally have questions on general appearance, body competence, others' reaction to appearance, value of appearance, and so forth. These tools have incorporated related concepts to body image, such as self-esteem and self-concept, and are able to measure affective, cognitive, and behavioral components of body image (Thompson & Van Den Berg, 2002).

Incorporating families into assessment is encouraged. This can be done by interviewing, observing, and taking note of both verbal and nonverbal interactions within the family system (Wright & Leahey, 2000). Assessing family meanings of the chronic illness, perceived losses, and stresses placed on the family due to the illness are important in planning interventions.

Body Image Issues Important to Chronic Illness

Chronic illness has many challenges, one of which includes the adaptation to changes in body image. The process of adaptation depends on many factors, but primary among those are the external changes to the person, functional limitations, the changes' significance and importance to the person, the time with which the change (and losses) occurred, social influences, and the impact of culture.

External Changes

Important external factors that influence body image are the visibility and functional significance of the part involved, the importance of physical appearance to the individual, and speed with which the change occurred (Rybarczyk & Behel, 2002). For example, epilepsy is a chronic disease that illustrates all of these factors. Epileptic seizures, such as a tonic–clonic seizure, can affect the entire body, are easily observed, and happen suddenly. Epilepsy may also prevent the client from maintaining a job, driving a car, or engaging in sports or popular activities such as swimming. Typically epilepsy's onset is acute. The person does not have time to prepare for accepting this chronic disease. A seizure occurs and the person's life is changed from that moment onwards. This can make it more challenging to accept and live "normally" with the image of "being an epileptic," and potentially having a very visible, sudden, and dysfunctional (possibly dangerous) experience. The severity of insult to appearance and functional sig-

nificance, and the degree of importance to the person, must be considered on an individual basis. For example, some persons may find epilepsy a minor nuisance but mild psoriasis traumatizing, because the latter is visible and mildly dysfunctional. It is essential to assess the meaning and significance of the change to the person.

Another common example is the obese client. Obesity is typically a non-acute, slowly progressing condition that may cause minimal, if any, dysfunction. The person may be able to minimize the appearance change by skillful dressing. Nonetheless, the person's body image can be strongly influenced in a negative manner without any obvious signs or symptoms of such.

It is also easy to overlook the body image influence from chronic mental illnesses. For instance, a person with schizophrenia may have a negatively altered body image as part of the disturbed thinking of the illness and/or from the perceived change the illness has on the behavior and presentation of the person. Furthermore, the medication used to treat schizophrenia can affect body image due to movement side effects, or in some cases, weight gain. Thus, overlooking the possible side effects on body image for the mentally ill would be a mistake for the health professional, and likely to affect medication compliance.

It is important for the healthcare professional to not make assumptions but always consider what this chronic illness and possible body image change means to the person. Each person is unique, and therefore each experience with chronic illness is unique.

Appearance

The physical appearance of a disease is frequently a change for which clients are unprepared. Given the possibility of perseverance, reformulation, or rejection of changes, body image and its accompanying variables affecting acceptance need to be studied further. Empirical evidence and anecdotal data exist to guide us in considering suitable interventions. For example, when the appearance also draws attention to its underlying cause, clients and their significant others are often ostracized, particularly when the disease is one that carries a stigma (see Chapter 3, on stigma). Many clients with AIDS develop Kaposi's sarcoma (KS), a common and sometimes disfiguring tumor of the human immunodeficiency virus (HIV). Because the skin is a common site for KS, the characteristic purple hue of KS is easily visible, and is considered by many patients as a "public signature" of HIV (Moore et al., 2000). In more severe cases of illness, in which the body is catastrophically debilitated, as in amyotrophic lateral sclerosis (ALS), Helman (1995) notes that the entire body image may accommodate the body as separated from the sense of self—that is, "It is my body that is diseased, but not me."

Visibility and Invisibility

Chronic illness and its treatment provide visible, outward changes in appearance and invisible internal changes. Both types of change can significantly affect individuals' perceptions of themselves. In an adult, it is suggested that the more visible or extensive the body alteration, the more likely it is to be perceived as a threat to one's body image. Loss of hair, scarring, edema, amputations, and disfigurement are common examples in the body image literature. In reading the life accounts of severely disfigured persons, many choose to work at unusual times (nights) and in jobs in which they have little contact with others (see Chapter 6, on social isolation).

The matter of body image and incorporation of changes seems to be more ambiguous in children. Children are strongly subject to the norms imposed by their peers with their self-image being readily influenced. A visible change or disfigurement in a child could ostracize the child from his or her peer group. Of particular importance to children, particularly for those with "stigmatized" body images, is the family member or health care professional who can support the child's acceptance of the body image changes.

When a change is not markedly visible, as when an ostomy is created, or its treatment (e.g., colostomy appliances) is introduced, chronically ill persons must take previously "invisible" body parts and make them "visible" (Helman, 1995). This dynamic is further compounded when the new intervention is preferentially hidden from others. Such procedures and the management of visible and hidden change likely lead to dramatic changes in an individual's life-style and self-image. For example, clients with a stoma must periodically empty the appliance bag, learn to change it, irrigate the stoma when needed, cope with social matters such as dressing to fit the appliance, and manage social etiquette with problems of leaking, odors, and the noises resulting from involuntary discharge into the appliance. The person dealing with such challenges may keep this hidden, and limit social functioning to avoid possible embarrassment (Kirkpatrick, 1986).

Functional Limitations

Functionality is something that is conceptualized as "external" in that functionality is usually a visible part of enactment of one's role. It may be that the function is carried out privately, as in a sexual function, but function is the ability of a body part to be able to be used to conduct its usual purpose. The ability to function in a meaningful way is essential to a sense of well-being; consequently, any limitation of functional ability may alter one's concept of body image. Most clients and their significant others are not prepared for the appearance and functional limitations associated with chronic illness.

The function of a body part and its importance and visibility are critical to one's body image. The leg, because of its functional importance in mobility and a person's life, is more likely to be a more important part of body image than, say, a toe (Brown, 1977). Loss of a toe, for example, is likely to be viewed as less problematic than loss of a leg, because much function can be retained by compensatory body parts and because a toe is less visible. Therefore, one might expect different accommodations in body image to such amputations, even as it is recognized that perception of loss and its impact vary from person to person and culture to culture. Indeed, the oldest prosthesis found has been that of a wooden large toe that was found attached by leather thongs to the foot of an ancient Egyptian female mummy. This well-carved prosthesis, unhidden by a sandal, aided the woman in walking and maintaining balance.

The roles of worker, gendered persona, and sexual being are three important facets of body image. Chronic illness or treatment can threaten the client's ability to perform each of these roles. Furthermore, the stage of one's life can make a major difference in the perception of the strength of the threat or its incorporation into one's body image. A teenager, perhaps, is likely to regard work or sexual function, and concomitant body image, differently than would a seasoned elder. However, each client is unique, and typifying elders as less interested in work and/or their sexual function is often incorrect.

Loss of sexual function for most persons, particularly those who are sexually active, is often perceived as a profound loss. Women with breast removal from cancer, or men and women with genital cancers frequently avoid sexual situations after treatments (Golden & Golden, 1986). The male client may feel especially vulnerable if he feels his sexuality or provider role is compromised by chronic illness. Testicular cancer is the most common cancer in young men ages 18 to 35 and typically results in the removal of the diseased testicle. Older men with prostate cancer may require the removal of both testicles, with a resultant loss of libido and virility, and compromised perception of "manhood." Though implants can be used, the perception of functional loss can strongly persist. The nurse can be, and may often be, the main source of professional support and education, and thus assist clients with the sensitive issues involved with body image.

■ Interventions

Interventions are used to help clients manage their own reactions and the reactions of others to changes in body structure, function, or appearance as the result of chronic illness. These changes are frequently interpreted as setting one apart and as different from one's peers (see Chapter 3, on stigma), leading to self-doubt, inhibited participation in social activities, and a disruption of perceptions of self. Finding appropriate interventions for clients experiencing an altered body image can aid the client in healing and adapting to changes in body image (Norris, Connell & Spelic, 1998).

Adapting to changes in body image resulting from chronic illness is a dynamic process. On a daily basis, clients are faced with thoughts and reminders of their illness and changes to their bodies. During periods of exacerbation, remission, and rehabilitation, clients are grieving the loss of their former selves, living with the uncertainty of their chronic illness, and learning to create new images of self (Cohen, Kahn & Steeves, 1998). Knowing that the process is continually changing, with steps forward and backward, helps the nurse to support clients as they adapt to changes in body image.

Specific Interventions

Interventions are chosen after careful assessment of the client. As mentioned previously, a therapeutic relationship with the client is an essential beginning to the process. Acknowledging barriers to communication, feelings about the illness, changes the illness caused, and personal biases on the part of the health care professional must be addressed before successful intervention may take place. Accurate knowledge about the disease process and the client's response are also necessary if the health care professional is to assist the client. Additionally, the health care professional must be able to recognize that body image changes will require a supportive, accepting, and consistent relationship that can withstand setbacks and emotional tension. It is important to be aware of the client's attitude and participation in the recovery process. This may involve professional rehabilitation, including physical and occupational therapy, or it may involve informal self or family directed interventions. The health care provider can be influential in acknowledging subtle progress which

Nurse as Patient

This time, Nancy, a nurse was the patient. She sat in the waiting room of a large clinic that provided mammograms and diagnostic testing. To pass the time, the nurse-patient watched the people in the waiting room, idly assigning names to those waiting.

Observing her companions in waiting, she watched a young, pretty white woman, around 35 years of age, whom she named "Jane," accompanied by a friend of about 40, "Ann." The nurse thought Jane was nervous: unsmiling, changing positions frequently, jiggling her foot, disinterestedly turning pages in her magazine, and occasionally talking distractedly to Ann.

Several seats away, sat "Ethel," an older white woman who sat quietly and said little. A few seats from her sat "Maddy," an African American woman in her mid 60s. Finally, quite near Maddy sat Nancy, a middle-aged white woman restlessly waiting for her doctor's call.

As they waited, Nancy asked Maddy who her doctor was. Finding they shared the same physician, Nancy exclaimed over his bedside manner, his education of his patients, and her own diagnosis. "I had a lumpectomy, and we talked about reconstruction. What do you think? Did you have that?"

Maddy looked at her and, expansively, around the room, announced: "I heard all about those things, but at my age; I said, I've done all that. I'm old, and I'm tired. I told my man he better not expect anything more, because there isn't going to be any more!"

Maddy's exchange brought a smile to everyone. Perhaps because it was such an open statement, other women waiting rushed in with their comments.

Jane announced what Nancy, the nurse-patient, had expected. Jane was there to hear the results of her breast cancer treatment. She, too, asked what the others had done about breast reconstruction. Her friend, Ann, held her hand supportively.

Ethel said that she wasn't sure what she was going to do just yet, as her diagnosis was in the process of confirmation. But, at her age, she just didn't know.

Nancy said, "I am having the breast implant, but I decided on the silicone variety. I don't want that stretch-the-skin stuff. It hurts, I was told by my friend, and I just didn't want to put up with weekly visits and stretching the pain out over a year. So, it's the implant for me. I'm just having him check them now."

Jane remarked that she had had a "tummy flap, but no one told me that my midsection would be permanently numb. I don't like the lack of feeling. On the other hand, my breast looks pretty real, which was important to my husband and me." Ann squeezed her hand supportively once more. Jane told everyone that this was her second post-op visit. She was terrified they would find a reoccurrence of her cancer. She had two young children, and she didn't know what she would tell them if they found a repeat of her cancer. She started to cry softly. Maddy looked at her and said, "Honey, you just hang in there. Did you have chemo and everything? This doc is good, I tell you. He'll do right by you."

the client may or may not be aware of, and supporting the benefit of rehabilitation as part of the overall recovery process.

Communication

Providing opportunities for clients to express feelings and thoughts about the changes they are experiencing can be beneficial to both clients and healthcare professionals. It allows clients to speak and be heard, and also allows careful assessment of the clients' thoughts and feelings directly. Assumptions should not be made about the meaning of experiences relating to changes in body image (Cohen, Kahn & Steeves, 1998). Additionally, ensuring client comfort in expressing both positive and negative feelings and emotions helps strengthen the therapeutic relationship and facilitate the journey to wholeness. Allowing family members to express their thoughts, feelings, and concerns is also beneficial and should be incorporated into the recovery process.

Talk therapy, cither individual or group, can be of much benefit in the recovery process. Cognitive-Behavioral Therapy has a proven record in assisting clients to change their dysfunctional thinking and related behaviors associated with chronic illness and negative body image (Peterson, et al., 2004; Rumsey & Harcourt, 2004; Rybarczyk & Behel, 2002; & Veale, 2004).

Self-Help Groups

Self-help groups for clients experiencing body image changes may help to buffer the stressors experienced by the changes. Providing clients with opportunities to share experiences with others in similar situations can be therapeutic for some individuals. Self-help or support groups can offer important emotional, social and spiritual fellowship. It is important to assess the willingness of individuals to participate in a group setting. Some individuals are not comfortable in a group setting, especially when they are dealing with a body image disruption. For

those who find it helpful, the benefits are many. Seeing others on the road to recovery, helping those who are struggling, and finding where they themselves are in the journey can help with the healing process (Corey & Corey, 1997). Additionally, these groups provide an opportunity for clients to begin socializing with others in a safe and non-threatening environment. It is important for the nurse to be aware of the self-help groups available and accessible to the client.

Self-Care

Encouraging clients to participate in the activities of daily living that are meaningful to them helps restore feelings of normalcy. Whether engaging in personal grooming activities, such as applying cosmetics, jewelry, or hair accessories, caring for oneself can be an effective intervention. Self-care will help the client incorporate the change into the normal functioning of daily living. This intervention may also help the client become less sensitive to physical appearances and learn to manage everyday activities (Norris, Connell & Spelic, 1998). Regular exercise can be helpful in improving body-image, along with supporting physical health and function (Wetterhahn, Hanson, & Levy, 2002).

Prostheses

Prostheses have been in use for centuries, helping to modify functionality, external appearances, and, most likely, body image. Because so much of chronic illness is visible or involves body parts with need for additional support, prostheses have varied in sophistication and availability. Most health care professionals are familiar with prosthetic eyes, hearing aids, various "limbs" (e.g., hand, foot, leg, arm), or breast, penile, or testicular implants.

For instance, in chronic disease involving amputations, the age of the client presents unusual concerns. The prosthetic hand, foot, or knee of a child, for example, may require, for the child's adequate social development, that the prosthetic stand up to repeated use in play, such as in swimming, with the effects of water, sand, and chlorine. Adults may wish to maintain a physically normal appearance and avoid the functional "hook" hand prosthesis. In the elderly, whose gait problems may be exacerbated by joint problems, the "fit" of a prosthesis, as in a hip replacement, is a special concern. The rehabilitation required after hip replacement is particularly necessary, and its success has much to do with subsequent body image improvement related to increased mobility.

Spinal cord injury has sparked research that focuses on current knowledge of spinal cord treatment, electrical stimulation, mechanisms of secondary damage, and possibilities for regeneration of nerves. Bioengineering, electric-powered prostheses, invasive and noninvasive sensors to control prostheses, or use of brain waves or eye pupil contraction to power computers for communication are currently being used or being tested. Their success is a huge event for the affected person, and this specialized area of knowledge typically requires focus and specialization by health professionals.

The use of prostheses and the unique technologies to power these prostheses will continue to grow in the future. It is important to understand the field of prosthetics requires knowledge about the illness as well as the care with which clients implement and maintain their prosthetics and the impact of prosthetics on body image.

Education and Anticipatory Guidance

This intervention is effective only when the client has indicated a readiness to learn. Knowledge of disease processes, information about symptoms, and methods of treatment are important educational topics for the client to understand. It is also helpful to consider the preferred learning style (e.g. visual, auditory, and/or practice) of the client, such as a visual or auditory learning style preference (Cohen, Kahn & Steeves, 1998). The benefits of client education and anticipatory guidance should be stressed in order to stimulate and support the client's readiness to learn. (see Chapter 15, on client and family education).

■ Outcomes

Body image, the physical aspect of self-concept, is closely linked with the concept of self-esteem in the *Nursing Outcomes Classification* (NOC) (Johnson & Maas, 1997). Disturbances of these along with personal identity disturbance, chronic low self-esteem, and situational low self-esteem are considered part of what Carpenito (2000) globally calls self-concept disturbance. These alterations can be a result of an immediate problem, such as sudden disfiguration from surgery or burns, or can be related to long-term changes from chronic illnesses such as cancer and its treatment effects, arthritis, Parkinson's disease, or a cerebrovascular accident.

Defining characteristics of this nursing classification can be multiple: denial, withdrawal of the individual, refusal to be part of the care required, refusal to look at the body part involved or let immediate family look at it, refusal to discuss rehabilitation efforts, signs and symptoms of grieving, self-destructive behavior such as alcohol or drug abuse, and hostility toward healthy individuals. One's sense of femininity or masculinity may also be threatened, which can lead to difficulty in sexual functioning, and combined, these changes can lead to social anxiety, self-consciousness, and depression (Carpenito, 2000; Otto, 1991; White, 2000).

The ten indicators for this outcome that are listed in the NOC are internal picture of self; congruence between body reality, body ideal, and body presentation; description of affected body part; willingness to touch the affected body part; satisfaction with body appearance; satisfaction with body function; adjustment to changes in physical appearance; adjustment to changes in body function; adjustment to changes in health status; and willingness to use strategies to enhance appearance and function. Other outcomes that could be closely tied to body image disturbance are coping, hope, well-being, caregiver–patient relationship, quality of life, will to live, grief resolution, self-esteem, and psychosocial adjustment: life change (NOC, 1997). However, the ultimate goal or outcome for individuals is adaptation to the change, a "positive perception of one's appearance and bodily functions," and an overall optimization of quality of life (Johnson & Maas, 1997, p. 86; Rybarczyk & Behel, 2002; Craig & Edwards, 1983).

Summary and Conclusions

Body image is one's perception image of self to include physical image, attitudes, state of health, skills and sexuality. The influence of one's body image cannot be underestimated when understanding an individual's psychosocial adjustment. The overlapping concepts of body image with self-esteem and self-concept are powerful in a client's outcome, both physically and emotionally. The astute healthcare professional is aware of the client's body image and intercedes appropriately to assure an optimal outcome for the client.

Study Questions

1. Name three concepts related to body image and explain their relationship.
2. What opportunities do you see for a nurse in the case study as described? What would you do?
3. If you could infer body images, what might you think was the likely stage of body image of Jane, Maddy, Ethel, and Nancy?
4. What meaning of her illness do you think you can find or infer from Jane's statements? From Maddy's?
5. What would you, as a nurse, have said to Jane as she cried? As a friend?
6. Describe how you would assess a client with a changed body image.
7. Discuss how age, gender, and culture can affect body image.

References

Altabe, M. (1998). Ethnicity and body image: Quantitative and qualitative analysis. *International Journal of Eating Disorders, 23,* 153–159.

Bello, L., & McIntire, S. (1995). Body image disturbance in young adults with cancer. *Cancer Nursing, 18* (2), 138–143.

Brown, M. S. (1977). The nursing process and distortions or changes in body image. In F. L. Bower (Ed.), *Distortions in body image in illness and disability* (pp. 1–19). New York: Wiley.

Byely, L., Archibald, A., Graber, J., & Brooks-Gunn, J. (1999). A prospective study of familial and social influences on girls' body image and dieting. *International Journal of Eating Disorders, 28,* 155–164.

Carpenito, L. (2000). *Nursing diagnosis: Application to clinical practice* (8th ed.). Philadelphia: Lippincott.

Cash, T. F. (2002). Cognitive behavioral perspectives on body image. In T. Cash & T. Pruzinsky (Eds.), *Body image: A handbook of theory, research, and clinical progress* (pp. 38–46). New York: Guilford Press.

Cash, T. F., & Fleming, E. C. (2002). The impact of body image experiences: Development of the body image quality of life inventory. *International Journal of Eating Disorders, 31,* 455–460.

Cash, T. F., & Pruzinsky, T. (1990). *Body images: Development, deviance, and change.* New York: Guilford Press.

Cash, T. F., & Pruzinsky, T. (2002). Understanding body image: Historical and contemporary perspectives. In T. Cash & T. Pruzinsky (Eds.), *Body image: A handbook of theory, research, and clinical progress* (pp. 30–37). New York: Guilford Press.

Cohen, M. Z., Kahn, D. L., & Steeves, R. H. (1998). Beyond body image: The experience of breast cancer. *Oncology Nursing Forum, 25* (5), 835–841.

Corey, M., & Corey, G. (1997). *Groups: Process and practice* (5th ed.). Boston: Brooks/Cole.

Corwyn, R. F. (2000). The factor structure of global self-esteem among adolescents and adults. *Journal of Research and Personality, 34,* 357–379.

Craig, M. M., & Edwards, J. E. (1983). Adaptation in chronic illness: An eclectic model for nurses. *Journal of Advanced Nursing, 8* (5), 397–404.

Dropkin, M. J. (1989). Coping with disfigurement and dysfunction after head and neck cancer surgery: A conceptual framework. *Seminars in Oncology Nursing, 5* (3), 213–219.

Erikson, E. (1963). *Childhood and society* (2nd ed.). New York: Norton.

Fisher, S. (1986). *Development and structure of the body image* (vol. 2). Hillsdale, NJ: Lawrence Erlbaum Associates.

Golden, J. S., & Golden, M. (1986). Cancer and sex. In J. M. Vaeth (Ed.), *Body image, self-esteem, and sexuality in cancer patients* (2nd ed.), (pp. 68–76). Basil: Karger.

Hayslip, B., Cooper, C. C., Dougherty, L. M., & Cook, D. D. (1997). Body image in adulthood: A projective approach. *Journal of Personality Assessment, 68* (3), 628–649.

Helman, C. G. (1995). The body image in health and disease: Exploring patients' maps of body and self. *Patient Education and Counseling, 26,* 169–175.

Jackson, L. A. (2002). Physical attractiveness: A sociocultural perspective. In T. Cash & T. Pruzinsky (Eds.), *Body image: A handbook of theory, research, and clinical progress* (pp. 13–21). New York: Guilford Press.

Johnson, M., & Maas, M. (Eds.). (1997). *Nursing outcomes classification (NOC).* St. Louis, MO: Mosby.

Kearney-Cooke, A. (2002). Familial influences on body image development. In T. Cash & T. Pruzinsky (Eds.), *Body image: A handbook of theory, research, and clinical progress* (pp. 99–107). New York: Guilford Press.

Kirkpatrick, J. R. (1986). The stoma patient and his return to society. In J. M. Vaeth (Ed.), *Body image, self-esteem, and sexuality in cancer patients* (2nd ed.) (pp. 24–27). Basil: Karger.

Krauss-Whitbourne, S. & Skultety, K. (2002). Body image development: adulthood and aging. In T. Cash & T. Pruzinsky (Eds.), *Body image: A handbook of theory, research, and clinical progress* (pp. 83–90). New York: Guilford Press.

Krueger, D. W. (2002). Psychodynamic perspectives on body image. In T. Cash & T. Pruzinsky (Eds.), *Body image: A handbook of theory, research, and clinical progress* (pp. 30–37). New York: Guilford Press.

Markus, H., & Wurf, E. (1987). The dynamic self-concept: A social psychological perspective. *Annual Review of Psychology, 38,* 299–337.

Mock, V. (1993). Body image in women treated for breast cancer. *Nursing Research, 42* (3), 153–157.

deMoore, G. M., Franzcp, N., Hennessey, P., Kunz, N. M., et al. (2000). Kaposi's sarcoma: The scarlet letter of AIDS. The psychological effects of a skin disease. *Psychosomatics, 41* (4), 360–363.

Nezlek, J. B. (1999). Body image and day-to-day social interaction. *Journal of Personality, 67* (5), 793–817.

Norris, J., Connell, M. K., & Spelic, S. S. (1998). A grounded theory of reimaging. *Advances in Nursing Science, 20* (3), 1–12.

Olivardia, R., Pope, H. J., & Hudson, J. I. (2000). Muscle dysmorphia in male weightlifters: A case control study. *American Journal of Psychiatry, 157,* 1291–1296.

Orr, D. A., Reznikoff, M., & Smith, G. M. (1989). Body image, self-esteem, and depression in burn-injured adolescents and young adults. *Journal of Burn Care and Rehabilitation, 10* (5), 454–461.

Otto, S. E. (1991). *Oncology nursing.* St. Louis, MO: Mosby.

Peterson, C., Wimmer, S., Ackard, D., Crosby, R., et al. (2004). Changes in body image during cognitive-behavioral treatment in women with bulimia nervosa. *Body Image, 1* (2), 139–153.

Pruzinsky, T. (2002). Body image adaptation to reconstructive surgery for acquired disfigurement. In T. Cash & T. Pruzinsky (Eds.), *Body image: A handbook of theory, research, and clinical progress* (pp. 440–449). New York: Guilford Press.

Pruzinsky, T. (2004). Enhancing quality of life in medical populations: A vision for body image assessment and rehabilitation as standards of care. *Body Image, 1,* 71–81.

Rhode Island Department of Health Office of Minority Health. (1998). *Minority health fact sheets.* Available on-line at http://www.health.state.ri.us/omh/mhfs.htm.

Rumsey, N. (2002). Body image and congenital conditions with visible differences. In T. Cash & T. Pruzinsky (Eds.), *Body image: A handbook of theory, research, and clinical progress* (pp. 226–233). New York: Guilford Press.

Rumsey, N., & Harcourt, D. (2004). Body image and disfigurement: Issues and interventions. *Body Image, 1,* 83–97.

Rybarczyk, B., & Behel, J. (2002). Rehabilitation medicine and body image. In T. Cash & T. Pruzinsky (Eds.), *Body image: A handbook of theory, research, and clinical progress* (pp. 387–394). New York: Guilford Press.

Schilder, P. (1950). *The image and appearance of the human body.* New York: International Universities Press.

Striegel-Moore, R., & Franko, D. (2002). Body image issues among girls and women. In T. Cash & T. Pruzinsky (Eds.), *Body image: A handbook of theory, research, and clinical progress* (pp. 183–191). New York: Guilford Press.

Thompson, J., & Gardner, R. (2002). Measuring perceptual body image in adolescents and adults. In T. Cash & T. Pruzinsky (Eds.), *Body image: A handbook of theory, research, and clinical progress* (pp. 142–154). New York: Guilford Press.

Thompson, J., & Van Den Berg, P. (2002). Measuring body image attitudes among adolescents and adults. In T. Cash & T. Pruzinsky (Eds.), *Body image: A handbook of theory, research, and clinical progress* (pp. 155–162). New York: Guilford Press.

Van Deusen, J. (1993). *Body image and perceptual dysfunction in adults.* Philadelphia: WB Saunders.

Veale, D. (2004). Advances in cognitive behavioural model of body dysmorphic disorder. *Body Image, 1* (1), 113–125.

Wetterhahn, K., Hanson, C., & Levy, C. (2002). Effect of participation in physical activity on body image of amputees. *American Journal of Physical Medicine and Rehabilitation, 81* (3), 194–201.

White, C. A. (2000). Body image dimensions and cancer: A heuristic cognitive behavioural model. *Psych-Oncology, 9,* 183–192.

White, C. A. (2002). Body image issues in oncology. In T. Cash & T. Pruzinsky (Eds.), *Body image: A handbook of theory, research, and clinical progress* (pp. 379–386). New York: Guilford Press.

Wright, L. & Leahey, M. (2000). *Nurses and families: A guide to family assessment and intervention* (3rd ed.). Philadelphia: F.A. Davis.

PART II

Impact on the Client and Family

CHAPTER 9

Quality of Life

Victoria Schirm

Introduction

The increased number of Americans who are living with chronic disabling conditions has shifted the emphasis from a health care system focused solely on cure and quantity of life to enhancement of the quality of life. Additionally, the greater emphasis on quality of life issues parallels the growth in medical knowledge and use of technology. Many fatal diseases of the past have become chronic in nature because of successful cure rates; and life-sustaining technologies have made it possible for people to live with many other chronic illnesses. Chronic illnesses are prevalent and costly, with more than 1.7 million people dying each year. Moreover, the course of chronic illness creates suffering and decreased quality of life for millions more Americans (National Center for Chronic Disease, n.d.).

These trends bring to the forefront the need to consider quality of life in chronic illness care and call attention to it as an important concept in nursing. Knowledge about a person's quality of life enables the nurse to plan holistic care. Nursing interventions can be planned and evaluated better with an understanding of the client's well-being. Treatment goals and responses to changes in therapy can be monitored in relationship to quality of life outcomes for clients.

In clinical practice, quality of life assessments provide an understanding of the impact that chronic illness has on clients and their families. The complex interrelationships of the associated burdens in chronic illness are appreciated more fully when the client's overall quality of life is known.

In nursing research related to chronic illness, quality of life is studied to identify and evaluate specific problems and needs of clients with illness or disability. Research is also conducted to test and compare the impact of interventions on clients' quality of life. Results of such investigations provide information for clinical practice and, ultimately, the nursing interventions that impact clients' quality of life.

Client participation in clinical decision making has also forced the issue of quality of life to the forefront. Equipped with an array of knowledge from the Internet, clients demand more information about how treatments and sequelae will affect the quality of their lives. They want to know if the positive outcomes of their treatments (improved health and function, pain and symptom control, or prolonged life) will outweigh the expected negative effects of their treatments (financial burdens, anxiety, or disrupted life-style). Satisfying these reasonable client needs requires that health care professionals be aware of the relationship of chronic illness and quality of life.

In the larger arena of the health care system, quality of life evaluations are used to monitor the extent to which delivered services address client needs. Outcomes that promote quality of life are valued, particularly when positive results are achieved with efficiency and cost savings.

A review of the Cumulative Index to Nursing and Allied Health Literature (CINAHL) shows that "quality of life" was first used as a subject heading in 1983. Since that time, scores of studies and reviews have been published about quality of life. The available CINAHL subheadings address several areas that are considered to influence quality of life. Included are economics, education, ethical issues, evaluation, organizations, psychosocial factors, standards, and trends. In this chapter, the literature related to quality of life as it is impacted by chronic illness is presented.

Defining Quality of Life

A subjective component is present in defining *quality of life*. Each individual's unique situation and experiences of the individual shape quality of life. The general or global meaning of quality of life to a person may be anchored to socioeconomic, demographic, and life-style factors; personality characteristics; aspects of social and community environments; and well-being in physical and mental health (Abeles, Gift & Ory, 1994). The more specific *health-related quality of life* is usually defined in relationship to health and physical function, emotional well-being, general health perceptions, and role and social function. However, the distinction between general quality of life and health-related quality of life is not made easily (Haas, 1999). Elements that contribute to global quality of life are not included necessarily in judgments about health-related quality of life, and reference to health-related quality of life may suggest preponderance on disease. Nurses, in particular, have a stake in understanding the distinctions and the overlaps in the dimensions of perceived quality of life because of the impact it has for nursing research and nursing practice in chronic illness.

Regardless of whether one is referring to global quality of life or health-related quality of life, the subjective or individual perspective is important to the definition. Rene Dubos's (1959) definition addresses the subjective nature and the multidimensionality of quality of life by saying, "Men naturally desire health and happiness. . . . The kind of health that men desire most is not necessarily a state in which they experience physical vigor and a sense of well-being, not even one giving them a long life. It is, instead, the condition best suited to reach goals that each individual formulates for himself" (p. 228). Haas (1999) recognizes the multidimensionality of quality of life and defines it as different from well-being, life satisfaction, and functional ability. It is a personal evaluation of "current life circumstances in the context of the culture and value systems in which they live and the values they hold" (p. 219).

An objective measurement of quality of life, including health-related quality of life, is well recognized in the literature (Abeles, Gift & Ory, 1994; Faden & German, 1994; Haas, 1999; Lawton, 1997). Standardized assessments are used to provide the objective indicators of what constitutes the "outside" judgments about quality of life. Ferrans' (1996) work provides an example of the development of a quality of life measure that offers an objective assessment and is connected to a person's judgments, values, life experiences, and satisfaction with aspects of life. The assessment tool includes four quality of life domains: health and functioning, psychospiritual, socioeconomic, and family. Evaluating an individual's quality of life can show how satisfying the person considers life in these domains. The assessment provides an understanding of the similarities and differences between the person's view and the views held by others. This information can be used to screen and monitor clients' progress and help care providers make treatment decisions (Faden & German, 1994). Nurses can use quality of life information to plan, implement, and evaluate interventions for clients with chronic illnesses.

Frameworks

Nurses use theories, frameworks, or models to explain the complex interrelationships among factors influencing the trajectory of chronic illness on quality of life. The use of such conceptualizations can enhance nursing practice by suggesting appropriate interventions in caring for persons with chronic illness.

Peplau's (1994) theory presents an interpersonal perspective toward quality of life, stating, "Human relationships are a major determinant of the quality of life" (p. 10). This theory emphasizes the importance of interpersonal relationships to a person's well-being and hence to the quality of life. Actions of the nurse using this interpersonal framework to promote quality of life would include active listening, facilitating coping skills, and enhancing support systems.

Parse's (1994) "human becoming" theory focuses on quality of life from the person's perspective. Parse (1996) used this conceptualization to explore meanings associated with quality of life in clients with Alzheimer's disease. In this study, early-stage Alzheimer's clients were asked to talk about their quality of life. Despite the difficulty for many in trying to put their thoughts into words, the 25 participants in the study were able to tell stories that reflected the quality of their lives. This story telling in the context of the human becoming theory provides nurses with an understanding about quality of life for clients with Alzheimer's disease.

Lee and Pilkington (1999) also used Parse's theory to gain a better understanding about quality of life for clients receiving palliative care. Openness to the experience of another as proposed in the human becoming theory allows the nurse to better understand the process of living with dying. Plank (1994) used the context of Parse's theory to guide nursing practice for counseling and information giving about treatment options to oncology clients. Recognizing that the goal of nursing is to enhance quality of life from the person's perspective, the nurse can use this conceptualization to individualize and structure informed consent for clients. This nursing intervention prepares clients to make better decisions about the kind of treatment options, supportive care, or chemotherapy that can maintain or promote their quality of life.

Watson's theory of human care (1985) provides an understanding of how individuals find meaning in their existence, particularly in the face of disharmony and suffering. Increased awareness of one's potential as a spiritual being opens up possibilities for becoming more fully human, surmounting physical limitations, and preserving meaning and quality of life. Similar to Watson's ideas, Benner and Wrubel (1989) also point out that a person's sense of well-being comes from the freedom to choose actions, outcomes, meanings, and relationships. Living with an illness does not mean that one's life is dominated by it, that one tries to conquer it, or that it can be mastered. Rather, the person goes forward with life and reaches the highest level of outcome possible by finding meaning and harmony in existence, even with chronic illness. Thus, meaning, harmony, and attaining the highest level of well-being possible can constitute quality of life.

One framework postulates that life satisfaction and happiness as viewed from the perspective of individuals are critical to quality of life (Oleson 1990). The individual's judgment about how satisfying life is or the extent of happiness is made within the context of quality of life domains. This anchoring, for example, could include the domains of health and function, psychosocial well-being, spirituality, or family ties. In this framework, an individual's subjectively perceived quality of life is important to decision making about health care treatments. Knowledge about a person's subjective quality of life can be used by nurses to plan appropriate nursing interventions.

Another model (Stuifbergen, Seraphine & Roberts, 2000) offers nurses a way to understand how health promotion interventions can be developed for persons with chronic illness, and thereby enhance an individual's quality of life. Components in this model of health-promoting behaviors for quality of life are the resources one has, barriers to achievement of quality of life, self-efficacy in performing health care behaviors, and acceptance of illness. These factors are interrelated and can influence the perceived quality of life in persons with chronic illness. The nurse's understanding of how these factors are associated can determine interventions to enhance quality of life in chronic illness. For example, knowing that improved social supports, decreased barriers, and increased self-efficacy enable better health promotion behaviors could assist the nurse in determining appropriate health-promoting behaviors for a person with chronic illness.

Health-promoting behaviors have been addressed also in Orem's self-care model (1990). This framework is a useful guide for nursing practice in chronic illness. For example, Nesbitt and Heidrich (2000) found that older women who had resources to deal with stressors and were provided information that promoted self-care had a high quality of life despite the health limitations of chronic illness.

The theory of self care management for vulnerable populations (Dorsey & Murdaugh, 2003) offers another model to help identify factors that can be used to understand quality of life for persons with chronic illness. Dorsey and Murdaugh cite the specific example of sickle cell disease to suggest that self-care is crucial to symptom management and maintaining control over chronic illness. The self care management theory provides direction for developing culturally sensitive interventions that can lead to improved quality of life for a vulnerable group such as adults with sickle cell disease.

Problems and Issues of Quality of Life in Chronic Illness

A discussion of the problems and issues surrounding quality of life in chronic illness is best done within the context of several domains. The work of Ferrans (1990, 1996) organizes the global concept of quality of life into four major domains: health and functioning, psychological/spiritual, social and economic, and family. Within each domain, the multiple dimensions of various aspects of life are considered. As shown in the following sections, considerable overlap exists among the relationships of the global concept quality of life, the major domains, and the specific aspects within each domain. Ferrans' conceptualization, however, offers a practicable way to organize the discussion of problems and issues that individuals living with chronic illness may confront.

Health and Function Issues

A client's perceived health, energy level, pain experiences, stress levels, independence, capacity to meet responsibilities, access to and use of health care, and usefulness to others are some aspects that contribute to quality of life in the health and function domain. Liao et al. (2000) pointed out there is reason to believe that even in the last year of life, persons 85 years and older are experiencing a better quality of life compared with elderly cohorts in previous times. The quality of life rating in this study was based on objective measures that included nursing home length of stay, cognitive and functional abilities, and an illness score.

That individual perceptions influence significantly a person's quality of life was upheld by Tang, Aaronson, and Forbes (2004) who studied terminally ill hospice clients. By virtue of their circumstances, hospice clients could be viewed as experiencing a mediocre quality of life, yet Tang and colleagues (2004) found above average quality of life ratings in their study group. Factors that contributed to these positive ratings were spiritual well-being, appropriate pain management, and social and emotional support. Promoting quality of life as a part of geriatric palliative care includes addressing pain, anxiety, and dyspnea (Sheehan & Schirm, 2003).

In chronic illness, assessments that rely solely on clinical parameters, such as laboratory results, functional ability, or physical health, may not capture the client's overall picture of health and well-being. In a study of health-related quality of life for rheumatoid arthritis clients, researchers (Kosinski et al., 2000) found that clients' and physicians' global quality of life and pain ratings corresponded more strongly with clients' perceived health quality of life than with physical measures of joint swelling or tenderness. These findings suggest that quality of life assessments can be used for determining treatment efficacy. Others have presented evidence that medication management for clients with hypertension or angina pectoris can be gauged by quality of life assessments that account for symptoms and the distress they cause (Hollenberg, Williams & Anderson, 2000).

Other researchers (Hudson, Kirksey, & Holzemer, 2004) found that quality of life in chronic illness is affected not only by the presence of symptoms but also by symptom intensity. Specifically, Hudson et al. reported that prevalent symptoms among HIV infected women included muscle aches, depression, thirst, weakness, fear, cognitive changes, and painful joints; and symptoms that proved more intense for this group were headaches, rash, insomnia, gynecological disturbances, anxiety, cramps, and painful joints. They suggested these findings have implications in the women's capacity to manage self care and to provide requisite care to their families.

Although people with chronic illness may have a "good" perceived quality of life, they can be affected profoundly by symptoms associated with their disease. Knowledge of how symptoms affect clients' health and function can lead to a better understanding of their quality of life in chronic illness. Typically, the presence of symptoms prompts an individual to seek health care—for example, weakness and poor coordination in the individual with multiple sclerosis or excessive thirst and frequent urination in a person with diabetes. Additionally, people with chronic illness are subjected to symptoms from the side effects of the treatments they undergo. Regardless of the origin, physically distressing symptoms affect health and function and, ultimately, one's quality of life.

The perceptions of symptoms and the distress they cause vary among clients, health care professionals, and family members, sometimes resulting in conflicting views about a person's quality of life and thereby impacting treatment decisions. Assumptions about quality of life in Alzheimer's disease (AD) clients, for example, have implications for the treatment decisions that caregivers make. Karlawish et al. (2003) found that older and more depressed caregivers who were caring for severely demented relatives were unwilling to consider risk-free treatments that may prolong the person's life. Karlawish et al., also reported that the higher a caregiver rated their relative's quality of life, the more inclined they

were to consider treatment that would slow the progress of AD. They noted that aspects of quality of life entered into decision making about using both risk-free and risky AD treatments. Decisions that care providers make to use available technology also has quality of life implications, especially when age is considered. Hamilton and Carroll (2004) found that younger clients who received an implantable cardioverter defibrillator had higher quality of life scores than older cardioverter recipients. Also, it is not unusual that care providers' and clients' quality of life evaluations are inconsistent (Fisch et al., 2003). These reports and findings suggest the importance of using quality of life assessments that consider clients' perspectives.

Psychological and Spiritual Issues

The complexity of health and function in chronic illness suggests that neither good health nor optimum function is a necessary or sufficient condition for quality of life. In Ferrans' (1996) quality of life model, the domain of psychological and spiritual includes life satisfaction, happiness, peace of mind, control, goal achievement, and a belief system. Kinney, Rodgers, Nash, and Bray, (2003) note that most quality of life models subsume the spiritual domain within psychological well-being, and rarely give attention to spiritual issues apart from mind or body. Kinney and colleagues' model includes theory-based nursing practice within a spiritually-based wellness program that provides holistic care to women with breast cancer. They assert that this integrative perspective is a guide for inclusion of spirituality in holistic care. Clearly, considerable overlap exists between psychological and spiritual well-being, and the separate discussion in this section is intended for better coverage of the problems and issues surrounding psychospiritual care in chronic illness.

Psychological Issues

Psychological well-being, as an essential component of health-related quality of life, influences overall adjustment to chronic illness. In addition to affective aspects such as happiness, satisfaction, goal achievement, or peace of mind (Ferrans, 1996), the psychological domain can include cognitive function (Patrick & Erikson, 1993). In fact, results of research have shown that loss of cognitive function was more detrimental to subjective and objective quality of life than were functional losses or severe pain (Lawton et al., 1999). In the Lawton et al. study, 600 subjects over 70 years old were presented hypothetical situations of different illness conditions and were asked to respond to how long they might wish to live. Despite the inherent difficulties of asking one to imagine circumstances of chronic illness and decline, Lawton and associates noted that the findings were similar to other quality of life research results, suggesting that people usually wish to live a shorter time if that time is of diminished quality.

Ryan (1992) showed that caring about the affective aspects of psychological well-being is important to promoting quality of life for homebound hospice clients and their primary caregivers. When asked to rate the most helpful behaviors that nurses did for clients, the primary family caregivers gave higher importance to meeting several psychosocial needs than they did to physical needs. Caregivers placed a high value on the nurse's presence and support, and listening to concerns and communicating information. Nurses also rated positively the importance of the psychosocial interventions they carry out for clients and families. Offering assurance, listening, helping the client feel safe, and providing consistent nursing services were mentioned among the most helpful nursing care activities.

The adjustments that a person living with a chronic illness must make influence the quality of life. Murdaugh (1998) reported that individuals with HIV/AIDS who maintained realistic expectations, modified job plans, or realigned goals that were congruent with their health and function had improved quality of life. Murdaugh commented that this "balance must be maintained between efforts and resources to ensure life quality" and "the process is not unique to HIV disease, as persons with other chronic illnesses experience a similar balancing act" (p. 69).

A close interplay exists between the affective aspects in the psychological domain and other quality of life domains. Findings from clients in a cardiac rehabilitation program showed that better physical function, increased energy, and improved perceived health are accompanied by decreased anxiety, depression, and negativity (Engebretson et al., 1999). A study about the quality of life of breast cancer survivors also demonstrated the close relationship of the psychological, spiritual, physical, and social domains (Wyatt, Kurtz & Liken, 1993). The women in this study described that coping with the physical concerns of cancer in their lives was dependent on psychological, spiritual, and social elements. For many, closer ties with families and friends became important, spiritual guidance served in making health decisions, and a fuller appreciation of life was more apparent. Clearly, the issues surrounding survival of breast cancer crossed over into more than one domain. The obvious interaction among quality of life domains suggests the importance of developing holistic treatment programs for clients with chronic illness.

Spirituality Issues

In the nursing literature, *spirituality* is generally defined broadly as embracing "love, compassion, caring, transcendence, relationship with God, and connection of body, mind, and spirit" (O'Brien, 2003, p. 6). Most definitions take into consideration that spirituality affects all aspects of a person's well-being. Spirituality is viewed as internal to each person, giving hope, promoting interconnectedness, and providing a sense of well-being. Most sources agree that spirituality is separate from religion, or that spirituality is composed of two dimensions: a religious orientation and an existential orientation (Landis, 1996). Hicks (1999) defines *spirituality* as the "dynamic principles developed throughout the lifespan that guide a person's view of the world" (p. 144). Berggren-Thomas and Griggs (1995) note that the spiritual aspect of an individual provides for meaningfulness in life and is a source of forgiveness and love. Spirituality is also described as the energy that either contributes to the individual's well-being or contributes to illness and diminished health through its effect on physical, mental, and emotional well-being (Isaia, Parker & Murrow, 1999). Clearly, spiritual well-being influences profoundly the quality of life. Not surprisingly then, spiritual distress can lead to physical and emotional illness (Heriot, 1992).

Individuals and their families, when faced with the crisis of a chronic illness, and especially with impending death, may look to others for spiritual support. For example, Wilson and Daley (1999) found that families appreciated any spiritual support that was provided, from having access to a chapel to a visit from clergy. Families also appreciated when staff prayed with them and when nurses cried with them. Prayers and tears made the families feel that the nurses cared for and about their loved one.

The existential part of spirituality is an important consideration for quality of life in HIV/AIDS clients. In their review of the literature, O'Neill and Kenny (1998) point out that people with AIDS struggle frequently with ways to find meaning and purpose in a life amid the myriad challenges of living with a chronic disease marked by misunderstandings, conflicts, and guilt. The resolve to live well requires inherent spiritual well-being. Landis (1996) found that the occurrence of chronic illness problems decreased in the presence of higher levels of spiritual well-being. Better spiritual well-being was also associated with decreased uncertainty in chronic illness.

Social and Economic Issues

The socioeconomic domain of quality of life includes specific aspects of emotional support, home, employment, finances, neighborhood, and friends (Ferrans, 1996). The components may also include social support and cultural influences (Patrick & Erickson, 1993). The problems and issues within this domain are varied and numerous.

Emotional Support

Emotional support offered by friends and confidantes contributes to quality of life in a variety of ways. It influences how meaning is ascribed to ill-

ness, alters the coping strategies used to manage stress, augments motivation to employ adaptive behaviors, promotes self-esteem, and protects individuals from the negative effect of stress by altering their mood (Wortman, 1984). Indeed, most people know the positive effect of having "moral support" and companionship at times of difficulty. Wilson, Hutchinson, and Holzemer (1997) found that for persons living with HIV/AIDS, social support, especially from people they know, is valued most. Others (Baxter et al., 1998; Landis, 1996) have shown that the social networks people have, such as friends and relatives, group activity participation, and time spent visiting, are associated with a higher quality of life, despite the presence of a chronic illness.

Cultural Aspects

Although quality of life appears as a worldwide concept, the unique cultural interpretations can influence perceived quality of life (Bullinger, 1997). Social conditions, expectations of individual behaviors, and cultural regulations determine the extent to which the domains or their components affect quality of life. However, in order to assess appropriately quality of life in various ethnic groups, it is necessary to understand its meanings across cultures.

An exploration of the meaning of comfort in immigrant Hispanic clients with cancer demonstrated two findings: feeling integrated and being nurtured. Feeling integrated meant a complex sense of inner peace and wholeness beyond the physical dimension. Being nurtured referred to care provided with patience and reciprocity by family or caregivers. Quality of life, one of the six categories of comfort needs that clients defined as important, was described as having things meaningful to them. *Amino*, another category of identified need, was described as having a positive mental disposition, drive, or energy in the face of the illness. Although *amino* is specific to Spanish-speaking clients, those reporting this need indicated that it is fundamental to being human (Arruda, Larson & Meleis, 1992).

Leininger (1994) points out that quality of life is dependent on one's culture, and is expressed in the actions of daily life and is influenced by individual values. For example, in the United States, the values of individuality, self-reliance, independence; emphasis on technology and competition; and assertiveness give rise to actions such as independent decision making, self-reliance whether sick or well, and individualism. These values and actions are in contrast to Mexican American cultural groups, in which the meaning of quality of life emphasizes values of filial love, respect for authority, and acceptance of God's will. Adherence to these cultural values for Mexican American groups is important to maintaining one's quality of life. Leininger's study of Native Americans shows the importance of values that maintain harmony between people and the environment. These values result in actions for maintaining quality of life, such as listening to and respecting elders and upholding life-care rituals and taboos that maintain mutuality between nature and people.

Employment and Finances

The economic impact of chronic illness on individuals and their families has a significant effect on financial resources. The negative impact causes financial burdens and drains financial resources. The reasons for financial strain and its effects vary. Frequently, a chronic illness requires individuals to decrease, suspend, or end their work, leading to a reduction or loss of income. Furthermore, if the care recipient requires much assistance or supervision, the primary family caregiver also may have to terminate employment. Thus, a family with a member who is chronically ill now faces an increased financial burden resulting from two members' unemployment. For people who retire from work early due to chronic illness, findings show that a smaller proportion of individuals with chronic conditions are very satisfied with retirement compared with those without chronic conditions. These situations contribute to an adverse quality of life through decreased workforce participation, and ultimately cause lost productivity, which further increases the overall cost of chronic illness (Workers & Chronic Conditions, 2000).

Persons with chronic illness also suffer financially due to the additional expenses incurred with medical insurance rates or out-of-pocket expenses for items not covered by insurance. Transportation to medical or treatment appointments, for example, or the extra cost of special dietary foods or supplements can add up quickly. The desperately ill person who has found little benefit from traditional therapies may spend large amounts of money on folk or alternative forms of treatment in an effort toward improvement (Cassileth et al., 1991). For HIV/AIDS clients, the financial burdens can be particularly acute. Wilson et al. (1997) note that not only must the client juggle treatments and side effects, but also must overcome financial and logistic hurdles that range from obtaining health care insurance to finding transportation to hospital and clinics.

The interrelatedness of quality of life domains and their aspects is shown in a study of working and nonworking mentally ill persons (Van Dongen, 1996). Results of the study suggested that for gainfully employed mentally ill persons, work may serve as a positive distraction from symptoms and worries. Moreover, workers with chronic mental illness had higher scores in all quality of life areas (except living situation) compared with similar nonworkers. Workers had significantly higher self-esteem, better family and social relationships, good health, and more financial security than did nonworkers.

The combined effect on quality of life associated with decreased income and increased expenses may not always be obvious. However, nurses must be aware of how this financial burden may contribute to decreased quality of life (Arzouman et al., 1991). Clients may take fewer medications because they cannot afford to take the prescribed amount, or the family caregiver may be overtaxed by the caregiving burden because the family cannot afford assistance. Despite the known positive relationship between a good quality of life and an adequate income (Artinian & Hayes, 1992), the nurse needs to be cautious in assuming that the situation is positive in all situations. The high degree of subjectivity in quality of life assessments suggests that other aspects may influence one's judgments about quality of life.

Family Issues

Family health, spousal relationships, family happiness, and children are aspects of quality of life within the family domain (Ferrans, 1996). Considerable attention has been given to the study of chronic illness and its impact on the family. Any illness affecting a family member will inevitably affect that individual's family and their quality of life. Factors that affect family quality of life include family structure and interaction patterns; the availability of social networks or support resources; the potential for adaptation; and family philosophy, such as beliefs, attitudes, values, and perceived stressors; and impact of illness (Jassak & Knafl, 1990).

When family members become primary caregivers of a chronically ill member, the role changes, additional responsibilities, and increased stressors influence quality of life for family members. The extent of this influence on particular domains and aspects of quality of life appears to vary. Artinian and Hayes (1992) found that spouses of clients undergoing a coronary artery bypass were more satisfied with family life than they were with the health, function, social, psychological, or spiritual components of quality of life. The varying effects on quality of life may be attributed in part to the caregiver's perception of the client's quality of life as it may be related to their own perceived health-related quality of life. For example, McMillan and Mahon (1994) found a positive association between family caregivers' ratings of their own health-related quality of life and the quality of life ratings they made of the hospice client for whom they were the primary caregiver.

Without a doubt, the overwhelming nature of chronic illness affects the quality of life not only for the client, but also for family members. Because of the importance of family caregiving to a chronically ill member, the effects on the primary caregiver's own health have been the focus of attention in quality of life research. End-stage renal disease, for example, has been shown to create stress in the client's family members. Wicks and colleagues (1998) found that mild and moderate burdens existed in caregivers of a family member who had end-stage renal disease

regardless of how well they were coping with the illness. Moreover, declines in burden and improvements in quality of life did not occur for caregivers despite decreases in care responsibilities when the family member had a transplant. Wicks et al. speculated that new concerns for the family about organ rejection and maintaining strict medication regimes created uncertainty that was as burdensome as the physical care required for dialysis in previous times.

A comparison of perceived quality of life for spouses of heart transplant clients showed findings similar to those of the Wicks et al. (1998) study. The ratings that spouses made of their own health declined significantly in the first year following their partner's heart transplant (Collins, White-Williams & Jalowiec, 2000). These spouses also indicated that they had more difficulty coping with stress post transplantation, especially if they were experiencing poor health. When caregivers are helped to manage their stress and anxiety, the evidence suggests that both the caregiver and the client realize better quality of life. Welk and Smith (1999) reported that failing to manage stress and anxiety in hospice clients contributes to a family member's stress and anxiety. Interestingly, when hospice workers paid attention to a caregiver's stress and anxiety, the care recipient reported a high level of satisfaction with the control of pain. This evidence illustrates how quality of life in chronic illness impacts *all* family members.

Interventions for Improving Quality of Life

An overview of nursing interventions focusing on the quality of life domains of health and function, psychological and spiritual, socioeconomic, and family is presented in this section. This organization around the quality of life domains includes examples of the ways that nurses can intervene effectively for clients and their families. Reports most often view the quality of life of a client as an important outcome measure across several domains. For organizational purposes, interventions that promote quality of life as an outcome are discussed within one of the four domains. Although this method is fitting for an organized discussion of nursing interventions, the assumption is made that interventions influence quality of life by affecting one or more domains.

Overall, a reasonable outcome of any nursing intervention is improved quality of life for clients. In chronic illness, this goal is even more salient. Nurses as essential health care professionals to clients with chronic illness can be instrumental in planning, carrying out, and evaluating care that promotes quality of life. For clients, finding ways to enhance their quality of life amid the debilitating effects of a long-term illness becomes an especially relevant outcome. Consequently, viewing quality of life from the client's context is a reasonable outcome measure of a clinical intervention's effectiveness.

Interventions for Health and Function

Traditionally, health and function assessments and the subsequent interventions have focused on outcomes more concerned with the stage of the disease, the extent of the disability, and the mortality rate (Cheater, 1998). This view of outcomes disregards care for other aspects of health and function in chronic illness, such as the client's perceived health, energy level, pain experiences, stress levels, independence, capacity to meet responsibilities, access to and use of health care, and usefulness to others. Clients want to know how interventions are going to influence these aspects of health and function, and want guidance in choosing the options that will produce the best outcomes. Moreover, when benefits of interventions are uncertain, the client's life-style and preferences should be considered in deciding on the treatment (Cheater, 1998).

Evidence suggests that client quality of life outcomes are dependent not only on appropriate nursing interventions, but also that outcomes are linked to client factors. Kreulen and Braden (2004) in a study of 307 women receiving breast cancer treatment found that nursing interventions to promote self care practice can influence positively physiological and functional quality of life outcomes. At the same time, client factors such as age, social support, disease severity, and uncertainty about the illness have an effect on these same outcomes. Kreulen and Braden reported that nursing interventions are linked to clients' self care behaviors and that self care practices lead to better outcomes relative to symptom management, role responsibilities, and mental well-being. They noted also that more severe illness may require higher intensity of nursing supportive interventions to ensure better client quality of life outcomes.

Client preferences about what they believe are important to their health and function can be used to develop interventions to enhance quality of life. Mowad (2004) found that engaging in health promotion behaviors and exercising control over personal choices are positive characteristics related to quality of life. Nursing interventions that empower clients to practice healthy behaviors and enable them to be self-directed in their care may contribute significantly to quality of life outcomes. Findings from other researchers (Sullivan, Weinert, & Cudney, 2003) also show that eliciting the lived experiences of women with chronic illness can enhance understanding of health and function that promotes quality of life. For example, knowing that fatigue and pain are major physical symptoms that impact quality of life is instructive for developing interventions that can be used to overcome limitations imposed by chronic illness.

Intervening appropriately in chronic conditions also includes paying attention to the effects of treatments. The quality of care that clients receive for symptom control, support during treatments, and information about medical care was found important to both clients' and family members' quality of life (Rieker, Clark & Fogelberg, 1992). Interventions that nurses can implement include preparing and monitoring clients for expected side effects of treatments, facilitating communication with other health team members, and supporting the individual needs of clients and families. Other research results suggest that proper medication management is essential to health and function quality of life outcomes. For example, improvements in physical symptom distress, and hence quality of life, occurred in clients with angina or hypertension who participated in a randomized drug trial (Hollenberg, Williams & Anderson, 2000). Compared with clients who received a placebo, the treatment group clients reported more symptom relief that was associated with better quality of life ratings. In a study of medication therapy for osteoarthritic elderly clients, researchers found that treated clients had better pain relief and improved physical functioning than the control group. These improvements enhanced clients' self-care abilities and independence, and produced positive views regarding their quality of life (Lisse et al., 2001). Nurses can use the many opportunities they have in their client encounters to intervene by discussing realistic self-care practices and safe medication use.

Intervening in situations in which conflicting views about quality of life exist among health care providers, clients, and family members is multifaceted. Clients with chronic illness may be confronted with choosing a life-extending treatment at the expense of irreversible and debilitating side effects, or they may refuse treatments likely to be successful because they are unwilling to face side effects. Dean (1990) suggests that nurses need to be well informed in order to "provide the highest quality of care we can that is aimed at providing clients the possibility of fulfilling their own goals for their lives" (p. 308).

Diabetes is a chronic illness that can be used to illustrate the complexity of assessing health and function as an indication of a client's quality of life. The literature in general shows a weak association between objective health status and a client's own views about their quality of life. This relationship holds true in diabetes wherein clients frequently rate their well-being positively despite the presence of diabetes-related complications or poor glycemic control (Snoek, 2000). These findings may be attributed to the coping style and ability of clients that are determined by other aspects that influence quality of life (i.e., social support, socioeconomic status, and personality characteristics). Snoek suggests that in addition to good health and medical

care, clients can benefit from educational and behavioral interventions that would facilitate coping with the illness.

The aspects of health and function as determinants of quality of life are used frequently with traditional clinical and disease indicators to evaluate outcomes in chronic illness conditions. For older adults, it is even more imperative that health and function assessments be conducted with traditional medical evaluations to form the basis for appropriate interventions to promote quality of life (Faden & German, 1994; Foreman & Kleinpell, 1990). In clinical practice, quality of life assessments can enhance understanding about treatment preferences. Considering the client's values with respect to their quality of life may improve decision making about treatment preferences and intensity (Faden & German, 1994). Foreman and Kleinpell (1990) summarize how information about quality of life can be used in clinical practice with elderly clients with cancer. The assessment data can be used to plan, carry out, and evaluate treatments. In situations in which treatments are known to cause extreme debility, changes should be considered for older clients based on quality of life outcomes. At the same time, it is important to have current information about treatments to assess accurately the potential effects on quality of life for elderly cancer clients. Nursing care for quality of life includes interventions for comfort, rest, pain and symptom management, and optimum function.

Findings from a study of participants in a cardiac rehabilitation program draw attention to the importance that specific personal and health factors, and adherence to physical activity have in quality of life (Sin et al., 2003). The results demonstrated that nurses need to consider a person's age and gender, as well as health and function status and ability to engage in physical activity when implementing interventions. Targeting interventions based on personal attributes and health status can make a significant impact on improving adherence to a rehabilitation program and thereby positively influence quality of life.

Quality of Life: Living with Dying

M. V. was a 70-year-old woman in seemingly good health when she was diagnosed with colon cancer. Prior to her diagnosis, she was experiencing some tiredness and frequent respiratory infections. However, on most days, she walked to church for daily Mass, worked part-time at a local grocery store, and visited with her daughter and grandchildren who lived nearby. She had been widowed for almost five years, and although she missed her husband greatly, she had adjusted to the loss by spending time with her children's families and visiting her siblings.

When surgery was performed to remove the cancerous colon, it was apparent that metastasis to nearby lymph nodes was extensive. Despite the serious nature of her illness, M. V., with the solicitous support of her daughter, proceeded undaunted with recommended treatments of chemo- and radiation therapy. Over the next several months, M. V.'s condition worsened. Realizing that it was becoming more difficult for her mother to manage alone. M. V.'s daughter made plans for her mother to move in with her family. M. V. enjoyed this arrangement, and spent quality time each day with her grandchildren.

Shortly after this move, it became evident that additional medical interventions were futile, and hospice was employed. Throughout this time, M. V. had frequent visits from her siblings, neighbors, and friends. Especially uplifting were visits from her parish priest, who was a spiritual support to her after the sudden death of her husband. M.V., likewise, found spiritual comfort in receiving communion at home, especially from her daughter-in-law, who was a Eucharistic minister. M.V. found satisfaction during these last months of her life through a supportive family, appropriate pain management and medical care, hospice care, and spiritual interventions.

Psychosocial and Spiritual Interventions

Psychological well-being during a chronic illness requires that a person have the capacity to view self in a positive manner. Foundational to an optimistic perspective is having a sense of control, self-esteem, and meaning and purpose. Nurses are in positions where they can assess the presence and efficacy of the strategies clients and families use to psychologically adapt to the chronic illness situation. Results from several studies are presented that provide examples of ways that nurses can intervene.

A study of individuals living with chronic leukemia offers insights into strategies that nurses can use to promote self-esteem and thereby improve the quality of life of clients (Bertero, Eriksson & Ek, 1997). When health care providers were open and honest about information given to clients about their illness, the clients, in turn, felt respected and valued. As a result, clients had better self-esteem, which contributed greatly to their feelings of well-being. Chronically mentally ill clients are another group that can benefit by nursing interventions that promote psychological well-being. Fisher and Mitchell (1998) reported that the nurses' exploration of meanings, relationships, and hopes with clients creates new self-perceptions for clients. These new insights can help clients clarify and choose options that can lead to an improved quality of life.

The relationship that health care professionals have with clients and families is important in developing interventions that can enable them to live with chronic illness in a way that maximizes health and well-being. Thorne et al. (2004) found that effective communication plays a critical role in promoting self-care and quality of life in individuals with multiple sclerosis. They cited specific actions that were helpful: Providing timely and accurate information that validates the client's experience; giving more information as opposed to less, and conceding that as care providers we do not have all the answers; and respecting the client, maintaining interest, and being willing to explore available options.

In a study of older adults, the concepts of mastery and self-confidence and the knowledge that resources are available to the individual are important to the one's health and well being (Forbes, 2001). These findings give importance to the psychological assessments that nurses should conduct, and the subsequent interventions that should be carried out. For example, it is important to first evaluate the resources needed by older persons that are congruent with their abilities. Specific interventions may include information and emotional assistance, developing service models that focus on self-reliance, enabling access to health care information, and addressing the needs of family caregivers. Results from a study of negative affect in chronically ill older adults show that the success of psychological interventions may depend, in part, on the clients' general disposition to stressful experiences (Kressin, Spiro & Skinner, 2000). Some clients experience distress by increased negative reactions expressed as anger, fear, guilt, or depression. These clients, despite the existence of satisfactory health and function, tend to have worse quality of life ratings. Such clients may benefit first from interventions that address the negative aspects. More education and reassurance about the client's state of health may overcome the negativity that is contributing to less than optimum quality of life. Correspondingly, clients whose clinical indicators of health and function suggest moderately good health, but instead report a diminished quality of life, may benefit from more attention to interventions that help them deal with their negative reactions to stress.

Psychological interventions to promote or, at the very least, maintain quality of life at the end of life pose special challenges to nurses. The assumption that quality of life deteriorates as death approaches for the chronically ill person may not be accurate. In one study, the presence of a terminal illness and awareness of the condition did not deter some clients from rating their quality of life as good (Waldron et al., 1999). This finding suggests that clients' values, goals, and preferences are important to making sense of and finding meaning in their lives. Nurses can use this information, unique to each individual, to help clients decide on treatment plans, make advance directives, or prioritize activities as they face death.

Spiritual Interventions

The emphasis on planning and carrying out interventions based on science and technology, in many instances, has overshadowed the inclusion of interventions related to spirituality (Donley, 1991). However, when technology is not the answer, as with chronic illness, the reality of facing suffering on a daily basis and the need to find meaning and purpose in living with a disability challenges health care providers to address a client's spiritual care needs (Muldoon & King, 1991). Donley outlined three components of spirituality that nurses should use in spiritual assessments. First, compassion on the part of the nurse is crucial to understanding the client's suffering and pain. Second, the nurse should help clients find and give meaning to their suffering. Third, the nurse should find ways to remove the suffering. This third component may not necessarily be done through traditional interventions, but rather may be carried out by a compassionate spiritual presence. In addition, the capacity to intervene in a spiritual way may be dependent on the individual nurse's spiritual perspective and practices (Cavendish et al., 2004). Self-knowledge and understanding about one's personal spirituality are essential. These attributes contribute to the ability to develop and use spiritual interventions in practice.

Spiritual interventions used in hospice care are appropriate in chronic illness care. These interventions include listening to clients talk about God, referring clients to clergy, praying with clients, sharing and exploring the meaning of spirituality, and reading scripture (Millison & Dudley, 1992). Larson and Koenig (2000) point out those clients with chronic illness are highly likely to rely on spiritual practices. Tactfully asking whether religion is important to them or how they manage tough times is a reasonable approach. When clients answer that, yes, religion is important or that religion and spiritual practices are helpful, the follow-up should be an active offer of support of the client's interests. Heriot (1992) suggested that assessment of spiritual well-being needs to include questions about how an individual expresses love, whether love is received, and the source of forgiveness. The goal of spiritual intervening is to help the client overcome feelings of guilt or regret and to emerge with a stronger sense of self-esteem. Intervening with AIDS clients is an example of the importance of this latter goal. Not only must these clients deal with guilt, angst, and rejection, but they must also transcend the illness to find meaning and purpose in their lives. Nurses can help AIDS clients face death and dying by gently guiding them in their search for meaning (O'Neill & Kenny, 1998).

Social and Economic Interventions

In the social and economic domain, the focus of interventions to promote quality of life is on social and emotional support and financial considerations. Considerations of the cultural aspects that may affect interventions for quality of life are also included in this section.

Social Interventions

The social and emotional support that people with chronic illness need can include practical things like support groups, offering ways to conserve energy, or encouraging maintenance of social relationships. Support groups such as telephone support, electronic on-line chat groups, and specially organized chronic illness groups can be helpful.

Helping clients and families through more complex issues around social and emotional aspects presents more of a challenge. Paterson (2001) offers guidance about the type of support clients may need for the duration of chronic illness. Chronic illness, because it encompasses periods of wellness and illness for clients, is ever-changing. At various points throughout the illness course, the illness may be in the forefront of a person's life; at other times, wellness may predominate. These shifting perspectives characterize how the person may appraise or react to their chronic illness. With illness in the foreground, a situation that occurs most often in newly diagnosed people, the focus is on the sickness, suffering, loss, and burden of the disease. These individuals are overwhelmed by the illness. When the focus is on wellness, clients respond to the illness situation as an opportunity. Paterson (2001) points out that people with wellness in the foreground come to this perspective by "learning as much as they can about the disease, creating supportive environments, developing personal skills such as negotiating, identifying the body's unique patterns of response, and sharing their knowledge of the disease with others" (pp. 23–24). The nurse who is aware of these shifts in chronic illness behavior is better equipped to support clients through appropriate interventions.

Economic Interventions

Nurses' responsibilities in financial interventions for quality of life vary with the circumstances of the position. The financial issues of chronic illness and quality of life are myriad. An awareness of the challenges that clients and families face is helpful to nurses. Knowledge about resources, services, and organizations for chronic illness conditions can help in making appropriate and timely referrals that will better maintain economic well-being of clients and families.

Cultural Interventions

Quality of life is influenced greatly by individuals' perceptions of what constitutes well-being. These perceptions are shaped by cultural interpretations of health and illness. Thus, it is important to have a full understanding of the meaning of the symptoms, patterns, and interactions in cultural groups when intervening to promote quality of life. For example, the meaning of pain may encompass more than physical pain in some cultural groups, and the salience of quality of life may not be as relevant in the presence of poverty or limited access to health care and treatments (Corless, Nicholas & Nokes, 2001). Nurses must also be aware of factors influencing choices that individuals from other cultures make for care in chronic illness. As an example, the Chinese concept that the body remain whole after death limits the supply of organs for transplantation. This view in turn affects the choices that persons with chronic renal failure are able to make. Organ scarcity creates a situation that may prevent more clients with chronic renal failure to experience improved quality of life, because with a transplant they are free from dialysis, have decreased medical expenses, and have improved social functioning (Luk, 2004).

Despite the existence of different and sometimes contradictory connotations about quality of life across cultures, it is the meaning that individuals ascribe to health or illness that is essential (Padilla & Kagawa-Singer, 1998). Therefore, knowledge of the personal meanings that are given to chronic illness within cultural groups is important to assessing, planning, and evaluating interventions aimed at promoting quality of life. Interventions from the spiritual domain may be applicable to cultural aspects, because such interventions address helping clients find meaning in suffering, transcending hopelessness, and developing inner strength.

Family Interventions

Chronic illness affects quality of life for the entire family. Therefore, family assessment and intervention is necessary. The level of the nurse's involvement with the family will determine the extent of the interventions. Most nurses can meet the basic need that families of clients with chronic illness have for factual information. This information may include education about the disease, treatments, and prognosis. Being available to answer questions and to give practical advice is important. Intervening at this fundamental level establishes trust with families that helps foster continued support. A safe and supportive environment can facilitate family sharing of feelings about the illness. Nurses can invite family members to participate in care activities as appropriate. Families with complex problems may need a referral to a specialist. Support groups can be suggested that would be appropriate for clients and their family caregivers. The nurse is one of the members of a collaborative health care team that is needed to maintain and promote optimum quality of life for clients with a chronic illness and their families.

The complex trajectory of chronic illness poses difficulties in making a strict separation of interventions for quality of life. It is reasonable to expect that nursing interventions with families can be as helpful as interventions that promote health and function. However, inclusion of the family may strengthen the adjustments that chronically ill clients must make during the course of illness. The situation of HIV clients is instructive about the interplay of interventions that can be used throughout the illness trajectory (Murdaugh, 1998). For example, knowing that support from loved ones and from other persons with HIV helps clients adjust to the illness suggests that nurses intervene in ways to promote family and other social supports. As family members increasingly are relied on to provide time-consuming health care, their health and well-being directly affects care outcomes for chronically ill members. Therefore assessments and interventions cannot be limited to the client, but should include promoting rest, respite, and support for caregivers as well (Schneider, 2004).

Women with breast cancer also reported a better quality of life when their family had abilities and skills to help and support them. Northouse et al. (1999) point out that including family members in care and helping them learn more about the illness should be part of nursing interventions. Moreover, assessing and promoting the health of the entire family has been shown to be important to quality of life for transplant clients and spouses alike (Collins et al., 2000).

Changing Roles: A. G.

A. G., a single, 40-year-old woman lives in the Southwest. Her parents retired some years earlier on the East Coast and decided that they wanted to be closer to her, so they moved within an hour's drive from her. She subsequently became the caregiver for her parents before she was prepared to take on this role.

Her father has a chronic cardiac condition that is poorly controlled. However, her mother's physical health, although frail, appears to be intact. Because her parents are less able to manage their own care, they let her take on the parental role. This was an uncomfortable role reversal for A. G. A couple of years after moving, her father's cardiac condition changed for the worse. A. G. consulted with her sister, who lived in another state, and they decided that her parents should move to a smaller home within walking distance of where she lived. A. G.'s sister served as an important part of her support network as she made decisions about their parents.

With the changes in living space and physicians, her father stabilized, but her mother became increasingly forgetful and was diagnosed as having Alzheimer's disease. The demands placed on A. G. affected her ability to maintain quality of life, both for herself and her parents.

Her mother's mental deterioration worsened, and her father became increasingly weak, again requiring realignment of family roles in an attempt to maintain quality of life for all concerned. A. G.'s support network increased in importance to her and helped her find resources that enabled her to cope with her parents' changing health status.

Outcomes

With the increase in chronic illness, it has become progressively more important not only to relieve symptoms and provide comfort, but also to intervene in ways that improve clients' quality of life. Moreover, evaluations of the extent to which interventions improve quality of life for clients are becoming ever more important. Decision-making about initiating, continuing, changing, or withdrawing treatments is made frequently based on quality of life outcomes. The efficacy of clinical interventions and practice behaviors, likewise, are evaluated on their contribution to clients' quality of life outcomes. In research, quality of life outcomes are used to test the effectiveness of interventions. Increasingly, the efficacy of interventions must consider cost effectiveness with quality of life considerations (Kliempt, Ruta & McMurdo, 2000).

Throughout this discussion, repeated emphasis has been given to the interrelatedness and overlap of the domains in quality of life. Health conditions, especially in the context of chronic illness, are a significant determinant of general quality of life. Indeed, in some instances, the characteristics of the social/environmental increase the threat of disease or disability. Alternatively, personal resources, community cohesion, educational opportunities, and access to social and health services, while primary components of general quality of life, encompass features of health-related quality of life (Albert, 1997).

Assessing the outcomes of nursing interventions using quality of life as a measure helps to explain the dynamics of well-being as experienced by clients. Knowledge of the individual circumstances that influence quality of life in chronic illness enables better care planning. This targeting of interventions to the specific quality of life for individuals can lead to successful preventive and therapeutic approaches in caring for people with chronic illness. At the same time, it is essential that nurses understand the meanings and values of their own lives, and how these values affect the care they give. With an ever-present awareness of the many components that influence quality of life in chronic illness, nurses can intervene more effectively.

Summary and Conclusions

Quality of life evaluations provide clinicians and researchers alike with information of the impact that chronic illness has on clients and their families. The complexity and burdens of chronic illness can more fully be understood within the context of subjective and objective evaluations of quality of life. Such evaluations account for the components that encompass quality of life that were discussed in this chapter: health and functioning, psychological/spiritual, social and economic, and family. These domains also provide a way to focus interventions that enable nurses to intervene effectively for clients and their families. Nurses as essential health care providers to clients with chronic illness can be instrumental in planning, carrying out, and evaluating care that promotes quality of life. Effectively intervening in care of clients and families with chronic illness is crucial to making quality of life a certain outcome.

Study Questions

1. Describe the relationship of quality of life to chronic illness. How is overall quality of life interrelated with health-related quality of life?
2. Identify a framework that is useful with quality of life issues in working with a client with chronic illness. Discuss how this framework would be useful in planning care for quality of life outcomes.
3. How does symptom control influence quality of life for the chronically ill client or the client's family?
4. What is the significance of using domains to describe quality of life in chronic illness? Discuss the interrelatedness of the several aspects within the quality of life domains.
5. Why is it essential to understand the care recipient's definition of *quality of life* and *meaning of illness*?
6. How does culture influence quality of life?
7. Describe outcomes that would indicate a good quality of life. How should decisions be made about quality of life issues?
8. What spiritual interventions can nurses use to promote client and family quality of life?

References

Abeles, R. P., Gift, H. C., & Ory, M. G. (Eds.). (1994). *Aging and quality of life*. New York: Springer.

Albert, S. M. (1997). Assessing health-related quality of life in chronic care populations. *Journal of Mental Health and Aging, 3* (1), 101–118.

Arruda, E. N., Larson, P. J., & Meleis, A. I. (1992). Comfort: Immigrant Hispanic cancer clients' views. *Cancer Nursing, 15* (6), 387–394.

Artinian, N. T., & Hayes, M. G. (1992). Factors related to spouses' quality of life 1 year after coronary artery bypass graft surgery. *Cardiovascular Nursing, 28* (5), 33–38.

Arzouman, J. M. R., Dudas, S., Ferrens, C. E., & Holm, K. (1991). Quality of life of clients with sarcoma postchemotherapy. *Oncology Nursing Forum, 18* (5), 889–894.

Baxter, J., Shetterly, S. M., Eby, C., Mason, L., et al. (1998). Social network factors associated with perceived quality of life: The San Luis Valley health and aging study. *Journal of Aging and Health, 10* (3), 287–310.

Benner, P., & Wrubel, J. (1989). *The primacy of caring.* Menlo Park, CA: Addison-Wesley.

Berggren-Thomas, P., & Griggs, M. J. (1995). Spirituality in aging: Spiritual need or spiritual journey? *Journal of Gerontological Nursing, 21* (3), 5–10.

Bertero, C., Eriksson, B., & Ek, A. (1997). A substantive theory of quality of life of adults with chronic leukaemia. *International Journal of Nursing Studies, 34* (1), 9–16.

Bullinger, M. (1997). The challenge of cross-cultural quality of life assessment. *Psychology and Health, 12,* 815–825.

Cassileth, B. R., Lusk, E. J., Guerry, D., Blake, A. D., et al. (1991). Survival and quality of life among clients receiving unproven as compared with conventional cancer therapy. *The New England Journal of Medicine, 324,* 1180–1185.

Cavendish, R., Luise, B. K., Russo, D., Mitzeliotis, C., et al. (2004). Spiritual perspectives of nurses in the United States relevant for education and practice. *Western Journal of Nursing Research, 26* (2), 196–212.

Cheater, F. (1998). Quality of life measures for the healthcare environment. *Nurse Researcher, 5* (3), 17–30.

Collins, E. G., White-Williams, C., & Jalowiec, A. (2000). Spouse quality of life before and 1 year after heart transplantation. *Critical Care Nursing Clinics of North America, 12* (1), 103–110.

Corless, I. B., Nicholas, P. K., & Nokes, K. M. (2001). Issues in cross-cultural quality-of-life research. *Journal of Nursing Scholarship, 33* (1), 15–20.

Dean, H. E. (1990). Political and ethical implications of using quality of life as an outcome measure. *Seminars in Oncology Nursing, 6* (4), 303–308.

Donely, R. (1991). Spiritual dimensions of health care: Nursing's mission. *Nursing and Health Care, 12* (4), 178–183.

Dorsey, C. J., & Murdaugh, C. L. (2003). The theory of self-care management for vulnerable populations. *The Journal of Theory Construction & Testing, 7* (2), 43–49.

Dubos, R. (1959). *Mirage of health: Utopias, progress, and biological change.* Garden City, NY: Doubleday.

Engebretson, T. O., Clark, M. M., Niaura, R. S., Phillips, T., et al. (1999). Quality of life and anxiety in a phase II cardiac rehabilitation program. *Medicine and Science in Sports and Exercise, 31* (2), 216–223.

Faden, R., & German, P. S. (1994). Quality of life: Considerations in geriatrics. *Clinics in Geriatric Medicine, 10* (3), 541–551.

Ferrans, C. E. (1990). Development of a quality of life index for clients with cancer. *Oncology Nursing Forum, 17* (3) (Suppl), 15–19.

_____. (1996). Development of a conceptual model of quality of life. *Scholarly Inquiry for Nursing Practice, 10* (3), 293–304.

Fisch, M. J., Titzer, M. L., Kristeller, J. L., Shen, J., et al. (2003). Assessment of quality of life in outpatients with advanced cancer: The accuracy of clinician estimations and the relevance of spiritual well-being – a Hoosier oncology group study. *Journal of Clinical Oncology, 21* (14), 2754–2759.

Fisher, M., & Mitchell, G. (1998). Patients' view of quality of life: Transforming the knowledge base of nursing. *Clinical Nurse Specialist, 12* (3), 98.

Forbes, D. (2001). Enhancing mastery and sense of coherence: Important determinants of health in older adults. *Geriatric Nursing, 22* (1), 29–32.

Foreman, M., & Kleinpell, R. (1990). Assessing the quality of life of elderly persons. *Seminars in Oncology Nursing, 6* (4), 292–297.

Haas, B. K. (1999). Clarification and integration of similar quality of life concepts. *Image: Journal of Nursing Scholarship, 31* (3), 215–220.

Hamilton, G. A., & Carroll, D. L. (2004). The effects of age on quality of life in implantable cardioverter defibrillator recipients. *Journal of Clinical Nursing, 13* (2), 194–200.

Heriot, C. S. (1992). Spirituality and aging. *Holistic Nurse Practice, 7* (1), 22–31.

Hicks, T. J. Jr. (1999). Spirituality and the elderly: Nursing implications with nursing home residents. *Geriatric Nursing, 20* (3), 144–146.

Hollenberg, N. K., Williams, G. H., & Anderson, R. (2000). Medical therapy, symptoms, and the distress they cause. *Archives of Internal Medicine, 160,* 1477–1483.

Hudson, A., Kirksey, K., & Holzemer, W. (2004). The influence of symptoms on quality of life among HIV-infected women. *Western Journal of Nursing Research, 26* (1), 9–23.

Isaia, D., Parker, V., & Murrow, E. (1999). Spiritual well-being among older adults. *Journal of Gerontological Nursing, 25* (8), 15–21.

Jassak, P. F., & Knafl, K. A. (1990). Quality of family life: Exploration of a concept. *Seminars in Oncology Nursing, 6,* 298–302.

Karlawish, J. H. T., Casarett, D. J., James, B. D., Tenhave, T., et al. (2003). Why would caregivers not want to treat their relative's Alzheimer's disease? *Journal of the American Geriatrics Society, 51* (10), 1391–1397.

Kinney, C. K., Rodgers, D. M., Nash, K. A., & Bray, C. O. (2003). Holistic healing for women with breast cancer through a mind, body, and spirit self-empowerment program. *Journal of Holistic Nursing, 21* (3), 260–279.

Kliempt, P., Ruta, D., & McMurdo, M. (2000). Measuring the outcomes of care in older people: A non-critical review of client based measures: I. General health status and quality of life instruments. *Reviews in Clinical Gerontology, 10,* 33–42.

Kosinski, M., Zhao, S. Z., Dedhiya, S., Osterhaus, J. T., et al. (2000). Determining minimally important changes in geriatric and disease-specific health-related quality of life questionnaires in clinical trials of rheumatoid arthritis. *Arthritis and Rheumatism, 43* (7), 1478–1487.

Kressin, N. R., Spiro, A., & Skinner, K. M. (2000). Negative affectivity and health-related quality of life. *Medical Care, 38* (8), 858–867.

Kreulen, G. J., & Braden, C. J. (2004). Model test of the relationship between self-help-promoting nursing interventions and self-care and health status outcomes. *Research in Nursing and Health, 27* (2), 97–109.

Landis, B. J. (1996). Uncertainty, spiritual well-being, and psychosocial adjustment to chronic illness. *Issues in Mental Health Nursing, 17* (3), 217–231.

Larson, D. B., & Koenig, H. G. (2000). Is God good for your health? The role of spirituality in medical care. *Cleveland Clinic Journal of Medicine, 67* (2), 80–84.

Lawton, M. P. (1997). Measures of quality of life and subjective well-being. *Generations, 21* (1), 45–47.

Lawton, M. P., Moss, M., Hoffman, C., Grant, R., et al. (1999). Health, valuation of life, and the wish to live. *The Gerontologist, 39* (4), 406–416.

Lee, O. J., & Pilkington, F. B. (1999). Practice with persons living their dying: A human becoming perspective. *Nursing Science Quarterly, 12* (4), 324–328.

Leininger, M. (1994). Quality of life from a transcultural nursing perspective. *Nursing Science Quarterly, 7* (1), 22–28.

Liao, Y., McGee, D. L., Coa, G., & Cooper, R. S. (2000). Quality of the last year of life of older adults: 1986 vs. 1993. *Journal of the American Medical Association, 283* (4), 512–518.

Lisse, J., Espinoza, L., Zhao, S. Z., Dedhiya, S. D., et al. (2001). Functional status and health-related quality of life of elderly osteoarthritic clients treated with celecoxib. *Journal of Gerontology: Medical Sciences, 56A* (3), M167–M175.

Luk, W. S. (2004). The HRQofL of renal transplant patients. *Journal of Clinical Nursing, 13* (2), 101–118.

McMillan, S. C., & Mahon, M. (1994). The impact of hospice services on the quality of life of primary caregivers. *Oncology Nursing Forum, 21* (7), 1189–1195.

Millison, M., & Dudley, J. R. (1992). Providing spiritual support: A job for all hospice professionals. *The Hospice Journal, 8* (4), 49–66.

Mowad, L. (2004). Correlates of quality of life in older adult veterans. *Western Journal of Nursing Research, 26* (3), 293–306.

Muldoon, M. H., & King, N. (1991). A spirituality for the long haul: Response to chronic illness. *Journal of Religion and Health, 30* (2), 99–108.

Murdaugh, C. (1998). Health-related quality of life in HIV disease: Achieving a balance. *Journal of the Association of Nurses in AIDS Care, 9* (6), 59–71.

National Center for Chronic Disease Prevention and Health Promotion. (n.d.). Chronic Disease Overview. Retrieved August 5, 2004, from http://www.cdc.gov/nccdphp/overview.htm

Nesbitt, B. J., & Heidrich, S. M. (2000). Sense of coherence and illness appraisal in older women's quality of life. *Research in Nursing and Health, 23,* 25–34.

Northouse, L. L., Caffey, M., Deichelbohrer, L., Schmidt, L., et al. (1999). The quality of life of African American women with breast cancer. *Research in Nursing and Health, 22,* 449–460.

O'Brien, M. E. (2003). *Spirituality in nursing: Standing on holy ground* (2nd ed.). Sudbury, MA: Jones & Bartlett.

Oleson, M. (1990). Subjectively perceived quality of life. *Image: Journal of Nursing Scholarship, 22* (3), 187–190.

O'Neill, D. P., & Kenny, E. K. (1998). Spirituality and chronic illness. *Image: Journal of Nursing Scholarship, 30* (3), 275–280.

Orem, D. (1990). *Nursing: Concepts of practice.* St. Louis: Mosby.

Padilla, G. V., & Kagawa-Singer, M. (1998). Quality of life and culture. In C. R. King & P. S. Hinds (Eds.), *Quality of life: From nursing and client perspectives,* (pp. 74–92). Sudbury, MA: Jones & Bartlett.

Parse, R. R. (1994). Quality of life: Sciencing and living the art of human becoming. *Nursing Science Quarterly, 7* (1), 16–21.

_____. (1996). Quality of life for persons living with Alzheimer's disease: The human becoming perspective. *Nursing Science Quarterly, 9* (3), 126–133.

Paterson, B. L. (2001). The shifting perspectives model of chronic illness. *Journal of Nursing Scholarship, 33* (1), 21–26.

Patrick, D. L., & Erickson, P. (1993). *Health status and health policy: Quality of life in health care evaluation and resource allocation.* New York: Oxford University Press.

Peplau, H. E. (1994). Quality of life: An interpersonal perspective. *Nursing Science Quarterly, 7* (1), 10–15.

Plank, D. M. P. (1994). Framing treatment options: A method to enhance informed consent. *Clinical Nurse Specialist, 8* (4), 174–178.

Rieker, P. P., Clark, E. J., & Fogelberg, P. R. (1992). Perceptions of quality of life and quality of care for clients with cancer receiving biological therapy. *Oncology Nursing Forum, 19* (3), 433–440.

Ryan, P. Y. (1992). Perceptions of the most helpful nursing behaviors in a home-care hospice setting: Caregivers and nurses. *American Journal of Hospice and Palliative Care, 9* (5), 22–31.

Schneider, R. A. (2004). Chronic renal failure: Assessing the fatigue severity scale for use among caregivers. *Journal of Clinical Nursing, 13* (2), 101–118.

Sheehan, D. K., & Schirm, V. (2003). Palliative nursing. End-of-life care of older adults: debunking some common misconceptions about dying in old age. *American Journal of Nursing, 103* (11), 48–59.

Sin, M., Sanderson, B., Weaver, M., Giger, J., et al. (2003). Personal characteristics, health status, physical activity, and quality of life in cardiac rehabilitation participants. *International Journal of Nursing Studies, 41* (2), 173–181.

Snoek, F. J. (2000). Quality of life: A closer look at measuring clients' well-being. *Diabetes Spectrum, 13* (1), 24–28.

Stuifbergen, A. K., Seraphine, A., & Roberts, G. (2000). An explanatory model of health promotion and quality of life in chronic disabling conditions. *Nursing Research, 49* (3), 122–129.

Sullivan, T., Weinert, C., & Cudney, S. (2003). Management of chronic illness: Voices of rural women. *Journal of Advanced Nursing, 44* (6), 566–574.

Tang, W., Aaronson, L. S., & Forbes, S. A. (2004). Quality of life in hospice patients with terminal illness. *Western Journal of Nursing Research, 26* (1), 113–128.

Thorne, S., Con, A., McGuinness, L., McPherson, G., et al. (2004). Health care communication issues in multiple sclerosis: An interpretive description. *Qualitative Health Research, 14* (1), 5–22.

Van Dongen, C. J. (1996). Quality of life and self-esteem in working and nonworking persons with mental illness. *Community Mental Health Journal, 32* (6), 535–548.

Waldron, D., O'Boyle, C. A., Kearney, M., Moriarty, M., et al. (1999). Quality-of-life measurement in advanced cancer: Assessing the individual. *Journal of Clinical Oncology, 17* (11), 3603–3611.

Watson, J. (1985). *Nursing: Human science and human care. A theory of nursing.* Norwalk, CT: Appleton-Century-Crofts.

Welk, T. A., & Smith, W. B. (1999). Family surveys: Measuring more than just satisfaction. *American Journal of Hospice and Palliative Care, 16* (3), 533–540.

Wicks, M. N., Milstead, E. J., Hathaway, D. K., & Cetingok, M. (1998). Family caregivers' burden, quality of life, and health following clients' renal transplantation. *Journal of Transplant Coordination, 8* (3), 170–176.

Wilson, H. S., Hutchinson, S. A., & Holzemer, W. L. (1997). Salvaging quality of life in ethnically diverse clients with advanced HIV/AIDS. *Qualitative Health Research, 7* (1), 75–97.

Wilson, S. A., & Daley, B. J. (1999). Family perspectives on dying in long-term care settings. *Journal of Gerontological Nursing, 25* (11), 19–25.

Workers and chronic conditions: Opportunities to improve productivity. (2000, August, Number 10). Washington, DC: National Academy on an Aging Society.

Wortman, C. B. (1984). Social support and the cancer client: Conceptual and methodological issues. *Cancer* (Suppl), *53,* 2339–2362.

Wyatt, G., Kurtz, M. E., & Liken, M. (1993). Breast cancer survivors: An exploration of quality of life issues. *Cancer Nursing, 16* (6), 440–448.

CHAPTER 10

Compliance

Jill Berg ▪ Lorraine S. Evangelista ▪
Donna Carruthers ▪ Jacqueline M. Dunbar-Jacob

Introduction

Compliance of patients to prescribed treatment by their health care providers has been examined for over 50 years. The lack of agreement between health care recommendations and client behavior has been defined as an issue of adherence or compliance (Haynes, 1979; Rand, 1993; World Health Organization, 2003). Early research identified this problem of discrepancy between an ordered treatment and the actual implementation of the treatment by the client (Sackett & Snow, 1979). In 2001, the World Health Organization (WHO) convened a meeting on treatment adherence and compliance. The magnitude of the problem identified poor adherence to treatment of chronic diseases at a rate of 50% in developed counties with lower rates of adherence in developing countries (World Health Organization, 2003). Compliance with medical recommendations is poor across all chronic disease regimens, which increases health care expenditures and prevents clients from achieving the full benefit of any intervention. In addition, most chronic disorders are treated with a plan of care that encompasses medication, diet, and exercise. Therefore, clients are often asked to self-manage a complex treatment regimen.

Compliance and Chronic Illness

The predominant pattern of illness has changed from acute illness to chronic illness as science and technology have advanced. Treatment regimens have become more complex. However, due to changes in managed health care, these complex regimens are implemented with limited or no supervision as the client and/or family caregivers carry out these prescribed regimens at home. Therefore, practitioners must be concerned with the extent to which clients can comply with the treatment plans they design, as well as the evaluation of the client's responses.

Client responsibility for managing chronic conditions has grown with concern for client compliance as it relates to medical outcomes and economic costs. For example, an individual who has insulin-dependent diabetes mellitus (IDDM) may have a computerized insulin pump and a blood-testing device. This individual may, at some point, be a candidate for hemodialysis or renal transplant. All of these treatment modalities require compliant behaviors to ensure maximal benefit and minimal harm to the client. According to DiMatteo (2004) the average rate of non-adherence to treatment across all diseases is 24.8%. If this rate was extrapolated to physician visits by individuals with diabetes, as many as 7.6 million visits would result in non-adherence.

The managed care environment has also had an impact on client burden in chronic illness. Managed care's influence on health care has been demonstrated by earlier hospital discharges, shortened office visits, and decreasing home health referrals. In addition, recent literature indicates that as many as 46% of health care professionals do not prescribe adequate therapy for their clients (McGlynn et al., 2003). Therefore, clients and family members have had to shoulder more of the responsibility for the treatment regimen, often in isolation. Although disease management programs are described by Health Maintenance Organizations (HMOs), few programs have been implemented and critically evaluated to date. Health care professionals working within a managed care system often have little time to address the management of chronic illness and compliance with the recommended regimen (Miller et al., 1997). More recent findings suggest that health care professionals and agencies can make a difference in medical outcomes by means of integrating multidisciplinary interventions specifically aimed at assisting the client to manage their chronic disease through education, self-management instruction, prevention, and outreach strategies (Feachem, Sekhri, & White, 2002).

Literally hundreds of studies have been conducted on compliance, but the research that has been done has not effected significant changes in compliance behavior (McDonald, Garg & Haynes, 2002; Dunbar-Jacob & Schlenk, 2001). Conrad (1985) asserted that it was reasonable to assume that a client with chronic illness attempts to self-regulate in order to gain some control over something that is not always controllable. Rosenstock (1988) noted that health care professionals should "encourage people to make informed decisions, but decisions of their own choice . . ." (p. 72). He also added that health professionals are not always right, and there is always the potential for untoward side effects from ordered treatment.

It is obvious that chronic illness regimens can be exceedingly complex, and resources to assist individuals with chronic illness are often limited. Therefore, it is important that the health care pro-

fessional who is working with a client with chronic illness understand the variables that affect the ability of the person to adhere to a regimen. To facilitate understanding, this chapter addresses factors that have an impact on compliance behavior. A discussion of the theories and a description of techniques are also presented to provide a context for the behavioral changes that are required in treatment regimens. Finally, interventions to improve compliance are presented.

Definition of Terms

Compliance is an umbrella term for all behavior consistent with health care recommendations (Holroyd & Creer, 1986). *Noncompliance* denotes behaviors that are not consistent with such recommendations. Physicians often make decisions about the effectiveness of treatments without regard to whether the client is actually following the treatment or in agreement with their health care provider (Cramer et al., 1989).

Adherence and *nonadherence* are generally used as synonyms for compliance and noncompliance. However, there is a growing trend to use the term adherence and nonadherence over the term compliance on the global stage of health care delivery. An example of a notable exception in the meaning of these words is presented by Barofsky (1978), who proposed a continuum of self-care with three levels of client response to health care recommendations: compliance, adherence, and therapeutic alliance. In his model, compliance is linked to coercion; adherence, to conformity; and self-care, to a therapeutic alliance with provider–client interactions. Misselbrook (1998) used the term *concordance* to indicate the partnership between practitioner and client in achieving health outcomes.

There are different schools of thought in the compliance literature. One school supports the notion that it is impossible to ever have clients completely comply with medical regimens. A contradictory school of thought suggests that it is possible through education or some other means to have clients comply with their regimen requirements. These contrary schools of thought may be dependent on how the health plan was formulated (Dunbar, 1980). If the plan is formulated by a partnership between client and health care professional, the possibility of the client "adhering" to the plan increases. Should the client be expected to follow a plan created exclusively by an expert provider, without input by the client, then the client may or may not "comply." The World Health Organization has adopted "adherence" as the term of choice for this topic and suggests that it is necessary to incorporate the agreement of the client with the prescribed treatment plan presented by the health care provider. (World Health Organization, 2003).

Creer and Levstek (1996) as well as Dunbar-Jacob (1993) question the extent to which we "blame the patient" for compliance behavior. Part of the responsibility, they assert, belongs to health care providers, and there are instances when client noncompliance is wise, given the regimen. Trostle (1997) argues that there is too much emphasis placed on the authority physicians have in recommending health care regimens. He further asserts that noncompliance is viewed as "nonconformity with medical advice" (p. 116) and suggests that we look broadly at the behaviors that are being engaged in by clients within the context of their illness. He also cautions that attempts to motivate clients to comply could be considered coercive and manipulative.

Components of Compliance

The relevance of compliance to the total wellness-illness continuum was first described by Marston in 1970. Marston considered compliance to be self-care behaviors that individuals undertake to promote health, to prevent illness, or to follow recommendations for treatment and rehabilitation in diagnosed illnesses.

It may be helpful to consider compliance as more than self-care behaviors; rather, it is behavior that is often shared, because clients cannot always implement their medical regimens without the participation of others, even though the delineation of responsibilities is not always clear. For example, Wade and colleagues (1999) noted that there are misunderstandings about the assumption of respon-

sibility for the asthma illness regimen in inner-city children with asthma, and that this misunderstanding often leads to noncompliance. This is especially true when there is a change in the dependence/independence status of the client, as with the teenager who assumes greater responsibility for management of his or her health care regimen or the older client who now requires more supervision and assistance by family members.

Strauss and associates (1984) noted that family members often take on assisting or controlling roles in influencing clients to adhere to medical regimens. Further study of how couples managed chronic disease revealed that coordination and collaboration between the couple were necessary to carry out the work of the medical regimen (Corbin & Strauss, 1984). Given that this shared responsibility exists, it seems reasonable to conclude that compliance-increasing strategies should be directed toward all those involved in the regimen, and that there may be a need for discussing the division of responsibility among family members.

Models and Theories of Compliance

Theoretical frameworks and conceptual models provide direction for health care professionals by guiding the focus and dimensions of assessment and providing structure to the interaction of client and provider. At this point in time, research needs to emphasize more theoretical frameworks as underpinnings for adherence studies. DiMatteo (2004) also suggests that adherence models should be developed and based on large sample studies that examine the interaction of variables.

Until recently, there has been a lack of organized effort for a unifying theoretical framework in studies that address the phenomenon of compliance (Brawley & Culos-Reed, 2000; Becker & Maiman, 1975; Dracup & Meleis, 1982; Connelly, 1984). Although, it is difficult to name specific theories that guide compliance research, client satisfaction with care is an underlying concept. Client satisfaction involves the relationship that exists with the provider as well as information given to the client and office staff and practice protocols (Ley, 1988; Goldstein et al., 1998; Dimatteo et al., 1993). Among the most commonly used frameworks in compliance research, many focus on client beliefs. Other models have focused upon self-management or self-regulation oriented models.

Health Belief Model

Motivation is clearly related to beliefs and attitudes held by an individual. The health belief model (HBM), developed by Hochman et al. (as cited in Rosenstock, 1974) was devised to explain health-related behaviors, especially preventive health behaviors, and contains a cluster of pertinent beliefs and attitudes (Becker & Maiman, 1975). It was modified to include a general health motivation (Becker, 1976) (Figure 10-1) and was again modified for sick-role behaviors (see Chapter 2, on illness behaviors and roles). Figure 10-2 shows modifying and enabling factors that reflect the individual's readiness to undertake sick-role behaviors that influence the likelihood of compliance in chronic illness.

FIGURE 10-1

The Health Belief Model as Predictor of Preventive Health Behavior

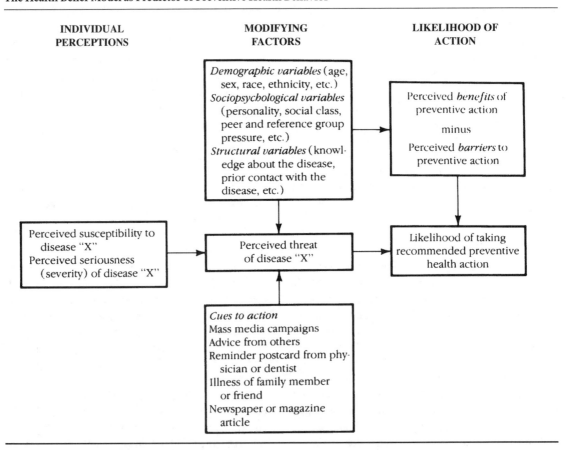

SOURCE: From Becker, M. H. (1974). A new approach to explaining sick-role behavior in low-income populations. *American Journal of Public Health, 64,* 205–216. Reprinted by permission of Sage Publications, Inc. Thousand Oaks, CA.

FIGURE 10-2

Summary of Health Belief Model for Predicting and Explaining Sick-Role Behaviors

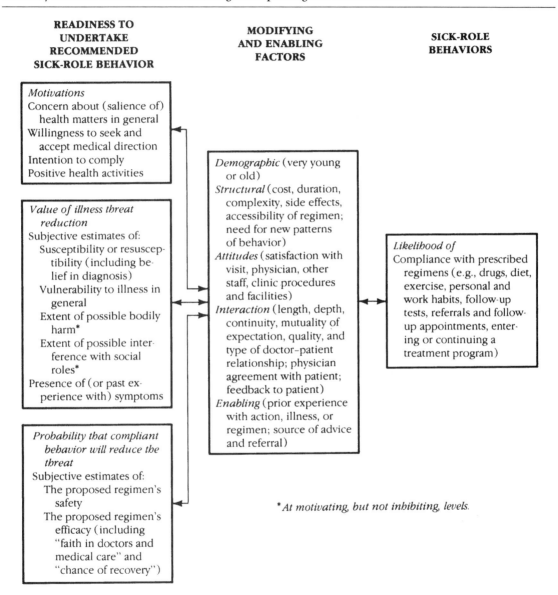

READINESS TO
UNDERTAKE
RECOMMENDED
SICK-ROLE BEHAVIOR

MODIFYING
AND ENABLING
FACTORS

SICK-ROLE
BEHAVIORS

Motivations
Concern about (salience of)
   health matters in general
Willingness to seek and
   accept medical direction
Intention to comply
Positive health activities

*Value of illness threat
   reduction*
Subjective estimates of:
   Susceptibility or resuscep-
      tibility (including be-
      lief in diagnosis)
   Vulnerability to illness in
      general
   Extent of possible bodily
      harm*
   Extent of possible inter-
      ference with social
      roles*
Presence of (or past ex-
   perience with) symptoms

*Probability that compliant
   behavior will reduce the
   threat*
Subjective estimates of:
   The proposed regimen's
      safety
   The proposed regimen's
      efficacy (including
      "faith in doctors and
      medical care" and
      "chance of recovery")

Demographic (very young
   or old)
Structural (cost, duration,
   complexity, side effects,
   accessibility of regimen;
   need for new patterns
   of behavior)
Attitudes (satisfaction with
   visit, physician, other
   staff, clinic procedures
   and facilities)
Interaction (length, depth,
   continuity, mutuality of
   expectation, quality, and
   type of doctor–patient
   relationship; physician
   agreement with patient;
   feedback to patient)
Enabling (prior experience
   with action, illness, or
   regimen; source of advice
   and referral)

Likelihood of
Compliance with prescribed
   regimens (e.g., drugs, diet,
   exercise, personal and
   work habits, follow-up
   tests, referrals and follow-
   up appointments, entering or continuing a
   treatment program)

*At motivating, but not inhibiting, levels.

SOURCE: From Becker, M. H. (1974b). The health belief model and sick-role behavior. *Health Education Monograph, 2,* 409–419. Reprinted by permission of Sage Publications, Inc.

The HBM's major proposition is that the likelihood of an individual taking recommended health actions is based on (1) the illness's perceived severity, (2) the individual's estimate of the likelihood that a specific action will reduce the threat, and (3) perceived barriers to following recommendations. The HBM is used frequently to explain the relationships of attitudes and behaviors to compliance. Research using this model has shown more predictive power in the explanation of compliance for preventive health behaviors rather than ordered regimens (Horne & Weinman, 1998). Although health beliefs and compliance are modestly correlated when measured concurrently, it is generally accepted that health beliefs do not predict compliance (Dunbar, 1990).

Health Promotion Model

A nursing model that evolved from the HBM is the health promotion model (HPM) (Pender, 1996). Pender conceptualizes health as a goal and believes that only the desire to be healthy leads to engagement of health promotion activities. Pender organized the concepts under the framework of individual characteristics and experiences, behavior-specific cognitions and affect, and behavioral outcomes (Figure 10-3). The Health Promoting Lifestyle Profile is an instrument for an assessment of health promotion behaviors.

Common Sense Model

Another model that discusses individual's beliefs about illness is the common sense model (CSM). Studies using this model are conducted primarily on individuals with asymptomatic illnesses, and there are no data available to determine whether this theory has any value in other populations. The CSM postulates that how an individual processes illness-related events shapes how that individual copes and complies with treatment (Leventhal, Meyer & Nerenz, 1980). Studies using the CSM demonstrated that subjects consistently look for symptoms, which match their view of the illness (Baumann et al., 1989; Meyer, Leventhal & Gutmann, 1985).

Self-Regulation Theory

Proposed by Leventhal and associates (1987), this theory departs from other theories because it incorporates a feedback loop. In this model, the client is an active participant in the process of managing health behaviors. Illness beliefs center around five components: identity, time-line, cause, consequences, and cure or control (Horne, 1998). This theory has been applied to a variety of chronic illnesses in studies that seek to explain illness management (Williams et al., 1995b; Christensen et al., 1996; Clark & Starr, 1994). There has been some criticism that the model is too complex to use (Horne & Weinman, 1998); however, the model is appealing because it takes into account client illness beliefs.

The Theory of Reasoned Action and the Theory of Planned Behavior

The theory of reasoned action (Fishbein & Ajzen, 1975) and the theory of planned behavior (Ajzen, 1985) have *intention* as a main component. Individuals engage in health behaviors intentionally based on attitudes toward a behavior and social influence. The theory of planned behavior adds a component to the model, called "perceived behavioral control," which captures the extent to which a person has control over any given behavior. Both of these theories have been useful in the examination of preventive behaviors, such as engaging in exercise programs (Norman & Smith, 1995), condom use (Chan & Fishbein, 1993), and smoking cessation (Norman, Conner, & Bell, 1999), where intention has been found to be an important component of engaging in the desired behavior. In chronic illness regimens, however, there has been limited use of these theories.

Cognitive Social Learning Theory

Cognitive social learning theory attempts to predict behavior that is dictated by outcome and efficacy expectancies. This theory helps bring together environment, cognition, and emotion in the

FIGURE 10-3

Health Promotion Model

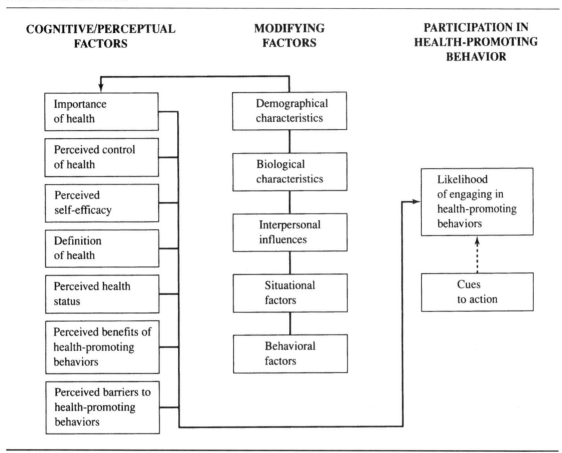

COGNITIVE/PERCEPTUAL FACTORS — MODIFYING FACTORS — PARTICIPATION IN HEALTH-PROMOTING BEHAVIOR

SOURCE: From Pender, N. J. (1987). *Health promotion in nursing practice* (2nd ed.), p. 58. © Reprinted by permission of Pearson Education, Inc., Upper Saddle River, NJ.

understanding of health behavior change (Perry, Baranowski, & Parcel, 1990). Three necessary pre-requisites to altering health behavior are a recognition that a life-style component can be harmful, the recognition that a change in behavior would be beneficial, and the recognition that one has the abil-ity to adopt a new behavior (self-efficacy) (Schwarzer, 1992). To effect any change then, each individual must be able to self-monitor and self-regulate health behavior. This aspect of self-regulation has

led to a variety of self-management strategies with which to cope with illness. The additional compo-nent of self-efficacy, defined as the client's expecta-tions or confidence in his or her *ability* to perform a recommended action, has also promoted research to test efficacy-enhancing strategies important in health behavior change. Self-efficacy has been found to be an important predictor of self-management behaviors useful for the treatment of AIDS (Chesney et al., 2000), cancer (Eiser, Hill & Blacklay, 2000), cardiac disease (Jenkins & Gortner, 1998), depression (Harrington et al., 2000), and diabetes (Ott et al., 2000).

Transtheoretical Model of Change (Stages of Change)

The stage of change, or transtheoretical model, was developed by Prochaska and DiClemente (1983). It is an eclectic model that encompasses various other theories and aims to examine and predict the process of change. This model contains three constructs: the stages of change; processes of change; and levels of change. The model's underlying premise proposes people are at different stages in their intentional desire to adopt certain health behaviors with or without assistance. The transtheoretical model of change also proposes that interventions should be matched to each categorical stage of change. Although presented hierarchically, the process of change is considered to be spiral with relapse from a healthy behavior placing an individual in a position to move backward toward contemplation of the healthy behavior. The model also incorporates self-efficacy and decision-making as key factors in the process of change, but these factors have an impact at different stages of change. The stages include the following:

1. Pre-contemplation: no intention of changing behavior
2. Contemplation: considering future action
3. Pre-action: have a timetable for action
4. Action: involved in behavior change
5. Maintenance: after change is adopted; relapse is a possibility

The stage model of health behavior was initially applied to the treatment of addictive behaviors and, although widely discussed, has had limited visibility for adherence behaviors in other chronic illnesses. This model has been widely pushed for clinical adoption for several health behaviors without a base of supportive research evidence. Within the last decade, it has been applied to asthma (Schmaling, Afari & Blume, 2000), chronic pain (Jensen et al., 2000), multiple sclerosis (Holland et al., 2001), depression (Tutty, Simon, & Ludman, 2000), and kidney failure (Welch, 2001). Exercise adherence studies suggest that this model has implications for initiation of a new behavior, but long term adoption/compliance is not maintained (Adams & White, 2003; Buckworth & Wallace, 2002). Therefore, more research with this model is needed before actively placing this strategy in a clinical setting as an intervention of choice.

Self-Management

Self-management refers to the "performance of preventative or therapeutic health care activities, often in collaboration with health care professionals" (Holroyd & Creer, 1986, Preface) and involves learning new skills and behaviors. The initiation of new behaviors, however, relies on certain assumptions: The individual must be motivated to change, only the individual can modify his or her own behavior, and difficult behaviors often cannot be monitored by anyone except the individual. These assumptions translate into three steps. First is *self-monitoring*, which involves deliberate attention to one's own behavior. Second is *self-evaluation*, in which the required behavior and the actual behavior are compared and evaluated. Third, *self-reinforcement* motivates the individual to correct any discrepancies in behavior to produce change. If the individual detects a discrepancy in the self-evaluation phase, there is sufficient motivation to produce change, but this is dependent on reinforcement from the individual's emotional and cognitive reactions during self-evaluation.

Self-management has been recognized as a fundamental basis for the tasks associated with chronic disease. Lorig et al. (1999) described the effectiveness of a self-management program that targeted individuals with a variety of chronic illnesses: cardiac, pulmonary, neurological, or musculoskeletal. For the 952 participants of the program, a seven-week self-management course reduced both disability and hospital days and demonstrated improvement in symptom control and other disease limitations. Clearly, attention to self-management capability for those with chronic disease needs to be integrated more widely.

Dimensions of Adherence/Compliance

A recently published model of adherence suggests there are five dimensions of adherence/compliance to include socio-economic, health system, therapy-related, condition-related, and patient-related dimensions (World Health Organization, 2003). The recent examination of treatment adherence by the World Health Organization led to the proposal of this model in their report and suggestion of its use in examining treatment adherence/compliance and developing strategies for enhancement. These dimensions also encompass areas that have been identified as barriers to compliance (Dunbar-Jacob, Schlenk, & Caruthers, 2002). Testing of this model is needed in future studies.

Prevalence of Noncompliance

Individuals suffering from chronic medical conditions face a variety of stressful life circumstances involving a range of adaptation demands. Individuals who are chronically ill must deal with a loss of independence, the threat of disease progression, and the challenge of modifying their behavior to meet the demands of a prescribed regimen. Lifestyle modifications may become necessary and include, but not be limited to, dietary changes, use of medications, and change in physical activity. Compliance with these modifications has substantial implications for treatment success and decreased disease progression.

For the client who is chronically ill, failure to comply can result in increased disease complications, increased hospitalizations, greater treatment costs, as well as disruptions in life-style, family dynamics, and coping skills. Although ascertaining the true picture of noncompliance in chronic illness is difficult, the consistency with which poor compliance rates are reported indicates that noncompliance is a major problem in health care. Recent studies indicate that compliance rates in chronic illness are approximately 50 percent (Dunbar-Jacob et al., 2000; (Haynes, McDonald, Garg, & Montague, 2002; World Health Organization, 2003). In the United States, medication compliance to antihyper-

tensive medications is 51% (Graves, 2000). This problem is not limited to the U.S. In developing countries, adherence to antihypertensive medications suggest compliance rates are less than 50% (van der Sande et al., 2000).

Different definitions of *compliance* have contributed to difficulties in comparing studies of particular disease groups, and make it impossible to generalize from studies with other diseases (Rapley, 1997). Compliance studies are typically disease-specific; that is, the study population is defined by the presence of a specific disease and shows high rates of noncompliance. However, more recent reviews of compliance behaviors in persons with chronic illness indicate that the nature and extent of compliance problems are similar across diseases, across regimens, and across age groups (Vermeire, Hearnshaw, Van Royen, & Denekens, 2001). A review of recent studies that examine medication compliance reported rates as low as 50 percent, with some differences in rates seen between settings and measurement methods (Dunbar-Jacob et al., 2000).

Medication compliance is one category of research that spans disease groups Unfortunately there is no gold standard to measure medication compliance, and current evidence suggests the use of several strategies besides disease outcomes to capture treatment compliance to medication (Krapek et al., 2004; Wagner & Rabkin, 2000; Wendel et al., 2001). Furthermore, polypharmacy in chronic disorders adds an additional dilemma in observing medication compliance (Vik, Maxwell, & Hogan, 2004). Electronic monitors have been used to assess medication compliance in many recent studies. Studies of treatment adherence in HIV populations have used both self-report, diaries, and electronic event monitors (MEMS caps). Not specific to HIV populations, electronic monitoring typically provides lower estimates of compliance than self-report data (Wagner & Rabkin, 2000). In a study of individuals with ankylosing spondylitis, only 22 percent strictly complied with prescribed medication (de Klerk & van der Linden, 1996). Although noncompliance rates were not as low among clients with epilepsy (34%) (Cramer et al., 1995), major depression (37% to 55%) (Demyttenaere et al., 1998; Carney et al.,

1995), schizophrenia (55%) (Duncan & Rogers, 1998), diabetes mellitus (47%) (Mason, Matsayuma & Jue, 1995), hypertension (30% to 47%) (Mounier-Vehier et al., 1998; Lee et al., 1996), and ischemic heart disease (38% to 45%) (Carney et al., 1998; Straka et al., 1997), these noncompliant behaviors were nonetheless significantly associated with poor control of symptoms.

Other methods for measuring medication compliance (drug dosing recall, pill counts, self-report surveys, and pharmacy refills) have been used and have yielded similar rates of compliance (DiMatteo, 2004; Dunbar-Jacob et al., 2002). In a study using subjects with chronic pain, paper and electronic diaries were compared. The electronic diaries offered a time-stamped variation on the paper diary and out performed the latter with regard to compliance of use by the subject (Stone, Shiffman, Schwartz, Broderick, & Hufford, 2003). Forty-eight percent of clients with tuberculosis were reported as having defaulted on their recommended medication prescriptions (Pablos-Mendez et al., 1997). Treatment compliance following renal transplant is associated with loss of the graft. In addition, a history of poor compliance prior to transplant has also been associated with graft loss (Butler, Roderick, Mullee, Mason, & Peveler, 2004). Self-reported medication noncompliance among renal transplant patients ranged between 13 and 36 percent (Hilbrands, Hoitsma & Koene, 1995; Greenstein & Siegal, 1998), while heart transplant patients showed noncompliance rates of up to 37 percent (Grady et al., 1996). Although persons with life-threatening disorders may comply somewhat better than others, researchers suggest that even moderate alterations in their treatment have significant clinical impact (Schweizer et al., 1990; De Geest, Abraham & Dunbar-Jacob, 1996).

Dunbar-Jacob and colleagues (2000) have also reported a summary of other behaviors that should be considered when assessing compliance:

■ Noncompliance with low-fat, low-cholesterol diets (15% to 88%)
■ Noncompliance with weight-reducing diets (greater than 50%)

■ Noncompliance with therapeutic exercise (50% dropping out of exercise during the first 3 to 6 months; leveling to a drop-out rate between 55% and 75% at 12 months)
■ Noncompliance with appointment keeping (8.5% to 63.4%)

Problems and Issues

Studies have demonstrated that large numbers of individuals do not follow health care recommendations completely. Although noncompliance is increasingly recognized as a problem, there is less consensus about appropriate or effective methods to increase compliance. Some of the difficulty lies in the inadequacies of research on compliance, some lies in differing role expectations of clients and providers, some relates to motivation, and some relates to conflict in values. As health care professionals prescribe, teach, and counsel clients about medical regimens, they must be cautious in making assumptions about compliance or noncompliance in a given situation before imposing any specific strategy on the client.

Barriers to the Study of Compliance

A comprehensive review of the compliance research is not appropriate to this chapter; however, discussions of some of the barriers that plague researchers and limit the confidence with which practitioners can apply findings are briefly presented. Methodological and conceptual problems in the study of compliance, and the lack of consistent results, lead one to the conclusion that there is no definitive basis for selecting and using one compliance-increasing strategy over another.

Methodological Barriers

Numerous methodological problems continue to plague compliance research (Miller et al., 1997). As early as 1979, Sackett and Snow highlighted the inadequacies of research design in their review of 537 original articles on compliance, which revealed only 40 studies meeting the methodological standards established for the review. This design concern has been highlighted in recent meta-analysis reviews and reports (Haynes et al., 2002; Vermeire, Hearnshaw, Van Royen, & Denekens, 2001; World Health Organization, 2003). They noted deficiencies in study design, specification of the illness or condition, compliance measurement, description of the therapeutic regimen, and definition of compliance:

1. Studies should use inception cohorts rather than cross-sectional samples. These samples would follow all clients who were started on a therapeutic regimen, and the study would encompass the least compliant individuals who "drop out."
2. Complete compliance distributions of all study patients would be published to reveal determinants of variance in distributions.
3. Description of the relationship between compliance levels and the achievement of treatment goals should be included.
4. The study design should be precisely described.

In a meta-analysis of interventions to improve adherence, Roter et al. (1998) stated that compliance intervention studies to date have been "too narrow and too limited" (p. 1153). They recommend that interventions be targeted both to improve compliance and to improve client outcomes. Additionally, it was difficult to advocate any particular compliance enhancing strategy because multiple interventions in the same study usually produced equivalent results (Roter et al., 1998; (Weingarten et al., 2002). However, the WHO proposed the need for more efforts with self-management approaches and integrated health care approaches that specifically address chronic disease care (World Health Organization, 2003).

Conceptual Barriers

Inadequate conceptualization of compliance has led to a lack of consistent findings. There is still debate about the appropriate terminology to use, whether it is *compliance, adherence,* or *concordance.* There is also discussion about who needs to be targeted to increase compliance with a recommended regimen (Dunbar-Jacob, 1993). The need for a multilevel approach for compliance improvement, which targets the client, the provider, and the health care system, has also been suggested (Miller et al., 1997). In an attempt to address this aspect of compliance, the WHO has initiated a database of best practice through research evidence. From the US, multilevel approaches encompass community-based outreach programming, integrated care for chronic disorders, self-management in chronic disease, and improving delivery of care in the primary health care setting (Bamberger et al., 2000; Feachem et al.; 2002; Gohdes, Rith-Najarian, Acton, & Shields, 1996; Lorig, Sobel, Ritter, Laurent, & Hobbs, 2001).

Variables of Noncompliance

Client Characteristics

Several client characteristics affecting compliance have been examined. These include demographic factors, psychological factors, social support, past health behavior, somatic factors, and health beliefs (Dunbar-Jacob et al., 2002). Ethnicity was addressed in a review by Schlenk and Dunbar-Jacob (1996) and Joshi (1998), indicating that more research is needed in this area. More recent literature has examined ethnicity as an influence upon compliance with diagnostic testing (Strzelczyk & Dignan 2002). Strzelczyk & Dignan (2002) reported that African American women were more likely to be noncompliant with mammography screening. With respect to retention in clinical trials, African American subjects were more likely to drop out of participation in a rheumatoid arthritis treatment adherence study than Caucasians (Dunbar-Jacob et al., 2004). Although these studies found disparity with study participation and detection screening, more research is needed to examine disparities with actual treatment adherence in chronic disease. In HIV populations, this has grave implications since poorer outcomes occur for HIV positive

African American women. In addition, this examination of disparity needs to be extended to whether treatment strategies for compliance should be tailored to ethnic and cultural differences.

So much inconsistency exists in studies that have been conducted that no overall statement can be made regarding age and compliance behaviors (Conn, Taylor & Stineman, 1992; Dunbar-Jacob, Burke & Puczynski, 1995; Weinstein & Cuskey, 1985). For example, one study (Grady, 1988) found that women over age 50 complied more with the practice of self-breast exam evaluation than did younger women. Conversely, Conn and associates (1992) found that increased age was associated with poorer health and lower adherence with the cardiac rehabilitation program under investigation. There are specific issues of compliance related to specific age groups that are associated with developmental stages rather than chronological age. However, in general, developmental issues have not been well addressed in the compliance literature (Dunbar-Jacob et al., 2000).

Psychological Factors

Intuitively, health care professionals believe that psychological factors may affect compliance behavior. However, results of studies are inconsistent with this assumption. Depressive and anxiety states have been associated with both decreased compliance (Conn, Taylor & Stineman, 1992; Blumenthal et al., 1982) and increased compliance (O'Leary, Rohsenow & Chaney, 1979; Nelson et al., 1978). Ford and associates (1989) found that asthmatic and hypertensive patients showed a negative correlation of medication taking when they were depressed and anxious, but that increased symptoms led to increased compliance. More recently, DiMatteo, Lepper, and Croghan (2000) completed a meta-analysis examining the relationship between depression and adherence and found that depressed clients were at threefold the risk for noncompliance. Other psychological factors, such as ambiguity, hostility, and general emotional distress, as single factors, are not predictive of compliance behavior but may, in fact, be components of motivation (Dunbar-Jacob et al., 1997).

Social Support

Social support is another variable that has frequently been explored in compliance research studies. However, social support has not been demonstrated to definitively increase compliance behavior. For example, pediatric asthma clients who received social support from family and friends demonstrated increased compliance (Spector, 1985). In contrast, implementing an asthma self-management program within a group setting only had limited effects on compliance (Bailey et al., 1987). More recently, it was found that social support was helpful for patients with AIDS (Brown et al., 1998).

Prior Health Behavior

It has been suggested that compliance to a particular health care regimen at a single point in time may predict subsequent adherence (Dunbar-Jacob et al., 1997). In the 10-year study of the Lipid Research Clinics Coronary Primary Prevention Trial, initial medication compliance accurately predicted compliance throughout the study; however, this did not extend to other health behaviors. In general, it was found that the more similar the initial behaviors to the behaviors that need to be predicated, the greater the likelihood of accuracy (Dunbar-Jacob et al., 1997). In a recent study examining HIV treatment adherence, compliance to attending clinic appointments was associated with medication treatment adherence (Wagner, 2003). In addition, Wagner (2003) used a placebo trial for highly active antiretroviral therapies (HAART) to examine treatment compliance prior to the initiation of HAART therapy. This method raises various issues of prediction of treatment and ethical issues.

Somatic Factors

It has been postulated that the presence of symptoms may lead to greater compliance with medical recommendations. For example, hypertensive individuals who are asymptomatic often believed they could tell when their blood pressure was high and complied with treatment at these times because of their belief that compliance relieved the symptoms (Meyer, Leventhal & Guttman, 1985). In another study, of individuals with lung disease, increased dyspnea predicted greater compliance with nebulizer therapy (Turner et al., 1995). Conversely, the severity of asthma did not predict increased compliance with inhaled medication (Berg, 1995).

Regimen Characteristics

Regimen type and regimen complexity have been linked to compliance behavior, with complexity being more important (Dunbar-Jacob, Burke & Puczynski, 1995). Complexity includes multiple medications, frequent treatments, multiple regimens (e.g., diet, exercise, and medications), duration of the regimen, complicated treatment delivery systems, as well as annoying side effects (Lemanek, 1990). A review of the literature (Wing et al., 1986) substantiated that complicated regimens lead to low compliance rates. This effect has also been documented in elderly clients, clients with renal disease, and those with asthma (Conn, Taylor & Stineman, 1992; Berg & Berg, 1990; Tashkin, 1995). Medical regimens often require life-style changes, which can be difficult for the client to accomplish.

Economic and Sociocultural Factors

Economic Factors Poverty, poor English-language proficiency, and limited access to health care are known predictors of noncompliance (Gonzalez, 1990). The burdens of financial costs alone may serve as a barrier to obtaining health care services, supplies, or medications needed to manage chronic illness. Another major economic barrier to compliance is a lack of resources, including inadequate or difficult transportation, inadequate availability of child care, loss of time from low-paying jobs, and little job security. Socioeconomic status has recently been associated with low compliance in those using hormone replacement therapy. This needs to be further examined with other studies of adherence (Finley, Gregg, Solomon, & Gay, 2001).

Some barriers to compliance are clearly related to an ineffective health care system for chronic disease management. For example, some individuals with chronic disease who come to emergency departments for non-urgent care have limited access to primary care services that would be more appropriate for chronic disease management (Mansour, Lanphear & DeWitt, 2000). Inefficient and inconvenient clinics serving the poor have long waiting lines and tend not to provide long-term relationships with the same provider (Hellenbrandt, 1983). Well known is the decreased availability of primary care services, particularly in inner cities and rural areas, to groups such as migrant workers, new immigrants, the homeless, and those with AIDS. In addition, the maze of governmental and third-party payers' policies and regulations often deny provider reimbursement for preventive or educational services, making these services less available to clients (see Chapters 27 and 26, on financial impact and politics and policy, respectively).

Cultural Factors More attention is being given to the ways in which culture influences health behaviors and the interactions of clients with health care providers. Cultural influences affect the way adults and children experience, interpret, and respond to illness and its treatment (Munet-Villaro & Vessey, 1990). Given this statement, it is surprising that few reviews have focused on culture and adherence behaviors. The studies that report culture or ethnic differences in adherence rates often focus on where there are discrepancies between African Americans and Caucasians.

Because of the influx of Latino and Asian immigrants into the United States, studies examining the behaviors of these groups have begun to appear in the literature. Some of these studies explore the dimension of being a minority group with a health problem. Newly immigrated persons may also lack financial and social support from an extended family, a major resource in many non-Western cultures (Kleinman, Eisenberg & Good, 1988). Language issues affect the utilization of health care and the ability to form relationships with health care professionals. Different cultural norms may also interfere with adherence behaviors. For example, in Latino families, the stigma of having tuberculosis may be a factor in poor adherence with medication taking (Morisky & Cabrera, 1997). Latinos have also been described as seeking health care late, if at all, and then using folk healers and medications for illness (Talamantes, Lawler & Espino, 1995; Zuckerman et al., 1996). Some of the delay in health care utilization relates to insurance issues, language barriers, and immigration status.

Asian immigrants may have difficulty accepting and actively engaging in regimen demands. Chinese immigrants were found to have ineffective self-care and coping strategies with diabetes, in a study by Jaynes and Rankin (2001). Similarly, in a study by Im and Meleis (1999), Korean women ignored the symptoms of menopause until symptoms became intolerable.

It will become increasingly important for health care professionals to interpret the effect of culture and ethnicity on adherence behavior. One of the issues that confounds the link between health behavior and culture is socioeconomic status. There is a need to distinguish if poor compliance is related to ethnicity, cultural, or socioeconomic factors, as opposed to the interaction of these factors.

Client–Provider Interactions

Of the variables associated with noncompliance, provider-client interactions are the most consistently mentioned (Jones, Jones & Katz, 1987). Hellenbrandt (1983) identified these variables in client-physician interactions that adversely influence compliance behavior:

1. Inadequate supervision
2. Client dissatisfaction
3. No explanation of illness given to the client
4. Physician disagreement with the client
5. Formality toward or rejection of the client

Poor communication is a common occurrence in client-provider interactions. For example, health care providers do not give enough health instruction

to asthma clients about the way to take medications (Creer & Levstek, 1996), leading to an estimation of less than 50 percent of asthma medications being taken as prescribed (Creer, 1993). There have been other studies that have examined the lack of clear and complete instructions that clients were to follow (Garrity & Lawson, 1989; Zahr, Yazigi & Armenian, 1989). Compliance rates are also affected by poor physician follow-up of instructions (Bender & Milgrom, 1996), because providers often assume that repeat instruction is unnecessary. Three specific aspects of client-provider interactions have been examined: differing expectations of the client and provider, personal control, and perspectives of the client and provider.

Differing Expectations Of importance to health care professionals and clients is how much active client participation is appropriate to interactions with providers. Both providers and clients have expectations about the appropriate level of participation. Both make judgments based on these expectations about their suitable behavior—expectations formed in large part from previous experiences.

Providers and clients have, by and large, been socialized to expect the client to exhibit sick role behaviors and the provider to use complementary role behaviors (Parsons, 1951). In the sick role, clients are expected to try to get well by seeking help and cooperating with the prescribed regimen (see Chapter 2, on illness behaviors and roles). The complementary role of the provider is that of dominance as the professional expert and manager of the condition. Parsons' view served to underline the asymmetry in doctor-client relationships and described an authority-to-subordinate relationship (Hingson et al., 1981).

Some decisions not to comply are rational when viewed from the client's perspective. Thorne (1990) identified two themes for noncompliance: self-protection and maintenance of services. Reasons for willful noncompliance included troublesome side effects of medications, disbelief in recommendations, and the necessity of juggling conflicting recommendations from different physicians. Often, clients misled health care professionals about their intentions, because they wanted to maintain relationships with the health providers for other needed services. Thorne suggests that health care professionals consider the chronically ill individual as the expert and aim for the role of consultant rather than assume expertise and moral authority.

Health care professionals might become more effective in their communication and interaction with clients if they viewed clients as occupying various positions on a passivity-to-autonomy continuum, rather than focusing on a preconceived notion of expected client behavior. The result would be increased sensitivity to each client's requirements for autonomy, guidance, and direction. Instead of questioning the extent of participation clients should have in interactions, a more appropriate question would be, "What is the optimal kind of participation for a particular client?" The answer can only evolve through the provider-client dyad as they communicate about expectations, goals, and perceived problems. There is a need for better models to address the importance of the provider-patient relationship (Trostle, 1997; Thorne, Nyhlin & Paterson, 2000). Adopting definitions of compliance and adherence that address the component of agreement to treatment by the client as an active participant have been promoted more recently in the literature (World Health Organization, 2003).

Personal Control The locus-of-control construct has been used to study client choices of self-care behavior. It focuses on individual expectancies about outcomes (rewards, reinforcements) and the perceived efficacy of behavior to modify outcomes. According to this construct, persons are at different positions on an internal-external continuum of orientation to perceived control. Internals believe in personal influence on future events, and externals attribute influence to others. The health locus-of-control construct modifies this generalized expectancy to specific expectancies of health and illness outcomes and health behaviors (Rotter, 1966; Wallston et al., 1976).

Research findings have been contradictory about the relationship of locus-of-control to com-

pliance (Wallston, Wallston & DeVellis, 1978; Dimond & Jones, 1983). In one study, externals were described as more compliant with treatment and less active in seeking information, whereas internals actively sought knowledge and manipulated treatment regimens (Oberle, 1991).

Perspectives of Client and Provider Clients and providers are likely to hold different perspectives of chronic illness, its treatment, and the relative merits of compliant behavior. The client lives with the disease, and treatment is only one aspect of that individual's life. Living with treatment consequences is vastly different from offering advice, counsel, education, or exhortation about health care recommendations. Clients rarely, if ever, seek help from health care professionals because they want to comply. Rather, they ask for help for other reasons: they feel ill, they are worried, they are responding to others' recommendations, they need evidence to validate claims for entitlement benefits, and so forth. Providers, on the other hand, are concerned about compliance, which may be seen as the desired outcome of the client-provider interaction (Anderson, 1985).

Anderson identifies two ways in which clients' perspectives of chronic illness—in this case, diabetes mellitus—differs from those of providers. First, there is a relative difference in understanding the treatment regimen, not just on the level of specificity, rationale, and consequences, but also with respect to the sources of problems. Clients may see treatment as part of the problem of having diabetes, whereas providers see treatment as a solution. Second, clients are more concerned about the "here and now" experience, in contrast to providers' concern over a problem that places future health at risk. For example, clients express more concerns about preventing hypoglycemic reactions than about managing higher than normal blood glucose levels. Providers, on the other hand, express more concern about the importance of achieving close to normal blood glucose levels because of their perceptions of serious long-term consequences if control of blood glucose levels is not achieved (Anderson, 1985).

Mrs. J.

Mrs. J., a 52-year-old woman of Latino descent had difficulty understanding the dietician's explanation of the two-gram low-sodium diet that was ordered for her newly diagnosed hypertension. Although she seemed intelligent, she focused more on her daughter's upcoming wedding. According to Mrs. J., the wedding was the "biggest event of my life." The wedding was to be in two weeks and had been planned for a while. This was the youngest of Mrs. J.'s four daughters. Her status as a good mother, future mother-in-law, and member of a newly extended family would be affirmed if the wedding was "flawless." As far as Mrs. J. was concerned, "It would be unthinkable for me not to join in the fiesta, where eating and drinking would last for hours." It was not until the dietician acknowledged the importance of the event and offered to work with Mrs. J. to plan the day's food intake, negotiating with her some compromise about avoiding foods particularly high in sodium, that Mrs. J. showed some willingness to incorporate the diet into her daily life.

Motivation

In the traditional medical model, noncompliance is often attributed to a lack of motivation. The provider interprets mastery of and continuation with the prescribed regimen as a result of client motivation and identifies a lack of motivation as an obstacle to compliance.

Most current models of motivation of health care decisions and behavior are derived from psychological cognitive theories that focus on attitudes, beliefs, intentions, and perceptions of the client's ability to initiate and maintain recommended health behavior (Bandura, 1997) Fleury, 1992). These models view individual motivation as related to beliefs and values held by the client about the outcome to be achieved, the client's intentions, and the client's perceived ability to initiate and maintain behavioral change.

Client's Life Perspective   Motivation for health care behaviors is understandable when the client's perspective of life is considered. Complying with a provider-recommended treatment regimen may compete with other valued tasks, roles, or relationships. Clients who are chronically ill must continue to manage their daily existence under specific sets of financial and social conditions (Strauss et al., 1984).

Consequently, the strength of motivation to carry out health care behaviors may vary with perceptions of current life demands ability.

The case study of Mrs. J. illustrates the necessity of learning the client's life perspective in order to understand apparent low-level motivation for assuming recommended health care behavior. This case study demonstrates the need to consider the client's primary motivating forces at a given time and to determine the way these forces affect the strength of motivation for specific health care behavior.

Labeling a client as poorly motivated without considering that person's perspective impedes the process of helping and provides no suggestions on intervening in an effective manner. However, taking the client's perspective into account can assist the health care provider in gaining clues about barriers to compliance as perceived by the client. Clients may be more motivated to learn when their perspective is considered and they are involved in planning, allowing them to achieve more complete compliance over longer time periods.

Ethical Issues in Compliance

Compliance or noncompliance with recommendations for health behavior is an increasingly important ethical issue in health care cost containment, because conflicts arise when health care resources are limited and decisions about the best use of time, money, and the energy of providers must be made. However, economic and ethical issues in compliance differ. Whereas economic issues are concerned with the most efficient distribution of resources, ethical issues are concerned with the most *equitable* distribution (Barry, 1982). Connelly (1984) believes that strategies that promote and improve a client's active and effective self-care are both ethically and economically significant.

There is also concern in providing resources to help those with chronic disorders in developing countries where treatment noncompliance is so high (World Health Organization, 2003). Ethical issues center on reciprocal rights and responsibilities of caregivers and clients, use of paternalism and coercion by caregivers, autonomy of the client, relative risks and benefits of proposed regimens, and the costs to society of noncompliance (see Chapter 18, on ethics in chronic illness). Again, the focus upon the clients' active participation with their health care providers appears to also raise ethical concerns (Bernardini, 2004; Rand & Sevick, 2000). This questions whether health care directed solely by the practitioner without input by the client is ethical and whether noncompliance should rest upon the shoulders of only the client.

Sackett (1976) described three preconditions for ethical practice that must precede strategies to change client behavior. These preconditions mandate the use of informed consent and the development of a partnership with responsibility for compliance equally shared.

1. The diagnosis must be correct.
2. Therapy must provide more benefit than harm.
3. The client who accepts the treatment regimen must be a partner in strategies used to increase compliance.

Jonsen (1979) added a fourth condition, the importance of client consent to the regimen, and emphasized that the ethics of compliance are based on freedom, mutual understanding, and mutual re-

sponsibility. Connelly (1984) incorporated both Sackett's and Jonsen's conditions in an ethical approach to compliance that has three phases:

1. Developing client competencies and reinforcing and supporting the client's self-care ability
2. Evolving a consensual regimen and outcome goals through a client-provider interaction based on mutuality
3. Focusing compliance-increasing strategies on joint exploration of problems and negotiation of conflicts in goals or implementation

Threats, pressure, and inappropriate fear-arousal tactics are not ethical (Jonsen, 1979; Connelly, 1984). Punitive responses that can be implemented by the provider for revealed or suspected noncompliance include decreased time and attention from the provider, less availability for crisis management, and limited access to services, resources, or supplies. The high incidence of noncompliance and the provider's frequent inability to differentiate clients who comply from those who do not, presents an argument against the withdrawal or diminution of services to clients who disclose noncompliance. If others may be equally noncompliant, punitive responses only to those who are honest about noncompliance constitute inequality of care, which is an issue of social justice.

If the client has been informed and understands that the consequence of noncompliance will be withdrawal by the provider, then termination of the relationship may be the right of the provider. If economic or social conditions preclude access to other caregivers, this termination raises serious questions about the ethical nature of withdrawing and abandoning the client (Wong et al., 2004). Assisting the client in finding another caregiver is ethically preferable to unilateral and abrupt termination (Jonsen, 1979).

Interventions to Attain Compliance

The complexity of the variables associated with noncompliance should not deter the health care practitioner from working with the client to achieve maximum possible integration of optimal health recommendations, given the client's needs, demands, and life-style. To accomplish maximum compliance, those who use compliance-increasing strategies have a responsibility to ensure the client's safety and comprehension. For the nurse, often working as liaison between client and physician, communicating with either or both is often necessary before matters are clear enough to select and begin specific compliance-increasing strategies. The WHO (2003) has suggested adopting the use of the five "A's" in an effort to assist clients with self-management aspects to their chronic disease, such as treatment compliance. The 5 "A's" include: assess, advise, agree, assist, and arrange (Locke & Latham, 2002). The interventions suggested in this chapter are adaptable within this framework. However, advising the client of the importance of treatment compliance, establishing agreement with a treatment plan and arranging adequate follow-up are also necessary steps for health care professionals interested in providing treatment compliance interventions to their clients.

Assessment

If we are to assume that any measurement of client compliance is an assessment of behaviors, then we must decide how to analyze those behaviors. Compliance behaviors can be assessed in many ways. Unfortunately, each measurement is prone to some error, usually consisting of a bias toward an overestimation of compliance (Dunbar-Jacob et al., 2002; Burke & Dunbar-Jacob, 1995). Unfortunately, there is no "gold standard" for measuring compliance. However, using a combination of methods to measure a specific compliance behavior is recommended to increase accuracy and reliability of the results, compared with a single method of measurement (World Health Organization, 2003). An assessment of the client's overall well-being and psychological structure is also essential to a better understanding of his or her compliance behaviors.

A systematic assessment of the client should include the client's family, sociocultural and economic factors, knowledge level, beliefs, attitudes, and current understanding of the proposed regimen. Attention should also be given to the client's perceptions of the illness threat, the efficacy of recommendations, and the client's ability to carry these out.

Enhancing compliance behaviors is not as simple as telling clients what to do and then telling them again when the desired effect is not achieved. In studying compliance, it is necessary to understand that it is not the length of their life that is of concern

Mr. A.

Mr. A., a 32-year-old man, was diagnosed with HIV 1 year ago and has been doing well on a complex medication regimen. He is a registered nurse on a busy medical-surgical unit in a hospital but has limited the number of days he works since his diagnosis. He recently was accepted into a nursing program to begin obtaining his BSN degree. When he shows up at clinical today, he has an increased viral load. When questioned, Mr. A. admits that he finds it difficult to follow the medication regimen given his work and school schedule.

Since school started, he has not been able to exercise at the local gym where he is a member. He also admits that he is very stressed since going back to school, is staying up late at night studying, and often skips meals. He asks you to help him strategize about organizing all of his activities and maintaining his necessary medication regimen. He acknowledges that he knows how important it is to comply, but needs your help.

to many people with chronic illness, but their perception that recommended behavior change will be worth the effort (Rapley, 1997). Understanding and respecting the social, cultural, and psychological factors affecting compliance behaviors may enhance efforts to manage the problem of noncompliance.

There should be a determination of the "rightness" of the prescriptions for the particular client, including an estimation of the relative harm or benefit that is expected. The assessment will allow the nurse to determine which aspects of the regimen management (1) are most unlikely to achieve compliant behavior, (2) are most important in attaining therapeutic goals, and (3) require the most learning to attain the desired behavioral change. The following questions should be asked in a compliance-oriented history (Hingson et al., 1981):

1. Have you been taking anything for this problem already?
2. Does anything worry you about the illness?
3. What can happen if the recommended regimen is not followed?
4. How likely is that to occur?
5. How effective do you feel the regimen will be in treating the disorder?
6. Can you think of any problems you might have in following the regimen?
7. Do you have any questions about the regimen or how to follow it?

Health care professionals are not infallible, and errors can occur in prescribing, in dispensing, in communicating with the client and family caregiver, or in maintaining updated written records, especially in settings in which multiple care providers are present. A second consideration is that the client/caregiver simply may not understand, or remember, instructions. If clients lack the knowledge or skills to undertake a recommended behavior or treatment, it is unlikely that they will do so. Instructions related to treatment regimens need to be reinforced continually over time to enhance compliance behaviors.

Enhancing a client's motivation requires careful assessment of his or her readiness to make and maintain behavioral changes. Building skills requires that he or she be ready to learn tasks such as reading food labels, selecting appropriate foods in restaurants, and incorporating taking medications into his or her daily routine. In other words, clients must learn new strategies to help them adopt and maintain new behaviors, especially when daily routines are interrupted (Bandura, 1997; Miller et al., 1997).

It is also important to be aware of a tendency among care providers to see compliant behavior as positive, admirable, and wise (being the "good patient") and noncompliant behavior as being negative, deplorable, and unintelligible (being the "problem patient"). It seems probable that health care professionals who have this view would be less likely to search out barriers to noncompliance.

Assessment should also lead to a determination of the proper focus of compliance-increasing strategies. It was said earlier that the notion of compliance as self-care may be too restrictive for situations in which compliance with medical regimens cannot be achieved without the assistance of others. For instance, the combination of marked disability and chronic illness makes the conceptualization of compliance as a self-care ability inappropriate. In such instances, social support networks may be the most important agents of compliance and, therefore, should become the focus of compliance-increasing strategies. However, the nurse should carefully assess the impact of social support on compliance. While social support—by significant others or support networks—may help clients cope with chronic illness and reinforce compliant behavior in some populations (Burke & Dunbar-Jacob, 1995), this may not be true for all, because there are clients who do not always want tangible help from others.

Measuring Compliance Behaviors

There are several common methodological approaches that focus on compliance. This chapter includes self-report, practitioner report, observation, physiological measures, medication monitoring, and electronic monitors. As mentioned in the preceding section, many researchers use multiple assessment measures and compare findings (Berg, 1995).

Self-Report

Client self-reports of compliance behaviors are the simplest and cheapest method of gathering noncompliance information and are feasible in virtually all care settings (De Geest, Abraham, & Dunbar-Jacob, 1996; Burke & Dunbar-Jacob, 1995). Self-reports also allow the collection of more detailed information on the circumstances surrounding poor compliance than any other types of measures (Burke & Dunbar-Jacob, 1995). They may be elicited through simple questions or through a more complex, structured interview schedule. Common self-report measures include medication and symptom diaries, structured questionnaires, and interviews.

Several studies have attempted to evaluate and define the accuracy of self-reported compliance. Many of these have compared client reports with pill counts, drug levels, or biological markers in body fluids. Most have found that individuals overestimate their compliance (Bender et al., 1998; Dunbar-Jacob et al., 2000). In spite of inherent problems, self-report is still the most common measure used in compliance behavior assessment.

Mr. M.

Mr. M., a 70-year-old business executive, was newly diagnosed with non-insulin dependent diabetes mellitus (NIDDM). He was educated, alert, and able to solve problems, and he attended classes on diabetes education so he could "learn why and how to follow his regimen." He decided to do home blood glucose monitoring, but he showed no interest in being compliant about diet and indicated little enthusiasm for changing food intake habits except to omit concentrated sugars.

Only when asked specific questions about his daily schedule, living conditions, and present concerns did he reveal that his attention, energy, and time were completely devoted to his business and to his ventilator-dependent wife. His business took most of his daytime hours, and he provided direct care to his wife seven nights a week and four evenings a week. Since her sudden respiratory failure six months earlier, he had learned to manage medicines and respiratory equipment and

oxygen and to perform other therapeutic tasks. He described the dinner hour as "precious time when we can talk about something besides sickness."

Mr. M. identified a number of factors that influenced his noncompliance with diet. First, breakfast was sometimes missed if he slept late. Second, it was difficult to be more consistent in eating lunch because his schedule revolved around his customers' needs, which led to missing this meal frequently. Third, dinner with his wife was the only time either could focus on family matters without interruption, and he did not want to be thinking about what he should be eating at that time. Fourth, he considered his wife's illness and care as more serious and having more immediacy than his own. Finally, it was determined that he received little reinforcement from the presence of symptoms, or from his physician contact, which was scheduled every three months.

Practitioner Report

Reports by health professionals are an indirect method of compliance assessment. However, studies indicate that this method is not accurate. Because there are no readily observable characteristics of the noncompliant client, clinicians rely on intuition and presumption (Steele, Jackson & Gutman, 1990). However, given that practitioner reports are fast, free, noninteractive, and consistent with the medical model, they are still used to assess compliance behavior.

Observation

Direct observation of the client is not always possible. Therefore, observation is not a practical method of assessing compliance. Theoretically, this method would be an ideal way to provide evidence of compliance behavior; however, individuals often "play to an audience," and the knowledge that someone is watching affects behavior. An example of this behavior for the individual with asthma is the demonstration/return demonstration of the correct method of using metered-dose inhalers (MDIs). Asthmatics are assessed on their ability to carry out the instructed regimen and compliance with teaching. Although nurses assess the clients' behavior in carrying out tasks related to health care management, the assumption cannot be made that this activity will continue at home.

Physiological Measures

Physiological measures of compliance include serum drug levels, heart rate monitoring, muscle strength, urine sample analysis, cholesterol levels, and glycosylated hemoglobin levels. The advantage of physiological methods is that these measures are not dependent on the client's memory or veracity.

Of all of the physiological measures, measurement of drug levels is most commonly used. While drug level measurements reflect a greater degree of accuracy than self-reports and practitioner reports, there are some difficulties with this type of assess-

ment. First, these measures do not reflect the level of compliance (Dunbar-Jacob, Burke & Puczynski, 1995). They merely classify a person as having followed or not followed some of the regimen (Burke & Dunbar-Jacob, 1995). Second, though assays offer a direct and objective approach to the measurement of noncompliance, this method is neither affordable nor available for every drug, is only applicable to medications with a long half-life, and may vary from individual to individual (De Geest, Abraham & Dunbar-Jacob, 1996). Third, physiological technologies are often unable to detect dosage levels. For example, many asthma medications are so rapidly absorbed systemically that it is not possible to detect them by biochemical assay (Rand & Wise, 1994). Finally, accurate detection of noncompliance through drug level testing offers no explanation or insight into the reasons for noncompliance (Besch, 1995).

Medication Monitors

Pill counts, pharmacy refill monitoring, and MDI canister weighing can all be used to measure medication compliance. In studies that use pill counts, the subject is given a vial each month that has a certain number of tablets, and this vial is exchanged for a new one each month. The medication left in the vial can be compared with the number that was supposed to be left if the medication were taken. Similarly, when a client requests a refill from the pharmacy, the time of the request is compared with the expected date of refill if the medication were taken as prescribed. This does not take into account whether clients are sharing medications with others or "dumping" pills prior to refill.

Metered-dose inhaler canister weighing is used with clients who have respiratory illnesses. The canister is weighed before it is given to the client and then at specific time frames during treatment. Although medication-monitoring methods appear highly accurate, they overestimate compliance behavior (Rand & Wise, 1994; Rudd et al., 1990). Recently, Simmons et al. (2000) described the phenomenon of canister dumping in the Lung Health Study. Only 30 percent of the sample triggered their MDI medications prior to a clinic visit. Other limitations of these methods include not knowing whether the client actually took the medication or being able to determine the timing of doses (Besch, 1995).

Electronic Monitoring

Electronic monitors are a newer technology for the assessment of compliance behaviors. The most common electronic monitoring device is the electronic medication monitor. Electronic monitors may also be used to capture heart rate and muscle movement with exercise adherence (Iyriboz et al., 1991) or to document nasal continuous positive airway pressure compliance for clients with sleep apnea (Kribbs et al., 1993).

Electronic monitors that assess medication adherence are used with tablets, eye drops, and MDIs (Dunbar-Jacob et al., 1997; Berg, Dunbar-Jacob & Sereika, 1997). These monitors function with the use of microprocessors placed in special bottle caps or blister packs and can monitor the date and time of day for each manipulation of the drug container and provide information on drug-taking behavior for days or weeks. Knowing the pattern of pill taking (or not taking) can be useful in evaluating clinical responses (or lack thereof) or side effects and provide guidance for interventions specifically tailored for each client (Besch, 1995).

Educational Strategies to Enhance Compliance

The primary purpose of client education is to assist with decision making regarding health promotion (Ungvarski & Schmidt, 1995). It is important to note that after education is provided, some clients may follow all the advice, some will select portions, and others will reject all the information. The ultimate decision belongs to the client and does not imply failure on the part of the nurse (Crespo-Fierro, 1997) (see Chapter 15, on client and family education).

Educational interventions should be individualized and include an assessment of the client's level of knowledge, cultural background, and particular goals. Educational information should be presented in manageable segments, with additional information and reinforcement at subsequent meetings. The nurse should focus on the key issues in the management of the regimen and should select the most important aspects necessary for health maintenance. Difficult skills should be demonstrated, and then the client should be allowed to practice and do a return demonstration. Difficult skills should also be reviewed each time the client visits.

Written material should be geared to the client's reading level and language. Glazer and colleagues (1996) evaluated printed materials to teach breast self-examination and found that, although the reading level of the materials being provided was at the ninth-grade level, the average reading level of the target population was at the sixth-grade level. Another study on health literacy found that 42 percent of clients could not understand even the most basic written medication instructions (Williams et al., 1995a). These findings underscore the need to prepare materials that can be used by the maximum number of clients. Other educational materials can be provided, such as videotapes, audiotapes, and computer-assisted instruction.

Often clients rely on family members to interpret regimen details at home. Therefore, when educating those with chronic illnesses, family members or significant others should be involved in the teaching session. Emphasis in teaching needs to be directed toward not only knowledge of the disease, but also the skills needed for the regimen (Burke & Dunbar-Jacob, 1995). In addition, the regimen should be simplified as much as possible.

Beyond Knowledge and Comprehension

Abilities beyond knowledge and comprehension are required. Therefore, educational goals must be broader than solely the acquisition of knowledge if compliance is to result. The outcome of compliance depends on participation of the learner beyond that of listening, reading, or assimilating information. Clinicians should also encourage participation in their own care. Flexible self-care regimens enable people to exercise a degree of autonomy that is not an option in standard regimens, even when these are adapted to some extent for individuals. The flexibility of instructions, such as *If you have this sign or this symptom, then try this activity,* allows people some freedom to make informed choices, and having choices fosters independence and a better quality of life (Rapley, 1997).

Behavioral Strategies to Enhance Compliance

Behavioral strategies are those procedures that attempt to influence specific noncompliant behaviors directly through the use of various techniques. These strategies may be used as a single intervention or in combination to achieve desired results.

It is generally believed that compliance is increased when clients actively participate in learning and deciding how to implement prescribed regimens. However, insistence by the health care provider on a preconceived or stereotyped notion of the most desirable level of participation may be inappropriate. A mismatch between an authoritarian provider and an assertive, active learner may influence compliance adversely. On the other hand, the provider who expects an active involvement process can overwhelm a passive and nonactive learner.

Tailoring

The minimal outcome of client participation with the nurse in developing a compliance strategy should be tailoring the treatment to the client's daily behaviors, because this process may help cue compliance (Burke & Dunbar-Jacob, 1995). Integrating treatment activities so that they coincide with routine activities, called rituals, is an important way of individualizing and enhancing the treatment plan. The daily schedule of eating, arising and retiring, hygiene, favorite television program, and so on, identifies rituals that may be used to incorporate health behaviors into daily life.

Simplifying the Regimen

As a result of discussion between client and nurse, it may become apparent that the client is unable to manage the complexity of the prescribed regimen. Negotiation with the prescribing source may result in better compliance if this barrier is cleared and the regimen is simplified. As a general rule, the number of times medications are taken and the number of pills should be held to a minimum.

Providing Reminders

Reminders or memory aids are useful when the problem is a failure of the behavior to occur because clients have forgotten to perform one or more aspects of the desired behavior. Calendars, clocks, and individually prepared posters with medication and food reminders can be very helpful. Separating a day's supply of medications can also help the person who has difficulty remembering if a particular dose was taken.

The health care provider can reinforce the importance of compliance at episodic visits. Such reinforcement may involve pill counting, attention to client diaries or to other reports of behavior, and self-monitoring; these are all methods that remind the client of the value of compliance and that elicit participation.

Telephone calls are also useful in reminding clients about health care recommendations, in encouraging compliance with medications in the elderly (Cargill, 1992), and as an effective intervention in enhancing compliance with making and keeping follow-up appointments after referral from emergency (Komoroski, Graham & Kirby, 1996). Friedman and colleagues (1996) tested a variation of telephone follow-up, which demonstrated a 17.7 percent improvement in medication adherence among those receiving automated telephone calls. Telephone reminders not only provide a personal touch, but also allow individuals who wish to reschedule an appointment the opportunity to do so at that time (Crespo-Fierro, 1997).

Enhancing Coping

The nurse should be very sensitive to clues from individual clients suggesting emotional responses that interfere with learning optimal health behaviors. Situational anxiety, marked depression, and denial are associated with low levels of compliance. These three emotional responses should be interpreted as signals that the client's coping skills are inadequate and that a modification in approach may be more effective.

Contracting

Contracting can be viewed as an educational strategy that engages clients' commitment to learn, to make changes, and to be accountable for their own behavior (see Chapter 14, on change agent, and Chapter 15, on client and family education). Contracting involves the nurse and client in a collaboratively developed written contract with specified goals and methods and explicitly identified incentives. Based on principles of behavioral modification, contracting uses reinforcements to establish and maintain new or changed behaviors. Contracting has been successfully used as a strategy to increase compliance in various settings and with different types of behavior (Crespo-Fierro, 1997). Contracting also creates a form of public commitment, which may foster the development of self-control over behaviors that have been identified in the written contract.

Ethnocultural Interventions

Recognition that the client's family patterns of communication may differ from the provider's is important for effective interactions. In addition, cultural components need to be integrated into any strategies that are proposed.

Sensitivity to ethnocultural beliefs of clients will promote an understanding of compliance behaviors of those who come from different cultures. Treatments prescribed within existing ethnocultural practices, as opposed to the traditional context of Western biomedical and nursing beliefs, is more likely to succeed in that they will represent the world view of the community served (Flaskerud, 1995). MacLachlan and Carr (1994) propose the importance of using both traditional healers and modern medical practitioners to promote health protection and behaviors.

For effective interaction with persons of a different culture, "cultural translation" is needed (Murphy, Anderson & Lyns, 1993). One requisite for a cultural translator is learning about the historical rituals and norms that relate to health of the particular group. Another requisite is evaluating health behaviors in the client's cultural context to determine competing priorities, environmental obstacles, or degree of knowledge and skills (Murphy, Anderson & Lyns, 1993).

Providers need to recognize that their belief system, values, and attitudes toward health care management also are culturally determined and may be responsible for their inability to recognize that the source of noncompliance might be ideological or philosophical differences. The emphasis on self-care in Western medical systems is ideologically quite consistent with the value of individual enterprise in Western cultures (Anderson, Blue & Lau, 1993). Persons of other cultures may find this value for self-care very foreign.

Knowing only an ethnic label is inadequate for understanding a particular individual's or group's beliefs (Friedman, 1990). Other cultural aspects that need to be assessed include whether traditional, folk, or alternative remedies are used by the client; whether ordered prescriptions interfere with important cultural practices; and what rituals, restrictions, meanings, and norms are associated with cultural use of items such as food.

Family communication and authority patterns are also influenced by culture. For African Americans, role obligations are seen as mandatory and family rights as strong. Therefore, family-centered care is more appropriate than the usual individual-centered approach seen in Western practice (Friedman, 1990). African American family patterns include strong kinship systems within the extended family; values for family, church, and religious life; active involvement of both parents in parenting; and assistance with child care by the maternal grandparent (Friedman, 1990).

Another example would be the Hispanic or Latino culture. Although current research disputes this (Friedman, 1990), the stereotypical image of the Latino culture is of a hierarchical family structure with male domination. Antonia Novello, Surgeon General of the U.S. Public Health Service from 1990 through 1993, contends that Western prevention and maintenance of health by self-care measures are not consistent with the fatalistic view of Hispanics, who often feel "what causes a disease, and its impact on you and your family, does not hold much weight when your sole purpose is just to live and, when God wills it, to die" (Ingle, 1993, p. 45). In addition, Hispanic women have an important role in controlling health care information and its use in the family and need to be included in discussion of compliance-increasing strategies (Ingle, 1993).

Outcomes

It is generally recognized that the success of medical treatment, in part, depends on the client's willingness to assume responsibility to carry out recommended regimens. Many important factors must be considered in the evaluation of treatment strategies for the individual with a chronic illness. One factor is the high cost of health care if clients are noncompliant with treatment regimens. Noncompliance can also increase the likelihood of complications (Schlenk & Dunbar-Jacob, 1996).

Another issue affecting outcomes may be our lack of knowledge about the "dose" of any therapy for treatment. The knowledge about the compliance dose-response curve is helpful for the provider so that compliance-enhancing strategies can be implemented (Schlenk & Dunbar-Jacob, 1996). If, in clinical trials testing the effects of new medication therapies for a given disease, the dose-response analysis is based on client self-reported adherence, it may or may not be accurate, resulting in possibly imprecise therapeutic dosages.

Our inability to ascertain "true" compliance behavior is also a barrier for the assessment of clinical outcomes, as is our limited ability to counsel clients about behaviors that are absolutely necessary for a given outcome to occur. Schlenk and Dunbar-Jacob (1996) assert that more research is needed to firmly establish that compliance leads to better outcomes. The fact that health care providers are unable to convey at what level a person needs to follow a regimen can be particularly important in chronic diseases, for which the regimen is extremely burdensome but critical.

Summary and Conclusions

Given the increasing number of individuals with chronic illness, the importance of compliance to treatment regimens is obvious. Responsibility for management falls to the client or family on a day-to-day basis. However, the provider is responsible for ensuring that the client or family has the needed knowledge, motivation, and skills, as well as for helping the client find ways to make compliance more feasible.

Study Questions

1. Why is trying to increase compliant behaviors important for clients who are chronically ill?
2. What factors are involved in compliance? Discuss them.
3. Do you agree that *compliance* and *noncompliance* are terms as acceptable as *adherence* and *nonadherence*? Why or why not?
4. How prevalent is noncompliance? What are the methodological barriers to the study of compliance? What is the relationship of single variables to compliance? What conceptual barriers exist?
5. What ethical issues arise when a provider tries to increase a client's compliance? Discuss an ethical approach.
6. Using your own or a client's culture, identify how norms, rituals, and practices affect compliance with health care recommendations.
7. How does motivation influence compliance?
8. What are the strengths and weaknesses of education as a means of increasing compliance?
9. How can you encourage client participation to increase compliance? Discuss tailoring, simplifying the regimen, and reminders.
10. How can you enhance coping to increase compliance?
11. What are the advantages and disadvantages of contracting? Of support groups?

References

Adams, J., & White, M. (2003). Are activity promotion interventions based on the transtheoretical model effective? A critical review. *British Journal of Sports Medicine, 37* (2), 106–114.

Ajzen, L. (1985). From intention to action: A theory of planned behavior. In J. Kuhl & J. Beckman (Eds.), *Action control: From cognition to behavior.* Heidelberg: Springer.

Anderson, J. M., Blue, C., & Lau, A. (1993). Women's perspectives on chronic illness: Ethnicity, ideology and restructuring of life. *Diabetes Spectrum, 6* (2), 102–115.

Anderson, R. M. (1985). Is the problem of noncompliance all in our head? *Diabetes Educator, 11,* 31–34.

Bailey, W. C., Richards, J. M., Manzella, B. A., Windsor, R. A., et al. (1987). Promoting self-management in adults with asthma: An overview of the UAB program. *Health Education Quarterly, 14* (3), 345–355.

Bamberger, J. D., Unick, J., Klein, P., Fraser, M., et al. (2000). Helping the urban poor stay with antiretroviral HIV drug therapy. *American Journal of Public Health, 90* (5), 699–701.

Bandura, A. (1997). *Self-efficacy: The exercise of control.* New York: W. H. Freeman and Company.

Barofsky, I. (1978). Compliance, adherence, and the therapeutic alliance: Steps in the development of self-care. *Social Science and Medicine, 12,* 369–376.

Barry, V. (1982). *Moral aspects of health care.* Belmont, CA: Wadsworth.

Baumann, L. J., Cameron, L. D., Zimmerman, R. S., & Leventhal, H. (1989). Illness representations and matching labels with symptoms. *Health Psychology, 8* (4), 449–469.

Becker, M. H. (1976). Socio-behavioral determinants of compliance. In D. L. Sackett & R. Haynes (Eds.), *Compliance with therapeutic regimens.* Baltimore: Johns Hopkins University Press.

Becker, M. H., & Maiman, L. A. (1975). Sociobehavioral determinants of compliance with health and medical care recommendations. *Medical Care, 13,* 10–24.

Becker, M. H., Drachman, R. H., and Kirscht, J. P. (1974). A new approach to explaining sick-role behavior in low income populations. *American Journal of Public Health, 64,* 205–216. Thousand Oaks, CA: Sage.

Bender, B., & Milgrom, H. (1996). Compliance with asthma therapy: A case for shared responsibility. *Journal of Asthma, 33,* 199–202.

Bender, B., Milgrom, H., Rand, C., & Ackerson, L. (1998). Psychological factors associated with medication nonadherence in asthmatic children. *Journal of Asthma, 35,* 347–353.

Berg, J. (1995). *An evaluation of a self-management program for adults with asthma.* Unpublished doctoral dissertation, University of Pittsburgh.

Berg, J., & Berg, B. L. (1990). Compliance, diet and cultural factors among Black Americans with end-stage renal disease. *Journal of National Black Nurses Association,* Sept/Oct, 16–28.

Berg, J., Dunbar-Jacob, J., & Sereika, S. (1997). An evaluation of a self-management program for adults with asthma. *Clinical Nursing Research, 6,* 225–238.

Bernardini, J. (2004). Ethical issues of compliance/adherence in the treatment of hypertension. *Advances in Chronic Kidney Disease, 11* (2), 222–227.

Besch, L. (1995). Compliance in clinical trials. *AIDS, 9,* 1–10.

Blumenthal, J. A., Williams, R. S., Wallace, A. G., Williams, R. B., et al. (1982). Physiological and psychological variables predict compliance to prescribed exercise therapy in patients recovering from myocardial infarction. *Psychosomatic Medicine, 44* (6), 519–527.

Brawley, L. R., & Culos-Reed, S. N. (2000). Studying adherence to therapeutic regimens: overview, theories, recommendations. *Controlled Clinical Trials, 21* (5 Suppl), 156S–163S.

Brown, M. A., Inouye, J., Powell-Cope, G. M., Holzemer, W. L., et al. (1998). Social support and adherence in HIV+ persons. *International Conference on AIDS, 12,* 590.

Buckworth, J., & Wallace, L. S. (2002). Application of the Transtheoretical Model to physically active adults. *Journal of Sports Medicine and Physical Fitness, 42* (3), 360–367.

Burke, L. E., & Dunbar-Jacob, J. (1995). Adherence to medication, diet and activity recommendations: From assessment to maintenance. *Journal of Cardiovascular Nursing, 9* (2), 62–79.

Butler, J. A., Roderick, P., Mullee, M., Mason, J. C., et al. (2004). Frequency and impact of nonadherence to immunosuppressants after renal transplantation: a systematic review. *Transplantation, 77* (5), 769–776.

Cargill, J. M. (1992). Medication compliance in elderly people: Influencing variables and interventions. *Journal of Advanced Nursing, 17* (4), 422–426.

Carney, R., Freedland, K., Eisen, S., Rich, M., et al. (1995). Major depression and medication adherence in elderly patients with coronary artery disease. *Health Psychology, 14,* 88–90.

Carney, R., Freedland, K., Eisen, S., Rich, M., et al. (1998). Adherence to a prophylactic medication regimen in patients with symptomatic versus asymptomatic ischemic heart disease. *Behavioral Medicine, 24,* 35–39.

Chan, D., & Fishbein, M. (1993). Determinants of college women's intention to tell their partners to use condoms. *Journal of Applied Social Psychology, 23,* 1455–1470.

Chesney, M. A., Ickovics, J. R., Chambers, D. B., Gifford, A. L., et al. (2000). Self-reported adherence to antiretroviral medications among participants in clinical trials: The AACTG Adherence Instruments. *AIDS Care, 12,* 255–266.

Christensen, A. J., Wiebe, J. S., Edwards, D. L., Michels, J. D., et al. (1996). Body consciousness, illness-related impairment and patient adherence in hemodialysis. *Journal of Consulting and Clinical Psychology, 64,* 147–152.

Clark, N. M., & Starr, N. S. (1994). Management of asthma by patients and families. *American Journal of Respiratory and Critical Care Medicine, 149,* S54–66.

Conn, V., Taylor, S. G., & Stineman, A. (1992). Medication management by recently hospitalized older adults. *Journal of Community Health Nursing, 9* (1), 1–11.

Connelly, C. E. (1984). Economic and ethical issues in patient compliance. *Nursing Economics, 2,* 342–347.

Conrad, P. (1985). The meaning of medications: Another look at compliance. *Social Science and Medicine, 20,* 29–37.

Corbin, J. M., & Strauss, A. L. (1984). Collaboration: Couples working to manage chronic illness. *Image: The Journal of Nursing Scholarship, 16* (4), 109–115.

Cramer, J., Scheyer, R., Prevey, M., & Mattson, R. (1989). How often is medication taken as prescribed? A novel assessment technique. *JAMA, 261,* 3273–3277.

Cramer, J., Vachon, L., Desforges, C., & Sussman, N. (1995). Dose frequency and dose interval compliance with multiple antiepileptic medication during a controlled clinical trial? *Epilepsia, 36,* 1111–1117.

Creer, T. L. (1993). Medication compliance and childhood asthma. In N. A. Krasneger, L. Epstein, S. B. Johnson, & S. J. Yaffe (Eds.), *Developmental aspects of health compliance behavior,* (pp. 303–333). Hillsdale, NJ: Erlbaum Associates.

Creer, T. L., & Levstek, D. (1996). Medication compliance and asthma: Overlooking the trees because of the forest. *Journal of Asthma, 33,* 203–211.

Crespo-Fierro, M. (1997). Compliance/adherence and care management in HIV disease. *Journal of the Association of Nurses in AIDS Care, 8,* 43–54.

De Geest, S., Abraham, I., & Dunbar-Jacob, J. (1996). Measuring transplant patients' compliance with immunosuppressive therapy. *Western Journal of Nursing Research, 18,* 595–605.

deKlerk, E., & van der Linden, S. (1996). Compliance monitoring of NSAID drug therapy in ankylosing spondylitis, experiences with an electronic monitoring device. *British Journal of Rheumatology, 35,* 60–65.

Demyttenaere, K., Van Ganse, E., Gregoire, J., Gaens, E., et al. (1998). Compliance with depressed patients treated with fluoxetine or amitriptyline. *International Clinical Psychopharmacology, 13,* 11–17.

DiMatteo, M. R. (2004). Variations in patients' adherence to medical recommendations: A quantitative review of 50 years of research. *Medical Care, 42* (3), 200–209.

DiMatteo, M. R., Lepper, H. S., & Croghan, T. W. (2000). Depression is a risk factor for noncompliance with medical treatment. *Archives of Internal Medicine, 160,* 2101–2107.

DiMatteo, M. R., Sherbourne, C. D., Hays, R. D., Ordway, L., et al. (1993). Physician's characteristics influence adherence to medical treatment. *Health Psychology, 12,* 93–102.

Dimond, M., & Jones, S. L. (1983). *Chronic illness across the life span.* Norwalk, CT: Appleton-Century-Crofts.

Dracup, K. A., & Meleis, A. I. (1982). Compliance: An interactionist approach. *Nursing Research, 31,* 32–35.

Dunbar, J. (1980). Adhering to medical advice: A review. *International Journal of Mental Health, 9* (1–2), 70–78.

_____. (1990). Predictors of patient adherence: Patient predictors. In A. Shumaker, E. Schron, & J. Ockene (Eds.), *The handbook of health behavior change.* New York: Springer.

Dunbar-Jacob, J. (1993). Contributions to patient adherence: Is it time to share the blame? *Health Psychology, 12,* 91.

Dunbar-Jacob, J., Burke, L. E., & Puczynski, S. (1995). Clinical assessment and management of adherence to medical regimens. In P. M. Nicassio & T. W. Smith (Eds.), *Managing chronic illness: A biopsychosocial perspective.* Washington, DC: APA.

Dunbar-Jacob, J., Erlen, J., Schlenk, E., Ryan, C., et al. (2000). Adherence in chronic disease. In *Annual Review of Nursing Research*, (pp. 48–90). New York: Springer.

Dunbar-Jacob, J., Holmes, J. L., Sereika, S., Kwoh, C. K., et al. (2004). Factors associated with attrition of African Americans during the recruitment phase of a clinical trial examining adherence among individuals with rheumatoid arthritis. *Arthritis Rheumatology, 51* (3), 422–428.

Dunbar-Jacob, J. & Schenk, E. (2001). Patient adherence to treatment regimen. In A. Baum & T. Revenson (Eds.) *Handbook of health psychology* (pp. 321–657), Mahwah, NJ: Lawrence Erlbaum Associates Publishers.

Dunbar-Jacob, J., Schenk, E. A., Burke, L. E., & Mathews, J. (1997). Predictors of patient adherence: Patient characteristics. In S. A. Schumaker, E. B. Schron, J. K. Ockens (Eds.), The handbook of health behavior change (2nd ed.). New York: Springer.

Dunbar-Jacob, J., Schenk, E., & Caruthers, D. (2002). Adherence in the management of chronic disorders. In A. Christensen & M. Antoni (Eds.), *Chronic physical disorders: Behavioral medicine's perspective.* (pp. 69–82), Malden, MA: Blackwell Publishers.

Duncan, J., & Rogers, R. (1998). Medication compliance in patients with chronic schizophrenia: Implications for the community management of mentally disordered offenders. *Journal of Forensic Sciences, 43,* 1133–1137.

Eiser, C., Hill, J. J., & Blacklay, A. (2000). Surviving cancer: What does it mean for you? An evaluation of a clinic based intervention for survivors of childhood cancer. *Psycho-Oncology, 9,* 214–220.

Feachem, R. G., Sekhri, N. K., & White, K. L. (2002). Getting more for their dollar: a comparison of the NHS with California's Kaiser Permanente. *British Medical Journal, 324* (7330), 135–141.

Finley, C., Gregg, E. W., Solomon, L. J., & Gay, E. (2001). Disparities in hormone replacement therapy use by socioeconomic status in a primary care population. *Journal of Community Health, 26* (1), 39–50.

Fishbein, M., & Ajzen, I. (1975). *Belief, attitude and intention: An introduction to theory and research.* Reading, MA: Addison-Wesley.

Flaskerud, J. (1995). Culture and ethnicity. In J. Flaskerud & P. J. Ungvarski (Eds.), *HIV/AIDS: A guide to nursing care* (3rd ed.), pp. 405–432. Philadelphia: Saunders.

Fleury, J. (1992). The application of motivational theory to cardiovascular risk reduction. *Image: The Journal of Nursing Scholarship, 24* (3), 229–239.

Ford, F., Hunter, M., Hensley, M., Gillieo, A., et al. (1989). Hypertension and asthma: Psychological aspects. *Social Science Medicine, 29* (1), 79–84.

Friedman, M. (1990). Transcultural family nursing: Application to Latino and Black families. *Journal of Pediatric Nursing, 5* (3), 214–221.

Friedman, R., Kazis, L., Jette, A., Smith, M., et al. (1996). A telecommunciation system for monitoring and counseling patients with hypertension: Impact on medication adherence and blood pressure. *American Journal of Hypertension, 9,* 285–292.

Garrity, T., & Lawson, E. (1989). Patient-physician communication as a determinant of medication misuse in older, minority women. *The Journal of Drug Issues, 19* (2), 245–259.

Glazer, H., Kirk, L., & Bosler, F. (1996). Patient education pamphlets about prevention, detection, and treatment of breast cancer in low literacy women. *Patient Education and Counseling, 27,* 185–189.

Gohdes, D., Rith-Najarian, S., Acton, K., & Shields, R. (1996). Improving diabetes care in the primary health setting. The Indian Health Service experience. *Annals of Internal Medicine, 124* (1 Pt 2), 149–152.

Goldstein, M. G., DePue, J., Kazura, A., & Niaura, R. (1998). Models for provider-patient interaction: Applications to health behavior change. In S. Shumaker & E. Schron (Eds.), *The handbook of health behavior change* (2nd ed.), (pp. 85–113). New York: Springer.

Gonzalez, J. (1990). Factors relating to frequency among low-income Mexican American women: Implications for nursing practice. *Cancer Nursing, 13,* 134–142.

Grady, K. E. (1988). Older women and the practice of self-breast exam. *Psychology of Women Quarterly, 12,* 473–487.

Grady, K. E., Lemkau, J. P., McVay, J. M., Carlson, S., et al. (1996). Clinical decision-making and mammography referral. *Preventive Medicine, 25* (3), 327–338.

Graves, J. W. (2000). Management of difficult-to-control hypertension.[see comment][erratum appears in *Mayo Clinical Proceedings 75* (5), 542]. *Mayo Clinic Proceedings, 75* (3), 278–284.

Greenstein, S., & Siegal, B. (1998). Compliance and non-compliance in patients with a functioning renal transplant: A multicenter study. *Transplantation, 66* (12), 1718–1726.

Harrington, R., Kerfoot, M., Dyer, E., McNiven, F., et al. (2000). Deliberate self-poisoning in adolescence: Why does a brief family intervention work in some cases and not others? *Journal of Adolescence, 23,* 13–20.

Haynes, R. (1979). *Determinants of compliance: The disease and the mechanics of treatment.* Baltimore, MD: Johns Hopkins University Press.

Haynes, R. B., McDonald, H., Garg, A. X., & Montague, P. (2002). Interventions for helping patients to follow prescriptions for medications.[update of Cochrane Database Syst Rev. 2000;(2):CD000011; PMID: 10796686]. *Cochrane Database of Systematic Reviews*(2), CD000011.

Hellenbrandt, D. (1983). An analysis of compliance behavior: A response to powerlessness. In J. F. Miller (Ed.), *Coping with chronic illness,* (pp. 215–243). Philadelphia: FA Davis.

Hilbrands, L., Hoitsma, A., & Koene, R. (1995). Medication compliance after renal transplantation. *Transplantation, 60,* 914–920.

Hingson, R., Scotch, N., Sorenson, J., & Swazey, J., (1981). *In sickness and in health.* St. Louis: Mosby.

Holland, N., Wiesel, P., Cavallo, P., Edwards, C., et al. (2001). Adherence to disease-modifying therapy in multiple sclerosis: Part II. *Rehabilitation Nursing, 26* (6), 221–226.

Holroyd, K. A., & Creer, T. L. (1986). *Self-management of chronic disease.* New York: Academic Press.

Horne, R. (1998). Adherence to medication: A review of existing research. In L. Myers & K. Midence (eds.), *Adherence to treatment in medical conditions.* Amsterdam: Harwood.

Horne, R., & Weinman, J. (1998). Predicting treatment adherence: An overview of theoretical models. In L. Myers & K. Midence (Eds.), *Adherence to treatment in medical conditions.* Amsterdam: Harwood.

Im, E., & Meleis, A. (1999). A situation-specific theory of Korean immigrant women's menopausal transition. *Journal of Nursing Scholarship, 31,* 333–338.

Ingle, K. L. (1993). Surgeon General broadcasts diabetes message to Hispanics. *Diabetes Forecast, 15* (8), 44–46.

Iyriboz, Y., Powers, S., Morrow, J., Ayers, D., et al. (1991). Accuracy of the pulse oximeters in estimating heart rate at rest and during exercise. *British Journal of Sports Medicine, 25,* 162–164.

Jaynes, R., & Rankin, S. (2001). Application of Leventhal's self-regulation model to Chinese immigrants with type 2 diabetes. *Journal of Nursing Scholarship, 31,* 333–338.

Jenkins L. S., & Gortner, S. R. (1998). Correlates of self-efficacy expectation and prediction of walking behavior in cardiac surgery elders. *Annals of Behavioral Medicine, 20,* 99–103.

Jensen, M., Nielson, W., Roman, J., Hill, M., et al. (2000). Further evaluation of the pain stages of change questionnaire: Is the transtheoretical model of change useful for patients with chronic pain? *Pain, 86,* 255–264.

Jones, P. K., Jones, S. L., & Katz, J. (1987, September). Improving follow-up among hypertensive patients using a health belief model intervention. *Archives of Internal Medicine, 147,* 1557–1560.

Jonsen, A. R. (1979). Ethical issues in compliance. In R. B. Haynes, D. W. Taylor, & D. L. Sackett (Eds.), *Compliance in health care,* (pp. 113–120). Baltimore: Johns Hopkins University Press.

Joshi, M. S. (1998). Adherence in ethnic minorities: The case of South Asians in Britain. In L. Myers & K. Midence (Eds.), *Adherence to treatment in medical conditions.* Amsterdam: Harwood.

Kleinman, A., Eisenberg, L., & Good, B. (1988). Culture, illness, and care. *Annals of Internal Medicine, 88* (2), 251–258.

Komoroski, E., Graham, C., & Kirby, R. (1996). A comparison of interventions to improve clinic follow-up compliance after a pediatric emergency department visit. *Pediatric Emergency Care, 12,* 87–90.

Krapek, K., King, K., Warren, S. S., George, K. G., et al. (2004). Medication adherence and associated hemoglobin A1c in type 2 diabetes. *Annals of Pharmacotherapy, 38* (9), 1357–1362.

Kribbs, N., Pack, A., Kline, L., Smith, P., et al. (1993). Objective measurement of patterns of nasal CPAP use by patients with obstructive sleep apnea. *American Review of Respiratory Disease, 147,* 887–895.

Lee, J. Y., Kusek, J., Greene, P., Bernhard, S., et al. (1996). Assessing medication adherence by pill count and electronic monitor in the African American Study of Kidney Disease and Hypertension. *American Journal of Hypertension, 9,* 719–725.

Lemanek, K. (1990). Adherence issues in the medical management of asthma. *Journal of Pediatric Psychology, 15* (4), 437–458.

Leventhal, H., Glynn, K., & Fleming, R. (1987). Is the smoking decision an 'informed choice'? Effect of smoking risk factors on smoking beliefs. *JAMA, 257,* 3373–3377.

Leventhal, H., Meyer, D., & Nerenz, D. (1980). The common sense representations of illness danger. In S. Rachman (Ed.), *Contributions to medical psychology,* (pp. 27–30). Oxford: Pergamon Press.

Ley, P. (1988). *Communicating with patients.* London: Crown Helm.

Locke, E. A., & Latham, G. P. (2002). Building a practically useful theory of goal setting and task motivation. A 35-year odyssey. *American Psychologist, 57* (9), 705–717.

Lorig, K. R., Sobel, D. S., Ritter, P. L., Laurent, D., et al. (2001). Effect of a self-management program on patients with chronic disease. *Effective Clinical Practice, 4* (6), 256–262.

Lorig, K., Sobel, D., Stewart, A., Brown, B., et al. (1999). Evidence suggesting that a chronic disease self-management program can improve health status while reducing hospitalization: A randomized trial. *Medical Care, 37* (1), 5–14.

MacLachlan, M., & Carr, S. (1994). Managing the AIDS crisis in Africa: In support of pluralism. *Journal of Management in Medicine, 8,* 45–53.

Mansour, M. E., Lanphear, B. P., & DeWitt, T. G. (2000). Barriers to asthma care in urban children: Parent perspectives. *Pediatrics, 106,* 512–519.

Marston, M. (1970). Compliance with medical regimens: A review of the literature. *Nursing Research, 19,* 312–323.

Mason, B., Matsayuma, J., & Jue, S. (1995). Assessment of sulfonylurea adherence and metabolic control. *Diabetes Educator, 21,* 52–57.

McDonald, H. P., Garg, A. X. & Haynes, R. B. (2002). Interventions to enhance patient adherence to medication prescriptions: Scientific review. *JAMA, 288* (22), 2868–79.

McGlynn, E., Asch, S., Adams, J., Keesey, J., et al. (2003). The quality of health care delivered to adults in the United States. *New England Journal of Medicine, 348* (26), 2635–2645.

Meyer, D., Leventhal, H., & Gutmann, M. (1985). Common-sense models of illness: The example of hypertension. *Health Psychology, 4* (2), 115–35.

Miller, N. H., Hill, M., Kottke, T., & Okene, I. (1997). The multilevel compliance challenge: Recommendations for a call to action. A statement for healthcare professionals. *Circulation, 95,* 1085–1090.

Misselbrook, D. (1998). Managing the change from compliance to concordance. *Prescriber, 19,* 23–33.

Morisky, D. E., & Cabrera, D. M. (1997). Compliance with antituberculosis regimens and the role of behavioral interventions. In D. Gochman (Ed.), *Handbook of health behavior research II: Provider determinants.* New York: Plenum.

Mounier-Vehier, C., Bernaud, C., Carre, A., Lequeyche, B., et al. (1998). Compliance and antihypertensive efficacy of amlodipine compared with nifedipine slow-release. *American Journal of Hypertension, 11,* 478–486.

Munet-Villaro, F., & Vessey, J. A. (1990). Children's explanation of leukemia. *Journal of Pediatric Nursing, 5* (4), 274–282.

Murphy, K. G., Anderson, R. M., & Lyns, A. E. (1993). Diabetes educators as cultural translators. *The Diabetes Educator, 19* (2), 113–118.

Nelson, E. C., Stason, W. B., Neutra, R. R., Solomon, H. S., et al. (1978). Impact of patient compliance with treatment of hypertension. *Medical Care, 16,* 893–906.

Norman, P., Conner, M., & Bell, R. (1999). The theory of planned behavior and smoking cessation. *Health Psychology, 18,* 89–94.

Norman, P., & Smith, L. (1995). The theory of planned behaviour and exercise: An investigation into the role of prior behaviour, behavioural intentions and attitude variability. *European Journal of Social Psychology, 12,* 403–415.

Oberle, K. (1991). A decade of research in locus of control: What have we learned? *Journal of Advanced Nursing, 16* (7), 800–806.

O'Leary, M. R., Rohsenow, D. J., & Chaney, E. F. (1979). The use of multivariate personality strategies in predicting attrition from alcoholism treatment. *Journal of Clinical Psychiatry, 40,* 190–193.

Ott, J., Greening, L., Palardy, N., Holderby, A., et al. (2000). Self efficacy as a mediator variable for adolescents' adherence to treatment for insulin dependent diabetes mellitus. *Children's Health Care, 29,* 47–63.

Pablos-Mendez, A., Knirsch, C., Barr, R., Lerner, B., et al. (1997). Nonadherence in tuberculosis treatment: Predictors and consequences in New York City. *American Journal of Medicine, 102,* 164–170.

Parsons, T. (1951). *The social system.* New York: Free Press.

Pender, N. J. (1996). *Health promotion in nursing practice* (2nd ed.). Norwalk, CT: Appleton-Century-Crofts.

Perry, C. L., Baranowski, T., & Parcel, G. S. (1990). How individuals, environments, and health behavior interact: Social learning theory. In K. Glanz, F. Lewis, & B. Rimer (Eds.), *Health behavior and health education theory, research and practice.* San Francisco: Jossey-Bass.

Prochaska, J., & DiClemente, C. (1983). Stages and processes of self-change of smoking: Toward an integrative model of change. *Journal of Consulting & Clinical Psychology, 51,* 390–395.

Rand, C. S. (1993). Measuring adherence with therapy for chronic diseases: implications for the treatment of heterozygous familial hypercholesterolemia. *Am J Cardiol, 72* (10), 68D–74D.

Rand, C. S., & Sevick, M. A. (2000). Ethics in adherence promotion and monitoring. *Controlled Clinical Trials, 21* (5 Suppl), 241S–247S.

Rand, C. S., & Wise, R. A. (1994). Measuring adherence to asthma medication regimens. *American Review of Respiratory and Critical Care Medicine, 149,* 289–290.

Rapley, P. (1997). Self-care: Re-thinking the role of compliance. *Australian Journal of Advanced Nursing, 15,* 20–25.

Rosenstock, I. M. (1974). Historical origins of the health belief model. *Health Education Monographs, 2,* 354–386.

_____. (1988). Enhancing patient compliance with health recommendations. *Journal of Pediatric Health Care, 2,* 67–72.

Roter, D. L., Hall, J. A., Merisca, R., Nordstrom, B., et al. (1998). Effectiveness of interventions to improve patient compliance: A meta-analysis. *Medical Care, 36,* 1138–1161.

Rotter, J. B. (1966). Generalized expectancies for internal versus external control of reinforcement. *Psychological Monographs, 80,* 1–28.

Rudd, P., Ahmed, S., Zachary, V., Barton, C., et al. (1990). Improved compliance measures: Applications in an ambulatory hypertensive drug trial. *Clinical Pharmacology and Therapeutics, 48,* 676–685.

Sackett, D. L. (1976). Introduction. In D. L. Sackett & R. B. Haynes (Eds.), *Compliance with therapeutic regimens,* (pp. 1–6). Baltimore: Johns Hopkins University Press.

Sackett, D. L., & Snow, J. C. (1979). The magnitude of compliance and noncompliance. In R. B. Haynes, D. W. Taylor, & D. L. Sackett (Eds.), *Compliance in health care,* (pp. 11–22). Baltimore: Johns Hopkins University Press.

Schlenk E., & Dunbar-Jacob, J. (1996). Ethnic variations in adherence: A review. Unpublished manuscript.

Schmaling, K. B., Afari, A., & Blume, A. W. (2000). Assessment of psychological factors associated with adherence of medication regimens among adult patients with asthma. *Journal of Asthma, 37,* 335–343.

Schwarzer, R. (1992). Self-efficacy in the adoption and maintenance of health behaviors: Theoretical approaches and a new model. In R. Schwarzer (Ed.), *Self-efficacy: Thought control of action,* (pp. 217–243). Washington, DC: Hemisphere.

Schweizer, R., Rovelli, M., Palmeri, D., Vossler, E., et al. (1990). Noncompliance in organ transplant recipients. *Transplantation, 49,* 374–377.

Simmons, M. S., Nides, M. A., Rand, C. S., Wise, R. A., et al. (2000). Unpredictability of deception in compliance with physician-prescribed bronchodilator inhaler use in a clinical trial. *Chest, 118,* 290–295.

Spector, S. L. (1985). Is your asthmatic patient really complying? *Annals of Allergy, 55,* 552–556.

Steele, D. J., Jackson, T. C., & Gutmann, M. C. (1990). Have you been taking your pills? *The Journal of Family Practice, 30* (3), 294–299.

Stone, A., Shiffman, S., Schwartz, J., Broderick, J., et al. (2003). Patient compliance with paper and electronic diaries. *Controlled Clinical Trials, 24* (2), 182–199.

Straka, R., Fish, J., Benson, S., & Suh, J. (1997). Patient self-reporting of compliance does not correspond with electronic monitoring: An evaluation using isosorbide dinitrate as a model drug. *Pharmacotherapy, 17,* 126–132.

Strauss, A. L., Corbin, J., Fagerhaugh, S., Glaser, B., et al. (1984). *Chronic illness and the quality of life* (2nd ed.). St. Louis: Mosby.

Strzelczyk, J. J., & Dignan, M. B. (2002). Disparities in adherence to recommended followup on screening mammography: interaction of sociodemographic factors. *Ethnic Disparities, 12* (1), 77–86.

Talamantes, M., Lawler, W., & Espino, D. (1995). Hispanic American elders: Caregiving norms surrounding dying and the use of hospice services. *The Hospice Journal, 19,* 35–49.

Tashkin, D. P. (1995). Multiple dose regimens: Impact on compliance. *Chest, 107,* 176s–182s.

Thorne, S. E. (1990, October). Constructive noncompliance in chronic illness. *Holistic Nursing Practice, 5* (1), 62–69.

Thorne, S. E., Nyhlin, K. T., & Paterson, B. L. (2000). Attitudes toward patient expertise in chronic illness. *International Journal of Nursing Studies, 37,* 303–311.

Trostle, J. A. (1997). The history and meaning of patient compliance as an ideology. In David S. Gochman et al. (Eds.), *Handbook of health behavior research II: Provider determinants.* New York: Plenum Press.

Turner, J., Wright, E., Mendella, L., Anthonisen, N., et al. (1995). Predictors of patient adherence to long term home nebulizer therapy for COPD. *Chest, 108,* 394–400.

Tutty, S., Simon, G., & Ludman, E. (2000). Telephone counseling as an adjunct to antidepressant treatment in the primary care system: A pilot study. *Effective Clinical Practice, 3* (4), 170–178.

Ungvarski, S., & Schmidt, J. (1995). Nursing management of the adult. In J. Flaskerud & P. J. Ungvarski (Eds.), *HIV/AIDS: A guide to nursing care* (3rd ed.), (pp. 143–184). Philadelphia: WB Saunders.

van der Sande, M. A., Milligan, P. J., Nyan, O. A., Rowley, J. T., et al. (2000). Blood pressure patterns and cardiovascular risk factors in rural and urban gambian communities. *Journal of Human Hypertension, 14* (8), 489–496.

Vermeire, E., Hearnshaw, H., Van Royen, P., & Denekens, J. (2001). Patient adherence to treatment: three decades of research. A comprehensive review. *Journal of Clinical Pharmacological Therapy, 26* (5), 331–342.

Vik, S. A., Maxwell, C. J., & Hogan, D. B. (2004). Measurement, correlates, and health outcomes of medication adherence among seniors. *Annals of Pharmacotherapy, 38* (2), 303–312.

Wade, S. L., Islam, S., Holden, G., Kruszon-Moran, D., et al. (1999). Division of responsibility for asthma management tasks between caregivers and children in the inner city. *Journal of Developmental and Behavioral Pediatrics, 20,* 93–98.

Wagner, G. (2003). Placebo practice trials: the best predictor of adherence readiness for HAART among drug users? *HIV Clinical Trials, 4* (4), 269–281.

Wagner, G., & Rabkin, J. G. (2000). Measuring medication adherence: Are missed doses reported more accurately then perfect adherence? *AIDS Care, 12* (4), 405–408.

Wallston, B., Wallston, K., Kaplan, G., & Maides, S. (1976). Development and validation of the health care locus of control scale. *Journal of Consulting and Clinical Psychology, 44,* 580–585.

Wallston, K., Wallston, B., & DeVellis, R. (1978). Development of the multidimensional health locus of control (MHLC) scales. *Health Education Monograph, 6,* 160–170.

Weingarten, S. R., Henning, J. M., Badamgarav, E., Knight, K., et al. (2002). Interventions used in disease management programmes for patients with chronic illness–Which ones work? Meta-analysis of published reports. *British Medical Journal, 325* (7370), 925.

Weinstein, A. G., & Clesky, W. (1985). Theophylline compliance in asthmatic children. *Annals of Allergy, 54,* 19–24.

Welch, J. L. (2001). Hemodialysis patient beliefs by stage of fluid adherence. *Research in Nursing and Health, 24* (2), 105–112.

Wendel, C. S., Mohler, M. J., Kroesen, K., Ampel, N. M., et al. (2001). Barriers to use of electronic adherence monitoring in an HIV clinic. *Annals of Pharmacotherapy, 35* (9), 1010–1015.

Williams, M. V., Parker, R. M., Baker, D. W., Parikh, N. S., et al. (1995a). Inadequate functional health literacy among patients at two public hospitals. *JAMA, 274,* 1677–1682.

Williams, S., Weinman, J., Dale, J., & Newman, S. (1995b). Patient expectations: What do primary care patients want from the GP and how far does meeting expectations affect patient satisfaction. *Family Practice, 12,* 193–201.

Wing, R., Epstein, L., Nowal, M., & Lamparski, D. (1986). Behavioral self-regulation in the treatment of patients with diabetes mellitus. *Psychological Bulletin, 99,* 78–89.

Wong, M. D., Cunningham, W. E., Shapiro, M. F., Andersen, R. M., et al. (2004). Disparities in HIV treatment and physician attitudes about delaying protease inhibitors for nonadherent patients. *Journal of General Internal Medicine, 19* (4), 366–374.

World Health Organization. (2003). *Adherence to long-term therapies: Evidence for action.* Geneva, Switzerland: World Health Organization.

Zahr, L. K., Yazigi, A., & Armenian, H. (1989). The effect of education and written material on compliance of pediatric clients. *International Journal of Nursing Studies, 26* (3), 213–220.

Zuckerman, M., Gerra, L., Dorssman, D., Foland, J., et al. (1996). Health-care-seeking behaviors related to bowel complaints: Hispanics versus non-Hispanic whites. *Digestive Diseases and Sciences, 41,* 77–82.

CHAPTER 11

Family Caregivers

Tama L. Morris ▪ Lienne D. Edwards

Introduction

The term *unpaid caregiver* refers to a range of kin and nonkin individuals who provide both functional (task-oriented) and affective (emotional) unpaid assistance to a dependent person with whom a long-term or life-long commitment usually exists (Shirey & Summer, 2000). The family and friends who provide care may also be referred to as *informal caregivers* (Mittelman, 2003).

The decisions about caring for a family member with chronic illness are complex and multifaceted for the caregiver. Each choice they make has advantages and disadvantages, both for the chronically ill family member and the family itself. Healthcare professionals who assist families find that no two situations are alike. Each and every situation needs to be individualized to best meet the needs of the entire family. This chapter focuses on the multiple aspects of coping and decision making that family caregivers face, often on a daily basis.

Current Family Caregiving

The incidence of chronic illness in the United States is increasing. Nearly one third of young adults aged 18 to 44 suffer from a chronic condition (Shapiro, 2002). The number of elders over the age of 65 is projected to increase to 20.3% of the US population by the year 2050 (US Bureau of the Census, 2000). With advances in healthcare, the number of elders living with debilitating and/or chronic diseases is expected to grow (Williams, Dilworth-Anderson, & Goodwin, 2003).

At the other end of the age spectrum are the growing number of children with chronic illness and/or disabilities. Advances in neonatal care are now saving increasing numbers of preterm and low birthweight infants. According to a 2003 report from the National Center for Health Statistics, the percentage of low birthweight infants (born weighing less than 2,500 grams) increased to the highest level in more than 30 years. In addition, the percent of preterm births (infants born at less than 37 weeks of gestation) increased to 12 percent of live births. Low birthweight and prematurity both lead to an increased incidence of chronic health problems in the pediatric population.

The Department of Health and Human Services (DHHS) Administration on Aging (2003) reports that 22.4 million households are involved in providing care to persons aged 50 or older. This number is expected to increase to 39 million by the year 2007 with caregivers providing an average of 20 hours of care per week.

Preferences for Family Care

It is important to clarify that some dependent individuals will always need the level of care provided in institutional settings and that not all families are willing or able to provide care over the long term. However, for all but the most severely impaired individuals, most chronically ill, dependent persons have their long-term care needs met in home or with community-based care arrangements. Approximately two thirds of dependent persons in the community rely solely on informal caregivers (Mittelman, 2003). For these arrangements to work, family members, friends, or neighbors must play central roles in long-term plans of care.

The decision about where and how to provide care for family members with chronic illness is emotionally charged and multifaceted. Home based care is financially cost effective for the health care system. However, the reliance on family members as care providers creates multiple stressors for the family (Hunt, 2003). When formal assistance is required, married persons prefer help in the home regardless of the level of disability of the care recipient; however, financial difficulty and the strain of extended caregiving often lead family caregivers to decisions for institutionalized care (Keysor, Desai, & Mutran, 1999).

Characteristics of Family Caregivers

Today, the title "family caregiver" extends beyond the traditional family boundaries. A "caregiver" is defined as anyone who provides assistance to another in need. The "informal caregiver" is anyone who provides care without pay and who usually has personal ties to the care recipient. The "family caregiver" is a term used interchangeably with the informal caregiver and can include family, friends or neighbors (DHHS Administration on Aging, n.d.c). "Caregiver coalition" is a term used to describe the addition of a support person or persons in traditional relationships when the caregiver/recipient arrangement is no longer sufficient (Haigler, Bauer, & Travis, 2004).

Motivations for caregiving, such as love, duty, or obligation, strongly influence a caregiver's willingness to accept primary caregiving status (Neufeld & Harrison, 1998). Additional reasons family caregivers report accepting their role are their expectations of themselves and others, religious training and spiritual experiences and role modeling (Piercy & Chapman, 2001).

Caregiver Dyads and Caregiver Systems

Early caregiving research identified caregiving dyads that are comprised of a care recipient and a caregiver with primary responsibility for the care and well-being of the care recipient. Caregivers today are most often part of caregiving systems or helping networks, consisting of many caregivers, rather than caregiving dyads (Weitzner, Haley, & Chen, 2000). For example, the helping networks that widowed and never-married individuals call on for assistance are often larger than those of married people (Barrett & Lynch, 1999). Therefore, many people now occupy positions as caregivers, especially in long-term care arrangements.

Because caregivers have varying degrees of responsibility for providing or arranging for care, the terms *care provider* and *care manager* are used to differentiate two types of caregivers (Stoller & Culter, 1993). This designation helps to clarify the previously invisible contributions of all family caregivers. If a son is close to his dependent parents, especially if he is not married, he is likely to be accountable for seeing that things get done, even if he does not provide all of the direct care that is required (Allen, Goldscheider, & Ciambrone, 1999; Keith, 1995; Thompson, Tudiver, & Manson, 2000). Similarly, an adult grandchild may help a grandparent in the absence of a nearby adult child, or children-in-law may find their relationships to relatives with chronic illness make them better suited to caregiving roles than the biological children (Peters-Davis, Moss, & Pruchno, 1999; Travis & Bethea, 2001).

Changes in the modern family social structure have resulted in more young parents working outside the home. Therefore this "sandwich generation" is often not available to provide care for family members. This has created a new level of caregivers—children and adolescents. These young caregivers assist with or even assume care of adults with chronic illness in their homes (Lackey & Gates, 2001).

Racial and Ethnic Diversity

The family caregiving experience is also shaped by race and ethnicity. These two factors influence one's life experiences in terms of socioeconomic status, education, marital status, health, living arrangements, and general life-style (Binstock, 1999). In chronic illness, access to programs and services and preferences for certain types of assistance are often sharply divided along racial and ethnic lines. The number of minority older adults is increasing at a faster rate than that of the Caucasian, non-Hispanic population, with the largest proportionate increases projected in the over 75-years group. While the number of African American elderly will increase slightly in the next 50 years, proportionately larger and more rapid increases will occur among Hispanic and Asian elders (Tripp-Reimer, 1999).

Comparative research indicates that patterns of family response to a family member with a chronic illness may be significantly different across ethnic groups (Chesla & Rungreangkulkij, 2001). Gerontological researchers are building a substantial body of literature on African American, Asian American, Native American, and Hispanic elders and their family caregiving experiences and preferences for support. Because this literature is extensive, only one example of diversity is provided to illustrate ethnic influences.

African American caregiving is shaped by cultural precedence, historical events, and the needs of extended kin and family structure. Documented barriers to formal programs and services include poverty and economic disparity, lower educational levels, ageism, and racial discrimination (Jones, 1999). As a result, persistent underutilization of formal assistance programs and a reliance on family and friends are typical patterns of long-term care for dependent African American elders (Cox, 1999).

While it is known that African American families have a strong sense of respect, duty, and obligation to elderly members of their communities, it may also be the case that generations have learned to be self- and family-reliant in the face of both overt and covert forms of racial discrimination (Binstock, 1999; Edmonds, 1999). As a result of this self-reliance, African American family caregivers, especially women, may be perceived to have a lower level of role strain than their white counterparts. Research demonstrates a large variation in the female African American caregiver's perception of role strain (Williams et al., 2003).

Gender Differences

The choice of who becomes the primary caregiver and what the family caregiving system looks like depends on many factors. In a spousal relationship, the unaffected spouse usually assumes the caregiving role. Often, both spouses are forced to cope with role reversal in addition to their new roles as the giver and receiver of care (Gordon & Perrone, 2004).

Among married adult children, daughters or daughters-in-law are most often the primary caregivers for aging parents (Shirey & Summer, 2000). Daughters are more likely to offer assistance to their father who is serving in a caregiving role than their mother. This may be because they are more comfortable with their mother in that role and feel that their father needs additional assistance performing the tasks required of a caregiver (Mittelman, 2003). Because the majority of elders who require assistance are women who have outlived their husbands, this partially accounts for the predominance of daughters as caregivers (Lee, Dwyer & Coward, 1993). It is also the case that caregiving is largely thought of as "women's work," because many of the needs of dependent persons are met by the "caring labor" that is most often done by women in families (Walker & Pratt, 1995). Therefore, in the majority of caregiving arrangements, it is a wife, mother, or adult daughter who is designated as the primary caregiver. The gendered nature of caregiving is certainly one important characteristic of long-term caregiving that is likely to continue in the future (Keysor et al., 1999; Walker & Pratt, 1995). All things being equal, the person who is closest to and the most involved in the daily life of the dependent person is usually the person most accountable for either doing or seeing that care is done.

Types of Care Provided by Family Caregivers

Over the long-term, a dependent person requires two types of care: social care and health-related care. Social care includes both *functional* and *affective assistance* in daily living while health-related care refers to specialized care by professionals and daily treatments that are done by family caregivers, such as medication administration.

Functional assistance is determined by the care recipient's ability to perform various tasks of daily existence, which are categorized as either instrumental or basic activities of daily living. *Instrumental activities of daily living* (IADLs) are the functions an adult would be expected to perform in the process of everyday life, including cooking, cleaning, buying groceries, doing yard work, and paying bills. For a child, these tasks might include getting to school, playing, or cleaning his or her room. *Basic activities of daily living* (ADLs) are the tasks required for personal care and basic survival. These tasks include eating, bathing, dressing, going to the bathroom, maintaining personal hygiene, and getting around (mobility).

Affective assistance, also called emotional support, includes behaviors that convey caring and concern to the care recipient. Affective assistance is most often linked with enhanced feelings of self esteem, contentment, life satisfaction, hope of recovery, dignity, and general well-being (Brody & Schoonover, 1986; Horowitz, 1985).

In the past, there was a somewhat clearer division between the formal and informal care network. The informal network, family caregivers or significant others, provided both emotional and functional aspects of care and monitored the care provided by formal providers. The formal network provided specialized care that was highly task-oriented and goal-directed. Today the roles of the formal and informal network reveal a more blended approach to caregiving. Family caregivers perform highly skilled tasks formerly reserved for the professional. Professional caregivers function as a team with the family in care decisions for the client (Haigler et al., 2004).

Caregiving Histories and Maturation over Time

Longitudinal studies of family caregiving have documented the many changes that occur in the role of family caregiver and note that family caregiving is not a static event. Pearlin (1992) equated caregiving to career development. There are two factors that contribute to this notion of a caregiving career or caregiving history: maturation of the caregiver over time, and ongoing role development associated with the inevitable transitions in care over the long term.

The expectations of the family caregiver are many. They often begin their roles with little or no training or support. In addition to the psychological aspects of caregiving, they are expected to provide competent, skilled healthcare for their loved ones (Elliot & Shewchuk, 2003). Most caregivers begin their experiences as novices with little or no experience or knowledge of how to navigate the long-term care system (McAuley, Travis, & Safewright, 1997; Skaff, Pearlin & Mullan, 1996). Over time, mature caregivers master a new language system of entitlements (Medicare, Medicaid) and treatments (medication administration, illness symptomatology), and learn how to incorporate the needs of a dependent person into their daily lives (Leavitt et al., 1999). Some caregivers mature more quickly and with greater ease than others, and some caregivers are never able to achieve adequate skill and/or confidence in the caregiver role. Thus, tremendous variability can be found in the levels, lengths, and forms of care provided by family caregivers, which are at least partially attributed to successful mastery of their roles (Seltzer & Wailing, 2000).

Transitions in care occur at three points: entry into a caregiving relationship, institutionalization (or transitions into other formal care arrangements), and bereavement (Seltzer & Wailing, 2000). Unlike acute or episodic care that has an end-point, the only natural end to long-term care is the death of the care recipient. Even families that ultimately opt for institutional placement of their dependent family members do not abandon their relatives over the long term. Most caregivers stay engaged as care managers following the institutional placement decision (Seltzer & Wailing, 2000).

Montgomery and Kosloski (n.d.) have identified a similar concept called a *caregiving trajectory*. Their seven markers of caregiving are: (1) performance of initial caregiving task; (2) self-definition as a caregiver; (3) provision of personal care; (4) seeking out or using assistive services; (5) consideration of institutionalization; (6) actual nursing home placement and (7) termination of the caregiver role. In this trajectory, Montgomery and Kosloski believe that the order and timing of the markers are indicative of the individual, culture and relationship of the caregiver to the care recipient.

One of the reasons why family caregiving that is precipitated by acute hospitalization is so stressful for new caregivers is that they have not had a period of maturation and development prior to the intense caregiving demands and the decision-making requirements that follow (Kane, Reinardy & Penrod, 1999). In addition, the transitions in care occur rapidly and over a highly compressed period of time. In a few days the caregiver may transition from having no care responsibilities to being fully engaged in post hospital rehabilitation, home or institutional long-term care (Kane et al., 1999).

Positive Aspects of Caregiving

In the past, research on stress, strain, burden, and burnout has overshadowed the positive aspects of providing care to a dependent family member. As a result, less is understood about how and why caregivers do as they do under difficult circumstances (Farran, 1997). Today the literature demonstrates an increased emphasis on the positive aspects of caregiving. In Kramer's (1997) review of research on

positive aspects of caregiving, it was noted that some caregivers experience *gain* when assisting others. Gain was conceptualized as "the extent to which the caregiving role is appraised to enhance an individual's life space and be enriching" (p. 219).

Caregivers report satisfaction with their role. Adults who functioned as caregivers during their childhood have reported that their participation taught them responsibility, allowed them to be 'part of the family', provided opportunities to be 'appreciated' and 'useful.' They also reported pride at learning skills at an early age (Lackey & Gates, 2001). Many couples feel that caring for their partner strengthened their relationship (Gordon & Perrone, 2004).

The understanding of what specific factors influence satisfaction in a caregiving experience is not clear at present. There are some indications that the quality of the prior relationship with the care recipient, the care recipient's degree of impairment, and relationship-focused coping strategies by caregivers may create a positive response to caregiving (Kramer, 1993a, 1993b). Additionally, caregiver motivations for helping and caregiver ideology have been associated with caregiver satisfaction (Lawton, Rajagopal, Brody, & Kleban, 1992). Family style, including receptivity has been suggested as an area for future study (Gilliss, 2002). Longitudinal research and research with caregivers in diverse arrangements are needed to provide a more comprehensive view of what contributes to a positive caregiving experience.

Future Caregiving

Looking to the future, it is likely that the next cohort of older adult Baby Boomers will be very different from their parents and grandparents and will further confound the current reliance on family caregivers. Divorce rates have soared and fertility rates have declined dramatically during the lifetimes of adult Baby Boomers (Dwyer, 1995). Parents of the Baby Boom generation have several children from whom to seek assistance, while elder Baby Boomers with smaller families will not be so fortunate. It remains to be seen what this societal trend will mean to this cohort.

The H. Family

Mrs. H. had coronary artery disease and congestive heart failure that caused increasing fatigue, dyspnea, and angina over a 5-year period. Frequent upper respiratory infections exacerbated her dyspnea.

Home Setting: Mrs. H. lived at home with her husband in a small rural town, in a home they had owned since their children were small. Mr. H. was four years younger than his wife.

Role Issues: Mr. H. assumed cooking tasks in the home and was the primary caregiver for his wife, assisting her to ambulate to the bathroom for toileting and bathing, making sure her clothes were clean and accessible, and making sure she took her medicine as prescribed.

Support: The H.s' married daughter and married son lived within a ten-minute drive of their parents' house. Both had children of their own, but assisted their parents at least once a week. The daughter did the major housecleaning for her parents, and drove them regularly to the grocery store,

the frequent doctor's visits, and the pharmacy. The son assisted his father with lawn work and household repairs; he was also called upon in cases of medical emergency to be the decision maker.

Transitions: Over several years, Mrs. H.'s health declined. Her upstairs bedroom became inaccessible, because stair climbing became exhausting. The living room was converted to her bedroom. She was hospitalized for a series of short-term stays for complaints of chest pain and/or difficulty breathing over this time span. Whenever she was hospitalized, the daughter and son took turns driving their father to the hospital, because he visited their mother daily.

During the next five years, these hospitalizations increased in frequency to several times yearly. She used portable oxygen at home. Initially it was only used for brief intervals during the night, and she was able to accompany her daughter for brief shopping trips or drives "to get out of

In the future, racial caregiving trends are likely to escalate. In particular, African American and Hispanic caregivers will be more available for long-term caregiving than will Caucasian caregivers. Furthermore, Caucasian caregivers are expected to purchase more services for dependent family members (Shirey & Summer, 2000). Most researchers agree, however, that any predictions about family caregiving in the future are tenuous because public policy is difficult to predict from one generation to the next. That policy will need to change to accommodate the caregiving needs of the aging Baby Boom cohort is the only certainty.

Problems and Issues

Family caregivers face multiple problems, issues, and concerns throughout their caregiving experiences. The case study of the H. family is typical of the effort most family caregivers put into fulfilling their responsibilities, attending to the wants and needs of the care recipient, and continuously adjusting their lives to the physical and emotional requirements of the caregiving situation.

Family caregiving experiences incorporate societal values and are shaped by governmental policy. Policies that affect family caregiving in the United the house." As her health declined, Mrs. H. used the oxygen continuously, remaining in her room. The family got a "medi-alert" call button that Mrs. H. always wore in case she needed emergency help.

With each hospitalization, Mrs. H. returned home weaker. Mr. H. began to worry that he could no longer care for his wife at home because of her increasing weakness. He moved her commode adjacent to her wheelchair; even so, Mrs. H. had difficulty transferring from her chair to the commode. Mrs. H. was heavier than her husband; he worried about her safety, fearing that she might fall and injure herself and he would be unable to assist her. The daughter had a part-time job, but visited her parents more frequently, twice weekly. She began to express concerns about both parents' health to her brother, her friends, and her husband.

Decisions: When Mrs. H. was hospitalized at the age of 78 for chest pain and difficulty breathing, the physician approached Mr. H. and his son and daughter with a request that they sign a Do Not Resuscitate (DNR) agreement. Mrs. H. had vehemently expressed, "I don't want them damn machines," so the family readily agreed to the DNR order. They were concerned for Mrs. H. because the DNR had never been brought up by the doctor before.

Mr. H. told his children that Mrs. H. would have to go to a nursing home when she was discharged from the hospital, as he could no longer care for her with her severely diminished abilities. Although the family discussed this problem, they did not resolve it. After visiting Mrs. H. one evening at the hospital, during which time she was alert and talkative, the family returned to their homes. That evening Mrs. H. died. The family expressed relief that her suffering was over, that she died the way she wanted to, without machines They were also relieved that the whole family did not have to struggle with the nursing home decision.

States have been created with the presumption that families are responsible for caring for their disabled members and will provide the majority of the care that is needed (Montgomery, 1999). For many years, these expectations were consistent with caregivers' resources and abilities.

Over the past decade, however, there has been a blurring of the lines of responsibility for long-term caregiving. Increased technology, greater acuity of those in need of assistance, and competing demands on available caregivers have created an imbalance between the demand for family care and the ability of family caregivers to provide care. Family caregivers are being asked to provide highly technical treatments; administer complex medication regimens; provide labor-intensive, hands-on care; and monitor the medical conditions of very ill family members.

The one responsibility that has remained constant over time, whether the family caregiver is a direct care provider or arranges care as a care manager, is the extensive decision-making demands placed on family caregivers. When the dependent family member cannot make decisions or has difficulty communicating choices, the responsibility for countless decisions associated with managing daily life falls to the caregiver. These decisions include the initiation, timing, and provision of assistance from informal and formal sources; integration of caregiving demands into work and family life, and planning for future long-term care needs (McAuley et al., 1997; Travis & Bethea, 2001).

The Influence of Public Policy on Family Caregiving

Containing the rising costs of health care services has become a national policy imperative. This goal is demonstrated through policies that promote prevention of premature or unwanted institutionalization of disabled elders in nursing homes, limit publicly funded home care services to individuals with the lowest incomes, and curtail the Medicare home health benefit. Such policies limit the amount and scope of services that are provided to persons who need ongoing assistance by formal caregivers as well as their family caregivers. Recent cost containment measures are occurring precisely when the demand for help in providing long-term care at home is increasing (Montgomery, 1999). These changes in government-sponsored services mean that many families, particularly low- and middle-income families, are faced with difficult choices about providing assistance while receiving minimal help from professional health care providers.

Several government initiatives have attempted to address the needs of family caregivers. In 1993, the Family and Medical Leave Act (FMLA) became law. This Act gives qualified caregivers the option of taking up to 12 weeks of unpaid leave from their jobs to care for a family member (U.S. Department of Labor, 1993). However, use of this benefit has been low, with only seven percent of those taking such leaves labeling them as pertinent to the FMLA (Scharlach & Grosswald, 1997). Most caregivers, who qualified for but did not use the FMLA, declined it on their inability to afford unpaid leave.

The Older Americans Act Amendments of 2000 established the National Family Caregiver Support Program (NFCSP). Federal funds are given to states based upon their proportionate share of the 70+ population. States, working in partnership with local agencies on aging and faith and community-service providers and tribes, offer five direct services to best meet the range of caregiver needs. The services include the provision of:

1. Information to caregivers about available services;
2. Assistance to caregivers in gaining access to supportive services;
3. Individual counseling, organization of support groups and caregiver training to assist caregivers in making decisions and solving problems relating to their roles;
4. Respite care to enable caregivers to be temporarily relieved from their caregiving responsibilities; and
5. Supplemental services, on a limited basis, to complement the care provided by caregivers.

Family caregivers eligible for the NFCSP are those who care for adults age 60 years or more and grandparents and relatives of children not more than 18 years of age, including grandparents who are sole caregivers of grandchildren and those individuals who are affected by mental retardation or have developmental disabilities. Priority is given to caregivers with social and economic need, particularly low-income and minority individuals, or older individuals providing care and support to persons with mental retardation and related developmental disabilities (DHHS Administration on Aging, n.d.a)

The lack of adequate monetary assistance for the family unit is a complex problem. Currently, there is no public financing of long-term care in a home setting, except for hospice programs with a time-limited period at the end of life. Many private insurers offer long-term care policies through employers, fraternal organizations, retirement communities, and health management organizations. Unfortunately, in the past, most of these policies did not cover many aspects of the personal care provided by family caregivers, leaving this in-home care as out-of-pocket expenses. Long-term care policies now on the market are more comprehensive.

Recently, individual states were authorized to craft their own programs to provide paid leave to workers who need to care for family members. The Clinton administration proposed relief to families in the form of a $1,000 annual tax credit for those receiving or providing long-term care in the home, but the proposal generated controversy among legislators. Many believed that government intervention would discourage people from purchasing long-term care insurance to cover nursing home care and health care services in the home (DuPont, 1999). The issue of the government's role in assisting caregivers remains a strongly debated one.

Emotional Effects of Being a Caregiver

Although not all persons experience stress when providing care, many do. There are a number of factors that influence caregiving and the stress it may cause. Factors include: the intensity of the care provided; types of care tasks performed; gender; personal characteristics of the caregiver; the relationship between the caregiver and the person receiving care; support from other family members; and competing obligations of the caregiver. Research on caregiver stress spans more than two decades, and researchers have labeled caregiver stress as either *strain* or *burden.*

Strain or Burden

Strain refers to "the extent to which the caregiving role is judged to infringe upon an individual's life space and be oppressive" (Montgomery, 1989, p. 204). Caregiver strain and burden are multidimensional concepts that include both subjective perceptions of caregivers, such as role overload; and objective factors, such as aggressive behavior of the care recipient. Factors reported by caregivers to cause higher levels of strain are when they perceive the patient to be manipulative, unappreciative or unreasonable (Nerenberg, 2002).

Burden is defined relative to the level of the care recipient's disability and the extent of care required.

According to this definition, as the level of disability increases, more care is required. Therefore, the caregiver will perceive a higher level of burden (Nerenberg, 2002).

One area of caregiver research that has focused heavily on caregiver strain is dementia care. In particular, it is known that caregiving is more stressful and produces more emotional and physical strain when the caregiver is caring for a person with dementia or Alzheimer's disease. These so-called dementia caregivers are more likely than non-dementia caregivers to say that they suffer mental or physical problems as a result of caregiving (Ory, Hoffman, Yee, Tennstedt, & Schulz, 1999).

Higher levels of depression have been found among dementia caregivers who cared for persons with moderate to severe functional impairment and greater amounts of behavioral disturbance (wandering and aggression) than among non-dementia caregivers (Meshefedjian, McCusker, Bellavance & Baumgarten, 1998). When caregivers' appraisals of the burden of caregiving are high, there is greater likelihood of caregiver depression and depressive symptoms (Clyburn, Stones, Hadjistavropoulos, & Tuokko, 2000). In fact, recent research reported that about 35 to 40 percent of dementia caregivers were at risk for developing a depressive disorder (Alspaugh, Stephens, Townsend, Zarit, & Greene, 1999). In addition to psychiatric disorders, caregiving is a risk factor for mortality in some dementia caregivers. One study reported that among spousal caregivers experiencing strain, there was a 63 percent higher mortality risk for family caregivers during a four-year period than among non-caregivers (Schulz & Beach, 1999).

There also appears to be a gender component associated with caregiver burden. Female caregivers experience more psychiatric disorders than do male caregivers (Yee & Schulz, 2000), and are much more likely than men to report being depressed or anxious and to experience lower levels of life satisfaction. The irony is that, while they report more caregiver burden, role conflict, or strain, women are more likely than are male caregivers to continue caregiving responsibilities over the long term. Women are less likely than men to obtain assistance from others with caregiving. Finally, women are less likely than men to engage in preventative health behaviors while caregiving, such as rest, exercise, and taking medications as prescribed (Burton, Newsom, Schulz, Hirsch & German, 1997).

Caregivers for spouses have reported a higher incidence of depression and stress than those caring for a disabled parent. The caregiving roles and responsibilities may have a major impact on the relationship itself. Health care professionals must realize that the relationship between the caregiver and the spouse receiving the care needs to be supported and nurtured in terms of love, affection and intimacy (Gordon & Perrone, 2004).

Children and adolescents who have functioned in the role of caregiver report difficulty watching their loved one progress with a chronic problem. They have memories of unpleasant smells and sights. They also report feeling helpless due to their lack of knowledge and fear that they would not be able to deal with a crisis (Lackey & Gates, 2001).

Burned Out and Giving Up

Burnout has been defined as a "state of physical, emotional, and mental exhaustion caused by long-term involvement in emotionally demanding situations" (Pines & Aronson, 1988, p. 9). For the caregiver, the term burnout can be used to describe exhaustion. This may be physical, emotional or mental exhaustion (Nerenberg, 2002).

Figley (1998) developed a model of burnout that explains caregiver and caregiver family situations quite well. In his model, burnout begins with a caregiver's stress response, i.e., *compassion stress,* which refers to "the stress connected with exposure to a sufferer" (Figley, 1998, p. 21). In this case, the sufferer is the care recipient. When compassion stress is accompanied by *prolonged exposure to the suffering* and/or *unresolved trauma, compassion fatigue* sets in. Compassion fatigue can also be exacerbated by a substantial *degree of life disruption.* These factors lead to caregiver burnout, which may be dealt with by placing the care recipient in an institution, having another family member assume primary

caregiver duties, or, in some cases, neglect or abuse of the care recipient. Parents caring for children with severe developmental disabilities or others caring for individuals with Alzheimer's disease are especially at risk for burnout due to prolonged exposure and high levels of life disruption.

Family Relationships When Long-Term Caregiving Is Required

Providing care to others, especially spouses and parents, often requires changes in the ways that family members interact with each other. For the care provider, this decision may be a life-long commitment to another family member (Elliot & Shewchuk, 2003).

Some researchers have called the changes in families "role reversal," and note that it can take many forms. For example, wives providing care to husbands are often required to make financial decisions or perform tasks to maintain their homes that have always been their husbands' responsibility. Adult children often speak of becoming "parents" to their frail parents. While most family caregivers handle these role changes over time, some caregivers struggle with changes in their family relationships (Brody, 1990; Harris, 1998).

There are some researchers who argue that the term *role reversal* is inaccurate and inadequate for describing family relationships in late life (Brody, 1990; Seltzer, 1990). They view the use of the term *role reversal* as a simplistic way of viewing a complex phenomenon and express concern that it reinforces negative stereotypes of dependency in general and old age in particular. If being a parent, child, or spouse is a social position in a family, these positions do not change during the lifetime of the family. A parent is always a parent. A spouse is always a spouse. While behaviors toward each other may change as health or functioning decline, the roles remain stable.

Support for this argument was offered in a study of adult child caregivers that found adult child caregivers respected traditional parental autonomy for as long as possible (Piercy, 1998). The caregivers in this study described sensitivity to the parents' wishes, even when they disagreed with the parent, and well beyond the point at which the parent experienced significant cognitive or physical decline.

Contradicting previous research, Lackey and Gates' (2001) found that child caregivers who provide care to their parents at times perceived a reversal of roles. When caring for a parent, children reported serving as the support person and confidant of the parent. In addition to the changed family dynamics, the child caregivers reported a pronounced effect on their school life and their friendships.

Elder Abuse and Neglect

The 2000 Survey of State Adult Protective Services stated there were 472,813 reported cases of elder or vulnerable adult abuse. For substantiated reports, the most common environment for abuse was in domestic settings. The typical abuser was a male between the ages of 26 and 50. Almost 62% of the perpetrators were family members (spouse, parents, children, grandchildren, siblings and other family members). The family member/perpetrator with the highest incidence of perpetration was the spouse or intimate partner, followed by an adult child (Teaster, 2003). Even with the impact of these statistics, one must realize that it is likely that the majority of elder or vulnerable adult abuses go unreported.

The DHHS Administration on Aging (n.d.d) defines the following types of abuse and neglect: physical, sexual, psychological, financial or material exploitation and neglect. *Physical abuse* is defined as the willful infliction of physical pain or injury. Examples of this are slapping, bruising, sexually molesting or restraining. *Sexual abuse* is the infliction of non-consensual sexual contact of any kind. *Psychological abuse* is infliction of mental or emotional anguish. Examples of psychological abuse are humiliating, intimidating or threatening. *Neglect* is the failure of a caretaker to provide goods or services necessary to avoid physical harm, mental anguish or mental illness. Examples of neglect include abandonment, denial of food or denial of health-related services.

It is important for healthcare professionals to recognize the precipitating factors for caregiver abuse of an elder. There appears to be a strong link between the likelihood for abuse and the caregiver's perception of their situation. Caregivers who have had a positive relationship with care recipients are less likely to become abusive. In certain situations, the risk of abuse increased in direct relationship to the amount of care required. The personality characteristics and behaviors of the care recipient have also been indicated in relationship to the caregiver's stress level. And finally, an abusive incident may be triggered by the use of alcohol, substance abuse or psychiatric illness (Nerenberg, 2002).

Although it is more common to think about the potential abuse of a dependent person by a family caregiver, it is also possible that a caregiver may be the victim of an abusive care recipient. Patterns of dysfunctional behavior in families can extend over decades. If a wife was abused by her husband before he became ill or dependent on her for assistance, there is no reason to believe that he would suddenly discontinue all forms of abusive behavior because of illness.

Family caregivers, especially women, who never know about the family finances and must always ask the care recipient or other family members for money, or who rely solely on the care recipients' families for other types of assistance, may be very vulnerable to neglect. In addition, self-neglect, behavior that threatens a person's own health or safety, can be an adverse consequence of profound caregiving stress and associated depression. Self-neglect usually manifests as refusal to provide oneself with adequate food, water, clothing, and shelter.

Excessive Caregiving

Although a very subjective notion, providing excessive care to an impaired adult occurs in some caregiving situations. One form of excessive care is assistance that puts the caregiver's physical or emotional health at risk. Excessive care may have deleterious effects on the health of spouse caregivers, as documented in the Caregiver Health Effects Study

(Schultz & Beach, 1999), in which persons who felt burdened while providing long-term care for demented spouses had a high risk of mortality over a four-year period.

Given and colleagues (1990) found that spouse caregivers who experienced a combination of negative care recipient behaviors, such as cognitive impairment and antisocial behaviors, were more likely to feel higher levels of responsibility and react negatively to the caregiver role than did persons caring for spouses not exhibiting such behaviors. Despite negative responses to the caregiver role, the greater levels of responsibility felt by these spouses may contribute to the provision of excessive care and the caregivers' rejection of or failure to take advantage of respite care opportunities.

A second type of excessive care occurs when caregivers assume responsibilities or perform tasks for their care recipients that they are capable of performing themselves. For example, a caregiver recently informed of her parent's heart disease may react by taking over responsibilities, such as paying bills or cooking, that her parent can still perform adequately. Such excessive care can rob parents of feelings of autonomy that may be beneficial to their health and emotional well-being. Caregiving is a delicate balance of providing for the care recipient's safety while preserving their autonomy to the fullest extent possible (Piercy, 1998). Albert and Brody (1996) found that greater feelings of burden on the part of caregivers were associated with viewing parent care as child care. These burdened caregivers also were less likely to encourage parental autonomy. Such findings suggest that promotion of care recipient autonomy to the greatest extent possible for as long as possible may be beneficial for both caregiver and care recipient.

Financial Impact of Caregiving

Caregiving has different degrees of financial impact on families, depending on their particular caregiving situations and financial resources. For elderly couples with a spouse as caregiver, the impact may range from minimal to considerable, depending on the extent to which other family help is available and formal services are used and how they are financed. For families of frail elderly relatives, reduced employment is most likely to occur when the caregivers are of ethnic minorities and for patients with specific clinical characteristics (Covinsky et al., 2001). When adult children are the caregivers, the picture becomes murky because it is the financial resources of the care recipient that are usually considered for public assistance.

The current public financing system for in-home and community-based services targets persons with the lowest incomes. Well-off family caregivers can afford to pay for home or community-based care out of pocket, regardless of the financial eligibility of the care recipient. However, families in the middle ranges of income may be unable to purchase in-home services or receive public financing for needed care. White-Means (1997) found that care recipients who were within 150 to 250 percent of established poverty levels and who were not receiving the Medicare home health benefit or state-financed programs were less likely to use in-home services than were individuals in other income ranges. In other words, these low-income care recipients were not financially eligible for assistance, nor were their family caregivers able to purchase services for them.

The cost of caregiving is associated with the level of need for the affected individual. Langa and colleagues (2001) estimated that the annual cost associated with the informal care of an elderly person with dementia was "$3,630 for mild dementia and up to $17,700 for severe dementia" (p. 774). In addition to overt costs, caregivers spend an average of 11% out-of-pocket for services not covered by Medicare (DHHS Administration of Aging, 2003b).

Research shows that relatively few adult children contribute financially to parent care; only 5 to 10 percent of adult children transfer money to parents in a year's time (Boaz, Hu & Ye, 1999). These "financial caregivers" tend to have higher levels of asset income and proportionally more women engaged in the paid labor force full time than those who do not offer any financial assistance to dependent parents. Furthermore, financial help almost always goes to single parents (usually widowed mothers) and for caregiving situations that require extensive personal assistance.

Employment

In the mid-1980s, the first national study of its kind revealed the shocking effects that being a caregiver had on the nation's workforce. About 14 percent of caregiver wives, 12 percent of daughters, 11 percent of husbands, and five percent of sons quit their jobs to care for elderly relatives. Of employed caregivers, 29 percent rearranged their work schedules, 21 percent reduced work hours, and 19 percent took time off without pay (Stone, Cafferata & Sangl, 1987). A second national survey of caregivers found that 34 percent lost time from work because of caregiving demands (Opinion Research Corporation, 1988).

Employees most in need of support are those who function as primary caregivers and those who care for elders with high care needs (Stone & Short, 1990). Being female, Caucasian, and in fair to poor health increased the caregiver's likelihood of needing some assistance to accommodate work and caregiving demands. There is also evidence to suggest that caregivers who have lower amounts of education and those less likely to view their work as a career are more likely than others to decide to leave paid employment altogether. Dautzenberg (2000) found that the nearest living daughter with the least competing demands was most vulnerable to being called upon for caregiving duties.

Clearly, there are hidden costs, both economic and non-economic, of informal care to older adults receiving care, their caregivers, and to other family members (Fast, Williamson & Keating, 1999). Unfortunately, these costs frequently are ignored by policy makers focused primarily on cost containment of services. The emotional well-being of the care recipient, who struggles with conflicting issues of dependency and burden to the family, and the emotional well-being of the family caregiver, who struggles with loss of control and independence in his or her daily life, can become very tenuous in

these situations (Pyke, 1999). The most dramatic economic costs to caregivers include giving up paid employment, lost income from unpaid leave or time off work, relinquishment of career advancement opportunities, and the prospect of out-of-pocket expenses to support home care. Employers need to consider flexible options to help the caregiver/employee meet the demands of their multiple roles.

■ Interventions

The Interface of Informal and Formal Caregiving Networks

The interface of a formal caregiving network with the family caregiver is important for the long-term emotional and physical health of the family caregiver. There are several diverse models currently in use to explain the ways in which informal and formal caregiving networks exist over the long term.

Dual Specialization Model. One model that is particularly useful for studying the shared care between formal and informal networks is the dual specialization or complementary model (Litwak, 1985). The model is based on the notion that formal and informal networks have certain kinds of caregiving responsibilities and abilities that are best suited to each particular network. Because of this specialized division of labor, there is the potential for friction and conflict among caregivers. Therefore, the networks work best when the amount of contact or level of involvement between them is minimized, and the groups perform only those tasks for which they are best suited.

This conceptualization of a clear division of labor worked well until the early 1990s when, as already described, highly technical aspects of care were expected of family caregivers. With a new emphasis on family caregivers receiving support and empowerment from formal providers to become competent caregivers, a somewhat less restrictive interpretation of the complementary model is required today. Still, the model is useful for thinking about potential stress and tension that family caregivers may feel toward formal caregivers.

Family Empowerment Model. A model that more appropriately reflects the current emphasis on support of the family caregivers and the inclusion of those caregivers as members of the care planning team is the Family Empowerment Model (see Figure 11-1). Families with members who have chronic health conditions, especially if those members are children, often feel a sense of powerlessness in satisfying the health care needs of that family member and in sustaining family life (Hulme, 1999). The Family Empowerment Model depicts an interactive intervention process that consists of phases corresponding to the amount of trust and decision making that a family shares with health professionals: professional-dominated, participatory, challenging, and collaborative (Hulme, 1999). Family members interact with each other, nurses and other health care professionals, the health care system, and their community as they participate in the family empowerment process.

In the *professional-dominated phase* there is a high level of trusting dependency on health professionals to direct health care while the family adjusts to the health care situation. This phase occurs during an initial diagnosis of the chronic illness and during a life-threatening situation or relapse (Hulme, 1999).

The participatory phase occurs as the family responds to the continuing chronic illness and its disruptive effect on family life. "Critical consciousness and action" (Hulme, 1999) become apparent and family members begin to perceive themselves as important members in the decision-making process about health care for their family member. During this phase, family members focus on learning about the care of their chronically ill family member and the rules of the health care system. They also seek support and try out changing roles and responsibilities to improve their family life (Hulme, 1999).

In the *challenging phase* the balance of power begins to shift from the health care professional to the family. Family members question aspects of care, sometimes triggering conflict with the health care professional over control of their family member's health care. Family frustration, uncertainty, disillusionment, and loss of trust in the health care professionals are not uncommon during this phase (Hulme, 1999).

The *collaborative phase* is entered as the family becomes more self-confident and assertive and less reliant on the health care professional. The family is now a full partner in the health care team (Hulme, 1999).

When using the Family Empowerment Model, it is important to remember that the phases are interdependent and overlapping, and that a family's progress through the phases may be delayed or reversed because of a prolonged or extremely challenging phase, a disruption in family life, or changes in the health care situation (Hulme, 1999). Health care professionals can help prevent these events by implementing Family Empowerment Interventions, such as guiding the family in assessing its own

FIGURE 11-1

Family Empowerment Model

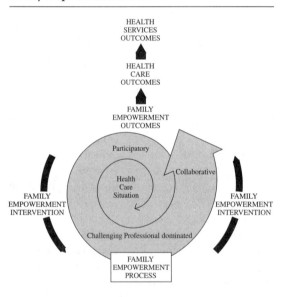

SOURCE: Hulme, P. A. (1999) Family empowerment: A nursing intervention with suggested outcomes for families of children with a chronic health condition. *Journal of Family Nursing, 5* (1), 33–50. Reprinted by permission of Sage Publications, Inc. Thousand Oaks, CA.

strengths and in mobilizing the use of those strengths for problem solving. The goal of such interventions is to recognize, promote, and enhance a family's ability to meet the health care needs of their family member with the chronic illness and to sustain their family life (Hulme, 1999). A valuable resource for nurses as well as family caregivers is the National Organization for Empowering Caregivers (www.nofec.org and www.care-givers.com).

Family Caregivers as Members of Care Planning Teams

Although the two terms are sometimes used interchangeably, *interdisciplinary* teams are very different from *multidisciplinary* models of care. The older concept of teaming included multidisciplinary teams. These teams typically included members from several different disciplines who shared common goals but worked independently from one another to propose and implement patient interventions. When a family caregiver interacts with a multidisciplinary team, he or she is more or less forced to compartmentalize caregiving needs, problems, or concerns into disciplines, such as a nursing problem, or a social need.

In contrast, the more contemporary concept of teaming calls for interdisciplinary teams. These teams work together to identify and analyze problems, plan actions and interventions, and monitor results of the care plan. Team meetings are used to make or negotiate assignments, share information, and evaluate the team's effort toward achieving client and caregiver outcomes. Lines of communication among team members are highly visible, while disciplinary boundaries are purposely blurred on interdisciplinary teams (Travis & Duer, 2000). Family caregivers who participate as members of interdisciplinary teams need only convey their problems, needs, issues, or concerns in order to activate a team effort for resolution.

Active inclusion as a member of the interdisciplinary team may help in overcoming a still common complaint of family caregivers: that of dissatisfaction with the level of their involvement in health care decision-making. Family caregivers have identified four markers of satisfactory involvement: feeling that information is shared; feeling included in decision-making; feeling that there is someone you can contact when you need to; and feeling that the service is responsive to your needs (Walker & Dewar, 2004). A goal of interdisciplinary teams should be to help family caregivers achieve these markers of involvement satisfaction. Use of the Family Empowerment Model (as previously discussed) can assist the interdisciplinary team in reaching that goal.

Interdisciplinary teaming works well in long-term care situations because it is virtually impossible to tease apart the ever-changing social and health care needs of dependent individuals and their family caregivers. If an elderly diabetic client and his spousal caregiver cannot afford to purchase appropriate food and medications in the same week, the health care plan will fail until the social needs of the couple are met. Similarly, a wheelchair-bound adult in a potentially neglectful situation will not be able to remain in community-based care with only health care support.

Life-Span Development and Developmentally Appropriate Care

Growth and development knowledge helps caregivers separate normal from disease-related changes in the dependent family member, regardless of the client's age. This knowledge helps caregivers deal more effectively with decision-making issues, obtain appropriate available community resources, and secure emotional support for themselves. Numerous specialty organizations, such as the March of Dimes, provide this type of educational material for families of recipients of different ages (e.g., children and adolescents). The case study of Andrew, the ventilator-dependent child, demonstrates the importance of support and education for the parent.

For families of chronically ill children, regardless of the type of chronic illness, certain developmental changes or times of transition trigger disequilibrium and stress in the family. Five principal periods of transition are: at the initial diagnosis; when symptoms increase; when the child goes to a new setting (such as the hospital); during a parent's absence; and during periods of developmental change (Meleski, 2002). Of the developmental milestones, five specific times are associated with increased stress: periods when most children learn to walk, talk, and enter school; the onset of puberty, and the child's 21st birthday. Nurses need to recognize these times of transition and to teach families how to foster the healthy development of their children as well as the family. The literature reveals several types of adaptation that parents use during times of transition: support, assigning meaning to the illness, managing the condition, role reorganization, and normalization. Nursing interventions should consider the type of adaptation, the family and its specific situation (Meleski, 2002).

Andrew's story illustrates some of the client and family needs that must be addressed. Andrew's growth, development, and social needs are addressed by his mother, her extended family, his nurses, and his therapists. As he grows older, his changing needs must be considered by individualizing the services he obtains and by treating him as normally as possible. His mother must learn about the changes he will undergo and how to interface effectively with institutions such as hospitals, clinics, and schools. To achieve this, she needs various supportive services. She also needs to have her own needs met so that she can more effectively deal with Andrew's chronic condition. Andrew's restructured family, without his father, has successfully incorporated him into a coherent unit and has not allowed his illness to be a major obstacle.

Helping Families Learn to Cope

Part of the maturation of individual family caregivers and caregiving systems involves the development of realistic expectations of the individual members' abilities and limitations, as well as an understanding of the anticipated trajectory of dependent care that lies ahead. In order to provide adequate care for a dependent relative and at the same time secure their own well being, family caregivers need support, aid, and understanding from their families and friends and from the health care system. To get that support, it is crucial that family caregivers learn to recognize when they need help, what kind of help to ask for, how to ask for the help they need, and whom to ask (Mittelman, 2003). Individual family caregivers and their caregiving systems may need assistance in learning how to cope with the positive and negative feelings and the emotional and social impacts of caregiving. Health care professionals need to promote family caregivers' well-being, which is a complex, multidimensional concept that includes personal meanings (George & Gwyther, 1986). In doing so, caregivers may need assistance in acquiring the information, support, and services to meet those needs (Elliott & Shewshuk, 2003; Piercy & Chapman, 2001).

Family caregivers need formal providers who have time and the training necessary to help them learn effective interventions. Because nurses with clinical training also understand behavioral and counseling techniques, they are often considered the most appropriate member of the team to work with family caregivers and to oversee educational programs. Stress-Point Intervention by Nurses (SPIN) (Kauffmann & Harrison, 1998) has proved useful in assisting families whose children have a chronic condition and are repeatedly hospitalized. A nurse helps the family develop a unique set of coping strategies, based on the family's own concerns and resources and the nurse's expertise. The nurse helps the family explore issues together. This helps the family to identify critical stress-points and in order to design a customized family intervention. A central strategy that nurses use in the SPIN process is to express realistic confidence in the family's ability to cope (Kauffmann & Harrison, 1998). While SPIN was developed for families with children who have chronic conditions, the SPIN process could be adapted for families of adult members with chronic illness.

In general, programs that build family caregiver confidence and skill and a feeling of support are more effective than those that simply impart knowledge (Piercy & Chapman, 2001). Problem-solving interventions that target the specific concerns of family caregivers are especially effective and can reduce caregiver depression and distress (Elliott & Shewshuk, 2003). Kaye and colleagues (2003) found that an early intervention screening for family caregivers of older relatives resulted in caregivers accessing sources of community support prior to a crisis and impending burnout. In all cases, intervention programs must be developmentally appropriate and tailored to be culturally relevant and learner-specific.

The types of intervention programs available range from individual or group caregiver counseling in the presence of a professional facilitator to self-paced, self-help computerized programs that can be completed in relative isolation from others. Software packages that provide caregivers with information and advice on promotion of personal psychological health, relaxation, and other coping strategies plus a carergiver self-assessment tool on coping with the caregiver role have proved useful to caregivers (Chambers & Connor, 2002). Caregivers report that the use of such software provides reassurance and emotional support and enables them to assess and enhance their own coping skills.

The time constraints of most contemporary family caregivers are now being addressed by such strategies as telephone conferencing, Internet chat rooms and e-mail. Link$_2$Care is an example of a successful innovative Internet-based program that combines high tech with traditional service to increase caregiver well-being and coping skills (Kelly, 2003-2004). Caregivers using Link$_2$Care rate the following as the top five valued features: updated news and research, information articles and fact sheets, online discussion groups, "Ask the Expert," and local educational event listings. It is no longer the case that an intervention program is only effective with direct face-to-face contact. The key is to make the interventions relevant, multi-component, tailored to caregivers' needs, and accessible when the caregiver needs it (Chambers & Connor, 2002; Elliott & Shewchuk, 2003; Gitlin et al., 2003; Mittelman, 2003).

Caregivers also need the opportunity for activities other than providing care to avoid a sense of entrapment and feelings of loss of self and burnout. Attention to self-help activities sustains one's sense of well-being and revitalizes energy that can later be used in providing care to the client, but many caregivers feel guilty about activities that focus on themselves (Medalie, 1994).

Spirituality and Caregiving

Spiritual beliefs and faith-based behaviors play multiple roles in caregivers' lives. Spirituality involves not only connectedness with a sacred other, but also with other people, perspectives, and sources of value and meaning beyond oneself (Faver, 2004). Such connectedness can produce happiness and energy to sustain a caregiver's ability to care for a chronically ill family member (Faver, 2004; Haley & Harrigan, 2004). Whether or not caregivers hold religious beliefs, they express needs for love, meaning, purpose, and sometime transcendence in their lives (Murray, Kendall, Boyd, Worth, & Benton, 2004). Caregivers draw strength from maintaining relationships with their families and value opportunities to give and receive love, to feel connected to their social world and to feel useful (Murray et al., 2004).

Religious beliefs and formal religious practices are essential aspects of caregiving. Heavy reliance on prayer to cope with adversity is reported by many caregivers (Paun, 2004; Stuckey, 2001). African American women caregivers describe their prayer as an ongoing dialogue that keeps them connected with their God rather than prayer as a formal religious ritual (Paun, 2004). Religiosity is also demonstrated by: the belief that God has a plan; belief in a loving God; hope in an afterlife; and a sense of the evidence of God all around (Stuckey, 2001). Reading the Bible and other religious materials and listening to music are also aspects of formal religion used by caregivers (Theis, Biordi, Coeling, Nalepka, & Miller, 2003). Churches provide an important source of encouragement and social support for caregivers (Faver, 2004; Murray et al., 2004; Theis et al., 2003). A strong connection with a caring community is what caregivers value

Caregiving for a Ventilator-Dependent Child

Ms. L. C. is a 29-year-old White female divorced from her husband. She lives with her two-year-old son Andrew, who has central hypoventilation syndrome (he does not breathe unassisted when asleep) and prolonged expiratory apnea (he has frequent hypoxic episodes when awake). It was Andrew's illness that led to the couple separating. After birth, Andrew was hospitalized for approximately three months with his mother remaining near the hospital rather than returning home, 70 miles away. Her absence was seen as inattentiveness and neglect by her husband. After they learned that the baby had a poor prognosis, the parents disagreed about his treatment, resulting in much conflict, domestic violence, and the eventual separation.

Home Setting. L. C. and Andrew live in a small, one-bedroom upstairs apartment on the outskirts of a small city. The living room is largely taken up with Andrew's crib and equipment: ventilator, apnea monitor, oxygen tanks, and suction equipment. Ms. C. keeps the apartment very clean to avoid respiratory irritants for her son. Toys are in every room.

Support System. Ms. C does not trust Mr. C. There is a restraining order to keep him out of the apartment, as he has stated he wishes to take Andrew off of life support. Mr. C.'s mother and sister do not acknowledge Andrew as part of the family. They visited once in the hospital after Andrew was born, but tried to take out the baby's tracheostomy tube, for in their culture only "normal" healthy babies are allowed to live.

L. C.'s mother comes to visit her daily. Her sister visits several times a week when she is off from work. Two nephews also visit once or twice weekly. Thus, there is extended family support for her from her family and much conflict from Mr. C.'s family. The consistent emotional support provided by her family keeps Ms. C. strong in her belief that her son deserves to live as normal a life as possible. She maintains a positive, almost stoic attitude about raising him at home.

SOURCE: This case study is provided by Allison M. Goodell, R.N., B.S.N., staff nurse in the Pediatric Intensive Care Unit of the Children's Hospital at Albany Medical Center Hospital, Albany, New York.

in their church relationships. Caregivers find that the consistent presence of fellow parishioners is a powerful sustaining force (Faver, 2004). Efforts to maintain chronically ill spouses' engagement in religious practices, such as church attendance, are important for caregivers. When church attendance is no longer possible, caregivers substitute televised or videotaped services and arrange for other formal religious practices like communion to be given at their home (Paun, 2004).

A spiritual or religious perspective seems to benefit caregivers in several ways. Caregivers report that attending religious services regularly is what keeps them going. Second to church attendance is prayer (Paun, 2004). Feelings of being supported and comforted by religious faith are associated with positive emotional experiences while caring for persons with Alzheimer's disease (Paun, 2004). A sense of sacred companionship with God or a sacred other acts as a sustaining force for many caregivers (Faver, 2004). Thus, a spiritual approach to caregiving may help caregivers cope with stressful situations and benefit those for whom they care. Strong faith-based beliefs, such as moral living and being of service to others, can motivate persons to become caregivers as well as to continue caregiving (Stuckey, 2001).

Growth and Development Issues. The developmental task for this family is to incorporate the child into the family unit. The family unit itself changed after Andrew's birth given the separation of the parents due to conflicts between their values of the child's right to live. Andrew is part of his mother's extended family system. L. C. has begun to date again, which has positive implications for her meeting her own needs as well as potential long-term implications for the family unit.

Andrew is played with in developmentally appropriate ways. He is frequently held and cuddled by his mother and her extended family. He is able to get around the apartment in his walker and is taken for age-appropriate excursions outside the home with his ventilator and the nurse.

Professional Assistance for the Child. Andrew has 24-hour-a-day nursing care. Importantly, Ms. C. refers to two of the nurses as part of the family, because they have cared for him for so long. In addition, he has a special education teacher once weekly, and a physical therapist and a speech therapist who come every other week.

Assistance for the Parent Caregiver. The mother identified her need for support and counseling services. She was provided with the following information: The American Red Cross offers support groups for parents of children at home on high-tech care. The New York State Department of Health Council on Child and Adolescent Health offers a *Directory of Self-Help/Mutual Support for Children with Special Health Needs and Their Families* (1992). The National Organization of Rare Disorders is also a reference for self-help groups. The local county Mental Health Association is an additional resource for parent caregivers. L. C. is fortunate that her family allows her respite from her parenting and caregiving responsibilities. She can therefore participate in such self-help and support groups.

While caregivers report the importance of spirituality and religion in their lives, they often are reluctant to initiate raising such issues with health care professionals. Murray and colleagues (2004) found that caregivers (as well as the care recipients) did not broach the subject of spiritual care need because they perceived the healthcare professionals to be busy and/or did not see spiritual care as part of healthcare professionals' role. Caregivers even actively tried to disguise their spiritual distress. Nurses need to be alert to caregivers' need for spiritual care and to create conditions where caregivers feel comfortable in discussing their spiritual needs. Giving caregivers this opportunity validates their concerns and needs and helps them feel connected and cared for. Spiritual support professionals, such as ministers and rabbis, should be included as an integral part of the interdisciplinary team.

Churches and Communities in Care Solutions

In addition to government-sponsored programs to help caregivers, churches have a potentially important role to play in caregivers' lives. Though little research has been conducted on the role of churches in eldercare, Stuckey (2001) found that churches supported caregivers by encouraging continued church participation whenever possible and by taking services to care recipient and caregiver when needed.

An example of a church collaboration is the Interfaith CarePartners (www.interfaithcarepartners.org) "Creating Caring Communities." An innovative aspect of this program is the Care Team model of caregiving implemented in 1985 to provide in-home support to individuals with chronic health conditions and to offer respite support to their caregivers. Volunteers are recruited from Jewish and Christian congregations, and are trained to provide companionship, meal preparation, transportation, light household chores, shopping assistance, spiritual, emotional, and physical support, and personal care to adults and children with debilitating illnesses and disabilities. A Second Family Care Team serves chronically ill and frail adults. As the title suggests, the vision of this Care Team is to be a "second family" for frail adults and their caregivers. As well as providing types of support and assistance for the chronically ill adult, the team provides caregivers with encouragement, hope, respite, emotional support, and physical assistance. Collaboration efforts like Interfaith CarePartners are generally perceived as very helpful resources for caregivers.

Communities also have a role in providing assistance to those in need of care. An excellent example of a community partnership to accomplish this goal is the Gatekeeper Model developed in Spokane, Washington (Substance Abuse & Mental Health Administration, 2004). Employees of community businesses and corporations who work with the public are trained to identify and refer community-dwelling older adults who may be in need of aid. Upon referral by these gatekeepers, home-based assessments are conducted by interdisciplinary teams provided by the local mental health services, with referrals made for additional services as needed. Another community example that benefits elderly persons and caregivers is the interfaith volunteer program organized by Faith in Action which administers 1000 community programs across the United States. The program, funded by the Robert Wood Johnson Foundation, aims to connect volunteers with older and disabled people who need help and to provide a source of respite for caregivers.

Programs, Services, and Resources for Family Caregivers

A Google internet search was performed using the key words *family caregiving* and 177,000 matches were found. The sites included information and referral links, products and services, educational sites, and on-line caregiver support groups. Clearly, there is no shortage of programs, services, and resources for family caregivers. The problem is in finding affordable programs that are accessible and convenient for hassled family caregivers. A comprehensive list of agencies and organizations with resources for family caregivers plus a list of books for caregivers and professionals can be found in the Winter 2003–2004 volume of *Family Caregiving* (Kelly, 2003–2004).

Utilization of community services by family caregivers provides a range of benefits for caregivers. Unfortunately, barriers to the services continue to exist. Benefits reported by caregivers include renewal, sense of community, and knowledge and belief that their family member also benefited from the service. Barriers include care recipient resistance, reluctance of the caregiver, hassles for the caregiver, concerns about quality, and concerns about finances (Winslow, 2003). Nurses and other health care professionals involved in community services need to work to decrease or eliminate the barriers faced by family caregivers.

Respite Programs and Services

Respite is temporary relief from caregiving responsibilities that provides intervals of rest and relief for the caregiver. Family members may provide respite for the primary caregiver by taking over some tasks; for example, daughters may assist their caregiving mothers by shopping, cleaning, and so forth. There are also formal sources of respite, such as adult day care, in-home companions, and special weekend respite programs.

It is important for caregivers to recognize the warning signs that indicate that their coping skills are overwhelmed and they are in need of outside help. For many caregivers, the hardest step is acknowledging that help is needed; the next most difficult step is extending the effort to seek this help. Caregivers often feel guilty about seeking respite and delay using formal respite services until they are exhausted and debilitated. Ambivalence on the part of caregivers to make use of respite services is illustrated by a study of family caregivers' experiences with in-hospital respite care for family members with dementia (Gilmour, 2002). Caregivers' feelings varied from acceptance to qualified acceptance to marked ambivalence. Caregivers were torn between the need to have a break and the worry over the impact of the in-hospital respite care on their family member. Nurses have the interpersonal skills to help decrease tensions and anxieties that caregivers have over respite care. Caregivers need to see respite services as a reasonable and appropriate action, not as a sign of personal failure, if they plan to continue caregiving without being overwhelmed by the physical and social demands.

When caregiving becomes too physically demanding or emotionally draining, short-term institutional placement of the client may be a care alternative. Planned short-term hospital admission provides in-facility professional care with relief for the caregiver. These programs can prevent the threshold of family tolerance being exceeded. To enhance family caregivers' comfort with this type of respite, nurses need to put themselves in a secondary and supporting care provider role and acknowledge the family caregiver as the authority on the care required by their family member (Gilmour, 2002). Family members are more fully able to relinquish care when they are confident that their relative is receiving care comparable to what is provided at home and that the relative is not negatively affected by the hospital stay (Gilmour, 2002).

Both Medicare and many long-term care insurance policies provide a short-term nursing home placement for a dependent family member (Elder Services of Worcester Area, 2003). Longer or more frequent temporary stays are also possible, if the family is able to pay the expenses out of pocket.

Adult Day Services

Adult day services (formerly known as adult day care) are congregate programs that provide opportunities for impaired adults to socialize and participate in organized activities, and for their families to receive respite time. Use of adult day care results in decreased caregiver worry and stress and improved psychological well-being (Ritchie, 2003). Caregivers appreciate the client socializing and improved health as well as the respite for themselves (Warren, Kerr, Smith, Godkin, & Schalm, 2003).

Great variation exists in the type and amount of services that these centers provide. In general, the centers are broadly classified as health or social models of care. Social models emphasize socialization and cognitive stimulation. Health models of care are often supported by a state's Medicaid program and include health care monitoring in the day program. In general, the major difference between the two types of programs is the presence or absence of a registered nurse on site in a center commonly called *adult day health care*. One example from the many programs throughout the United States is the San Francisco Senior Citizen Adult Day Services provided in the city's 17 neighborhood-based centers (http://www.sfms.org/sfm/sfm699j.htm). Some day health programs with advanced rehabilitation/restorative programs are certified by Medicare as day treatment hospitals and include rehabilitation specialists on staff.

Work by Campbell and Travis (1999) highlights the interesting ways in which family caregivers integrate formal programs and services into their informal caregiving routines. In their study of spousal caregivers, these researchers concluded that weekends were a time when other caregivers were not at work and were more readily available to help. Thus, better support to the primary caregiver appeared to have contributed to low interest in paying for additional adult day services during the weekend.

Social day programs have a variety of funding options, but most reimbursement sources are limited to low-income families or those with long-term care insurance (DHHS Administration on Aging, n.d.b). Day health programs are primarily Medicaid programs or those skilled, rehabilitation programs that are Medicare reimbursed. The out-of-pocket cost of day care to the family caregivers varies widely depending on the region of the country and the type of program offered. In an analysis of cost implications of adult day services for persons with dementia, Gaugler (2003) found that the daily costs to reduce caregivers' role overload and depression decreased with adult day utilization over one year. Apparently the adult day programs are most cost-effective for caregivers who use them consistently and for longer periods of time.

Home Care Programs

Home care has expanded in recent years as a result of earlier hospital discharge and the increase in technically more complex therapies. The home represents a different context for provision of care than the medical office or community clinic. Toth-Cohen and colleagues (2001) discuss four key factors that must be considered when providing care within the home setting: understand the personal meaning of the home for the family; view the caregiver as a "lay practitioner;" identify the caregiver's beliefs and values; and recognize the potential impact of the interventions on caregiver well-being.

Multiple benefits as well as challenges for the caregiver and the health care professional are present in home care (Toth-Cohen et al., 2001). Benefits for the caregiver include: (1) saving of time, and mental and physical energy; (2) remaining in control and guiding interaction with the provider; (3) being more comfortable and at ease in own surroundings; (4) practicing newly learned skills in the context in which they will be used. Benefits for the health care professional include: (1) gaining an in-depth understanding of the client, the caregiver, and the home context; (2) designing interventions tailored to specific home situations; (3) identifying

safety issues that caregivers may be unaware, (4) observing performance in the context in which it occurs. Challenges and potential solutions are presented in Table 11-1. Nurses can work more effectively with families in their homes by being aware of the benefits, challenges, and possible solutions to those challenges. The nurse's ability to meet whatever challenges are encountered will influence a caregiver's response to interventions and recommendations.

Some home care programs provide respite services for families. Services can include homemaking, monitoring of both client and caregiver health status, and performing various skills, such as taking vital signs or changing catheters. Unfortunately, reimbursement for these programs is increasingly limited to those families with the greatest financial need. Paying out of pocket can be very expensive over the long term.

Psychotherapeutic Approaches

Individual, couple, group, or family counseling may be needed to help families respond to the demands of caregiving. Individual counseling is directed toward enhancing the caregiver's capacity to deal with the day-to-day rigors of caregiving. As described by Montcalm (1995), counseling for couples can be complex because of the multiple issues involved, such as dependency, grief over the losses in the relationship, and fear. When peer interaction and feedback seem appropriate, group therapy can be effective in steering a family caregiver toward more positive resolutions of internal conflict over the caregiving role.

Family treatment often includes a strategy called the "family meeting," at a time when all affected family members meet face to face. A family-based therapy, found effective for caregivers of family members with dementia, is the Structural Ecosystems Therapy (SET) (Mitrani & Czaja, 2000). The aim of SET is to address the entire family's needs within a "cojoint context" (p. 201). SET views the behavior of family members as interdependent and repetitive. Sometimes the repetitive patterns are maladaptive and cause symptoms such as caregiver

TABLE 11-1

Summary of Challenges and Recommendations for Providing Services in the Home

Challenge	Recommendations
Building rapport	■ Identify caregiver's goals for intervention. ■ Use and respect caregiver's language. ■ Validate caregiver's existing strategies. ■ Involve and collaborate with family members and other supportive persons.
Incorporating needs of both caregiver and person with dementia into interventions	■ Use holistic approach that addresses needs of both caregiver and person with dementia. —Involve person with dementia in meaningful activities. —Consider effects of education and home modification on both caregiver and person with dementia.
Obtaining assessment data	■ Actively involve care receiver in intervention, when feasible. ■ Ask permission of care receiver to discuss ways of helping caregiver. ■ Schedule telephone contacts to discuss sensitive issues. ■ Obtain assessment data when person with dementia is not present.
Ensuring optimal fit between intervention and family	■ Reflect on possible differences between self and caregiver. ■ Review caregiver's management practices step by step. ■ Refocus on the caregiver's needs and priorities. ■ Discuss and try out possible strategies.
Matching the intervention to caregiver expertise and knowledge of dementia	■ Recognize that caregiver may need more time to accept family member's condition and use provider's strategies. ■ Ensure that recommendations fit the caregiver's perspective and priorities. ■ Address quality-of-life issues in master caregivers. ■ Obtain information on specific strategies from master caregivers that may be helpful for other caregivers. ■ Follow up on how recommended strategies are working; if necessary, modify strategies. ■ Reinforce value of strategies. ■ Photograph physical adaptations or develop pre-post photos to reinforce positive changes.
Working within the family system of roles and relationships	■ Role play using simple language and validation of care receiver's feelings. ■ Recognize roles of multiple caregivers and reflect on how they fit into the caregiving situation. ■ Facilitate communication and collaborative problem solving between caregivers.
Helping caregivers access and use resources	■ Be aware of existing resources available to caregiver. ■ Educate caregiver about appropriate resources. ■ Help caregiver identify tasks that others could perform. ■ Role play with caregiver ways of asking for help.

SOURCE: Toth-Cohen, S., Gitlin, L. N., Corcoran, M. A., Eckhardt, S., Johns, P., & Lipsitt, R. (2001). Providing services to family caregivers at home: Challenges and recommendations for health and human service professions. *Alzheimer's Care Quarterly, 2* (1), 23–32. Reprinted with permission of Lippincott Williams & Wilkins.

stress. Other interaction patterns are adaptive and relieve caregiver burden. SET focuses on improving the caregiver's interactions within her whole social ecosystem, i.e., family, community, health care providers, etc., thus, increasing the extent to which the caregiver's emotional, social and instrumental needs are met. SET is particularly appropriate for minority families because it acknowledges the importance of culture as a contextual variable which can have a marked influence on family interaction (Mitrani & Czaja, 2000).

Support Groups

Also called self-help groups, these forums focus on specific client populations and related caregivers' needs. Self-help groups for caregivers have been established in many communities throughout the United States. Some are self-directed or run by volunteers; others are led by health care professionals who act as group facilitators. These groups provide information, emotional support, advocacy, or a combination of these services. They address such areas as skills in the care and maintenance of the disabled person and managing problems in the family; information regarding the aging process; emotional needs for recognition and support from caring people; and concrete service needs for referral and information regarding resources. Telephone support networks and Internet chat rooms are simply contemporary versions of the traditional face-to-face support group.

The Need for Culturally Sensitive Interventions

During the past century, the United States and Canada experienced massive waves of immigration, as well as a growing population of native-born minorities. Given the diversity of racial, ethnic, and religious groups in North America, there is a need for helping professionals to learn more about the many cultural groups with which they work so that they can provide interventions that are sensitive to the client's culture. To that end, there has been a rapid rise of multicultural consciousness in the United

States. However, cultural awareness among health care professionals continues to be inadequate to serve those of other cultures.

Awareness that the definition of *family* differs from one cultural group to another is important. For example, the dominant Caucasian definition focuses on the intact nuclear family. However, African Americans focus on a wider network of kin and community, and often include fictional kin, who are not biological family members, in their family networks. The Chinese culture includes all of a person's ancestors and descendants in the definition of *family* (McGoldrick & Giordano, 1996). Who the client considers to be family and who is providing care will influence who should be included in interventions.

Cultural groups vary greatly in how they respond to problems and their attitudes toward seeking help. For example, Hispanic elders typically want to have problems addressed only by the family, not by outsiders. The family may not want the outside world to know a problem exists (Rittman, Kuzmeskus & Flum, 1998). To assist an Hispanic family, a helping professional will have to work on *personalismo*, knowing the elder and her caregiver as total persons, before focusing on personal matters; *dignidad*, developing a working relationship that reflects dignity and self-worth; *respeto*, respect between the helping professional and Hispanic elder; and *confianza*, trust between the two parties (Applewhite & Daley, 1988).

Ethnic differences exist in attitudes toward caregiving and caregiving responsibilities. For example, Cuban Americans often have a hierarchical relational orientation and adhere to traditional family roles. Because of this, female caregivers may have difficulty in adopting the leadership role of caregiving (Mitrani & Czaja, 2000). Other cultural characteristics of Cubans are collectivism, giving precedence to the needs of the family over the individual, and the high degree of emotional and psychological closeness or enmeshment between caregiver and the care recipient. Enmeshment, observed more frequently in Cuban families than Caucasian Americans families, can produce a lack of objectivity and an unwillingness to delegate care tasks, making it difficult for the caregiver to be an effective care manager (Mitrani & Czaja, 2000). To work effectively with families from varied ethnic and cultural heritages, the nurse must tailor family interventions to be culturally congruent.

Providing assistance to family caregivers of minority elders for any number of issues is most effective when the members of the targeted minority group are represented in the provider or intervention group. For this reason, neighborhood-centered services, in which minority caregivers can interact with bilingual professionals, tend to be highly effective. These programs are well suited to respecting the values and customs of families in need of help and to offering culturally relevant solutions to the caregivers (Spector, 2000).

Outcomes

Care Recipient, Caregiver, and Caregiving System Outcomes

Providing care to another person has both positive and negative outcomes for the primary caregiver and the caregiver system. Because caregiving is a very personal journey, it is almost impossible to predict how each caregiver or care recipient will respond to the demands of dependency and caregiving support. Therefore, all of the interventions provided by an interdisciplinary team are ultimately directed toward supporting family caregivers when the situation is going well, and to helping caregivers correct practices that will lead to potentially negative outcomes.

Much of the caregiving literature reflects a focus on the negative aspects of caregiving. Less available are the positive aspects of the caregiver role. The literature continues to need studies that identify the potential benefits of caregiving (Hudson, 2004), for the purpose of increasing our understanding of the caregiving experience (Tarlow et al., 2004) as well as preventing the likelihood of viewing caregiving only from a pathological perspective and thus socializing caregivers to expect burden (Gaugler, Kane & Langlois, 2000). The study of caregiver benefits can also provide data for the development of evidence-based supportive care strategies for families and family caregivers (Harding & Higginson, 2003).

Despite the paucity of information regarding the benefits derived from the caregiver role, studies available indicate that most caregivers find some element of satisfaction in the caregiving experience (Nolan, 2001; Scott, 2001). Hudson (2004) reported 60% of caregivers readily identified positive aspects of the caregiver role. Given what is known about long-term family caregiving, there are three outcomes that are commonly monitored. Together, these outcomes form a gold standard by which caregiving experiences can be measured. Outcomes for both the family caregivers and their care recipients include improved quality of life and meaning in life, enhanced autonomy and control, and reduced family stress and enhanced coping ability.

Quality of Life and Meaning in Life

It has been written that human beings "can be at their best when they are behaving with altruism and commitment to a person they love" (Lattanzi-Licht, Mahoney & Miller, 1998, p. 31). Finding enhanced quality of life and meaning in life associated with the caregiving experience is one of the most positive outcomes of caregiving for the care recipient and the caregiver (Sheehan & Donorfio, 1999). Evidence of enhanced meaning of life can be seen in caregivers' comments about positive aspects of caregiving: "Love doing it—we've been given an opportunity we'd never thought we'd have" (Hudson, 2004, p. 62).

Until recently, systematic assessments of these positive outcomes of caregiving have been limited because of the difficulty clinicians have encountered in finding and accessing psychometrically sound measures of these abstract constructs (Farran, Miller & Kaufman, 1999). The new generation of measurement tools allows interdisciplinary teams to tap into the day-to-day meaning and ultimate meaning of caregiving relationships so that these aspects of caregiving become a visible outcome of the experiences (Farran et al., 1999). One such measurement tool is the Positive Aspects of Caregiving (Tarlow et al., 2004).

Perceived Autonomy and Control

Autonomy, as an outcome of family caregiving, means that the choices of long-term caregivers and their care recipients are self-determined. Consistent with the principles of self-determination is the need to have some control over events and decisions. In chronic care situations, autonomy and control are interrelated and both are affected by the ability of professional providers to support family caregivers in the choices they make and the care that they give. It follows that autonomy and control may need to be renegotiated with the formal network and within the informal caregiving system as the caregiving situation changes.

Those caregivers who are able to feel most relaxed and confident in managing their caregiving situations have reported that being successful does not mean being in total control (Karp & Tanarugsachock, 2000). Learning to "go with the flow" is how caregivers frequently describe their approach to control issues (Travis et al., 2000). If interdisciplinary teams respect the values and goals of the caregivers and their care recipients and help to translate these into real world plans of care, then perceived autonomy and control for both caregivers and care recipients are enhanced. Evidence of an enhanced sense of autonomy and control can be seen in caregivers' comments about positive aspects of caregiving: "Taking responsibility for things I had not previously been responsible for;" "I feel like I'm a stronger person now;" and "I've been able to undertake much more than I thought I could" (Hudson, 2004, p. 62).

Reduced Family Stress and Coping

As previously discussed, the many adverse effects of caregiving include an array of affective responses by caregivers to the demands of long-term caregiving. The goal of most care teams is to reduce this distress to a level that is perceived to be manageable for the caregivers. Caregivers are able to voice positive aspects in the role despite the negative aspects, such as stress and burden (Hudson, 2004; Roff et al., 2004). Perhaps caregivers use positive emotions to augment and maintain their coping strategies when faced with an ongoing stressor like caregiving (Folkman, 1997). Because family stress and coping are global, multidimensional, and multifaceted, interventions are often designed to address a specific aspect of stress and coping, such as perceived burden, depression, or fatigue (Buckwalter et al., 1999).

Societal Outcomes

A number of studies have examined the cost effectiveness of community-based home services to groups of individuals at risk for nursing home use. Even though the most consistent justification for delivering long-term care services in home- and community-based environments is cost containment, such claims have not been supported in the research (Weissert & Hedrick, 1999). Part of the problem is the way that costs of care are compared across settings. For example, while nursing home care appears to be more costly than community-based care, the calculations do not take into consideration the out-of-pocket expenses and subsidized programs and services that family caregivers must use in order to make community-based care a viable long-term care option for them and their dependent family members.

Delayed or Diverted Episodes of Institutional Care

Despite the fact that home- and community-based care may not be cost effective, providing such care remains a goal for many families and a priority of policy makers. This is because institutional care is *perceived* as more expensive by most policy makers, and less desirable than home care by older adults and policy makers alike, who clearly *prefer* noninstitutional solutions to long-term care.

In their study of the influence of service use on consequences for caregivers, Bass, Noelker, and Rechlin (1996) conceptualized services as a type of social support. They found that certain services, such as health care, personal care, and homemaker services, reduced the adverse effects of heavy or burdensome care on the family caregivers. These types of programs serve a clientele that may not be at imminent risk of nursing home placement, but their needs for assistance in the home or community are real (Weissert & Hedrick, 1994).

Instead of looking to home and community-based services as a cost-effective alternative to nursing home placement, a better outcome of success may be measures of diverted hospital stays (Weissert &

Hedrick, 1994). Advanced death planning and decisions about when to institutionalize, as well as working with clinicians and families as dependent persons transition from active treatment to palliation, can reduce inappropriate and expensive care (Weissert & Hedrick, 1994). This outcome requires more discussions and decision making among care recipients and their family members regarding care decisions and increased communication with their physicians to ensure that the decisions are respected and carried out. Nurses can foster this decision making by encouraging families to talk openly with one another about care and by assisting families to put the plans into place in advance of the need to make decisions about hospitalizations or other unwanted aggressive measures.

■ **Summary and Conclusions**

As the incidence of chronic illness continues to increase, it is imperative that family caregivers be prepared for the challenges of their role. By working through the challenges, both the caregiver and the care recipient benefit. The nurse is in a position to support and intervene with the caregiver to maximize the family's strengths and abilities in caring for their loved one.

Acknowledgement: The authors of this chapter would like to acknowledge Shirley S. Travis and Kathy Piercy for their original work on the chapter "Family Caregivers" in the 5th edition.

Study Questions

1. What are the advantages and disadvantages of the client being cared for at home? For the family? For the caregiver?
2. What factors influence the cost effectiveness of home care versus institutionalization?
3. Who are the primary providers of home care? What are some of the providers competing demands?
4. How does ethnicity influence family caregiving? .
5. What are some of the emotional responses to family caregiving?
6. What is the financial impact of caregiving on the caregiver?
7. How does public policy affect caregiving?
8. How can health professionals assist family caregivers?
9. Where can family caregivers go for assistance/information?
10. As an advocate for family caregivers, what would facts would you present to lawmakers related to supportive legislation?

References

Albert, S. M., & Brody, E. M. (1996). When elder care is viewed as child care. *American Journal of Geriatric Psychiatry, 4,* 121–130.

Allen, S. M., Goldscheider, F., & Ciambrone, D. (1999). Gender roles, marital intimacy, and nomination of spouses as primary caregivers. *The Gerontologist, 39,* 150–158.

Alspaugh, M. E. L., Stephens, M. A. P., Townsend, A. L., Zarit, S. H., et al. (1999). Longitudinal patterns of risk for depression in dementia caregivers: Objective and subjective primary stress as predictors. *Psychology and Aging, 14,* 34–43.

Applewhite, S. R., & Daley, J. M. (1988). Cross-cultural understanding of social work practice with the Hispanic elderly. In S. Applewhite (Ed.), *Hispanic elderly in transition,* pp. 3–16. New York: Greenwood Press.

Barrett, A. E., & Lynch, S. M. (1999). Caregiving networks of elderly persons: Variation by marital status. *The Gerontologist, 39,* 695–704.

Bass, D. M., Noelker, L. S., & Rechlin, L. R. (1996). The moderating influence of service use on negative caregiving consequences. *Journal of Gerontology, Social Sciences, 51B,* S121–S131.

Binstock, R. H. (1999). Public policies and minority elders. In M. L. Wykle & A. B. Ford (Eds.), *Serving minority elders in the 21st century,* (pp. 5–24). New York: Springer.

Boaz, R. F., Hu, J., & Ye, Y. (1999). The transfer of resources from middle-aged children to functionally limited elderly parents: Providing time, giving money, sharing space. *The Gerontologist, 39,* 648–657.

Brody, E. M. (1990). Role reversal: An inaccurate and destructive concept. *Journal of Gerontological Social Work, 15,* 15–22.

Brody, E. M., & Schoonover, C. B. (1986). Patterns of parent-care when adult daughters work and when they do not. *The Gerontologist, 26,* 372–381.

Buckwalter, K. C., Gerdner, L., Kohout, F., Hall, G. R., et al. (1999). A nursing intervention to decrease depression in family caregivers of persons with dementia. *Archives of Psychiatric Nursing, 13,* 80–88.

Burton, L. C., Newsom, J. T., Schulz, R., Hirsch, C. H., et al. (1997). Preventative health behaviors among spousal caregivers. *Preventative Medicine, 26,* 162–169.

Campbell, D. D., & Travis, S. S. (1999). Spousal caregiving when the adult day services center is closed. *Journal of Psychosocial Nursing, 37,* 20–25.

Chambers, M., & Connor, S. L. (2002). User-friendly technology to help family carers cope. *Journal of Advanced Nursing, 40* (5), 568–577.

Chesla, C. A., & Rungreangkulkij, S. (2001). Nursing research on family processes in chronic illness in ethnically diverse families: A decade review. *Journal of Family Nursing, 7* (3), 230–243.

Clyburn, L. D., Stones, M. J., Hadjistavropoulos, T., & Tuokko, H. (2000). Predicting caregiver burden and depression in Alzheimer's disease. *Journal of Gerontology, Social Sciences, 55B,* S2–S13.

Covinsky, K. E., Eng, C., Lui, L., Sands, L. P., et al. (2001). Reduced employment in caregivers of frail elders. *The Journals of Gerontology Series A: Biological Sciences and Medical Sciences, 56,* M707–M713.

Cox, C. (1999). Race and caregiving: Patterns of service use by African American and white caregivers of persons with Alzheimer's disease. *Journal of Gerontological Social Work, 32,* 5–19.

Dautzenberg, M. G. H. (2000). The competing demands of paid work and parent care. *Research on Aging, 22,* 165–188.

DHHS Administration on Aging (n.d.a). About NFCSP. Retrieved September 21, 2004 from http://www.aoa.gov/prof/aoaprog/caregiver/overview/overview_caregiver_pf.asp

DHHS Administration on Aging (n.d.b). Because We Care. Retrieved September 21, 2004 from http://www.aoa.dhhs.gov/prof/aoaprog/caregiver/carefam/taking_care_of_others/wecare/hire_pf.asp

DHHS Administration on Aging (n.d.c). Common Caregiving Terms. Retrieved September 21, 2004 from http://www.aoa.gov/prof/aoaprog/caregiver/careprof/progguidance/resources/caregiving_terms_pf.asp

DHHS Administration on Aging (n.d.d.) Fact Sheets Elder Abuse Prevention, Retrieved September 24, 2004 from http://www.aoa.gov.press/fact/alpha/fact_elder_abuse_pf.asp

DHHS Administration of Aging (2003a). Family caregivers: Our heroes on frontlines of long-term care. Retrieved September 20, 2004 from http:///www.aoa.gov/prof/aoaprog/caregiver/careprof/TownHall/townhall_12_16_03.asp

DHHS Administration of Aging (2003b). National Family Caregiver Support Program Townhall Meetings. Retrieved September 20, 2004 from http://www.aoa.gov/prof/aoaprog/caregiver/careprof/TownHall/townhall_12_16_03.asp

DuPont, P. (1999). The short term problem facing long-term care. *National Center for Policy Analysis.* Available on-line at http://www.ncpa.org/oped/dupont/dup010699.html

Dwyer, J. (1995). The effects of illness. In R. Blieszner & V. Bedford (Eds.), *Handbook of aging and the family,* (pp. 401–421). Westport, CT: Greenwood Press.

Edmonds, M. M. (1999). Serving minority elders: Preventing chronic illness and disability in the African American elderly. In M. L. Wykle & A. B. Ford (Eds.), *Serving minority elders in the 21st century,* (pp. 25–36). New York: Springer.

Elder Services of Worcester Area (2003). *Nursing home placement.* Retrieved August 30, 2004 from http://www.eswa.org/faq/nursing

Elliot, T. R., & Shewchuk, R. M. (2003). Social problem-solving and distress among family members assuming a caregiving role. *British Journal of Health Psychology, 8,* 149–163.

Farran, C. J. (1997). Theoretical perspectives concerning positive aspects of caring for elderly persons with dementia: Stress/adaptation and existentialism. *The Gerontologist, 37,* 250–256.

Farran, C. J., Miller, B. H., & Kaufman, J. E. (1999). Finding meaning through caregiving: Development of an instrument for family caregivers of persons with Alzheimer's disease. *Journal of Clinical Psychology, 55* (9), 1107–1125.

Fast, J. E., Williamson, D. L., & Keating, N. C. (1999). The hidden costs of informal elder care. *Journal of Family and Economic Issues, 20,* 301–326.

Faver, C. A. (2004). Relational spirituality and social caregiving. *Social Work, 49* (2), 241–249.

Figley, C. R. (1998). Burnout as systemic traumatic stress: A model for helping traumatized family members. In C. R. Figley (Ed.), *Burnout in families: The systemic costs of caring,* (pp. 15–28). Boca Raton, FL: CRC Press.

Folkman, S. (1997). Positive psychological states and coping with severe stress. *Social Science & Medicine, 45* (8), 1207–1221.

Gaugler, J. E. (2003). Evaluating community-based programs for dementia caregivers: The cost implication of adult day services. *Journal of Applied Gerontology, 22* (1), 118–133.

Gaugler, J., Kane, R. & Langlois, J. (2000). Assessment of family caregivers of older adults. In R. Kane & R. Kane (Eds.), *Assessing older persons: Measures, meaning and practical applications, (*pp. 321–359), New York: Oxford University Press.

George, L. K., & Gwyther, L. P. (1986). Caregiver well-being: A multidimensional examination of family caregivers of demented adults. *The Gerontologist, 26* (3), 253–259.

Gilliss, C. L. (2002).There is science, and there is life. *Families, Systems & Health, 20* (1), 49.

Gilmour, J. A. (2002). Dis/integrated care: family caregivers and in-hospital care. *Journal of Advanced Nursing, 39* (6), 546–553.

Gitlin, L., Burgio, L., Mahoney, D., Burns, R., et al. (2003). Effect of multicomponent interventions on caregiver burden and depression: The REACH Multisite Initiative at 6-month follow-up. *Psychology and Aging, 18* (3), 361–374.

Given, B., Strommel, M., Collins, C., King, S., et al. (1990). Responses of elderly spouse caregivers. *Research in Nursing and Health, 13,* 77–85.

Gordon, P. A. & Perrone, K. M. (2004). When spouses become caregivers: Counseling implications for younger couples. *Journal of Rehabilitation, 70* (2), 27–32.

Haigler, D. H., Bauer, L. J., & Travis, S.S. (2004). Finding the common ground of family and professional caregiving: The education agenda at the Rosalynn Carter Institute. *Educational Gerontology, 30,* 95–105.

Haley, J., & Harrigan, R. C. (2004). Voicing the strengths of Pacific Island parent caregivers of children who are medically fragile. *Journal of Transcultural Nursing, 15* (3), 184–194.

Harding, R. & Higginson, I. (2003). What is the best way to help caregivers in cancer and palliative care? A systematic literature review of interventions and their effectiveness. *Palliative Medicine, 17,* 63–74.

Harris, P. B. (1998). Listening to caregiving sons: Misunderstood realities. *The Gerontologist, 38,* 342–352.

Horowitz, A. (1985). Sons and daughters as caregivers to older parents: Differences in role performance and consequences. *The Gerontologist, 25,* 612–617.

Hudson, P. (2004). Positive aspects and challenges associated with caring for a dying relative at home. *International Journal of Palliative Nursing, 10* (2), 58–64.

Hulme, P. A. (1999). Family empowerment: A nursing intervention with suggested outcomes for families of children with a chronic health condition. *Journal of Family Nursing, 5* (1), 33–50. Thousand Oaks, CA: Sage.

Hunt, C. K. (2003). Concepts in caregiver research. *Journal of Nursing Scholarship, 35* (1), 27–32.

Interfaith Care Partners (n.d.) Retrieved September 20, 2004 from http://www.interfaithcarepartners.org

Jones, S. (1999). Bridging the gap: Community solutions for black-elderly health care in the 21st century. In M. L. Wykle & A. B. Ford (Eds.), *Serving minority elders in the 21st century,* (pp. 223–234). New York: Springer.

Kane, R. A., Reinardy, J., & Penrod, J. D. (1999). After the hospitalization is over: A different perspective on family care of older people. *Journal of Gerontological Social Work, 31,* 119–141.

Karp, D. A., & Tanarugsachock, V. (2000). Mental illness, caregiving, and emotion management. *Qualitative Health Research, 10,* 6–25.

Kauffmann, E. & Harrison, M. B. (1998). Stress-point intervention for parents of children hospitalized with chronic conditions. *Pediatric Nursing, 24* (4), 362–366.

Kaye, J., & Robinson, K. M. (1994). Spirituality among caregivers. *Image, 26,* 218–221.

Kaye, L. W., Turner, W., Butler, S. S., Downey, R., et al. (2003). Early intervention screening for family caregivers of older relatives in primary care practices. Establishing a community health service alliance in rural America. *Family Community Health, 26* (4), 319–328.

Keith, C. (1995). Family caregiving systems: Models, resources, and values. *Journal of Marriage and the Family, 57,* 179–190.

Kelly, K. (2003–2004). Link$_2$Care: Internet-based information and support for caregivers. *Family Caregiving,* Winter, 87–88.

Keysor, J. J., Desai, T., & Mutran, E. J. (1999). Elders' preferences for care setting in short- and long-term disability scenarios. *The Gerontologist, 39,* 334–344.

Kramer, B. J. (1993a). Marital history and the prior relationship as predictors of positive and negative outcomes among wife caregivers. *Family Relations, 42,* 367–375.

_____. (1993b). Expanding the conceptualization of caregiver coping: The importance of relationship-focused coping strategies. *Family Relations, 42,* 383–391.

_____. (1997). Gain in the caregiving experience: Where are we? What next? *The Gerontologist, 37,* 218–232.

Lackey, N. R., & Gates, M. F. (2001). Adults' recollections of their experiences as young caregivers of family members with chronic physical illnesses. *Journal of Advanced Nursing, 34* (3), 320–328.

Langa, K., Chernew, M. E., Kabeto, M. U., Herzon, A. R., et al. (2001). National estimates of the quantity and cost of informal caregiving for the elderly with dementia. *Journal of General Internal Medicine, 16,* 770–778.

Lattanzi-Licht, M., Mahoney, J. J., & Miller, G. W. (1998). *The hospice choice: In pursuit of a peaceful death.* New York: Simon & Schuster.

Lawton, M. P., Rajagopal, D., Brody, E., & Kleban, M. (1992). The dynamics of caregiving for a demented elder among black and white families. *Journal of Gerontology: Social Sciences, 47,* S156–S164.

Leavitt, M., Martinson, I. M., Liu, C. Y., Armstrong, V., et al. (1999). Common themes and ethnic differences in family caregiving the first year after diagnosis of childhood cancer: Part II. *Journal of Pediatric Nursing, 14,* 110–122.

Lee, G. R., Dwyer, J. W., & Coward, R. T. (1993). Gender differences in parent care: Demographic factors and the same-gender preferences. *Journals of Gerontology, Social Sciences, 48* (1), S9–S16.

Litwak, E. (1985). *Helping the elderly: The complementary roles of informal networks and formal systems.* New York: Guilford Press.

McAuley, W. J., Travis, S. S., & Safewright, M. P. (1997). Personal accounts of the nursing home search and selection process. *Qualitative Health Research, 7,* 236–254.

McGoldrick, M., & Giordano, J. (1996). Overview: Ethnicity and family therapy. In M. McGoldrick, J. Giordano, & J. K. Pearce (Eds.), *Ethnicity and family therapy* (2nd ed.), (pp. 1–30). New York: Guilford Press.

Medalie, J. H. (1994). The caregiver as the hidden patient. In E. Kahana, D. E. Biegel, & M. L. Wykle (eds.), *Family caregiving across the lifespan,* (pp. 312–330). Thousand Oaks, CA: Sage.

Meleski, D. D. (2002). Families with chronically ill children. *American Journal of Nursing, 102* (5), 47–54.

Meshefedjian, G., McCusker, J., Bellavance, F., & Baumgarten, M. (1998). Factors associated with symptoms of depression among informal caregivers of demented elders in the community. *The Gerontologist, 38,* 247–253.

Mitrani, V. B. & Czaja, S. J. (2000). Family-based therapy for dementia caregivers: Clinical observations. *Aging & Mental Health, 4* (3), 200–209.

Mittelman, J. S. (2003). Community Caregiving. *Alzheimer's Care Quarterly, 4*(4), 273–285.

Montcalm, D. M. (1995). Caregivers: Resources and services. In Z. Harel & R. E. Dunkle (Eds.), *Matching people with services in long term care,* (pp. 159–179). New York: Springer.

Montgomery, R. J. V. (1989). Investigating caregiver burden. In K. S. Markides & C. L. Cooper (Eds.), *Aging, stress and health,* (pp. 201–218). New York: John Wiley & Sons.

_____. (1999). The family role in the context of long-term care. *Journal of Aging and Health, 11,* 383–416.

Montgomery, R. J. V. & Kosloski, K. D.(n.d.). *Change, continuity and diversity among caregivers.* Retrieved September 24, 2004 from http://www.aoa.gov/prof/aoaprog/caregiver/careprof/progguidance/background/program_issues/Fin-Montgomery.pdf

Murray, S. A., Kendall, M., Boyd, K., Worth, A., et al. (2004). Exploring the spiritual needs of people dying of lung cancer or heart failure: A prospective qualitative interview study of patients and their carers. *Palliative Medicine, 18,* 39–45.

National Center for Health Statistics. (2003). U.S. birth rate reaches record low. Retrieved September 20,

2004, from http://www.cdc.gov/nchs/pressroom/03news/lowbirth.htm

Nerenberg, L. (2002). *Preventing elder abuse by family caregivers.* Washington, DC: National Center of Elder Abuse.

Neufeld, A., & Harrison, M. J. (1998). Men as caregivers: Reciprocal relationships or obligation? *Journal of Advanced Nursing, 28,* 959–968.

Nolan, M. (2001). Positive aspects of caring. In S. Payne & C. Ellis-Hill (Eds.), *Chronic and terminal illness: New perspectives on caring and carers,* (pp. 22–44). Oxford: Oxford University Press.

Opinion Research Corporation. (1988). A national survey of caregivers. Final report submitted to the American Association of Retired Persons. Washington, DC: American Association of Retired Persons.

Ory, M. G., Hoffman, R. R. III, Yee, J. L., Tennstedt, S., et al. (1999). Prevalence and impact of caregiving: A detailed comparison between dementia and nondementia caregivers. *The Gerontologist, 39,* 177–185.

Paun, O. (2004). Female Alzheimer's patient caregivers share their strength. *Holistic Nursing Practice, 18* (1), 11–17.

Pearlin, L. I. (1992). The careers of caregivers. *The Gerontologist, 32,* 647.

Peters-Davis, N. D., Moss, M. S., & Pruchno, R. A. (1999). Children-in-law in caregiving families. *The Gerontologist, 39,* 66–75.

Piercy, K. W. (1998). Theorizing about family caregiving: The role of responsibility. *Journal of Marriage and the Family, 60,* 109–118.

Piercy, K. W. & Chapman, J.G. (2001). Adopting the caregiver role: A family legacy. *Family Relations, 50,* 386–393.

Pines, A. M., & Aronson, E. (1988). *Career burnout: Causes and cures.* New York: The Free Press.

Pruchno, R. A., Burant, C. J., & Peters, N. D. (1997). Understanding the well-being of care receivers. *The Gerontologist, 37,* 102–109.

Pyke, K. (1999). The micropolitics of care in relationships between aging parents and adult children: Individualism, collectivism, and power. *The Journal of Marriage and the Family, 61,* 661–673.

Ritchie, L. (2003). Adult day care: Northern perspectives. *Public Health Nursing, 20* (2), 120–131.

Rittman, M., Kuzmeskus, L. B., & Flum, M. A. (1998). A synthesis of current knowledge on minority elder abuse. In T. Tatara (Ed.), *Understanding elder abuse in minority populations,* (pp. 221–238). Philadelphia: Brunner/Mazel.

Roff, L., Burgio, L., Gitlin, L., Nichols, L., et al. (2004). Positive aspects of Alzheimer's caregiving: The role of race. *Journals of Gerontology Series B: Psychological Sciences and Social Sciences, 59B* (4), 185–190.

San Francisco Medical Society (n.d.) San Francisco senior citizen services: Adult day services. Retrieved September 1, 2004 from http://www.sfms.org/sfm/sfm699j.htm

Scharlach, A. E., & Grosswald, B. (1997). The family and medical leave act of 1993. *Social Service Review, 71,* 335–360.

Schulz, R., & Beach, S. R. (1999). Caregiving as a risk factor for mortality: The caregiver health effects study. *Journal of the American Medical Association, 282,* 2215–2219.

Scott, G. (2001). A study of family carers of people with a life-threatening illness 2: The implications of the needs assessment. *International Journal of Palliative Nursing, 7* (7), 323–330.

Seltzer, M. M. (1990). Role reversal: You don't go home again. *Journal of Gerontological Social Work, 15,* 5–14.

Seltzer, M. M., & Wailing, L. (2000). The dynamics of caregiving: Transitions during a three-year prospective study. *The Gerontologist, 40,* 165–178.

Shapiro, E. R. (2002). Chronic illness as a family process: A social-developmental approach to promoting resilience. *JCLP/in session: Psychotherapy in practice, 58* (11), 1375–1384.

Sheehan, N. W., & Donorfio, L. M. (1999). Efforts to create meaning in the relationship between aging mothers and their caregiving daughters: A qualitative study of caregiving. *Journal of Aging Studies, 13,* 161–176.

Shirey, L., & Summer, L. (2000). *Caregiving: Helping the elderly with activity limitations.* Washington, DC: National Academy on Aging Society.

Skaff, M. M., Pearlin, L. I., & Mullan, J. T. (1996). Transitions in the caregiving career: Effects on sense of mastery. *Psychology and Aging, 11,* 247–257.

Spector, R. E. (2000). *Cultural diversity in health and illness* (5th ed.). Upper Saddle River, NJ: Prentice Hall Health.

Stoller, E. P., & Cutler, S. J. (1993). Predictors of use of paid help among older people living in the community. *The Gerontologist, 33* (1), 31–40.

Stone, R., Cafferata, G. L., & Sangl, J. (1987). Caregivers of the frail elderly: A national profile. *The Gerontologist, 27,* 616–626.

Stone, R. I., & Short, P. F. (1990). The competing demands of employment and informal caregiving to disabled elders. *Medical Care, 28,* 513–526.

Stuckey, J. C. (2001). Blessed assurance: The role of religion and spirituality in Alzheimer's disease caregiving and other significant life events. *Journal of Aging Studies, 15* (1), 69–84.

Substance Abuse and Mental Health Service Administration (2004). SAMHSA Model Programs. Retrieved September 20, 2004 from http://model programs.samhsa.gov

Tarlow, B., Wisniewski, S., Belle, S., Rubert, M., et al. (2004). Positive aspects of caregiving. *Research on Aging, 26* (4), 429–453.

Teaster, P. B. (2003). *A response to the abuse of vulnerable adults: The 2000 survey of state adult protective services.* Retrieved September 25, 2004 from http://www.elderabusecenter.org/pdf/research/apsreport030703.pdf

Theis, S. L., Biordi, D. L., Coeling, H., Nalepka, C., et al. (2003). Spirituality in caregiving and care receiving. *Holistic Nursing Practice, 17* (1), 48–55.

Thompson, B., Tudiver, F., & Manson, J. (2000). Sons as sole caregivers for their elderly parents. How do they cope? *Canadian Family Physician, 46,* 360–365.

Toth-Cohen, S., Gitlin, L. N., Corcoran, M. A., Eckhardt, S., et al. (2001). Providing services to family caregivers at home: Challenges and recommendations for health and human service professions. *Alzheimer's Care Quarterly, 2* (1), 23–32.

Travis, S. S., & Bethea, L. S. (2001). Medication administration by family members of elders in shared care arrangements. *Journal of Clinical Geropsychology, 7,* 231–243.

Travis, S. S., Bethea, L. S., & Winn, P. (2000). Medication administration hassles reported by family caregivers of dependent elders. *Journal of Gerontology, Medical Sciences, 55A,* M412–M417.

Travis, S. S., & Duer, B. (2000). Interdisciplinary management of the older adult with cancer. In A. S. Luggen & S. E. Meiner (Eds.), *Handbook for the care of the older adult with cancer,* (pp. 25–34). Pittsburgh, PA: Oncology Nursing Press.

Tripp-Reimer, T. (1999). Culturally competent care. In M. L. Wykle & A. B. Ford (Eds.), *Serving minority elders in the 21st century,* (pp. 235–247). New York: Springer.

U.S. Department of Commerce Bureau of the Census 2000, Population Division. Statistical Brief. Sixty-five plus in the United States. Washington, D.C.

U.S. Department of Labor. (1993). *The family and medical leave act of 1993.* Washington, DC: U.S. Department of Labor, Wage and Hour Division.

Walker, E. & Dewar, B. J. (2004). How do we facilitate carers' involvement in decision making? *Journal of Advanced Nursing, 34* (3), 329–337.

Walker, A. J., & Pratt, C. C. (1995). Informal caregiving to aging family members: A critical review. *Family Relations, 44,* 402–411.

Warren, S., Kerr, J., Smith, D., Godkin, D., & Schalm, C. (2003). The impact of adult day programs on family caregivers of elderly relatives. *Journal of Community Health Nursing, 20* (4), 209–221.

Weissert, W. G., & Hedrick, S. C. (1994). Lessons learned from research on effects of community-based long-term care. *Journal of the American Geriatrics Society, 42,* 348–353.

_____. (1999). Outcomes and costs of home and community-based long-term care: Implications for research-based practice. In E. Calkins, C. Boult, E. H. Wagner, & J. T. Pacala (Eds.), *New ways to care for older people,* (pp. 143–157). New York: Springer.

Weitzner, M. A., Haley, W. E., & Chen, H. (2000). The family caregiver of the older cancer patient. *Hematology and Oncology Clinics of North America, 14,* 269–281.

White-Means, S. L. (1997). The demands of persons with disabilities for home health care and the economic consequences for informal caregivers. *Social Science Quarterly, 78,* 955–972.

Williams, S. W., Dilworth-Anderson, P. & Goodwin, P. Y. (2003). Caregiver role strain: The contribution of multiple roles and available resources in African-American women. *Aging and Mental Health, 7* (2), 103–112.

Winslow, B.W. (2003). Family caregivers' experiences with community services: A qualitative analysis. *Public Health Nursing, 20* (5), 341–348.

Yee, J. L., & Schulz, R. (2000). Gender differences in psychiatric morbidity among family caregivers: A review and analysis. *The Gerontologist, 40,* 147–164.

CHAPTER 12

Sexuality

Margaret Chamberlain Wilmoth

Introduction

Humans are sexual beings from birth until death. Sexuality is an integral aspect of our personalities and is more than sexual contact and the ability to function to reach sexual satisfaction. Sexuality includes views of ourselves as male or female, feelings about our body, and the ways we communicate verbally and nonverbally our comfort about ourselves to others. It also includes the ability to engage in satisfying sexual behaviors alone or with another. Sexuality does not end when one reaches a certain age, nor does it end with the diagnosis of a chronic illness. In fact, sexuality and intimacy may become *more* important after such a diagnosis as a way of reaffirming human connections, aliveness, and continued desirability and caring. Sexuality is a critical aspect of quality of life that, unfortunately, is often ignored by health care professionals.

This chapter briefly reviews standards of nursing practice as they relate to sexuality, sexual physiological functioning, alterations in sexuality caused by common chronic illnesses and their treatments, and nursing interventions. This chapter also provides nurses with suggestions to incorporate discussions of sexuality into their practice.

Definitions

Sexuality is a complex construct with terminology that has yet to be defined in a manner that is accepted by all. When discussing sexuality with other professionals or with clients, it is important to be sure that everyone has the same frame of reference for the many descriptors that are used for aspects of sexuality. The definitions used in discussing sexuality in this chapter are found in Table 12-1.

Standards of Practice

Standards of practice imply a legal standard of practice as well as an ethical responsibility that must be adhered to (Andrews, Goldberg & Kaplan, 1996). Standards of practice for the profession, published by the American Nurses Association (ANA) (2004), include six standards of care that encompass significant actions taken by nurses when providing care to their clients. These standards include the components of the nursing process. These standards also assume that all relevant health care needs of the client will be assessed and appropriate care provided, including needs surrounding sexuality.

TABLE 12-1

Definitions

Sexuality	Everything that makes us man or woman, including the need for touch, feelings about one's body, the need to connect with another human being in an intimate way, interest in engaging in sexual behaviors, communication of one's feelings and needs to one's partner, and the ability to engage in satisfying sexual behaviors
Sexual behaviors	Specific activities used to obtain release of sexual tension alone or with another in order to achieve sexual satisfaction; refers also to the multiple ways one verbally and nonverbally communicates sexual feelings and attitudes to others
Sexual functioning	The physiological component of sexuality, including human sexual anatomy, the sexual response cycle, neuroendocrine functioning, and life-cycle changes in sexual physiology
Sexual dysfunction	Characterized by disturbances in the processes of the sexual response cycle or by pain associated with sexual intercourse; is a DSM-IV diagnosis and should not be used by nurses unless they are specially trained in treating sexual dysfunctions

---

SOURCES: From Wilmoth, 1998, and the American Psychiatric Association, 1994.

Specialty organizations may have derived standards of nursing practice from those published by the ANA that are specific to their practice. For example, the Oncology Nursing Society (2004) published nursing practice standards that specifically identified sexuality as one potential area of client concern. These standards include both Assessment Criteria and Outcome Criteria. Nurses who care for cancer patients then are expected to follow each of these standards in the provision of patient care. (see Figure 12-1).

Nurses and physicians are legally obligated to ensure that clients have the necessary information to make decisions regarding treatment. The provision of informed consent also requires that all risks, benefits, and side effects of diseases and their treatments be provided to clients as they choose treatments for any illness. This includes information about potential sexual side effects of proposed treatments. Failure to provide this information could potentially lead to legal action by the client.

The Sexual Response Cycle and Sexual Physiology

Kaplan (1979) identified three phases of the sexual response cycle that are used in delineating components of sexual physiology: desire, arousal, and orgasm. Physical changes that occur in both men and women as a result of sexual stimulation are vasocongestion and myotonia. Vasocongestion occurs in the penis in men and in the labia in women, and is an essential requirement for orgasm and subsequent sexual satisfaction. *Myotonia* refers to the involuntary muscular contractions that occur throughout the body during sexual response (Kolodny, Masters, Johnson, & Biggs, 1979).

Desire is the prelude to engaging in satisfying sexual behaviors and is the most complex component of the sexual response cycle. Desire is often affected by factors such as anger, pain, and body image, as well as disease processes and medications (Kaplan, 1979). Desire can be enhanced through touch, visual imagery, and fantasy (Friday, 1973). This may partially explain why psychic factors modify sexual interest, particularly in women (Guyton, 1992).

Arousal, manifested by erection in males, is mediated by the parasympathetic nervous system and is the result of either psychic or somatic sexual stimulation (Masters & Johnson, 1966). Somatic sensations pass through the pudendal nerve, through the sacral plexus, and into the sacral portion of the spinal cord (Guyton, 1992). A second center between T11 and L2 appears to mediate the response to psychic stimulation (Sands, 1995). In men, these impulses cause di-

FIGURE 12-1

Oncology Nursing Society *Statement on the Scope and Standards of Oncology Nursing Practice (2004).*

Standard I Assessment	Standard III Outcome Identification
The oncology nurse systematically and continually collects data regarding the health status of the patient.	The oncology nurse identified expected outcomes individualized to the patient.
Measurement Criteria	**Measurement Criteria**
The oncology nurse collects data in the following 14 high-incidence problem areas that may include but are not limited to: (j) sexuality.	The oncology nurse develops expected outcomes for each of the 14 high-incidence problem areas within a level consistent with the patient's physiology, psychosocial, spiritual capacities, cultural background, and value system. The expected outcomes include but are not limited to (j) sexuality. The patient and/or family:
1. Past and present sexual patterns and expression.	1. Identifies potential or actual changes in sexuality, sexual functioning or intimacy related to disease and treatment.
2. Effects of disease and treatment on body image.	2. Expresses feelings about alopecia, body image changes, and altered sexual functioning.
3. Effects of disease and treatment on sexual function.	3. Engages in open communication with his or her partner regarding changes in sexual functioning or desire, within cultural framework.
4. Psychological response of patient and partner to disease and treatment.	4. Describes appropriate interventions for actual or potential changes in sexual function.
	5. Identifies other satisfying methods of sexual expression that provide satisfaction to both partners, within cultural framework.
	6. Identifies personal and community resources to assist with changes in body image and sexual functioning.

SOURCE: Oncology Nursing Society. (2004). *Statement on the scope and standards of oncology nursing practice.* Pittsburgh, PA: Author.

lation of the arteries in the penis, resulting in vasocongestion and, subsequently, an erection (Guyton, 1992). Swelling of the testes and scrotal sac also occurs secondary to vasocongestion. Alternately, activation of the sympathetic nervous system will lead to loss of an erection through vasoconstriction.

It was previously thought that an analogous process of parasympathetic nervous system stimulation led to arousal in women. However, recent ev-

idence suggests that it is stimulation of the sympathetic nervous system that is responsible for female arousal (Meston, 2000). Data also suggest that stimulation of the SNS may enhance arousal in women with low sexual desire (Meston & Gorzalka, 1996) and that induction of relaxation may negatively affect arousal (Meston, 2000).

Vaginal lubrication is the initial indication of arousal in women and is believed to be caused by vasocongestion. This is accompanied by lengthening and widening of the vagina, elevation of the cervix and uterus, and initial swelling of the labia minora (Guyton, 1992; Masters & Johnson, 1966). These changes are caused by vasocongestion and are secondary to a parasympathetic response mediated to S2 and S4 through the pudendal nerve and sacral plexus (Guyton, 1992).

Impending orgasm is determined by the presence of an intense color change in the labia minora in women and full elevation of the scrotal sac to the perineal wall in men, all a result of intense vasocongestion (Masters & Johnson, 1966). Orgasm is mediated by the sympathetic nervous system and is the physical release and peak of pleasurable expression, followed by relaxation (Guyton, 1992). The sympathetic nerves between T12 and L2 control ejaculation (Koukouras et al., 1991). The intensity of orgasm in women is dependent upon the duration and intensity of sexual stimulation.

The Grafenberg spot (G-spot) plays an important role in sexuality for many women but has not been incorporated into the sexual response cycle. The G-spot is located in the anterior wall of the vagina, about halfway between the back of the pubic bone and the cervix along the course of the urethra (Ladas, Whipple & Perry, 1982). When stimulated, this tissue swells from the size of a bean to greater than a half dollar (Ladas et al., 1982). Stimulation of this area appears to cause a different orgasmic sensation, which may be due to the fact that this response is mediated by the pelvic nerve, causing the uterus to contract and descend against the vagina rather than elevate, as with stimulation mediated by the pudendal nerve (Ladas et al, 1982). Approximately 40 percent of women will experience expulsion of a fluid upon orgasm caused by G-spot stimulation (Darling, Davidson & Conway-Welch, 1990). Research indicates that this is a prostatic-like fluid that is released during orgasm (Zaviacic & Whipple, 1993). Knowledge that this is not urine but a normal release of fluid that occurs during sexual response can lead to a reduction in embarrassment for many women.

The neurohormonal system influences sexual functioning through its effect on hormone production. The hypothalamic–hypophysial portal system has an important role in sexual functioning in both genders through production of gonadotropin-releasing hormone (GnRH) and subsequent stimulation of gonadotropin production by the anterior pituitary gland. The anterior pituitary gland secretes six hormones, two of which play an essential role in sexual functioning. Follicle-stimulating hormone (FSH) and luteinizing hormone (LH) control growth of the gonads and influence sexual functioning. In men, LH influences production of testosterone by the Leydig cells in the testes through a negative feedback loop (Guyton, 1992). Production of GnRH is reduced once a satisfactory level of testosterone has been attained. A negative feedback loop also exists in the woman, although it is much more complex due to the concurrent production of estrogen and progesterone by the ovary and the production of androgens by the adrenal cortex.

Psychic factors appear to play a larger role in female sexual functioning than in that of men, particularly in relation to sexual desire. Multiple neuronal centers in the brain's limbic system transmit signals into the arcuate nuclei in the mediobasal hypothalamus. These signals modify the intensity of GnRH release and frequency of the impulses (Guyton, 1992). This may explain why desire in women is more vulnerable to emotions and distractions than it is in men.

Aging affects the sexual response cycle in predictable ways, but it does not signal the end of sexuality. In fact, the old adage, "Use it or lose it," is applicable to continued sexual activity throughout life (Masters & Johnson, 1981). The general impact of aging on the sexual response cycle is a slower, less intense sexual response. The frequency of sexual activity in earlier years is predictive of frequency as one ages. The quality of the sexual relationship appears to be the greatest influence on the frequency and satisfaction of sexual activity (Masters & Johnson, 1981). As in younger adults, the quality of communication in a relationship, degree of mutual intimacy, and level of commitment to the relationship are vital to a satisfying sexual relationship and to achieving sexual satisfaction.

In men, the primary change with aging is an increase in the time it takes to achieve a full erection.

Masters and Johnson (1966) found that in men between 51 and 90 years of age, the time to achieve erection was two to three times longer than in younger men. Achieving erection also required more tactile stimulation than in younger years. However, once achieved, older men can maintain a full erection for a longer time period before ejaculation. Scrotal vasocongestion is reduced, with a subsequent decrease in testicular elevation. The ability to attain orgasm is not impaired with aging, but there is an overall decrease in myotonia and fewer penile and rectal sphincter contractions. There is an increase in time from hours to days before older men can achieve another erection once they have ejaculated and achieved an orgasm.

Women also experience sexual response cycle changes primarily after completing the menopausal transition. Vaginal changes include a thinning of the mucosa, with a decrease in vaginal lubrication. In women who abstain from sexual intercourse, narrowing and stenosis of the introitus and vaginal vault can occur (Leiblum & Segraves, 1989). Older women experience a decrease in the vasocongestion of the labia and other genitalia analogous to the decrease in penile tumescence experienced by men. Orgasm in sexually active women is not impaired; however, there is some decrease in the degree of myotonia experienced. Intense orgasm may lead to involuntary distension of the external meatus, leading to an increase in frequency of urinary tract infections in older women.

Sexuality and Chronic Illness

The presence of a chronic illness affects all aspects of an individual's life, including their sexuality. There are numerous chronic illnesses, and discussion of the impact of each on sexuality is beyond the scope of this chapter. Therefore, this chapter is limited to discussing the effects that coronary artery disease, diabetes mellitus, cancer, and multiple sclerosis have on sexuality.

Coronary Artery Disease

The heart is linked to romance and to the soul, so any threat to cardiac functioning is emotionally linked to matters of the self, sexuality, and intimacy. Cardiovascular disease, that includes coronary ar-

tery disease (CAD) and stroke, causes more death in both genders and all racial and ethnic groups in the United States than any other disease (Centers for Disease Control, 2004). More men and women are living longer and continue to lead productive lives after experiencing a myocardial infarction (MI) than ever before; however recent data suggests that women experience a lower degree of quality of life than men (Agewall, Berglund & Henareh, 2004; Svedlund & Danielson, 2004). Thus, having adequate and accurate knowledge about sexuality post-diagnosis may have a positive impact on an individual's self-concept, to their sexuality, and to their sexual relationships.

The Princeton Consensus Conference was convened to address issues related to sexuality and cardiovascular disease (DeBusk et al., 2000). The relative safety at which clients can engage in sexual activity is dependent on their degree of cardiac disease. This panel recommended a classification system that would stratify clients into a risk category based on the extent of their cardiac disease. These categories and management recommendations are found in Table 12-2. With MI, all clients less than two weeks post-MI are considered to be at high risk for coition-induced reinfarction, cardiac rupture, or coition-induced arrhythmias. All clients should, therefore, be encouraged to refrain from sexual activity during this period. Between 2 and 6 weeks post-MI, all clients are considered to be at intermediate risk for a cardiac event and should be encouraged to have a post-MI stress test before engaging in sexual activity (DeBusk et al., 2000).

Counseling of all clients regarding life-style changes and activity restrictions should begin as soon as the client is stabilized. Discussions regarding sexual activity should be included in the counseling. Potential fear of cardiac arrest during sexual activity should be eradicated as soon as possible by assuring clients and their partners that this risk is only 1.2 percent and that sex only accounts for 0.5 to 1.0 percent of all acute coronary incidents (DeBusk, 2000).

Recent reports continue to validate the appropriateness of the stair-climbing tolerance test for successful return to sexual activity after six weeks

TABLE 12-2

Management Recommendations Based on Graded Cardiovascular (CV) Risk Assessment

Grade of Risk	Categories of CVD	Management
Low risk	Asymptomatic, < 3 risk factors for CAD Controlled hypertension Mild, stable angina Post–successful coronary revascularization Uncomplicated post-MI (> 6 weeks) Mild valvular disease LVD/CHF (NYHA class I)	Primary care management Consider all first-line therapies Reassess at regular intervals
Intermediate risk	< 3 major risk factors for CAD Moderate, stable angina Recent MI (> 2, < 6 weeks) LVD/CHF (NYHA class II) Noncardiac sequelae of atherosclerotic disease (e.g., CVA, PVD)	Specialized CV testing Restratification into high or low risk based on results of CV testing
High risk	Unstable or refractory angina Uncontrolled hypertension LVD/CHF (NYHA class III/IV) Recent MI (< 2 weeks), CVA High-risk arrhythmias Hypertrophic obstructive and other cardiomyopathies Moderate/severe valvular disease	Priority referral for specialized CV management Treatment for sexual dysfunction deferred until cardiac condition stabilized and dependent on specialist recommendations CAD, coronary artery disease; CHF, congestive heart failure; CVA, stroke; CVD, cardiovascular disease; NYHA, New York Heart Association.

CAD, coronary artery disease; CHF, congestive heart failure; CVA, stroke; CVD, cardiovascular disease; NYHA, New York Heart Association.

SOURCE: From DeBusk, R., Drory, Y., Goldstein, I., Jackson, G., Kaul, S., & Kimmel, S. E. (2000). Management of sexual dysfunction in patients with cardiovascular disease: Recommendations of the Princeton consensus panel. *The American Journal of Cardiology, 86* (2), 175–181. Reprinted with permission from Excerpta Medica Inc.

post-MI. Sexual activity conceptualized simply as arousal is unassociated with physical exertion. It is not until exertion is coupled with arousal that energy expenditure occurs. Data indicate that the man in the top position results in greater responses of heart rate and VO_2, and thus greater energy expenditure that may or may not reflect both heightened arousal and exertion. If sexual activity is conceptualized as exertion, then the capacity to climb two flights of stairs without limiting symptoms is a clinical benchmark of exercise tolerance and subsequent

ability to engage in sexual activity without symptoms (DeBusk, 2000).

Depression has been indicated as a psychological cause of sexual dysfunction and may increase the risk of cardiac mortality in both genders (Roose & Seidman, 2000). An 18 percent incidence of major depression and a 27 percent incidence of minor depression has been documented in post-MI clients (Schliefer et al., 1989). Others have shown that at six months post-MI, depressed clients have a cardiac mortality of 17 percent (Frasure-Smith, Lesperance

& Talajic, 1993). Roose and Seidman (2000) indicate that the male client with ischemic heart disease who is depressed is also likely to have erectile difficulties. This is also a predisposing factor for other adverse cardiac events. Therefore, it appears prudent that all post-MI clients be evaluated for depression and receive appropriate therapy. It is also important to note that medications frequently used in treating depression, namely the selective serotonin reuptake inhibitors, can lead to a variety of sexual dysfunctions (Gitlin, 1995).

Clients should be counseled regarding the effects of medications on sexuality. For example, thiazide diuretics and sympatholytic drugs can cause erectile dysfunction (Weiner & Rosen, 1997). Calcium channel blockers reduce peripheral vascular resistance, and thus have few to no negative effects on sexual functioning (Lehne, 1998). Use of sildenafil is absolutely contraindicated in men taking nitrates due to its action on vasodilation (DeBusk et al., 2000).

Counseling and education about return to pre-infarct activities, including sexuality, should be a part of a comprehensive cardiac rehabilitation program. Age and marital status should not be a factor in determining who receives information about resuming sexual activity. Data indicate that married women may actually engage in sexual activity less frequently than single women with heart disease (Baggs & Karch, 1987). If clients have a spouse or regular partner, they should be included in education and counseling sessions unless the clients request otherwise. Discussions about sexual activity should include talking about anxieties concerning resumption of sexual activities with one's partner, scheduling sexual encounters after periods of rest, avoiding sex after heavy meals or alcohol ingestion, and keeping nitroglycerin at the bedside as a form of reassurance (Steinke, 2000). An integral part of successful resumption of sexual activity is engaging in regular exercise based on physician recommendations. Partners of cardiac clients also experience distress due to the disease that may manifest as decreased intimacy and may require intervention to assist them in adjusting to disease-related stressors (O'Farrell, Murray & Hotz, 2000).

Diabetes Mellitus

The incidence of diabetes mellitus in the United States is on the increase with an estimated 18 million Americans living with this chronic disease (Mokdad et al., 2001), and with it, the number of persons who have alterations in their sexuality will increase. Nurses must be prepared to assist these individuals with the multiple life changes they will experience due to this disease, including changes in sexual functioning. It is well known that diabetes mellitus has serious effects on sexual functioning in men. Prevalence rates of erectile dysfunction (ED) in diabetic males range from 33–75% depending on age, glycemic control and presence of other behaviors such as smoking (Jackson, 2004). Less is known about the effects of diabetes on women (LeMone, 1996) and there is great variability in reports on the effect of diabetes on the sexual response cycle in women (Sarkadi & Rosenquist, 2004).

Men with diabetes typically experience minimal changes in their desire for sexual activities. Any changes in desire may be attributable to difficulties in achieving satisfactory arousal. Arousal difficulties are manifested by the lack of adequate penile erection, typically referred to as erectile dysfunction (ED). The term *impotence* has multiple negative psychological connotations and is no longer used by health professionals (NIH, 1992). Approximately 50 percent of all men with diabetes will experience ED (Tilton, 1997). Acute onset of ED may reflect poor glycemic control of the disease; however, ED may be reversible if control is regained. Acute onset of ED reflects accumulation of sorbitol and water in autonomic nerve fibers and is generally a temporary condition. Chronic ED is primarily reflective of neuropathy of the autonomic parasympathetic nervous system, with some varying degree of influence by microangiopathy, and becomes a permanent condition (Tilton, 1997).

Treatment options for erectile dysfunction in diabetic men include use of sildenafil or similar medications, intracavernosal injection therapy or placement of a penile prosthesis (Jackson, 2004). Men who experience ED should be referred to a urologist for work-up prior to making a decision about treatment options. (See Table 12-3 for treatment options.) Couples should be referred for counseling to help them adjust to the strains this chronic illness will place on their sexual relationship.

Men with diabetes are capable of experiencing orgasm and ejaculation even after developing erectile dysfunction because the disease has lesser effects on the sympathetic autonomic nervous system. Men may experience a retrograde ejaculation due to autonomic system disruption of the internal vesical sphincter (Tilton, 1997). Fertility may also be impaired in diabetic men secondary to ED, low semen volume, and lowered sperm counts. Couples desiring children should be referred to a fertility specialist.

Despite recent efforts in identifying and quantifying the prevalence of sexual problems in women with diabetes, data continue to be inconsistent and conflicting. Hypoactive sexual desire in diabetic women has been reported to range from 0 percent (Kolodny, Rostlapid & Kabshelova, 1971) to 45 percent in these women (Zrustova, 1978). Other prevalence data suggest that all phases of the sexual response cycle are negatively affected in women with IDDM with diabetic women reporting 27% dysfunction as compared with 15% of those in a control group (Enzlin et al., 2002). Additionally, there was a significant difference between diabetic women and the control group on vaginal lubrication, with diabetic women reporting decreased lubrication (Enzlin et al., 2002). Data are scarce in comparing levels of desire between women with insulin-dependent (IDDM) and non-insulin-dependent diabetes (NIDDM). LeMone (1996) reports interview data that indicate that women do experience decreased desire for sexual activity after diagnosis with diabetes.

Vaginal lubrication is a manifestation of sexual arousal and can be viewed as analogous to erection in men. As such, women would experience alterations in vaginal capillary dilation and loss of transudate formed in the vagina. Data are somewhat more consistent about degree of difficulty in achieving arousal by women with diabetes, with diabetic women reporting twice the rate of arousal problems

as do healthy women (Enzlin et al., 1998). Women self-reported alterations in vaginal lubrication, with those with IDDM reporting greater changes in lubrication based on phase of the menstrual cycle and blood glucose levels (LeMone, 1996). Women also reported that it took longer to reach a level of arousal necessary to be orgasmic, but that there were no discernible changes in their orgasms since the onset of diabetes. Other research reports varying frequencies of orgasmic difficulties. Kolodny (1971) found that 35 percent of his sample reported complete loss of orgasm, while Jenson (1981) had only 10 percent report decreased or absent orgasm.

Although the data cannot pinpoint the exact percentage of diabetic women and men with sexual difficulties or identify exactly when in the course of the disease sexual problems occur, nurses still have an obligation to address this aspect of care. Factors influencing sexual dysfunction in diabetic women include depression, marital dissatisfaction, difficulty adjusting to the diagnosis and low satisfaction with diabetic treatment options. Sexual dysfunction in men also appears to be related to depression, as well as poor adjustment to the diagnosis and negative appraisal of the disease (Enzlin, Matieu & Demyttenaere, 2003). Nurses should assume that all clients with diabetes will experience a sexual difficulty at some point in time after diagnosis and *routinely* assess the sexual concerns of their clients. Women who report vaginal dryness can be encouraged to use over-the-counter water-soluble vaginal lubricants. Eating yogurt with active cultures may help in reducing the frequency of yeast infections. Maintaining close control over fluctuations in their blood glucose levels will also reduce the frequency of yeast infections. Couples should be referred to counseling as issues arise related to the strains of living with a chronic illness in order that better communication may occur about these issues.

Cancer

Cancer occurs in people of all ages. Cancer happens to a couple and to a family. A complete discussion of the multiple ways cancer can have an impact

TABLE 12-3

Treatments for Erectile Dysfunction

Treatment	Mechanism of Action	Side Effects	Pro/Con
Sildenafil citrate (Viagra) Vardenafil	Blocks enzyme phosphodiesterase-5 and allows for persistent levels of cyclic GMP. This chemical is produced in the penis during sexual arousal and leads to smooth muscle relaxation in penis and increases blood flow, leading to erection.	Headache, flushing of face, GI irritability, nasal congestion, muscle aches	Pro: Allows for some degree of spontaneity Con: Cannot be taken if the client also takes nitrates for cardiac disease
Intracavernosal injections	Medications act on sinusoidal smooth muscle to induce relaxation and enhance corporal filling.	Penile pain during injection Priaprism in 1% Hematoma in 8%	Pro: Allows for some degree of spontaneity Con: Requires office visits to ensure proper technique; can only use qod; expense
Vacuum extraction device (VED)	Places negative pressure on corporal bodies of the penis to allow for blood flow into the penis and cause an erection. A constriction band is placed around the base of the penis to prevent loss of erection until the sex act is completed.	Penile hematoma; injury to erectile tissue or penile skin necrosis may lead to pemanent penile deformity. Painful erections due to impairment of blood flow by the constriction band at the base of the penis.	Pro: Allows for penile–vaginal penetration Con: Loss of spontaneity; erection only involves a part of the penis
Malleable device	Straightens the penis for intercourse	Potential for postoperative infection; may place prolonged pressure on corporal bodies and cause tissue damage	Pro: May be used in patients with neurological disease Con: Surgical procedure
Inflatable penile prosthesis	Inflate erectile cylinders from reservoir. As fluid moves from the reservoir into corporal bodies, the penis becomes erect.	Infection in first few months after implanted; may have failure of device, requiring removal and replacement	Pro: Allows intercourse to continue Con: Reports of sexual dissatisfaction due to loss of girth and length of erection Surgical procedure
External prosthetic penis	A strap-on dildo made of silicone rubber. Shaft of dildo is mounted at angle on flanged base, which holds it in the harness. Cleaning: soap/water	No physiologic implications; may require counseling with partner to overcome hesitancy	Pro: allows intercourse to continue; enhances partner satisfaction Con: Personal inhibition may make this appear as a non-legitimate option

on sexuality is beyond the scope of this chapter; for more detailed information, the reader is referred to any of the major cancer nursing textbooks and publications by the Oncology Nursing Society. This discussion is limited to the general ways that cancer and cancer treatments affect sexuality.

In general, surgical treatments for cancer have an impact on body image and the ability to function sexually. Surgical procedures for cancers of the gastrointestinal system can lead to sexual difficulties secondary to damage to nerves that enervate sexual organs or cause alterations in body image that affect sexuality. Other procedures may involve removal of or alterations in organs that directly impact the ability to function sexually. For example, invasive cervical cancer is commonly treated by radical hysterectomy with pelvic and periaortic lymphadenectomy (DiSaia & Creasman, 1997). Radical hysterectomy renders a woman unable to bear children and will lead to a surgically induced menopause if oophorectomy is included in the procedure. Due to removal of the upper portion of the vagina, women and their partners may be concerned that having a shortened vagina may preclude satisfactory sexual intercourse. The postoperative clinic or office visit is an ideal time to discuss resumption of sexual activity. In addition to reassuring the woman that the vagina is elastic and that hysterectomy does not end sexual intercourse, the nurse should also suggest use of sexual positions that allow the woman to control the rate and depth of penile penetration, such as the woman-on-top position (Wilmoth & Spinelli, 2000).

Men also suffer sexual side effects from surgical intervention. Characteristics associated with postoperative sexual recovery after radical prostatectomy include younger age, use of nerve-sparing techniques, smaller prostate at time of surgery, pretreatment erectile ability, presence of a sexually functional partner and absence of androgen deprivation (Hollenbeck, Dunn, Wei, Sandler & Sanda, 2004). Specific information regarding the effects of other surgical procedures on sexual functioning is found in Table 12-4.

Radiation therapy can cause alterations in organ functioning, primary organ failure resulting in either permanent or temporary alterations in fertility, as well as side effects that are not directly related to sexual functioning (Table 12-5). For example, radiation therapy for invasive cervical cancer may include a combination of external and internal radiation therapy. Side effects include fatigue, diarrhea, vaginal dryness, and vaginal stenosis (Hilderley, 2000). Vaginal dryness will definitely occur; however, vaginal stenosis can be prevented. A patent vagina is important in maintaining sexual function as well as allowing for adequate follow-up evaluations. Women must be educated about the need to either use a vaginal dilator or have vaginal intercourse on a regular basis (Wilmoth & Spinelli, 2000). Likewise, men who receive either external beam or brachytherapy for prostate cancer are at increased risk of sexual dysfunction (Hollenbeck et al, 2004).

Chemotherapy has a major impact on sexual functioning, may lead to infertility, or lead to altered ovarian failure (McInnes & Schilsky, 1996). The extent of the impact on fertility varies based on the patient's gender, type of cancer, and the type and dosage of chemotherapy. Combination chemotherapy that includes alkylating agents and being a woman older than age 35 appear to be the primary factors related to altered fertility. In addition to altered fertility, chemotherapy can lead to altered ovarian function and subsequent menopause (McInnes & Schilsky, 1996). Menopausal symptoms such as hot flashes, vaginal dryness, and skin changes in addition to chemotherapy side effects can be traumatic for women, particularly if they are not aware of the potential for menopause (Wilmoth, unpublished data). The nurse could suggest use of vitamin E, use of water-soluble vaginal lubricants, and doing Kegel exercises to reduce symptoms (Wilmoth, 1996).

The use of alkylating agents in men has a major impact on their sexuality and fertility. Men who receive cumulative doses greater than 400 mg are always azoospermic, as are those treated with cisplatin (Krebs, 2000; Viviani et al., 1991). Adult men, regardless of age, are likely to experience long-term side effects of chemotherapy. However, age, total dose, and time since therapy are key to recovery of fertility. If fertility is to recover, normal sperm counts should return to normal within three years

TABLE 12-4

Effects of Cancer Surgery on Sexual Functioning

Type of Surgery	Effects on Sexual Functioning	Client Education
Colorectal surgery with colostomy	Varies; depends on type and extent of surgical procedure; major impact on body image, self-concept	Encourage expression of feelings and communication with partner.
Abdominoperineal resection	Females: shortening of vagina; vaginal scarring may cause dyspareunia; decreased lubrication if ovaries also are removed Males: erectile dysfunction; decrease in amount/force of ejaculate or retrograde ejaculation because of interruption of sympathetic and parasympathetic nerve supply. Amount of rectal tissue removed appears to determine degree of dysfunction. Capacity for orgasm not altered.	Use water-soluble lubricant prior to intercourse; allow more time for pleasuring prior to attempting penetration; with shortened vagina, use coital positions that decrease depth of penetration (e.g., side-to-side lying, man on top with legs outside the woman's, woman on top). Erectile dysfunction may be temporary or permanent; encourage use of touch, other means of communication.
Transurethral resection of bladder/partial cystectomy	Mild pain or dyspareunia	Encourage more time for pleasuring.
Radical cystectomy	Females: surgery usually includes removal of bladder, urethra, uterus, ovaries, fallopian tubes, and anterior portion of vagina. Males: surgery involves removal of bladder, prostate, seminal vesicles, pelvic lymph nodes, and possibly urethra. May cause retrograde or loss of ejaculation and decrease in or loss of erectile ability.	Vaginal reconstruction is possible; use water-soluble lubricant; encourage self-pleasing and use of dilators; encourage use of touch and other means of sexual communication. Explore possibility for penile implant.
Radical prostatectomy	Involves removal of prostate, seminal vesicles, and vas deferens. Damage to autonomic nerves near prostate may cause loss of erectile ability; loss of emission and ejaculation.	Desire, penile sensations, and orgasmic abilities not altered. Explore possibility for penile prosthesis.
Transurethral resection of prostate	Causes retrograde ejaculation because of damage to internal bladder sphincter	Reassure that erection and orgasm will still occur but that ejaculate will be decreased or absent; urine may be cloudy.
Bilateral orchiectomy	Results in low levels of testosterone; causes sterility, decreased libido, impotence, gynecomastia, penile atrophy, and decreased growth of body hair and beard	Discuss option of sperm banking prior to surgery; discuss optional ways of expressing sexuality with patient and partner.
Retroperitoneal lymph node dissection	Damages sympathetic nerves necessary for ejaculation; results in temporary or permanent loss of ejaculation; patient maintains potency and orgasmic ability	Discuss option of sperm banking.

continues

TABLE 12-4

Continued

Type of Surgery	Effects on Sexual Functioning	Client Education
Total abdominal hysterectomy with bilateral salpingoooophorectomy	Loss of circulating estrogens; decrease in vaginal elasticity, decrease in vaginal lubrication; some women report decreased desire, orgasm, and enjoyment.	Use water-soluble lubricants; intercourse may be resumed after 6-week post-op check; encourage discussion about meaning of loss of uterus to self-identity.
Mastectomy	Decrease in arousal associated with nipple stimulation; affects body image, self-concept	Encourage communication with partner.
Radical vulvectomy	Removal of labia majora, labia minora, clitoris, bilateral pelvic node dissection; loss of sexually responsive tissue with concomitant loss of vasocongestive neuromuscular response	Possibility of perineal reconstruction with split-thickness skin graft or gracilis muscle grafts. Intercourse is still possible; explore ways of achieving arousal other than genital stimulation. Preoperative and postoperative counseling are essential.
Penectomy	Degree of sexual limitation depends on length of remaining penile shaft. Glans will be removed; remainder of shaft of penile tissue will respond with tumescence and will allow ejaculation and orgasm.	Discuss possibility of artificial insemination if children are desired.

SOURCE: Wilmoth, M. C. (1998). Sexuality. In C. Burke (Ed.), *Psychosocial dimensions of oncology nursing care*, pp. 102–127. Pittsburgh: Oncology Nursing Press.

after completion of treatment. Data also suggest that if FSH levels do not return to normal within two years of completing therapy, it is unlikely that fertility will return (Kader & Rostom, 1991). Men and their partners should be counseled about the effects of chemotherapy on fertility and sexuality and offered the option of semen cryopreservation (Krebs, 2000).

Currently, there are no published studies describing the impact, if any, that biologic response modifiers or gene therapies have on sexuality (Krebs, 2000). Anecdotal data suggest that systemic effects such as fatigue will cause alterations in sexuality (Krebs, 2000).

Multiple Sclerosis

Multiple sclerosis (MS) has the potential to have a profound impact on the sexual relationships of couples due to the resulting motor, sensory and cognitive alterations. The prevelance of sexual difficulties ranges between 60-80% in males and 20-60% in women (McCabe, 2002). Sexual difficulties in persons with multiple sclerosis (MS) can be classified as being primary, secondary or tertiary in origin (Kalb & LaRocca, 1997). Primary sexual problems are those that are caused directly by the neurologic changes caused by the disease; secondary issues are caused by the debilitating symptoms of the disease and tertiary concerns arise from the psychosocial sequellae of MS.

Neurological changes caused by MS can affect sexual feelings as well as sexual response. Both men and women can experience a decrease in sexual desire, altered genital sensitivity and response to stimulation, reduced vasocongestion of the genitalia, and diminished or absent orgasmic experience (Kalb &

TABLE 12-5

Site-Specific Effects of Radiation Therapy on Sexuality

Radiated Site	Effect on Sexuality	Client Education
Testes	Reduction in sperm count begins in 6 to 8 weeks and continues for 1 year. Doses 2 Gy will result in temporary sterility for about 12 months. Doses ± 5 Gy result in permanent sterility. Libido and potency will be maintained.	Discuss sperm banking prior to therapy and continued use of contraceptives.
Prostate	External beam: temporary or permanent erectile dysfunction because of fibrosis of pelvic vasculature or radiation damage of pelvic nerves Interstitial: less incidence of impotency	Age is variable—men older than age 60 have higher incidence of impotence. Erectile dysfunction—may experience pain during ejaculation because of irritation of urethra. Potency preserved in 70%–90% of men who were potent before treatment.
Cervix/vaginal canal	External beam: vaginal stenosis and fibrosis, fistula, cystitis Intracavitary: vaginal stenosis, dry, friable tissue, loss of lubrication. Both result in decreased vaginal sensation and dyspareunia.	Use of water-soluble lubricant; empty bladder before and after sex; encourage pleasuring prior to attempting penetration; use dilators or frequent intercourse to lessen amount of stenosis. Explore new positions for intercourse to allow woman control over depth of penile penetration.
Pelvic region	Women: temporary or permanent sterility dependent on dose of radiation, volume of tissue irradiated, and woman's age; the closer to menopause, the more likely permanent sterility will result. A single dose of 3.75 Gy will cause complete cessation of menses in women older than age 40. Men: temporary or permanent erectile dysfunction secondary to vascular or nerve damage	Oophoropexy and shielding may help to maintain fertility in women; continue use of contraceptives; use of water-soluble lubricant Both genders: encourage alternate means to express sexuality, such as touch.
Breast	Skin reactions, changes in breast sensations	Explore alternate pleasuring techniques and good communication techniques; breastfeeding should only occur on nonradiated side.

SOURCE: Wilmoth, M. C. (1998). Sexuality. In C. Burke (Ed.), *Psychosocial dimensions of oncology nursing care*, pp. 102–127. Pittsburgh: Oncology Nursing Press.

LaRocca, 1997). Counseling for underlying emotional concerns as well as depression may affect treatment of desire problems as well. Changes in genital sensations can be troubling, because something that used to feel good may now be noxious. Teaching couples to communicate about these changes and to try new techniques can be of help. Vaginal dryness can be improved with the use of water-soluble lubricants. Unfortunately, treatment of ED in men is not as easily remedied. Treatments for ED in MS are the same options for men with other chronic illnesses and can be found in Figure 12-2.

Secondary sexual alterations caused by MS are a result of the physical symptoms that accompany the disease. These include spasticity, bowel and bladder problems, fatigue, and cognitive impairment (Kalb & LaRocca, 1997). Spasticity during sexual activity appears to affect women more than it does men and may be controlled by baclofen, chemical nerve blocks, and surgery. Bowel and bladder problems can cause significant alterations in sexuality and can severely impair spontaneity of sexual activity. Engaging in sexual activity successfully requires open communication as well as aggressive symptom management. Limiting fluid intake for several hours prior to and urinating immediately before sexual activity can help with bladder control. Medications are available for incontinence; however, these medications may also increase vaginal dryness. Intermittent catheterization or taping a permanent catheter out of the way can allow successful activity. Bowel problems may be either ones of constipation, no control, or lack of predictability of function. A regular bowel regimen consisting of laxatives, enemas, or disimpaction can allow stress-free sexual interactions.

Fatigue is a pervasive symptom of MS as well as other chronic illnesses. In MS, fatigue can be managed with several pharmacological agents and energy-conserving techniques. Medications include amantadine or pemoline. Use of wheelchairs or motorized carts or regular naps during the day can allow clients to conserve energy for activities they enjoy, including sexual activity. Cognitive impairment can also have a pervasive impact on a relationship. Memory loss, impaired judgment, and other prob-

lems can impair the interpersonal communication that is integral in any intimate relationship.

The psychosocial changes that accompany MS cause tertiary sexual dysfunctions. Decreased self-concept, grieving for loss of self, and role changes affect both the client and the partner. Persons with MS report lower levels of sexual activity, sexual satisfaction and relationship satisfaction than those without MS (McCabe, McKern, McDonald & Vowels, 2003). Ongoing counseling and participa-

---

FIGURE 12-2

PLISSIT Model

Permission (P):	(Assessment) Actions taken by the nurse to let the patient/partner know that sexual issues are a legitimate aspect in providing nursing care. This could include questions about sexuality that are incorporated into the general admission assessment or questions specifically related to their disease process or treatment.
Limited Information (LI):	(Education) Sharing of information regarding the effects of disease, treatments, and medications. Examples of limited information include discussing when sexual intercourse may be resumed after surgery, the possibility of menopause occurring in conjunction with chemotherapy, or medications leading to erectile dysfunction.
Specific Suggestions (SS):	(Counseling) This level of care requires specialized knowledge about specific conditions and their relationship to sexual functioning. Various techniques, positions, and alternate techniques useful in achieving sexual satisfaction are examples of counseling concerns.
Intensive Therapy (IT):	(Referral) Treatment of sexual dysfunction requires specialized training in psychotherapy, sex therapy techniques, crisis intervention, and behavior modification.

SOURCE: Based on information from Annon, 1976.

tion in support groups can help couples deal with these sexual and relationship issues caused by MS (McCabe, 2002).

Interventions

Sexual Assessment

Sexuality should be a routine part of every physician- or nurse-initiated assessment for nearly every client diagnosed with a chronic illness (Wilmoth, 2000). Assessing sexuality as routinely as other body systems serves two purposes. First, it decreases embarrassment on the part of the client and practitioner if it is accepted as a normal aspect of health care. Second, routine inclusion will give the client permission to mention sexual difficulties to the practitioner and give the practitioner permission to ask specific questions when it is suspected that the client might be experiencing a sexually related side effect of the disease or treatment.

The nurse should keep in mind the same principles when discussing sexuality as any other topic with a client and/or partner. These include the need for privacy, confidentiality, and use of appropriate verbal and nonverbal cues and language (Woods, 1984). Communication about sexual issues is facilitated if the practitioner uses bridge statements to transition from comfortable topics to those that are less comfortable (Lefebvre, 1997). These statements emphasize the professional nature of these discussions, clarify the content component of communications, and reinforce permission to include sexuality in the plan of care. An example of a bridge question is, "Has anyone talked to you about how your (injury/illness/treatments) can affect your ability to have sex?" "Unloading" a topic is another technique that is useful in discussing sexuality and can ease a client's concern once he or she learns that others have experienced this problem (Woods, 1984). An example of unloading is, "Many women who have received chemotherapy have had problems with vaginal dryness. Have you experienced this problem?"

The inclusion of questions on sexuality in the admission assessment is an excellent way to legit-imize the role of the nurse in addressing sexuality. Woods (1984) suggests that such questions should proceed from less intimate questions, such as role functioning, to more personal ones on sexual functioning. Closed (yes/no) questions should be avoided, as they eliminate opportunities for further discussion. Questions for an initial assessment include the following (Woods, 1984; Wilmoth, 1994a):

- How has (diagnosis/treatment) affected your role as wife/husband/partner?
- How has (diagnosis/treatment) affected the way you feel about yourself as woman/man?
- What aspects of your sexuality do you believe have been affected by your diagnosis/treatment?
- How has your (diagnosis/treatment) affected your ability to function sexually?

A more medically focused sexual evaluation might include determination of chief complaint, sexual status, medical status, psychiatric status, family and psychosexual history, relationship assessment, and summary with recommendations (Auchincloss, 1990). A complete sexual history is not usually indicated unless initial assessment indicates the presence of a sexual problem. Most nurses are not adequately prepared to conduct a full sexual assessment; therefore, referral to a more appropriate practitioner is appropriate.

Including Sexuality into Practice

Four areas of competency must be achieved for nurses to successfully include sexuality into practice to attain the published standards of practice: comfort with one's own sexuality and comfort in discussing sexuality with others; excellent communication skills; a knowledge base about sexuality in health and illness; and role models to demonstrate integration of sexuality into practice (Woods, 1984; Wilmoth, 1994b).

Comfort with sexuality and enhancement of communication skills can be attained through reading, values clarification exercises, and participation in courses on sexuality. Some options include semester-long college courses related to sexuality or shorter weekend courses, often referred to as "SARs." Sexual attitude reassessment, or SAR, programs combine explicit films with small group discussions over a 2- or 3-day period to allow for analysis of one's personal values surrounding sexuality. Knowing one's own values and attitudes toward a variety of other sexual practices and sexual orientation is the first step in becoming comfortable with sexuality (Wilmoth, 1994a). Values clarification exercises can assist in this process. The outcome of clarifying one's values about sexuality is knowing what one believes is acceptable sexual behavior. It is important to remember that there is no right or wrong set of behaviors or values, just different ones.

Comfort in discussing sexuality and enhancing the ability to communicate clearly about sexuality can be achieved through a variety of methods. One option is to form a discussion group or journal club among colleagues. This group could engage in discussion of values clarification exercises or articles related to human sexuality in general or disease-focused articles on sexuality. Sharing with a peer group, particularly an interdisciplinary peer group, is a non-threatening way in which to become comfortable talking about sexuality. This approach also assists with increasing knowledge about a variety of illnesses, their treatments, and their effects on sexuality.

Nurses are skilled communicators, but they initially may find initiating discussions with clients about sexuality anxiety provoking. Nurses should assume that their clients have some form of sexual experience rather than none at all, and should also assume that they have questions about the impact of their disease or its treatments on their sexuality. Data are available that indicate that clients are waiting for nurses to initiate these discussions (Waterhouse & Metcalfe, 1991; Wilson & Williams, 1988). Nurses should use terminology, including slang that their clients understand, and should not hesitate to use appropriate humor in seeking clarification. For example, 'That's a new one for me. . . . What is that?" This can help diffuse a tense situation for both client and nurse.

Participation in each of the aforementioned processes will add to the nurse's knowledge base about normal sexual functioning. The professional nurse should also engage in independent study within their specialty regarding the effects that the illnesses, treatments, and medications have on sexuality. Engaging in discussions with other health care providers, such as physicians or pharmacists, or through participation in interdisciplinary journal clubs and research projects can add depth to the nurses' knowledge. Such interdisciplinary efforts will have large payoffs for clients and their partners.

Nurses who are comfortable with their own sexuality, are proficient communicators, and have knowledge about sexuality possess the foundation necessary to include sexuality into their practice. However, many are still reluctant to do so. Peers who can role-model the incorporation of sexuality into nursing practice may be influential in helping others incorporate it into their practices. Role models can assist in this process by relating positive experiences with clients about discussions surrounding sexuality, by role-playing ways of initiating discussions about sexuality, and by acting as a resource for staff. However, there is little research documenting the effectiveness of role models in teaching others to incorporate sexuality into practice.

Grand rounds and presentations of individual cases that exemplify typical sexual concerns associated with a particular treatment, medication, or diagnosis are other strategies for enhancing comfort in including sexual discussions into practice. Physicians and pharmacists could discuss a particular disease process and treatment options, including medications and their effect on sexual functioning. A social worker or clinical nurse specialist skilled in assessing and educating about sexual issues could lead practitioners through the sexual assessment and educational process. Finally, a clinician or sex therapist could discuss interventions that the majority of practitioners could use in their counseling of persons with sexual issues.

Many health professionals use the PLISSIT model (Annon, 1976) to assist them in their sexual assessments. In this model, P stands for *permission;* LI, for *limited information,* SS, for *specific suggestions,* and IT, for *intensive therapy* (Figure 12-2). Mims and Swenson (1978) suggest that all nurses should be able to intervene at all levels except for provision of intensive therapy. If assessment suggests a problem beyond the level of needing specific suggestions, the client and partner should be referred to a sex therapist.

Outcomes

Desired client and partner outcomes that may be anticipated after nursing intervention include:

- The ability to identify possible changes in sexuality as a result of the disease process or as a result of treatment side effects and to make appropriate modifications in their behavior to accommodate these alterations.
- The ability to express their feelings about the impact of these changes and to discuss the impact of these changes with their significant other.
- The ability to engage in satisfying sexual activity. (Carpenito, 2000).

Summary and Conclusions

Nursing research in the area of sexuality is still at the level of identifying sexual concerns among persons with chronic illnesses and in describing the occurrence of these concerns in the disease trajectory. Research identifying nursing interventions in the area of sexuality is in its infancy. Much of what is known about interventions related to sexual concerns comes from medical research and knowledge about pharmacology. Furthermore, research follows

funding streams, and until adequate levels of funding are available in the area of sexuality, knowledge will remain limited.

Nursing education programs have focused little, if any, attention on quality-of-life issues such as sexuality. Nurses enter the workforce woefully undereducated about a major component of their own humanness. Nurses know very little about the effects of most diseases and medications on sexuality, and they are not provided role models who can guide them in incorporating sexual information into their practices. Nurse educators have a responsibility and are accountable to ensure that graduates can provide care according to the profession's standards of practice, including the area of sexuality.

Nurses who include discussions of sexuality in their practices will find that their clients and their partners are relieved to *finally* find someone who will address these very real concerns that have serious implications for the quality of their relationships. Many times, clients suffer in silence, believing that they are the only ones experiencing sexual difficulties since their diagnosis. Too often, they end the sexual aspect of their relationships—or end the relationships altogether—thinking that there are no options for them. Nurses have an obligation to include discussions of sexuality and will find that doing so is really not as difficult as they think, and may actually find that they add a new dimension to their practice that has a major positive effect on the quality of life of their clients.

References

Agewall, S., Berglund, M. & Henareh, L. (2004). Reduced quality of life after myocardial infarction in women compared with men. *Clinical Cardiology, 27* (5), 271–274.

American Nurses Association (2004). *Nursing: Scope and standards of practice.* Washington, DC: Author.

American Psychiatric Association. (1994). *Diagnostic and statistical manual of mental disorders* (4th ed.). Washington, DC: Author.

Andrews, M., Goldberg, K., & Kaplan, H. (Eds.). (1996). *Nurse's legal handbook* (3rd ed.). Springhouse, PA: Springhouse Corporation.

Annon, J. S. (1976). *The behavioral treatment of sexual problems: Volume I: Brief therapy.* New York: Harper & Row.

Auchincloss, S. S. (1990). Sexual dysfunction in cancer patients: Issues in evaluation and treatment. In J. C. Holland & J. H. Rowland (Eds.), *Handbook of psy-*

chooncology, (pp. 383–413). New York: Oxford University Press.

Baggs, J. G., & Karch, A. M. (1987). Sexual counseling of women with coronary heart disease. *Heart and Lung, 16* (2), 154–159.

Carpenito, L. J. (2000). *Nursing Diagnosis: Application to Clinical Practice* (8th ed.). Philadelphia: Lippincott.

Centers for Disease Control, Office of Minority Health. (November 1, 2004). Eliminate Disparities in Cardiovascular Disease. Accessed November 3, 2004 from: http://www.cdc.gov/omh/AMH/factsheets/cardio.htm

Darling, C. A., Davidson, J. K., & Conway-Welch, C. (1990). Female ejaculation: Perceived origins, the Grafenberg spot/area, and sexual responsiveness. *Archives of Sexual Behavior, 19,* 29–47.

DeBusk, R. (2000). Evaluating the cardiovascular tolerance for sex. *The American Journal of Cardiology, 86* (2A), 51F–56F.

DeBusk, R., Drory, Y., Goldstein, I., Jackson, G., et al. (2000). Management of sexual dysfunction in patients with cardiovascular disease: Recommendations of the Princeton consensus panel. *The American Journal of Cardiology, 86* (2), 175–181.

DiSaia, P. J., & Creasman, W. T. (1997). *Clinical gynecologic oncology* (5th ed.), (pp. 1–50). St. Louis: Mosby.

Enzlin, P., Matieu, C., & Demyttenaere, K. (2003). Diabetes and female sexual functioning: A state-of-the-art. *Diabetes Spectrum, 16,* 256–259.

Enzlin, P., Mathieu, C., Van den Bruel, A., Bosteels, J., et al. (2002). Sexual dysfunction in women with Type 1 diabetes: A controlled study. *Diabetes Care, 25*: 672–677.

Enzlin, P., Mathieu, C., Vanderschueren, D., & Demyttenaere, K. (1998). Diabetes mellitus and female sexuality: A review of 25 years' research. *Diabetic Medicine, 15,* 809–815.

Frasure-Smith, N., Lesperance, F., & Talajic, M. (1993). Depression following myocardial infarction: Impact on 6-month survival. *Journal of the American Medical Association, 270,* 1819–1825.

Friday, N. (1973). *My secret garden: Women's sexual fantasies.* New York: Pocket Books.

Gitlin, M. J. (1995). Effects of depression and antidepressants on sexual functioning. *Bulletin of the Menninger Clinic, 59* (2), 232–248.

Guyton, A. C., & Hall, J. E. (1992). *Basic neuroscience: Anatomy and physiology* (10th ed.). Philadelphia: Saunders.

Hilderley, L. J. (2000). Principles of radiotherapy. In C. H. Yarbro, M. H. Frogge, M. Goodman, & S. L. Groenwald (Eds.), *Cancer nursing: Principles and practice* (5th ed.), (pp. 286–299). Sudbury MA: Jones and Bartlett.

Hollenbeck, B. K., Dunn, R. L., Wei, J. T., Sandler, H. M., et al. (2004). Sexual health recovery after prostatectomy, external radiation or brachytherapy for early stage prostate cancer. *Current Urology Reports, 5*: 212–219.

Jackson, G. (2004). Sexual dysfunction and diabetes. *International Journal of Clinical Practice, 58*(4), 358–362.

Jensen, S. B. (1981). Diabetic sexual dysfunction: A comparative study of 160 insulin-treated diabetic men and women and an age-matched control group. *Archives of Sexual Behavior, 10,* 493–504.

Kader, H. A., & Rostom, A. Y. (1991). Follicle-stimulating hormone levels as a predictor of recovery of spermatogenesis following cancer therapy. *Clinical Oncology, 3,* 37–40.

Kalb, R. C., & LaRocca, N. G. (1997). Sexuality and family planning. In J. Halper & N. J. Holland (Eds.), *Comprehensive nursing care in multiple sclerosis,* (pp. 109–125). New York: Demos Vermande.

Kaplan, H. S. (1979). *Disorders of sexual desire and other new concepts and techniques in sex therapy.* New York: Simon & Schuster.

Kolodny, R. C. (1971). Sexual dysfunction in diabetic females. *Diabetes, 20,* 557–559.

Kolodny, R., Masters, W., Johnson, V., & Biggs, M. (1979). *The textbook for human sexuality for nurses.* Boston: Little, Brown.

Koukouras, D., Spiliotis, J., Scopa, C. D., Dragotis, K., et al. (1991). Radical consequence in the sexuality of male patients operated for colorectal carcinoma. *European Journal of Surgical Oncology, 17,* 285–288.

Krebs, L. U. (2000). Sexual and reproductive dysfunction. In C. H. Yarbro, M. H. Frogge, M. Goodman, & S. L. Groenwald (Eds.), *Cancer nursing: Principles and practice* (5th ed.), (pp. 831–854). Sudbury, MA: Jones & Bartlett.

Ladas, A. K., Whipple, B., & Perry, J. D. (1982). *The G-spot.* New York: Dell.

Lefebvre, K. A. (1997). Performing a sexual evaluation on the person with disability or illness. In M. L. Sipski & C. J. Alexander (Eds.), *Sexual Function in People with Disability and Chronic Illness: A Health Professional's Guide* (pp. 19–46). Rockville: Aspen Publishers, Inc.

Lehne, R. A. (1998). *Pharmacology for nursing care* (3rd ed.). Philadelphia: WB Saunders.

Leiblum, S. R., & Segraves, R. T. (1989). Sex therapy with aging adults. In S. R. Leiblum & R. C. Rosen (Eds.), *Principles and practice of sex therapy: Update for the 1990s* (2nd ed.), (pp. 352–381). New York: Guilford Press.

LeMone, P. (1996). The physical effects of diabetes on sexuality in women. *The Diabetes Educator, 22* (4), 361–366.

Masters, W. H., & Johnson, V. E. (1966). *Human sexual response*. Philadelphia: Lippincott-Raven.

Masters, W. H., & Johnson, V. E. (1981). Sex and the aging process. *Journal of the American Geriatrics Society, 24* (9), 385–390.

McCabe, M. P. (2002). Relationship functioning and sexuality among people with multiple sclerosis. *The Journal of Sex Research, 39* (4), 302–309.

McCabe, M. P., McKern, S., McDonald, E., & Vowels, L. M. (2003). Changes over time in sexual and relationship functioning of people with multiple sclerosis. *Journal of Sex & Marital Therapy, 29* (4), 305–321.

McInnes, S., & Schilsky, R. L. (1996). Infertility following cancer chemotherapy. In B. A. Chabner & D. L. Longo (Eds.), *Cancer chemotherapy and biotherapy* (2nd ed.), (pp. 31–44). Philadelphia: Lippincott-Raven.

Meston, C.M. (2000). Sympathetic nervous system activity and female sexual arousal. *The American Journal of Cardiology, 86* (2) Suppl. 1, 30–34.

Meston, C. M. & Gorzalka, B. B. (1996). The differential effects of sympathetic activation on sexual arousal in sexually functional and dysfunctional women. *Journal of Abnormal Psychology, 105*, 582–591.

Mims, F., & Swenson, M. (1978). A model to promote sexual health care. *Nursing Outlook, 26* (2), 121–125.

Mokdad, A. H., Bowman, B. A., Ford, E. S., Nelson, D. E., et al. (2001). The continuing epidemics of obesity and diabetes in the United States. *Journal of the American Medical Association, 286* (10), 1195–200.

National Institutes of Health (NIH). (1992). Impotence. *NIH Consensus Statement, 10* (4), 1–31.

O'Farrell, P., Murray, J., & Hotz, S. B. (2000). Psychologic distress among spouses of patients undergoing cardiac rehabilitation. *Heart and Lung, 29* (2), 97–104.

Oncology Nursing Society. (2004). *Statement on the scope and standards of oncology nursing practice*. Pittsburgh, PA: Author.

Robert Wood Johnson Foundation. (1996). *Chronic care in America: A 21st century challenge*. Princeton, NJ: Author.

Roose, S. P., & Seidman, S. N. (2000). Sexual activity and cardiac risk: Is depression a contributing factor? *The American Journal of Cardiology, 86* (2A), 38F–40F.

Sands, J. K. (1995). Human sexuality. In W. J. Phipps, V. L. Cassmeyer, J. K. Sands, and M. K. Lehmen (Eds.). *Medical surgical nursing: Concepts & clinical practice* (5th ed.), (pp. 262–284). St. Louis: Mosby.

Sarkadi, A. & Rosenquist, U. (2004). Intimacy and women with Type 2 diabetes: An exploratory study using focus group interviews. *The Diabetes Educator, 29* (4), 641–652.

Schliefer, S. J., Macari-Hinson, M. M., Coyle, D. A., Slater, W. R., et al. (1989). The nature and course of depression following myocardial infarction. *Archives of Internal Medicine, 149*, 1785–1789.

Steinke, E. E. (2000). Sexual counseling after myocardial infarction. *American Journal of Nursing, 100* (12), 38–44.

Svedlund, M. & Danielson, E. (2004). Myocardial infarction: Narrations by afflicted women and their partners of lived experiences in daily life following an acute myocardial infarction. *Journal of Clinical Nursing, 13* (4), 438–446.

Tilton, M. C. (1997). Diabetes and amputation. In M. L. Sipski & C. J. Alexander (Eds.), *Sexual function in people with disability and chronic illness: A health professional's guide*, (pp. 279–302). Rockville, MD: Aspen Publishers.

U.S. Department of Health and Human Services, Centers for Disease Control and Prevention. (1999). *Chronic diseases and their risk factors: The nation's leading causes of death*. Atlanta: Author.

Viviani, S., Ragni, G., Santoro, A., Perotti, L., et al. (1991). Testicular dysfunction in Hodgkin's disease before and after treatment. *European Journal of Cancer, 27*, 1389–1392.

Waterhouse, J., & Metcalfe, M. C. (1991). Attitudes toward nurses discussing sexual concerns with patients. *Journal of Advanced Nursing, 16*, 1048–1054.

Weiner, D. N., & Rosen, R. C. (1997). Medications and their impact. In M. L. Sipski & C. J. Alexander (Eds.), *Sexual function in people with disability and chronic illness: A health professional's guide*, (pp. 85–114). Rockville, MD: Aspen Publishers.

Wilmoth, M. C. (1994a). Strategies for becoming comfortable with sexual assessment. *Oncology Nursing News* (Spring), 6–7.

_____. (1994b). Nurses' and patients' perspectives on sexuality: Bridging the gap. *Innovations in Oncology Nursing, 10* (2), 34–36.

_____. (1996). The middle years: Women, sexuality and the self. *Journal of Obstetric, Gynecologic, and Neonatal Nursing, 25,* 615–621.

_____. (1998). Sexuality. In C. Burke (Ed.), *Psychosocial dimensions of oncology nursing care,* pp. 102–127. Pittsburgh: Oncology Nursing Press.

_____. (2000). Sexuality patterns, altered. In L. J. Carpenito (Ed.), *Nursing diagnosis: Application to clinical practice* (8th ed.), (pp. 837–857). Philadelphia: Lippincott.

Wilmoth, M. C., & Spinelli, A. (2000). Sexual implications of gynecologic cancer treatments. *Journal of Obstetrics, Gynecologic and Neonatal Nursing, 29,* 413–421.

Wilson, M. E., & Williams, H. A. (1988). Oncology nurses' attitudes and behaviors related to sexuality to patients with cancer. *Oncology Nursing Forum, 15,* 49–52.

Woods, N. F. (1984). *Human sexuality in health and illness* (3rd ed.). St. Louis: Mosby.

Zrustova, M., Rostlapid, J., & Kabshelova, A. (1978). Sexual disorders in diabetic women. *Ceska Gynekologie, 43,* 277.

Zaviacic, M., & Whipple, B. (1993). Update on the female prostate and the phenomena of female ejaculation. *The Journal of Sex Research, 30,* 48–151.

CHAPTER 13

Powerlessness

Lisa L. Onega

Introduction

Mrs. Petrouski, a 45-year-old woman who was diagnosed with multiple sclerosis one year ago, often misses health care appointments. She appears quiet, withdrawn, and tired when she sees the advanced practice nurse, and periodically says, "No matter what I do, nothing makes a difference with this disease." Mr. Lamb, a 26-year-old recently diagnosed with insulin-dependent diabetes mellitus, often yells at health care professionals about their "incompetence," blames his wife for "trying to control" his dietary intake, and periodically tells health insurance employees that he is "going to come down there and make them pay" for his diabetes-related expenses. Ms. McGuire, a 72-year-old diagnosed ten years ago with congestive heart failure, complains of sleeplessness, says that she doesn't understand the reasons for her medications, and states that she doesn't know "why I'm living if I can't do anything anymore."

Although each of these individuals is demonstrating different behavior, they all are experiencing a feeling of powerlessness in response to a chronic illness. Mrs. Petrouski's feelings of powerlessness are manifested by apathetic behavior. Mr. Lamb's feelings of powerlessness are demonstrated by angry behavior. Ms. McGuire's feelings of powerlessness are evident in her depressed behavior.

Historical Perspectives

Powerlessness was initially described in relationship with social learning by Seeman (1959). Seeman argued that *alienation,* a classic term in sociological theory, had five variants: powerlessness, meaninglessness, normlessness, value isolation, and self-estrangement. Seeman's first study examining powerlessness compared the learning outcomes in a sample of 86 hospitalized men with tuberculosis. Men possessing high alienation scores, signifying a high degree of powerlessness, were compared with those with low alienation scores, signifying a low degree of powerlessness. The study used the I-E scale to measure internal locus of control (low degree of powerlessness) versus external locus of control (higher degree of powerlessness) (Rotter, 1966). Powerlessness was associated with poorer learning of health-relevant information among the hospitalized men (Seeman & Evans, 1962).

Other terms associated with a sense of low control or powerlessness evolved in the 1960s and 1970s. Terms included *helplessness* (Seligman, 1975), *locus of control* (Rotter, 1966), and *loss of freedom* (Worthman & Brehm, 1975).

Rodin and Langer (1977) described the relationship between powerlessness, more control, and choices given to clients, and the resulting outcomes on health status. An intervention of choice and personal control was used in an experimental group of elderly residents in a nursing home. Residents who were given more choices, personal control, and personal responsibility had better health outcomes and statistically significant less mortality than the control group (Rodin & Langer, 1977).

The early research of Seeman and Evans in the 1960s was followed with a longitudinal study in which an individual's low sense of control was significantly associated with less preventive health behavior, less optimism concerning the efficacy of early treatment, poorer self-rated health, and more acute illness episodes (Seeman & Seeman, 1983, p. 144). Seeman and Seeman acknowledge that any causal relationship is difficult to support because a sense of control can be a *product* of one's health experience, as well as a *determinant* of it (p. 155).

In 1995, Seeman and Lewis evaluated the relationship of powerlessness, health status, and mortality using nationally representative samples of men and women from the National Longitudinal Surveys (NLS). The NLS were conducted by the United States Department of Labor using a multistage probability sampling method. The initial surveys began in 1966 with men aged 45 to 59. Surveys with women 30 to 44 years of age began in 1967, with data collection continuing over a decade.

Findings revealed significant relationships between powerlessness and health status and between powerlessness and mortality. These relationships included the following:

- Powerlessness was associated with activity limitations and psychosocial symptoms.
- Initial powerlessness was predictive of health problems five and ten years later.
- Increasing powerlessness was associated with deteriorating health status.
- Initially high powerlessness scores were associated with mortality in men.

The study used the Rotter I-E measure of internal versus external control to measure powerlessness (the sense of mastery versus powerlessness). It should

be noted that there is not clear acceptance that individuals with external control are powerless or that those having internal control possess power; however, this is the premise of these particular researchers. A pattern of high powerlessness (as measured by I-E scores) and greater health problems was evidenced for both males and females regardless of the individual's earlier health status (Seeman & Lewis, 1995). Although Seeman and Lewis have "linked" powerlessness with chronic illness, they state that powerlessness is only one form of alienation, and one among many potentially significant social psychological variables affecting health (Seeman & Lewis, 1995, p. 524).

An early description and analysis of powerlessness appeared in the nursing literature in 1967. Dorothy Johnson's analysis was based on Seeman's work that powerlessness was a variant of alienation. In her work, Johnson defined powerlessness as a "perceived lack of personal or internal control of certain events or in certain situations" (p. 40). Her view equated powerlessness with perceived external control. She further elaborated that nursing care should be planned around this concept when establishing priorities of care, particularly when it came to client education, as she felt that if a client felt powerless, the education would not be effective.

Roberts and White (1990) associated loss of personal control with powerlessness in their work with clients with myocardial infarction (MI). Loss of control occurs in four areas that affect powerlessness in MI clients: physiological, cognitive, environmental, and decisional.

Richmond and colleagues (1992) studied powerlessness and its relationship with health status in a sample of 50 spinal cord injured clients. Powerlessness was measured using the current, at that time, indicators of powerlessness that were derived from the Fifth Conference on Classification of Nursing Diagnoses in 1984. There was a statistically significant correlation between the presence of powerlessness and the increased acuity of the client. Additionally, quadriplegics and individuals over the age of 60, in general, had a higher occurrence of powerlessness.

Significant concept development and analysis of powerlessness has been accomplished with the work of Judith Miller (1983, 1992, 2000). Miller delineates powerlessness from similar constructs such as helplessness, learned helplessness, and locus of control. Miller concurs with an earlier idea of Lewis (1982), that helplessness and locus of control are based on a reinforcement paradigm, whereas powerlessness is an existential construct. Miller (2000) categorizes locus of control as a personality trait as opposed to powerlessness which she believes is situationally determined.

Defining Powerlessness

Powerlessness is often experienced by clients with chronic illness at some time during the course of their illness. Powerlessness may be a *real* loss of power or a *perceived* loss of power by the client. Miller defines *powerlessness* as "the perception that one lacks the capacity or authority to act to affect an outcome" (Miller, 2000, p. 4). Accompanying this definition, Miller identifies the power resources that may be decreased or lost in chronic illness: physical strength, energy, hope, motivation, knowledge, positive self-esteem, psychological stamina, and social support (Miller, 2000). If a client's power resources are significantly affected, the outcome for the client may be a feeling of powerlessness.

Miller's definition of *powerlessness* is one of several found in the literature. Table 13-1 presents other definitions that may be considered.

It is also helpful to differentiate powerlessness from other concepts. Although there are some similarities, there are differences as well (Table 13-2).

■ Issues Related to Powerlessness

Illness has been described as the ultimate out-of-control experience (McDaniel, Hepworth & Doherty, 1997, p. 7). Chronic illness provides many out-of-control experiences and influences that may affect a feeling of powerlessness in a client and family. If one views powerlessness as a situational attribute, as Miller (2000) does, then it is logical that during the different phases of the illness trajectory, a client may experience a variety of feelings. A client may feel powerless when an exacerbation of the disease is present but may feel in control when the disease is in remission.

Physiological Factors

Strauss and colleagues' classic framework of viewing chronic illness (1984) is still relevant today. In particular, the framework addresses two physiological components that may cause feelings of powerlessness:

1. Prevention of medical crises and their management once they occur
2. The control of symptoms

TABLE 13-1

Definitions of Powerlessness

- "Thinking one has no control over events" (Davidhizar, 1994, p. 156)
- "The perception that one lacks the capacity or authority to act to affect an outcome"(Miller, 2000, p. 4)
- "Feelings of lacking influence over their own life" (Nyström & Segesten, 1994, p. 128)
- "Expectancy that one's own behavior cannot determine the outcome one seeks" (Roberts & White, 1990, p. 85)
- "Feeling of lack of power over your life or situation. . . . the extent of power varies by the situation" (White & Roberts, 1993, p. 127)
- "Loss of control over one's life as a whole, with all that this implies" (Bright, 1996, p. 1)
- "Expectancy or the probability held by the individual that his own behavior cannot determine the outcome or reinforcements he seeks" (Seeman, 1959, p. 784)

TABLE 13-2

Differentiating Powerlessness from Other Concepts

Concept	Differs from Powerlessness
Alienation	■ Alienation is the ***lack of a relationship*** in work settings, social institutions, with family, or with other persons. A person may feel powerful while remaining apart. With powerlessness the key issue is a ***lack of control***; however, often people who feel powerless feel misunderstood and alone (Maddi, Kobasa, & Hoover, 1979).
Hopelessness	■ Hopelessness is a global despair that corresponds with a belief that ***everyone*** lacks the power to effect change unlike the more focused perspective associated with powerlessness where a person believes that ***he or she*** lacks the power to effect change (Schorr, Farnham, & Ervin, 1991).
Locus of Control —External —Internal	■ Internal locus of control means that an individual believes that ***he or she has control*** over the situations that they encounter. On the other hand, external locus of control is when an individual believes that he or she has limited power and that ***other forces*** such as people, institutions, the weather, and God ***have control***. This differs from powerlessness because the powerless person believes that ***he or she does not have control*** and is unconcerned if other forces have control (Gibson & Kenrick, 1998).
Vulnerability	■ Vulnerability is synonymous with being ***disadvantaged***. A person may be disadvantaged by virtue of a variety of reasons including lack of education, language barrier, or poverty but may not feel a sense of powerlessness. Just because a person is ***disadvantaged***, it does not mean that he or she ***lacks the power*** to effect change (powerlessness) (Hildebrandt, 1999).

Each of these components may include pain, both acute and chronic, nausea, vomiting, anorexia, fatigue, altered functioning, shortness of breath, and so forth. Within each chronic illness, the physiological symptoms of the disease are different, some with more intensive symptomatology than others.

Management of the Medical Regimen

Strauss and colleagues (1984) identify the carrying out of prescribed regimens and the problems associated with these regimens as one component of their framework of chronic illness (p. 16). Initially, one might not see the medical regimen as a factor related to the powerlessness of the client; however, adherence to a medical regimen may cause other physical symptoms. For example, the client with cancer, who may be undergoing chemotherapy or radiation therapy, has an entirely new set of symptoms with which to deal, in addition to the ones provided with the original disease.

The time involved with carrying out a medical regimen may significantly limit other activities. An individual's life centers around the disease and all of the accompanying activities of adhering to the prescribed regimen. One example is a client who chooses to do peritoneal dialysis at home. That client's time is highly structured to ensure that the procedures are carried out appropriately. By following the medical regimen step by step, the client and family experiences a loss of control over their time, their choices, and their quality of life. The disease and medical regimen are in control but powerlessness may occur if the client does not see that attention to this activity is making a difference in his or her condition or function. Health care providers, however, expect that the treatment regimen will be followed, giving little thought to how that might be accomplished. The following excerpt from Strauss and associates (1984) typifies how health care providers see adherence to the regimen.

Regimens are either followed by obedient, sensible patients or ignored at their peril.

Indeed physicians and other health personnel tend to regard patients (or their families) as not only foolish if they do not carry out the prescribed regimens, but downright uncooperative. They talk approvingly or disapprovingly about the adherence or lack of adherence to regimens. (p. 34)

Loss

It is important to remember that the diagnosis of a chronic illness for most individuals is a loss, and for some individuals, it may be as significant as the death of a loved one. With a loss, the individual and family experience grief. The diagnosis of a chronic illness may indicate the loss of hope for the future, decreased income, decreased sexual ability or intimacy, disability, decreased quality of life, dependence on others, or even a loss of self (Clarke & James, 2003).

Others may see chronic illness as a sign of aging and loss of their youth. In our youth-oriented society, little value has typically been placed on the elderly population. The individual may fear that he or she will become dependent, not able to live alone, and that placement in a nursing home is possible. These multiple losses give many individuals a feeling of powerlessness. Bright (1996) refers to powerlessness as both a consequence of being in grief, in this case due to diagnosis of a chronic illness, and is itself a cause for grief (p. 4).

Losses are a prominent feature of chronic illness. It should also be noted that chronic illness may be only *one* of the losses that the client is facing. The client may be experiencing the death of a loved one, a change in roles, retirement, financial loss, and so forth. These multiple losses over time adversely influence an individual's self-confidence to address problems associated with his or her health.

Lack of Knowledge

The physiological factors of the disease may be affected by the client's lack of knowledge or skills about the disease. Education may have occurred during a hospitalization, but both client and family may have been unable to grasp the concepts at the time the education was provided. The newness of the diagnosis and the unfamiliar surroundings may have decreased learning. The client "heard" the instruction but could not comprehend it. Also, the client may have already discovered that even if the treatment regimen is followed accurately, there isn't any perceivable difference in how he or she feels. This further intensifies a feeling of powerlessness.

Health Care System

While designed to assist individuals and families, the health care system often contributes to a client's feelings of powerlessness. It is well known that the health care system, or nonsystem as some have called it, was designed for clients with acute illness. Frustration and inability to overcome obstacles in accessing, receiving, and paying for services add to feelings of powerlessness (Dunn, 1998; Walker, Holloway & Sofaer, 1999). The traditional health care system is unable to cure chronic disease and often little help can be offered to significantly increase one's activities of daily living or improve physiological functioning. Due to the unpredictable nature of most chronic illnesses, health care providers may not furnish needed education about the disease or potential complications until after an exacerbation or problem has occurred. At times, in an attempt to contain costs, needed occupational or physical therapy referrals may not be initiated.

Another significant problem is that health care providers often fail to listen to the unique needs of individuals and family members. Part of this problem may be related to the limited time the health care provider has with the client, but part may be due to the inability of the provider to *actively listen* to a client and provide individualized care. Additionally, when individuals with a chronic illness decide that their treatment is not satisfactory, they may receive patronizing care, have their concerns minimized, or be labeled difficult clients (Clarke & James, 2003; Dunn, 1998; Walker, Holloway & Sofaer, 1999).

Pervasiveness of the acute care model of care indicates to clients with chronic illness that the system doesn't know what to do with them. Clients may be confused about caring for themselves long term, but the system, or "non-system" is similarly confused. Individuals become clients in the acute care system and repeat the same information and share their insurance cards repeatedly with three or four different people. Individuals wonder if anyone even knows who they are in this system, or, more importantly, who cares. It has been said that the health care system is organized for the convenience of the health care professionals and not for the consumers of those services.

Gibson and Kenrick (1998) summarize the powerlessness felt by clients within the health care system.

Powerlessness can be seen in the context of becoming a patient, the expectations of individuals, and the ways in which they "play by the rules." It is also a key to understanding the ways in which their horizons change, both as fact—the loss of mobility and contacts—and as metaphor—acceptance, control and changing outlook. It is a response to the limits of the conditions itself, and to the power which is perceived to be vested in the health care system. (p. 743)

Societal Issues

The Americans with Disabilities Act became effective in 1990; clients in wheelchairs, however, may find that little has changed. The ability to access public buildings, shopping centers, and church remains difficult. Where are the curb cuts for one's wheelchair? Where is the ramp? Where is the elevator? Where are the handicapped parking spaces?

Societal stigma remains an issue as well. Persons with chronic disease, particularly those with visible disabilities, present examples of deviations from the "norm." The values and overriding culture of the United States emphasize youth, personal attractiveness, and athleticism. These societal values are in direct conflict with chronic illness (see Chapter 3, on stigma).

Lack of Resources

Lack of resources often contributes to feelings of powerlessness. Money, transportation, health insurance, material resources, and social support are only a few of the resources that are needed for individuals with chronic illness (Israel et al., 1994; Nyamathi et al., 1996; Strehlow & Amos-Jones, 1999). Lack of resources may limit an individual's ability to access needed services and treat physical health problems. The lack of human resources, family, friends, and caregivers further affects the client and may lead to social isolation or withdrawal from society (see Chapter 6, on social isolation).

Uncertainty

Uncertainty is a common concept in chronic illness and affects an individual's feeling of powerlessness. The uncertain and unpredictable nature of chronic illness adds to the sense of powerlessness that individuals and their family members experience (Mishel, 1999). Three aspects of the illness seem to cause uncertainty: (1) severity of the illness, (2) erratic nature of symptomatology, and (3) ambiguity of symptoms (Mishel, 1999). Uncertainty regarding physical functioning and recurrence of pain may cause an individual to avoid any activity. Uncertainty regarding access to both financial and human resources may create an environment of constant fear and worry for the client and family members. All of these issues are tied to the future, and the client realizes how unpredictable the illness is. What power or control does he or she have in the illness? If I'm a good client and adhere to my medications and treatments, will it affect my health outcomes? Will it improve my health? Will it decrease my exacerbations? Does anything I do have an effect on my health?

Culture

Little research has been done examining culture and powerlessness. In the past a few small studies of nurses from various cultural groups, such as Dutch community nurses (n = 21) and female nurses in South Africa (n = 17), used qualitative methods to understand nurses' feelings of power and powerlessness (deSchepper, Francke, & Abu-Saad, 1997; van der Merwe, 1999). More recently research has been done examining non-nursing cultural groups and their experiences of power and powerlessness. Mok, Martinson, and Wong (2004) used grounded theory to understand the experiences of empowerment in Chinese cancer patients living in Hong Kong (n = 12). Their research revealed that the process of empowerment is "embedded in a relational context, which was described as connection with others, including family, friends, and health care professionals, and those in the patients' cultural, religious, and personal belief systems" (p. 63). In this study the Chinese cultural beliefs of loyalty to the family, letting go, harmony with the universe, and the cycles of life and nature were essential to the development of feelings of empowerment.

Green et al. (2004) surveyed African-Americans in Alabama churches (n = 1,253) and found that:

■ Women who believed in fate or destiny were less likely than those who did not to have breast exams.

■ More women believed in fate or destiny than men.

■ Surprisingly, more educated individuals believed in fate or destiny more than less educated individuals.

■ Surprisingly, individuals with incomes above $50,000/year believed in fate or destiny more than individuals with incomes below $50,000/year.

Denner and Dunbar (2004) interviewed Mexican-American girls between 12 and 14 years of age (n = 8) in order to understand what it means to be a girl and how Latina girls think about power in their relationships. Interviews revealed that power is complex and occurs in the context of relationships, not in isolation.

Nurses working with individuals who have chronic illnesses need to understand the cultural context and belief system that frames each person's life. By taking an interest in individuals and developing a relationship that helps to bridge cultural differences; healing, mutually respectful, and empowering experiences can result (Mok et al., 2004).

■ Interventions

Assessment

Comprehensive assessments of the individual with chronic illness and significant family are necessary to identify whether powerlessness exists and develop appropriate interventions. Client strengths or power resources are identified in this process. These resources include physical strength, energy, hope, motivation, knowledge, positive self-concept, psychological stamina, and social support (Miller, 2000).

Family functioning and ability to balance multiple demands and stresses should be identified as well. Nurses must be cognizant of an individual's developmental stage as well as his or her values and beliefs. The health care professional needs to be aware that the current chronic illness with its deficits may be only one of several losses the client has suffered. Taking the time to *listen* and *observe* individuals and their families will enable the nurse to accurately identify whether powerlessness is being experienced.

Another aspect of assessment is knowing an individual's usual response to an illness situation or a stressful situation in general. This information is important in facilitating effective coping measures. How does the client usually respond? Denial? Anger? Helplessness? Sadness?

The assessment process may also identify a client who is potentially suicidal. Identification of suicidal ideation and referral to a psychiatric health care professional for treatment and follow-up are essential. To help individuals who are suicidal gain control over an overwhelming situation, medication and short-term therapy may be needed (Bright, 1996; Lunney, 1997).

One model that may be used in identifying strengths of a client and the development of nursing interventions is the Personal Control Model. White and Roberts (1993) developed a model that links personal control with powerlessness. The Personal Control Model postulates that four types of loss of control are associated with powerlessness:

1. *Physiological loss of control* is related to the problematic biological changes associated with a chronic illness.
2. *Cognitive loss of control* is indicative of the inability to correctly interpret the effects of a chronic illness and is categorized as *sensory loss of control* and *appraisal loss of control*. Sensory loss of control is related to the misinterpreta-

tions of visual, auditory, touch, smell, and taste sensations. Appraisal loss of control occurs when individuals are unable to focus their attention on the threatening situation, identify potential harm, and understand their emotions associated with the event.

3. *Environmental loss of control* occurs when individuals are unable to control where they are and what they are experiencing.
4. *Decisional loss of control* is when individuals are unable to make decisions for themselves or for their care.

The Personal Control Model can be used to design specific interventions for each of the four types of loss of control that are associated with powerlessness (Table 13-3). *Physiological control* can be fostered by minimizing fatigue and assisting with energy conservation. Specific strategies include pacing and sequencing activities and educating individuals and their families about managing illness-related events. *Cognitive control* can be facilitated by preparing in-

TABLE 13-3

Nursing Interventions Based on the Personal Control Model

Type of Control Loss	Description	Nursing Interventions
Physiological	Occurs with the biological changes associated with a chronic illness	Minimize fatigue by pacing and sequencing activities and educating individuals about managing illness-related events.
Cognitive	Means used to interpret the effects of chronic illness; categorized as *sensory loss of control* and *appraisal loss of control*	Prepare individuals for common sensory experiences associated with their illness, diagnostic procedures, and treatments. Refocus their attention on resources and goals.
Environmental	Happens when people are unable to control where they are and what they are experiencing	Personalize the environment and facilitate meaningful relationships with loved ones, friends, others with similar chronic illnesses, and health care professionals.
Decisional	When individuals are unable to make decisions for themselves or for their care	Provide a repertoire of options that are realistic and personally relevant.

Source: Developed from White & Roberts, 1993.

Experiencing Powerlessness

Mrs. Estes is a 68-year-old widow who has been diagnosed with obesity, diabetes mellitus, and osteoarthritis in her hips and knees. She says that no matter what she does, she is unable to lose weight. She feels overwhelmed and discouraged. She states that she eats "whatever I want" and does not exercise routinely because she is "tired all of the time." She has poor eye contact, sighs frequently, does not initiate conversation with health care providers, and does not ask questions. The nurse identifies that Mrs. Estes is experiencing feelings of powerlessness. The nurse sits down with Mrs. Estes, holds her hand, and empathetically states that it can feel overwhelming and discouraging to have several chronic illnesses. The nurse asks Mrs. Estes how she feels about her situation. Mrs. Estes starts to cry and says that her situation is hopeless. The nurse gives Mrs. Estes a tissue and sits with her quietly for a few minutes. When Mrs. Estes stops crying, the nurse asks her what her biggest concern is. Mrs. Estes comments that not being able to exercise is discouraging.

The nurse acknowledges Mrs. Estes' concern. The nurse asks her what type of exercise she most enjoys. Mrs. Estes says that she likes to walk and that she even has a treadmill but she gets "bored" when she uses her treadmill. The nurse asks her if she would enjoy walking on her treadmill more if she were to watch television or listen to music while walking. Mrs. Estes says that she likes jazz music and would enjoy walking more if she listened to jazz music. Together they plan that she will walk on her treadmill while listening to jazz music for five minutes three times this week. The nurse offers to call her the following week to discuss how successful Mrs. Estes has been at meeting this goal. Mrs. Estes looks at the nurse, smiles, and says "I think that I can do this!"

---

dividuals for common sensory experiences that may be associated with their illness, various diagnostic procedures, and treatments and by refocusing their attention on resources and goals. Interventions to improve *environmental control* include helping clients personalize their environments and fostering meaningful relationships with loved ones, friends, others with similar chronic illnesses, and health care professionals. *Decisional control* can be encouraged by providing a repertoire of options that are realistic and personally relevant (White & Roberts, 1993; Wetherbee, 1995).

Some individuals with chronic illness have other concerns in their lives that may be contributing to feelings of powerlessness (Hildebrandt, 1999). Health care providers often believe that the client's illness is the primary focus of the client and family.

Certainly this can be the case, but there may be other issues more important to the client at the time. An example might be a client that is newly diagnosed with breast cancer, and while she is concerned about her own health, her focus is on her 16-year-old daughter's admission to a psychiatric hospital.

Client and Family Education

Creating mechanisms whereby uncertainty and unpredictability can be minimized will help reduce feelings of powerlessness. Client and family education can facilitate understanding of symptoms associated with the chronic illness. Additionally, maintaining a familiar and routine environment and having knowledge about the typical disease trajectory enable individuals and their families to reduce feelings of powerlessness (Mishel, 1999). An individualized educational plan is needed for each client with chronic illness (see Chapter 15, on client and family education).

Diversional Experiences

Meaningful diversional experiences may enable individuals to clearly identify their feelings, reframe their chronic illness, and thereby view their illness as one aspect of their life instead of the condition that consumes their entire life. Music is one tool that can be used in a therapeutic manner for diversion. Nurses can work with individuals to plan meaningful musical sessions, facilitate enjoyment in listening to music, and foster discussion of feelings after the session (Bright, 1996).

Empowerment

Nurses may identify the *empowerment* of persons and families coping with a chronic illness as the goal of their care. The term *empowerment* is broad and has a variety of meanings (Clarke & Mass, 1998) (Table 13-4). Identifying specific and measurable outcomes associated with empowerment enables nurses to evaluate client progress in reducing their feelings of powerlessness. Helping individuals with chronic illnesses perceive that their ability to cope is greater than their problems is critical.

It must be noted that it might be difficult for health care providers working in an acute care setting or a clinical site using a medical model paradigm to develop strategies to empower clients. The medical model does not view client involvement as salient to care. Within the acute care setting, the health care provider, not the client, is in "control" or has power. A paradigm shift may need to occur for the health care provider to be able to empower the client.

Specific nursing strategies used in empowering individuals with chronic illnesses and their family include the following: (Clarke & Mass, 1998; Davidhizar, 1994; Falk-Rafael, 2001; Landau, 1997; Mok et al., 2004; Ruhl, 1999; Stapleton, 1978)

- Being willing to try innovative approaches
- Listening to individuals; asking them to describe their experience
- Displaying a kind and helpful attitude and being approachable
- Respecting people and fostering individualized decision making

---

TABLE 13-4

Definitions of Empowerment

- "An individual's ability to make decisions and have control over his or her personal life" (Israel et al., 1994, p. 152)
- "Process [that] will lead to a positive self-concept, personal satisfaction, self-efficacy, a sense of mastery, a sense of control, a sense of connectedness, self-development, a feeling of hope, social justice and improve quality of life" (Nyström & Segesten, 1994, p. 127)
- "Process through which internal feelings of powerlessness (helplessness/hopelessness) were transformed and actions initiated to change the physical and social living conditions that created or reinforced inequalities in power" (Clarke & Mass, 1998, p. 218)
- "Active, internal process of growth that was rooted in one's own cultural/religious/personal belief systems, reached toward actualizing one's full potential, and occurred within the context of a nurturing . . . relationship" (Falk-Rafael, 2001, p. 4)
- "An individual can be made stronger or gain more confidence through the facilitative process of a relationship, or through changes in one's beliefs and views....an enabling process...help individuals develop the capacity to change their situations, to believe that they can have influence in their life situations" (Mok et al., 2004, pp. 82 & 83)

- Being flexible and responding to the client's and family's needs
- Providing individuals and their family members with education, training, and support
- Preparing individuals and their families to accept that health care providers cannot cure chronic illnesses and that unexpected events will occur
- Helping individuals and their families focus on supports and resources rather than on feeling overwhelmed by deficits
- Simplifying goals and tasks so that they are realistic, understandable, and manageable; focusing on small achievements
- Maintaining collaboration between health care systems
- Initiating and monitoring community partnerships and needed referrals to ensure that problems are successfully resolved

Establishing a Sense of Mastery

Empowerment is facilitated by the development of a sense of mastery. A sense of mastery reduces feelings of powerlessness that individuals with chronic illness experience. *Mastery,* as defined by Younger (1991) is:

a human response to difficult or stressful circumstances in which competency, control, and dominion are gained over the experience of stress. It means having developed new capabilities, having changed the environment, and/or reorganized the self so that there is a meaning and purpose in living that transcends the difficulty of the experience. (p. 81)

Four defining characteristics are needed to develop a sense of mastery (Younger, 1991):

1. Achieving a sense of control over a threatening situation
2. Instituting problem-solving measures to prevent a similar event from happening again

3. Feeling good about oneself
4. Finding new sources of satisfaction for losses associated with the threatening situation

The development of a sense of mastery is a process that occurs over time. The stages leading to the development of a sense of mastery are as follows (Younger, 1991):

- *Certainty:* assigning causes to an event and understanding the significance of that event; certainty enables a person to plan and make decisions
- *Change:* instituting problem-solving measures and actions to reduce the negative impact of a situation
- *Acceptance:* completing a process of suffering as a person grieves losses and comes to realize that he or she must adapt because the valuable things lost will not be regained
- *Growth:* acquiring new skills and relationships, finding meaning in life, and moving forward with life

Additionally, nurses need to recognize that assessing and intervening with individuals and their families with a chronic illness is an intense experience that can be invigorating yet exhausting. Throughout the illness trajectory, nurses need to take the time necessary to examine their feelings related to the suffering that they are witnessing (McDaniel, Hepworth & Doherty, 1997). Taking the time and effort to address their feelings will enable nurses to accurately and objectively address the needs of individuals and their families.

Services

Clients with chronic illness may find a sense of control and loss of powerlessness with their involvement with a professional health care organization. Services provided by these organizations may include health promotion, illness prevention, rehabilitation, support groups, and other supportive services. These organizations provide accessible and affordable services, often can coordinate and integrate health services, and foster self-care and participation in care (Clarke & Mass, 1998). Examples include the American Cancer Society, the American Diabetes Association, the Arthritis Foundation, and the National Multiple Sclerosis Society.

Nonprofessional services include self-help groups, mutual support groups, and peer group programs. These programs offer unique benefits for individuals and families coping with chronic illnesses (Swayze, 1991). Group members meet on a regular basis and offer empathy and support to each other. Communication is open and nonjudgmental, enabling members to share vulnerable feelings and intimate concerns. Members report that powerlessness diminishes and is replaced by feelings of being cared for, being understood, belonging, and confidence (Hildingh, Fridlund & Segesten, 1995).

Recommendations for Further Conceptual and Data-Based Work

Powerlessness is not an isolated concept in chronic illness. A number of other concepts are related to it, but currently there is little data-based research that links powerlessness to these concepts. Greater clarity of powerlessness may be gained by examining how powerlessness relates to alienation, hopelessness, locus of control, and vulnerability (Table 13-2). Additional concepts that may be related to powerlessness and merit further comparative analysis include Antonovsky's generalized resistance resources (1985), coping style, dependence, hardiness (Maddi, 2002), and helplessness.

Research using empowerment as an independent variable and as a dependent variable will yield data-based information that will enable nurses to assist individuals in reducing feelings of powerlessness. When powerlessness is an independent variable, outcomes related to empowerment may include increased self-efficacy, perceived control, and improved health and quality of life. When powerlessness is a dependent variable, factors leading to empowerment may include support, participatory decision making, and education (Vander Henst, 1997). In the last year or two,

a few researchers have begun to use qualitative methods to understand powerlessness; however, additional work is needed to further explain the concept from the individual's perspective.

Philosophical Considerations

Powerlessness in the absolute sense is the inability to affect an outcome. Is anyone ever completely powerless? As long as a person is living, does that mean that he or she has some level of power? Although people with chronic illnesses do not have the power to cure their disease, are there aspects of their situation that they may have power to control? The individual is likely to feel overwhelmed, exhausted, and discouraged at times; therefore, one of the most important challenges for nurses working with these clients is to help them overcome feelings of powerlessness. Nurses typically have two major ways of helping individuals with chronic illnesses overcome feelings of powerlessness: by providing physical assistance and guidance and by offering emotional and mental assistance often through motivation and education.

Outcomes

Outcomes associated with powerlessness in clients with chronic illness may be monitored in three categories: 1) self, 2) relationships with others, and 3) behaviors. Specifically, changes in self include increased self-confidence and self-esteem, which facilitate coping with chronic disease. Changes in relationships include improved relationships with family, friends, and health care providers. And, changes in behavior include health and goal oriented decisions, which promote personal responsibility for health (Falk-Rafael, 2001).

Summary and Conclusions

Powerlessness is defined as having the belief that one cannot control an event or situation. Power and control are absent when a person experiences feelings of powerlessness. Individuals often experience feelings of powerlessness in response to a chronic illness. These feelings may manifest in a variety of ways, including displaying apathy, anger, or depression. Nurses need to be able to identify feelings of powerlessness that individuals experience.

The Personal Control Model can be used as a framework in designing specific interventions based on the four types of loss of control that are associated with powerlessness: physiological, cognitive, environmental, and decisional. Diversional activities may provide meaning and facilitate exploration of feelings. Educating individuals about the common symptoms associated with their chronic illness, outlining the typical disease trajectory, and explaining the importance of maintaining a familiar and routine environment enable individuals and their families to reduce feelings of powerlessness. Additionally, both professional and nonprofessional services may assist clients in experiencing some control over their illness.

Note: The author would like to thank David C. Wood for his input, comments and editing to this chapter.

Study Questions

1. Describe the ways in which individuals with chronic illnesses display feelings of powerlessness.
2. Describe the relationship between powerlessness and chronic illness.
3. Define *power* and *personal control.*
4. What physiological and psychosocial factors are associated with powerlessness?
5. What are some of the key factors that need consideration when assessing individuals and families for feelings of powerlessness?
6. How can the Personal Control Model be used to design interventions to reduce powerlessness?
7. Describe empowerment of the client with a chronic illness.
8. What nursing interventions can reduce powerlessness in individuals with chronic illness?
9. What is a sense of mastery? How does developing a sense of mastery enable individuals with a chronic illness to reduce feelings of powerlessness?

References

Antonovsky, A. (1985). *Health, stress, and coping.* San Francisco: Jossey-Bass.

Bright, R. (1996). *Grief and powerlessness: Helping people regain control of their lives.* Bristol, PA: Jessica Kingsley Publishers.

Clarke, H. F., & Mass, H. (1998). Comox valley nursing centre: From collaboration to empowerment. *Public Health Nursing, 15* (3), 216–224.

Clarke, J. N., & James, S. (2003). The radicalized self: The impact on the self of the contested nature of the diagnosis of chronic fatigue syndrome. *Social Science and Medicine, 57* (8), 1387–1395.

Davidhizar, R. (1994). Powerlessness of caregivers in home care. *Journal of Clinical Nursing, 3* (3), 155–158.

Denner, J., & Dunbar, N. (2004). Negotiating femininity: Power and strategies of Mexican American girls. *Sex Roles, 50* (5/6), 301–314.

deSchepper, A. M., Francke, A. L., & Abu-Saad, H. H. (1997). Feelings of powerlessness in relation to pain: Ascribed causes and reported strategies. *Cancer Nursing, 20* (6), 422–429.

Dunn, J. D. (1998). Powerlessness regarding health-service barriers: Construction of an instrument. *Nursing Diagnosis: The Journal of Nursing Language and Classification, 9* (4), 136–143.

Falk-Rafael, A. (2001). Empowerment as a process of evolving consciousness: A model of empowered caring. *Advances in Nursing Science, 24* (1), 1–16.

Gibson, J., & Kenrick, M. (1998). Pain and powerlessness: The experience of living with peripheral vascular disease. *Journal of Advanced Nursing, 27* (4), 737–745.

Green, B. L., Lewis, R. K., Wang, M. Q., Pearson, S., et al. (2004). Powerlessness, destiny, and control: The influence on health behaviors of African Americans. *Journal of Community Health, 29* (1), 15–27.

Hildebrandt, E. (1999). Focus groups and vulnerable populations: Insight into client strengths and needs in complex community health care environments. *Nursing and Health Care Perspectives, 20* (5), 256–259.

Hildingh, C., Fridlund, B., & Segesten, K. (1995). Social support in self-help groups, as experienced by persons having coronary heart disease and their next of kin. *International Journal of Nursing Studies, 32* (3), 224–232.

Israel, B. A., Checkoway, B., Schulz, A., & Zimmerman, M. (1994). Health education and community empowerment: Conceptualizing and measuring perceptions of individual, organizational, and community control. *Health Education Quarterly, 21* (2), 149–170.

Johnson, D. (1967). Powerlessness: A significant determinant in patient behavior? *Journal of Nursing Education, 6* (2), 39–44.

Landau, J. (1997). Whispers of illness: Secrecy versus trust. In H. McDaniel, J. Hepworth, & W. J. Doherty (Eds.), *The shared experience of illness: Stories of patients, families, and their therapists.* New York: Basic Books.

Lewis, R. (1982). Experienced personal control and quality of life in late-stage cancer patients. *Nursing Research, 31,* 113–119.

Lunney, A. T. (1997). Case study: Response to a diagnosis of chronic illness when confounded by other life events. *Nursing Diagnosis, 8* (2), 48, 79.

Maddi, S. R. (2002). The story of hardiness: Twenty years of theorizing, research, and practice. *Consulting Psychology Journal: Practice and Research, 54* (3), 173–185.

Maddi, S. R., Kobasa, S. C., & Hoover, M. (1979). An alienation test. *Journal of Humanistic Psychology, 19* (4), 73–76.

McDaniel, S. H., Hepworth, J., & Doherty, W. J. (1997). The shared emotional themes of illness. In S. H. McDaniel, J. Hepworth, & W. J. Doherty (Eds.), *The shared experience of illness: stories of patients, families, and their therapists.* New York: Basic Books.

Miller, J. F. (Ed.). (2000). *Coping with chronic illness: Overcoming powerlessness* (3rd ed.). Philadelphia: FA Davis.

———. (1992). *Coping with chronic illness: Overcoming powerlessness* (2nd ed.). Philadelphia: FA Davis.

———. (1983). *Coping with chronic illness: Overcoming powerlessness.* Philadelphia: FA Davis.

Mishel, M. H. (1999). Uncertainty in illness. *Annual Review of Nursing Research, 19,* 269–294.

Mok, E., Martinson, I., & Wong, T. K. (2004). Individual empowerment among Chinese cancer patients in Hong Kong . . . including commentary by Buchanan D and Chiu L with author response. *Western Journal of Nursing Research, 26* (1), 59-84.

Nyamathi, A., Flaskerud, J., Leake, B., & Chen, S. (1996). Impoverished women at risk for AIDS: Social support variables. *Journal of Psychosocial Nursing and Mental Health Services, 34* (11), 31–39.

Nyström, A. E., & Segesten, K. M. (1994). On sources of powerlessness in nursing home life. *Journal of Advanced Nursing, 19,* 124–133.

Richmond, T., Metcalf, J., Daly, M., & Kish, J. (1992). Powerlessness in acute spinal cord injury patients: A descriptive study. *Journal of Neuroscience Nursing, 24* (3), 146–152.

Roberts, S. L., & White, B. S. (1990). Powerlessness and personal control model applied to the myocardial infarction patient. *Progress in Cardiovascular Nursing, 5* (3), 84–94.

Rodin, J., & Langer, E. (1977). Long-term effects of a control-relevant intervention with the institutionalized aged. *Journal of Personality and Social Psychology, 35* (12), 897–902.

Rotter, J. B. (1966). Generalized expectancies for internal vs. external control of reinforcement. *Psychology Monographs, 80* (1), 1–28.

Ruhl, K. B. (1999). Rehabilitation considerations for the client with chronic, nonmalignant pain. *Nursing Case Management, 4* (2), 90–101.

Seeman, M. (1959). The meaning of alienation. *American Sociological Review, 24* (6), 783–791.

Seeman, M., & Evans, J. (1962). Alienation and learning in a hospital setting. *American Sociological Review, 27,* 772–783.

Seeman, M., & Lewis, S. (1995). Powerlessness, health and mortality: A longitudinal study of older men and mature women. *Social Science in Medicine, 41* (4), 517–525.

Seeman, M., & Seeman, T. (1983). Health behavior and personal autonomy: A longitudinal study of the sense of control in illness. *Journal of Health and Social Behavior, 24* (2), 144–160.

Seligman, M. (1975). *Helplessness: On depression, development and death.* San Francisco: Freeman.

Schorr, J. A., Farnham, R. C., & Ervin, S. M. (1991). Health patterns in aging women as expanding consciousness. *Advances in Nursing Science, 13* (4), 52–63.

Stapleton, S. R. (1978). *Powerlessness in individuals with chronic renal failure.* Unpublished master's thesis. Milwaukee, WI: Marquette University.

Strauss, A., Corbin, J., Fagerhaugh, S., Glaser, B., et al. (1984). *Chronic illness and the quality of life* (2nd ed.). St. Louis: Mosby.

Strehlow, A. J., & Amos-Jones, T. (1999). The homeless as a vulnerable population. *Nursing Clinics of North America, 34* (2), 261–274.

Swayze, S. (1991). Helping them cope: Developing self-help groups for clients with chronic illness. *Journal of Psychosocial Nursing, 29* (5), 35–37.

Vander Henst, J. A. (1997). Client empowerment: A nursing challenge. *Clinical Nurse Specialist, 11* (3), 96–99.

van der Merwe, A. S. (1999). The power of women as nurses in South Africa. *Journal of Advanced Nursing, 30* (6), 1272–1279.

Walker, J., Holloway, I., & Sofaer, B. (1999). In the system: The lived experience of chronic back pain from the perspectives of those seeking help from pain clinics. *Pain, 80*, 621–628.

Wetherbee, L. L. (1995). Powerlessness and the hospice client. *Home Healthcare Nurse, 13* (5), 37–41.

White, B. S., & Roberts, S. L. (1993). Powerlessness and the pulmonary alveolar edema patient. *Dimensions of Critical Care Nursing, 12* (3), 127–137.

Worthman, C., & Brehm, J. (1975). Responses to uncontrollable outcomes: An integration of reactance theory and the learned helpless model. In L. Berkowitz (Ed.), *Advances in Experimental Social Psychology* (vol. 8), (pp. 278–336). New York: Academic Press.

Younger, J. B. (1991). A theory of mastery. *Advances in Nursing Science, 14* (1), 76–89.

PART III

Impact of the Health Professional

CHAPTER 14

Change Agent

Patricia A. Chin

Introduction

Change is an intensely personal experience (Duck, 1988). Clients with chronic illness, and their families, experience continuing and often overwhelming change on a regular basis. These clients are required to make major changes in their knowledge level, attitudes and behaviors, or life-styles. When a client changes one aspect of their life, everyone around them-family, significant others, and friends-is affected by that change. Suffering, dysfunction, premature mortality, and medical costs can be reduced by positive changes in health practices and behavior. An understanding of how change occurs, the best time for initiating the change process, and the skills necessary to facilitate the change process are essential for nurses working with clients with chronic illness.

The Concept of Change

The term *change* has many meanings and uses within the English language. *Change* can be used as a noun, to mean the movement from one state of being to another, an act or process, or the result of changing. *Change* can be used as a verb, to indicate the action of making or becoming different, to alter,

modify, substitute, adapt, or adjust. It can also be used as an adjective: *changed,* changeable, or transformed. The list of synonyms for the term is endless. Antonyms for *change* include stability, constancy, immutability, and firmness.

Change is an experience associated with all organisms, situations, and processes (Lippitt, 1973). Change is any planned or unplanned alteration (Chin, Finocchiaro & Rosebrough, 1998). Change implies an essential difference, sometimes amounting to the loss or substitution of one thing or state for another. Change has been described as the creating, maintaining, breaking down, and recreating of form (Lewin, 1951). Change involves modification of not only behavior, but also feelings, emotions, attitudes, and values. In fact, change cannot occur and be maintained successfully without alterations in all domains, cognitive, affective, and behavioral.

While many aspects of one's life cannot be intentionally changed, individuals can exert power to bring about change in their own lives (Prochaska, Norcross & DiClemente, 1994). In the following discussion, change implies both action and process. Change will indicate the deliberate alteration in the behavioral, cognitive, and affective patterns of individuals, groups, or organizations. This intentional alteration in behavior is the result of deliberate choices by the individual, group, or organization. Change occurs from the process of "going out there and doing it" (Durrant & Kowalski, 1993).

Change affects people both positively and negatively. People are more comfortable with life stability and consistency. Many people find it uncomfortable and threatening to deal with the ambiguity and conflict that are inherent with change. Change often means giving up control and moving into unfamiliar and uncertain territory; that, in turn, creates uncertainty and doubt (Geraci, 2004). While change can be stressful, it also creates opportunities for growth, personal development and progress.

Assumptions

Three key assumptions are important within the concept of change: (1) Change is inevitable, (2) only small change is necessary for success, and (3) clients have the plasticity, ability, and resources to change.

Change Is Inevitable

Change is an inevitable and inescapable process. Buddhists profess that change is a continuous process and stability is only an illusion (Mitchell, 1988). While most individuals share the assumption that change is inevitable, few see change as something that is within the control of the individual. Many perceive change to be controlled by external forces, something outside the self, such as fate, karma, or more powerful individuals. However, when there is an expectation that a client can and will change, that expectancy will have a positive influence on the client's behavior. Nurses need to work with clients, families, and other groups to create positive, self-fulfilling prophecies regarding the ability to bring about change. When talking about change, the discussion should focus on *when* the change will occur, not *if* the change will occur (Gingerich & de Shazer, 1991). A belief in the client's ability to change will be a significant determinant of treatment outcomes (Selekman, 1993).

Only Small Change Is Necessary for Success

An individual's realization of self-potential is achieved mainly through a series of progressive changes that can have a snowball effect on client behavior (Gordon & Meyers-Anderson, 1981). All efforts to change should be encouraged, and clients should be encouraged to value even minimal change. Once clients have been able to effect some change, their expectations about their ability to change are enhanced (Bandura, 1986; Erikson, 1963). Plans for facilitating client change should include manageable, concrete, incremental changes, ensuring goal attainment and success to increase a sense of self-efficacy.

Clients Have the Plasticity, Ability, and Resources to Change

Individuals have the potential for being more purposeful in life, being more actualized, and being more competent in managing their health by developing their unique personal resources (Pender, 1996). Clients have strengths and resources that can be capitalized on for developing constructive approaches to change. Clients are more likely to cooperate in the change process when their personal strengths and resourcefulness are emphasized. Any past successes with change should be used as a model for present and future success. Families and significant others can be power allies for facilitating change. Everyone who has contact with the person engaged in a behavioral change will be affected by the change. It is important that nurses assess the impact of change on members of the client's support system and alert them to the fact that the change, and any potential behavioral alterations, will have significant impact on their lives.

Planned and Unplanned Change

Change is traditionally categorized as *unplanned* or *drift change* and *planned change* (Chin et al., 1998). There are distinct differences between the two categories of change. Unplanned change is random in nature. Often the change occurs in small increments, with a cumulative effect that is only perceived as a rapid, sudden event. Because change is not planned, its occurrence may not even be perceived or is perceived only as "drift" (Reinkemeyer, 1970). Outcomes of unplanned change are neither deliberate nor predictable and are always negative. An example of unplanned change is deciding to stop smoking "cold turkey."

Planned change is a deliberate, controlled, and conscious (Geraci, 2004; Huber, 2000) systematic process. It is directed toward producing an improvement in function, some output, or a solution to a problem. Because planned change is intentional, it requires problem solving, decision making, and interpersonal skills. The outcomes of planned change are deliberate and predictable. An example of planned change is developing a weight-reduction program.

Issues Related to Change

Resistance to Change

A common reaction to change is resistance. Opposition to change is often based on a threat to security as change disrupts normal patterns of behavior (Swansburg & Swansburg, 2002). Many clients are well aware of their problems and the cost to themselves and others, but they feel overwhelmed, powerless, or unable to bring about a resolution to the problem. Their resistance can be either passive or active. When resistance occurs, the client will oppose, obstruct, or block movement toward change. New and Couillard (1981) identified five reasons for the development of resistance in the change process:

1. Threats to self-interest
2. Inaccurate perceptions about the nature or implications of the change
3. Disagreements in the understanding of information related to the change

4. Psychological reactance: a strong motivation to maintain a sense of autonomy and resist coercion by other (O'Connell, 1997)
5. Feelings of alienation

Resistance to change can be dealt with as follows: (New & Couillard, 1981)

■ Including those involved in the change process in the design and implementation of change techniques
■ Using formal authority or power judiciously to implement and enforce change
■ Using information to reinforce the benefits of change and logic of change
■ Using external agents, those with expertise and trustworthiness, not affected by the change to introduce the recommended change
■ Using selective incentives and rewards
■ Being supportive and empathic while gradually introducing change

Clients Who Choose Not to Change

Change can be a challenging experience. Individuals with a chronic illness will be faced with multiple changes as they cope and adapt to their health state. Even though a change may be perceived as beneficial, there may still be a sense of threat or a loss of control or autonomy. Some individuals make conscious decisions to disregard recommended health promotion, disease prevention or health maintenance behavioral changes.

There may be numerous reasons why a client chooses not to make a change, not to make a change at that time, or not to change in the way recommended. Clients have a right not to change or not to change directly in the manner their health care professional may desire. A decision not to make a recommended health behavior change may have either negative or neutral consequences for the client.

If the client chooses not to make a recommended change and there are no negative or harmful consequences, the nurse should continue to establish and maintain the therapeutic nurse-patient relationship, assist the client to simplify and prioritize goals, identify alternative behavioral patterns and be alert for consciousness raising and insight development opportunities regarding the recommended behavior or behavioral pattern change. This approach allows the nurse to use the marketing strategy of "the foot-in-the-door." The client should be asked to agree to minimal participation in the change process continuing to discuss the possibility of change, being receptive to accepting materials on the proposed behavioral change. Minimal participation will result in a gradual increase in involvement. Maintaining an open supportive relationship with repetitive and consistent messages sets the stage for potential future change (Ryan, 2000).

If the client chooses not to make a recommended change and there are significant negative consequences, effective interventional strategies include negation, graduated regimen recommendations, and contracting (Ryan, 2000). Graduated regimens are based on the assumption that only small change is necessary for change. The individual successfully masters one phase of a behavioral change leading to willingness to advance to another phase. Contracting is a negotiation process in which the nurse and the client select a behavior change and specify the conditions of change and identify the rewards for completing the contract. Contracting is most effective when committed to in writing and stated positively (Steckel, 1982).

Barriers to Change

During the process of change, two types of forces are at work that can either promote or thwart the change process. Forces that promote the change process by moving the individual in the direction of positive outcomes are identified as *driving forces*. In opposition to the driving forces are *restraining forces* that thwart the change process (Lewin, 1947). Nature is constantly striving to maintain a state of equilibrium. When restraining and driving forces are equal, referred to as a steady state, the status quo

is maintained. In a steady state, the individual will not perceive the need for change, and change will not occur. Change occurs when driving forces or restraining forces are in a state of imbalance. To be effective in facilitating change, it is essential to identify both types of forces so that maximum benefit can be derived from the power of the driving forces while averting or modifying the restraining forces (New & Couillard, 1981).

Change is difficult for people under normal conditions, but it is particularly difficult for those who are stressed, feel out of control or powerless (Seligman, 1991), or are experiencing attacks on their self-esteem or self-worth (Chin et al., 1998). Restraining forces can take the form of external barriers, factors existing in the environment, or internal barriers within the individual. External forces may include the lack of adequate facilities, materials, financial resources, or social support or the erosion of support systems (Bailey, 1990). The client's support system, consisting of the client's established personal and professional relationships, is one of the most significant influences on the client and the change process. The client's established relationships can be supportive, non-supportive, neutral, or apathetic. The degree of impact of the support system on the change process involves several issues:

- The relevance of the disagreeing persons or groups to the client
- The attractiveness of the disagreeing persons or groups to the client
- The extent of the disagreement of relevant persons or groups
- The number of persons relevant to the client who are in disagreement with the change
- The extent to which the client is self-directed rather than dependent on others

Internal barriers influencing the client's progress through the change process may include the lack of necessary knowledge and/or skills, appropriate affective state, or insufficient motivation necessary for change. Change is also difficult when the client is experiencing pain, anxiety, inconvenience, deterioration of vigor, immobility, or the stress of the day-to-day management of chronic illness (Farley, 1992; Bailey, 1990). Clients who are highly anxious about change or are mourning a loss created by a change will learn little or apply little about the desired change, blocking the process (Bushnell, 1979). The desire to maintain the status quo (Farley, 1992), competing multiple problems, or the inability to detach from negative perceptions (Chin et al., 1998) can also impede change.

It is futile to encourage the client's efforts to change when actions are likely to be blocked or frustrated by internal or external barriers (Pender, 1987). That might occur when

- goals are unclear,
- there are insufficient skills to follow through with self-modification,
- there are perceptions of lack of control over contingencies related to targeted behaviors,
- there has been inadequate planning or preparation for decision making and implementing the change process.

Emotional Response to Change

Responses to change are widely variable and often inconsistent (Yoder-Wise, 2003). Responses to change can range from enthusiastic acceptance, to little or no outward reaction, or to outright rejection. How the person will respond to change is often influenced by the degree to which the person is cognitively and emotionally involved in the change. The emotional response to change has been characterized as similar to the response associated with the process of health and dying (Geraci, 2004: Perlman & Takacs, 1990).

Perlman and Takacs (1990) describe the stages of emotional response to change based on Kubler-Ross's (1969) stages of death and dying.

- Equilibrium: balance and comfort with personal goals in sync.
- Denial: emotional energy spent on denying reality of the change

- Anger: active resistance to the change expressed through anger and frustration
- Chaos: energy diffused with a loss of direction scattered thought and emotions
- Depression: energy is spent leaving emotional emptiness and lack of will
- Resignation: no energy or enthusiasm, resigns to the change
- Openness: renewed energy ready to explore options
- Readiness: can let go of the old and adopt changes
- Reemergence: renewed energy the result is comfort with change and full re-engagement with the new behavior.

Ethical Issues

It is an individual's creativity, problem-solving ability, and self-directed nature that make intentional change possible (Pender, 1987). An awareness and recognition of human dignity, autonomy, capabilities for self-management, and the right to choose how life will be lived are important considerations for health care providers engaged in intentional change.

Many clients with chronic illness are vulnerable, especially during times when critical decision making is required. Children, the frail elderly, or debilitated adults must often be dependent on family members and others to assist them in making significant life decisions. Conflicts can arise among the client's, significant other's, and professional's value and belief systems. These conflicts need to be resolved before decisions are made. There can also be instances when decisions about change are in the best interest of the client, but the client may not agree. In such situations, it may be necessary to use formal authority or power to protect the client's status (Bailey, 1990; Dixon, 1998). This should be permitted only in rare instances or when the client is in a state of total dependence.

The nurse should be certain that power remains with the client. As an advocate for the client, the nurse should intervene only when others impede on the client's autonomy and right of free choice. The nurse should also be certain that the client has adequate information to make informed choices about change and the strategies employed to facilitate the change process. It is unprofessional and irresponsible to allow clients to make decisions or engage in activities when they have not weighed all the consequences and risks involved. The legitimate goal of change is the elimination of ignorance and enhancing of adherence (Dixon, 1998).

The focus of planning and interventions should be on enhancing clients' strengths for decision making and goal attainment. The client is an "active producer" (Pender, 1987; Prochaska, Norcross & DiClemente, 1994) rather than a passive entity. The client must be willingly and actively engaged in the change process. All affected by the planned change must mutually plan and design goals and outcomes and willingly accept changes necessary to achieve those goals and outcomes. Because autonomy is the focal point, authoritarian, coercive, and manipulative strategies should be avoided. Because modification is the goal of intentional change, nurses should be certain that knowledge of the change process is not used to manipulate the client or deprive the client of the right to make independent decisions. Ultimately, the client has the right to choose to change or not change (Bailey, 1990), to choose when to change, and to determine what form change will take.

"Slipping" and Relapsing

Relapse begins with a "slip" from the action plan. A relapse is a norm for any single attempt to change (O'Connell, 1997; Prochaska et al., 1994). A slip involves engaging in a behavior that had been diminished or eliminated, or not engaging in a desired new behavior. When a slip has occurred, the client may again talk and act in a manner similar to that of an earlier stage of change, or the client may reenter periods of resistance and avoidance (precontemplation) or may see change as a future event (contemplating) (Prochaska et al., 1994).

Research indicates that it may take individuals in smoking cessation programs as long as seven years to progress from the precontemplation state to the maintenance stage. During that time, they may experience as many as three relapses when they return to earlier smoking behavior (O'Connell, 1997; Prochaska et al., 1994). Often, these clients can successfully resume progression though the change process because they have previously made a determination that change was needed and have experienced some success with change. One key in assisting clients who relapse is that the nurse not make the client feel ashamed. A relapse will have a demoralizing effort on the client because they have invested a great deal of personal resources into the efforts to change. The client needs support for successful efforts and encouragement to reaffirm their commitment to change.

Clients who relapse have complex stories, explanations, and rationales for why the relapse has occurred. These stories, explanations, and rationales should be investigated in detail and analyzed. Often, this information can be used to modify the change plan to bring about the desired outcomes.

Health care providers often harbor an unwarranted sense of their own importance in creating change. Health care providers may ignore outside variables that have an impact on a client's life. If health care providers overestimate their role in creating change, there can be a diminishing of a client's sense of accomplishment rather than client empowerment. In those situations, the possibility will exist for the negating, or nonutilization, of client resources. A major function of the nurse change agent is to interact with clients in ways that help them broaden their perspective and clarify their thinking about the situation. The change agent needs to create an accepting, respectful climate for doing so. This climate will be unique for each client and in each situation (Lippitt, 1973).

The key intervention for dealing with a relapse is the "reframing" of the relapse into an opportunity for learning. What can the client learn from the present attempt to change for use in a subsequent attempt to change? A comprehensive assessment of factors that might have caused the slip or relapse to occur needs to be discussed. This information will be used in planning the next effort to change. It is important that the client answer the question, "What is the next step toward change?" (O'Connell, 1997).

Change During Times of Crisis

Stressful events and emergencies are a part of life for clients with chronic illness. Without effective life skills and strategies, these events have the potential for becoming crises. If stress becomes overwhelming and the client is unable to problem-solve, a crisis may result. Whether the crisis experience results in client growth and enrichment or in a lower level of client functioning depends on previous problem-solving abilities and current levels of support. Increased stress and psychic "dis-ease" can actually create a state in which the client experiences heightened awareness and is open to change as a means of decreasing stress and distress.

Stress is a common denominator as people move through life (Hoff, 1978). Clients with chronic illness experience crises related to both developmental and situational issues. People generally experience higher levels of anxiety during developmental transition states. During those periods, there are natural changes in roles, body image, and functions, and in ways of relating to others. The successful completion of developmental tasks (Erikson, 1963) requires additional energy and nurturing that may not be available to individuals who are already debilitated by a chronic disease.

Situational crises occur as a result of some unanticipated traumatic event or unforeseen occurrence beyond one's control. Common situational crises include loss of a loved one through death or divorce, unemployment, urban dislocation, natural disaster, or the diagnosis of a chronic or life-threatening illness. During these times, people are very vulnerable. The increased levels of anxiety and psychic "dis-ease" makes them more vulnerable to potential crisis, but may also make them more open to learning and change.

Crises do not occur instantaneously. Several authors have developed models for understand crises and their interventions (Caplan, 1964; Greenstone

& Levitson, 1993; Roberts & Burgess, 1997). Each of these models describes crisis as a linear stage process. Recognition of the stages of the process of crisis aids in prevention of crisis and provides understanding on how change can be hindered or facilitated during a time or crisis.

The emphasis in working with a client in crisis is on the here and now (Roberts & Burgess, 1997). Efforts are focused on learning new approaches or changing approaches to problem solving and stress reduction. Resolution will be either adaptive, growth promoting, or maladaptive, resulting in less functioning for the client than existed in the pre-crisis period. Nurses who care for clients with chronic illness should be alert to the potential for crises, and use that state as an opportunity to facilitate positive change. With guidance, the client will integrate adaptive change and be able to meet future situations more effectively.

Cultural Influences

The rationale for targeted intervention programs arises from the growing ethnic and racial diversity in the U.S. population, health disparities in disease, differences in mortality across racial and ethnic groups, and differences in the prevalence of behavioral risk factors across groups. Culturally tailored health behavior change programs arise from differences in the predictors of health behaviors across groups (Resnicow, Braithwaite, Dilorio, & Glanz, 2002; Kreuter & Skinner, 2000).

Designing health behavior change interventions requires an understanding of the intended audience. Planning change begins by "starting where the people are" (Resnicow, et al., 2002). Targeted and tailored health behavior change programs must evolve from an awareness of race or ethnicity, socioeconomic status, age, location or language to name a few factors.

In every nurse-client relationship, there must be positive regard and sensitivity for a client's cultural heritage. When nurses demonstrate cultural competency, a better understanding of particular life situations is demonstrated. When cultural beliefs and life-style are considered when working with the client, the result is a better "cultural fit," which is more apt to be maintained over time (Spector, 2000; Sue, 1999). This is especially true when working with clients in the process of change. Factors requiring identification and clarification include the following:

- Potential conflict between indicated change and traditional folkways, beliefs, and values
- Potential conflicts between indicated change and traditional religious beliefs or healing arts
- Potential conflicts between indicated change and familial traditions
- Perceived benefits or value for taking, or not taking, suggested actions
- Impact of making a change on traditional social roles and lifeways
- Similarities and dissimilarities between the care provider encouraging the behavioral change and the client
- Degree of acculturation, assimilation into the predominant culture, and heritage consistency
- Time orientation: past, present, and future
- Expectations of health care providers
- Expectations of clients as receivers of care and self-care agents
- Client's perceptions of personal power or lack of power (self-efficacy)
- Beliefs about attribution (i.e., self, chance, luck, karma, fate)

Interventions

Change Agent

A *change agent* is defined as a person who deliberately promotes a change process (Mauksch & Miller, 1981). A change agent may also be considered an advocate or sponsor of planned change (Geraci, 2004). An effective change agent strives to empower the client and family members. Effective change agents are partners and catalysts for change. Establishing a helping relationship with others engaged in the change process may be either a formal or informal contract for services, indicating a mu-

tual commitment by all involved parties to work toward identified outcomes. The nurse-client relationship for creating effective change is similar to that in other areas of nursing practice; it is a time-limited therapeutic relationship. Nurses should be aware of their "helping" style and evaluate its effect and influence on others with differing personalities, backgrounds, and life-styles (Pender, 1987).

Change agents should be helpers, not enablers. There are significant differences between enablers and helpers. Enablers avoid discussion and confrontation of the client's behaviors. They diminish the consequences of actions and behaviors by minimizing the importance of interactions and events. The enabler often makes excuses for, covers for, and defends the client's problem behaviors. They rarely recommend behavioral change (Prochaska, Norcross & DiClemente, 1994).

Helpers are specific and address disruptive or distressing client behaviors. They assist the client by relating negative behavior with negative outcomes and/or consequences. They insist that the individual accept responsibility for actions and directly and frequently recommend behavior change (Prochaska, Norcross & DiClemente, 1994).

Effective change agents have been described as possessing integrity, optimism, self-confidence, sincerity, and charisma (Lippitt & Lippitt, 1978). Change agents are flexible, self-motivated, and sensitive toward others; possess cultural sensitivity; are able to deal with ambiguity; are able to adapt to unfamiliar situations; and are genuine. Successful change agents have expertise in problem-solving, decision-making, and interpersonal communication skills (Geraci, 2004).

Rogers (1972) identified the following functions of the change agent:

Assists in the development of a perception of a need for change

Establishes the change relationship

Assists in labeling the problem

Examines the goals and alternative courses of action

Translates intent into action

Stabilizes change and attempts to prevent discontinuance of the changed behaviors

Facilitates closure

The change agent is responsible for creating an environment that facilitates change. That environment is open, stable, goal directed, and supportive. Interrupting, personal meaning, and the importance of language serve as media for creating the effective change environment. An effective change agent encourages the client's self-authoring capacities. By shifting the responsibility for identifying and evaluating capacities from the health care provider to the client, the nurse facilitates cognitive restructuring and enhances self-efficacy.

Effective change agents engage in "change talk." Change talk involves spending time eliciting what is working for the client, amplifying client expectations, and having clients imagine hypothetical solutions. Strategies include the use of play and humor, the context for change, establishing what change the client desires to focus on first, establishing what small signs of progress toward the goal will look like, and establishing what degree of change will be considered as acceptable. Change talk can also help to establish what Fanger (1993) describes as the "possibility frame."

The possibility frame shifts the therapeutic focus from a problem orientation to a probability orientation. First, a well-specified future action (to stop smoking) is elicited from the client: "What do you want to change?" "What is your goal?" "What is wanted and how?" Then, past unsuccessful attempts to reach that goal are identified. The nurse seeks ways to interrupt and reframe that past unsuccessful attempt. This reframing can be accomplished through words or actions. The reframed approach provides the client with new and expanded perspectives that support new effective action toward achieving the goal (Fanger, 1993; Friedman & Fanger, 1991).

Assessing and Planning for Change

Successful attempts to modify client behavior depend on an accurate assessment of the client's readiness for change. It is important to remember that stages of change are specific to problem behaviors and are not aspects of the client's personality (O'Connell, 1997; Prochaska et al., 1994). When a client's stage of change has been determined, strategies can be selected to better assist the client.

Planned change considers the entire system (Chin et al., 1998). Intentional change can be achieved only through progressive change and when guided by relevant goals that are meaningful to the client (Pender, 1996). To design interventions that best assist clients with chronic illnesses to change behaviors requires that the nurse have an understanding of the determinates of human behavior (Resnick, 2004). A comprehensive assessment is necessary to identify intrapersonal, interpersonal, and external barriers to change and the possible development of resistance to change.

A comprehensive format for obtaining baseline data (Table 14-1) for a client with chronic illness contemplating change includes the following areas:

■ History of presenting problem
■ Health history, including chronic illness history
■ Assessment of health beliefs and perceptions
■ Assessment of activities of daily living and functional level
■ Assessment of interpersonal relationships
■ Assessment of personal values and beliefs
■ Assessment of readiness for change

Developing a plan for change should be specific for the client's stage of change and the nature of the desired change. Generally, however, the following plan outlines the basics:

1. Identify the problem area of change.
2. Identify the client's goals and short-term expectations and outcomes.
3. Identify the nurse's role in the change process.
   Areas of collaboration
   Experiential strategies
   Behavioral strategies
   Empowerment strategies
4. Create a positive environment for change.

TABLE 14-1

Comprehensive Client Assessment

Personal and Family Health History	Chronic Illness	Health Beliefs and Perceptions	Activities of Daily Living
Demographics	Illness behaviors/roles	Perceptions of susceptibility to illness	Nutrition
Family genetic history	Impaired behaviors/role	Perceptions of seriousness of illness	Sleep
Religion and spirituality	Illness trajectory	Perceived threats to health	Exercise
Treatment and medications	Perceptions of stigma	Perceived threats to self	Play and hobbies
Drug use/abuse	Altered mobility	Perceived benefits of health practices	Mobility
	Chronic pain	Perceived barriers to health practices	Functional level
	Social isolation	Attribution of control (internal/external)	
	Nonadherence issues	Willingness to seek assistance	
		Information-seeking behaviors	

Interpersonal Relationships	Significant Others	Personal Values and Beliefs	Family Functional Level
Coping mechanisms	Nature of relationship	Level of self-esteem	What is the goal and how successful is the family in keeping to the goal?
Defense mechanisms	Existing or potential conflicts	Perceptions self-worth	How invested are family members in the goal?
Problem-solving style	Availability and willingness to assist client	Perceptions of self-efficacy	How does the family make decisions?
Family or relationship roles	Perceptions of client's problem	Satisfaction with life-style	What underlying barriers and negative dynamics exist?
Family or relationship communication patterns	Perceptions of client's intention and commitment to change	Meaning of life	Do members participate equally in family tasks and assignments?
Emotional regulation (affect, feelings)	Perceptions of potential disruption resulting from client's planned change		How do members feel about the family and its effectiveness
Situational supports/ resources	Coping mechanisms		Who heads the family?
Availability of helping relationships	Defense mechanisms		What is the power structure of the family, do inequities exist?
	Problem-solving style		

TABLE 14-1

Continued

Interpersonal Relationships	Significant Others	Personal Values and Beliefs	Family Functional Level
			Do struggles with autonomy exist? Do differences in perceptions and interpretation of others behavior and messages exist?

Communication Patterns	Readiness for Change: Preparation		
Individual member's verbal and nonverbal communication Spatial and seating arrangements Common themes expressed by members Quality of listening Problem-solving ability and capabilities	Degree of understanding that change is needed Degree of commitment to change process Perceptions of obstacles and barriers to change Alteration in self-image following change		

Readiness for Change: Precontemplation	Readiness for Change: Contemplation		
Level of awareness of problem and need for change Level of denial regarding problem and need for change Willingness to discuss possible change	Level of openness to discuss problem or need for change Perceptions regarding pros and cons of change Prior experience with change process Successes Failures Perceived factors leading to success or failure		

5. Enhance the change process.
6. Mitigate or remove barriers to change.
   Weaken restraint forces.
   Strengthen drive forces.
   Decrease pain.
   Reduce anxiety and emotional distress.
   Increase mobility.
   Assist in access to resources.
   Foster adherence.
   Increase socialization.
7. Plan for family change.
   Review family effectiveness assessment with family members.
   Determine consensus with the assessment findings.
   Mutually identify problems that the family desires to address.
   Suggest corrective measures or a new direction that needs to be taken.
   Assist in the identification of skills and resources necessary to achieve goals and desired outcomes.
   Create a supportive climate to promote effective problem solving.
   Promote member involvement.
   Promote empathy and mutual problem solving.
   Provide and elicit feedback.
   Reduce competition and promote individual achievement.
   Provide rewards for accomplishments.
   Keep the family focused on goals.
   Model good group communication skills.
   Send clear messages, and speak clearly and thoughtfully.
8. Evaluate and modify.
   Evaluate the plan of change.
   Deal with slips and relapses.
   Modify plan as necessary.
9. Develop a plan to maintain change.

Theoretical Frameworks

There are a number of theoretical frameworks that may be used to develop interventions for change. Considerable effort has been devoted to developing techniques that change behavior. Many early frameworks focused on how to bring about change. These approaches "pushed" people to change and were perceived by clients as manipulative, reducing choice and giving unbalanced power to the change agent. Recent approaches have shifted from behavioral strategies and are based on reducing the restraints against change. These newer approaches promote informed decision making (Glanz, Rimer & Lewis, 2002). Each change theory, model, or framework has its own merit; however, it seems unlikely that a single approach is appropriate for all individuals, problems, or situations. Instead of attempting to fit clients into a specific theoretical model, strategies need to be shaped to meet the unique needs of each client. The right set of internal and external conditions needs to be created to support the desired change.

The action paradigm dominating behavioral change programs over the past four decades has supported the view that change occurs dramatically and discretely. Various approaches in explaining the change process discuss two general categories of intervention strategies: behavioral (behavioral domain) and experiential (cognitive and affective domains).

Behavioral domain intervention strategies involve factors external to the client and focus directly on the client's behaviors. Strategies involve stimuli response, stimuli response modification, response extinction, and reinforcement of responses. Change occurs through a learning process called conditioning. The client is seen as a passive reactor to the environment. The goal of behavioral interventions is to shape or modify behavior.

Experiential domain intervention strategies involve thinking. They focus on internal processing that links emotions, attitudes, values, ideas, and thoughts. The client is seen as an active processor of information. The goal of experiential interventions is to assist the client in acquiring and developing new ways of thinking about change, and the need for change, and creating expectations about outcomes.

Programs developed following the frameworks of these two paradigms enroll individuals in time-limited programs aimed at behaviors such as reducing body weight, stopping smoking, overcoming dependency to alcohol or other substances, and adopting healthier life-styles. However, the programs address change from the perspective of only one or two domains, not all three domains. Program interventions reflect the specific framework upon which the program is developed. Seldom are these programs individualized, nor do they take into account the individual variables that might influence an individual's ability to change. In addition, these programs do not consider the individual's readiness for change. When individuals complete these programs and fail to maintain the change, the failure is attributed to the client, not to any limitation of the program. The individual is blamed for a relapse because of a lack of willpower or motivation.

Lewin Force-Field Model of Change

One of the traditional models for understanding, implementing, and predicting change is the field model of change. Nurses frequently use this approach to implement individual, family, group, and organizational change. According to this model, change is conceptualized as an interaction between the environment and personality (experiential). Lewin (1951) conceptualized change as a three-phase formative process. The framework characterizes change as occurring in three distinct phases: unfreezing, change (movement), and refreezing.

During the unfreezing phase, there is an increased awareness of a need for change. This increased awareness may occur because of discomfort with the present situation, questioning of the status quo, or a change in a relationship. The perception of need increases the individual's desire for change. This phase may be the most difficult for some clients because it requires planning and movement (Laughlin, 1989). During the change, or movement, phase, the individual makes a commitment to change, engages in decision making, and problem-solves regarding changing actions. During the refreezing phase, the focus is on maintaining new behaviors over time and incorporating supportive attitudes and values into the self-system. The three phases with appropriate action and nursing interventions are presented in Table 14-2.

Psychoanalytic Theories

Psychoanalytic theoretical approaches are effective for raising awareness. These approaches are internally focused and are the preferred approaches for raising awareness of conscious and unconscious motivations. The strategies of transference, dream interpretation, and free association are helpful for creating a state of "dis-ease," prompting the individual to the need for change. Techniques used with this approach are useful for raising awareness and emotional arousal and include clarification of the meaning of events (insight), uncovering past conflicts, transference, and working through countertransference issues.

Behavioral Modification Theory

Strategies based on behavior modification are particularly effective for changing discrete behaviors and shaping behavior. These approaches focus on the behavior itself and not the "whys" of behavior. Behavioral approaches are based on the general premise that behaviors are determined by consequences (Shumaker, Schron & Ockene, 1990) and focus on actual behaviors and reinforcement management. Behavior modification strategies use reinforcement to change and shape behavior (operant conditioning). The underlying assumption of operant conditioning is that behavior followed by a favorable consequence is apt to be repeated in the future when the same conditions occur. Positive reinforcement, rather than negative reinforcement or punishment, provides the most effective motivation for change.

Behaviorists believe that responses are shaped by conditioning to positive reinforcement and are extinguished by either negative punishment or the absence of rewards. Reinforcers are categorized as tangible (objects or activities), social (interactions with others), or self-generated (self-praise, positive self-statements).

Timing is very important in reinforcement management. In the early phases of change, immediate and continuous reinforcement is highly beneficial for moment-by-moment control over behavior. Continuous reinforcement also facilitates

TABLE 14-2

Lewin Force-Field Model of Change

Phase	Action	Intervention
Unfreezing	Development of awareness of the need and desire for change to solve the problem or cope with the situation Beliefs and perceptions are disturbed Movement from a steady state to an unsteady state, ready for change. Assessing the motivation and capacity for change	Assist client with identification of the problem Assist client with the identification of factors promoting or preventing change
Change (Movement)	Assessment and labeling of the problem Selecting progressive change objectives Identification of options and alternative actions Establishment of goals and outcomes Action is taken to facilitate change in perceptions, views, actions, values, and standards Evaluation of outcome of action Identification Internalization	Provide appropriate information Provide support Provide encouragement for movement toward desired change Evaluate effectiveness of outcomes
Refreezing	Integration and stabilization of learning New behavior and responses integrated into life-style Modification of relationships Change is adopted and maintained	Review the change and its effects on the client and family Plan for anticipated future change

SOURCES: Bailey, 1990; Farley, 1992; Geraci, 2004; Lewin, 1951.

rapid learning of the new or modified behavior. During the latter phases of change, intermittent reinforcement helps to stabilize the behavior and increase resistance to behavioral extinction (Fordyce, 1977).

Primary behavioral modification strategies include reinforcement management, manipulation of the environment, treatment of overt behavior, scheduling, and desensitization. The process of change occurs through a series of actions that result in client conditioning. The interventions reflect the mainly passive role of the client. The goal of these behavioral interventions is to shape or modify client behavior. Table 14-3 presents the major behavioral modification process, client activities, nursing interventions, and possible resources to accomplish the process goals.

While behaviorism is effective for making discrete behavioral change, the model does not address cognitive or affective domains. This limits its usefulness in the change process.

Experiential Theories

Experiential strategies evolve from various theories, including social cognitive theory (Bandura, 1986), rational-emotive theory (Ellis & Grieger, 1977), and reasoned action theory (Shumaker, Schron & Ockene, 1990). Three processes that are important for facilitating successful change include consciousness raising, self-evaluation, and cognitive restructuring. These three processes are the focus of this discussion because of their effectiveness in change process and their fit with the Spiral Model of

TABLE 14-3

Key Behavioral Strategies

Process	Client Activities	Nursing Interventions	Resources
Reinforcement management (Behavior modification)	Select behavior to be changed Select how change will occur Select: • Motivational aids • Positive reinforcement (rewards) • Negative reinforcement (removal or an aversive condition) • Punishment (aversive experience) Self-observation and monitoring	With patient, clearly identify exact behavioral change With patient, design a plan for managing clearly delineated reinforcement Base reinforcement strategies on patient's selection of behavior, positive/negative reinforcement, and punishment Establish behavioral frequency count (baseline) Monitor patient's progress to established outcomes and target rates Provide support for positive progress	Behavior record account (daily record) Tangible reinforcement (objects or activities) Social reinforcement (interaction involving others) Self-generated reinforcement (self-praise, self-compliments, positive statements) Intrinsic motivation (feeling relaxed, feeling energetic, improved breathing, increased mobility)
Modeling	Acquire new skills or behaviors Observe models engaging in desired behavior Observe how to relate to others	Help patient identify appropriate models Facilitate observations or interaction with selected models while engaged in the focus behavior Assess patient's ability to correctly perform focus behavior Assess patient's perceived self-efficacy Provide opportunities for patient to rehearse focus behavior	Models • Age-specific • Gender-specific • Culture-specific, etc. • Self-help groups
Counterconditioning	Break bond between a stimulus and a conditioned response Replace undesirable stimulus response bond with more desirable one	Help patient to identify undesirable stimulus-response bond Suggest appropriate alternative counterconditioning strategies	Imagery Relaxation techniques Desensitization

continues

TABLE 14-3

Continued

Process	Client Activities	Nursing Interventions	Resources
		Help patient to generalize new stimulus-response bond to other situations	
Controlling stimuli	Learn to identify precipitating verbal and nonverbal cues	Restructure internal and external cues that trigger behavior or response	Reminder letters and postcards
	Learn to control response to precipitating verbal and nonverbal cues	• Cue restriction (reduction to zero)	Personal phone calls
	Develop sensitivity to appropriate verbal and nonverbal cues	• Cue elimination (reduced, localization of cues)	Reminders from family members or supportive others
	Develop a system of internal cues to trigger desired behavior or response	• Cue expansion (cue combinations)	Reminders from models
	Learn to identify where and when desired behavior or response could occur	Identify personally relevant verbal and nonverbal cues for reinforcement	
	Learn to identify conditions that result in undesired behavior or response	Design a reinforcement program	

Adapted from: Bandura, 1986; Deci & Ryan, 1985; Dixon, 1998; Glanz, Rimer & Lewis, 2002; O'Connell, 1997; Pender, 1996; Prochaska, Norcross & DiClemente, 1994; Shumaker, Schron & Ockene, 1990. Reprinted with permission of Springer Science and Business Media.

Change (Prochaska et al; 1994). Table 14-4 presents experiential processes, client activities, nursing interventions, and potential resources for accomplishing desired process outcomes. Goals of interventions focus on the client's internal processing, linking emotions, attitudes, values, ideas, and thoughts. The objective of these interventions is to make the client an active processor of information and assist the client in acquiring and developing new ways of thinking about change and the need for change.

From a cognitive theory perspective, a person's behavior is determined by intentions to perform behavior and a combination of cognitive activities. Client intention is determined by assigning weight to attitudes toward the behavior and the value of anticipated outcomes. Attitude is formed by beliefs that

the behavior will lead to certain outcomes and that those outcomes have value to the client. It also results from application of subject standards, or norms, held by the client that others do or do not want the client to engage in certain behavior and the motivation of the client to comply with the wishes of others.

Increasing Awareness Initial desire and commitment to change results from an increased awareness that change is necessary. Increased awareness of needed change and the client perceptions of self-efficacy significantly influence the initiation and early phases of the change process. The client will engage in risk-appraisal and risk-reduction evaluation and compare this evaluation with perceptions of the benefit to be gained if expending energy in the change

TABLE 14-4

Key Experiential Strategies

Process	Client Activities	Nursing Interventions	Resources
Consciousness raising	Seek information Process information Interpret information Observe and interact with others who have changed or who engage in focus behavior	Provide information discussing the change being contemplated; to include pro and con information Provide information discussing short- and long-Books and other references term consequences of making contemplated change or failure to make the change Appraise values beliefs and emotions associated to the change Risk appraisal and risk reduction counseling Appraise how change alters the trajectory of the illness Appraise how health potential can be maximized as a consequence of the change Appraise amount of interpersonal support available Appraise real and perceived barriers to change and means to overcome them Discuss perceptions regarding targeted change Discuss the degree of involvement of other, amount of time available to assist the patient, and what type of assistance will be available Catharsis/dramatic relief	Culturally relevant materials Newspaper and magazine articles Posters Audio- and videotapes Computer programs Testimonials Involvement in self-help groups Journaling

continues

TABLE 14-4

Continued

Process	Client Activities	Nursing Interventions	Resources
Cognitive reevaluation and confrontation	Reevaluate self-standards (values and beliefs) Recognize inconsistencies between self-standards and behavior Announce plan to change	Assist in the identification of the patient's inconsistencies between values, standards, and behaviors Compare and contrast patient's behavior with some patient-identified ideal or role model Help patient to identify ways life would be enhanced if change occurred and the negative influences on quality of life without change Contrast what is, or will be, with what could be Dramatic relief Self-liberation Contingency management	Role models Respected individuals Reference groups Pro and con lists Available self-evaluation scales and questionnaires
Cognitive restructuring	Reflect on self-thoughts, self-imagery, and self-attitudes Analyze self-generated thoughts	Teach patient to think more rationally Increase incidence of positive emotions and self- appraisal Augment perceptions of self-efficacy and control Help patient to recognize positive and negative self-messages Help patient to correct problematic patterns of thinking and dysfunctional beliefs Rehearsal of positive self-statements Change irrational statements to rational statements	Self-statement Self-dministered praise Meditation Imagery Journaling

TABLE 14-4

Continued

Process	Client Activities	Nursing Interventions	Resources
		Help patient to increase perceptions of self-efficacy	
		Assist the patient to reduce self-criticism	
		Correct illogical or irrational ideas	
		Distinguish skills deficit in executing a new behavior from self-inhibition due to negative self-messages	

Adapted from: Bandura, 1986; Deci & Ryan, 1985; Dixon, 1998; Glanz, Rimer & Lewis, 2002; O'Connell, 1997; Pender, 1996; Prochaska, Norcross & DiClemente, 1994; Shumaker, Schron & Ockene, 1990. Reprinted with permission of Springer Science and Business Media.

process. This entire analysis is strongly influenced by the client's own values, beliefs, and perceptions of available internal and external resources. Client self-efficacy and perception of capability can be enhanced during this process. Clients derive a sense of self-esteem and feelings of satisfaction and pride from adherence to internalized standards and behavioral consistency based on those values. Personal values and beliefs are internalized during early developmental stages. These values and beliefs are derived from the value and belief systems of significant others and society. Violation of those internalized standards results in negative self-assessment, decreased self-esteem, and negative feelings of guilt and shame (Chin, Finocchiaro & Rosebrough, 1998; Rokeach, 1973).

Self-evaluation Self-evaluation is a change process intervention that is based on the assumption that change results from affective arousal. Clients are motivated to make a necessary change to achieve internal equilibrium when an awareness of disturbing inconsistency between self-standards and behaviors is perceived (Rokeach, 1973). Strong intentions of meeting personal standards lead to actual performance of the behavior (Pender, 1996). It is important that the client, not the nurse, make the determination of the inconsistency between standards and behavior. Mod-

eling of behavior is an excellent intervention both for self-evaluation and for enhancing self-efficacy. Models provide a comparison standard. Appropriate models should be identified from the client's reference group and should be individuals that the client admires. When a change in self-standards occurs, there will be a corresponding change in behavior as the client strives to achieve internal equilibrium.

Cognitive Restructuring The phenomenon of cognitive restructuring arises from rational-emotive theory (Ellis & Grieger, 1977). Its focus is a synthesis of affect and cognition. Interventions focus on the modification of thinking, imagery, and attitudes toward self worth, self-efficacy, and self-competency. From this perspective on change, key factors include appraisals, attributions, and evaluation in the form of self-statements and self-images. Frequently, dysfunctional thinking, imagery, attitudes, and punitive self-criticism result in diminished perceptions of self-efficacy and the inability to initiate and maintain behavioral change. Interventions facilitating cognitive restructuring include assessing the nature of the client's self-statements and self-image, assisting the client to recognize irrational or illogical statements and images, and replacing or correcting irrational or illogical statement and images.

Using the Spiral of Change Process

Stage 1: Contemplation

The Client Contemplating Change

The nurse is interviewing John, a 47-year-old client newly diagnosed with hypertension. He has been smoking a pack of cigarettes a day since he was 19 years old. He states that he started the habit because of peer pressure. When questioned further by the nurse, John can state several pros and cons of smoking. John also admits that his wife and teen-aged children have been pressuring him about the effects of second-hand smoke. He understands and values their desire not to be exposed to second-hand smoke. John thinks that his habit is both expensive and "stupid," but feels that smoking is one of the few ways that he finds to relax at work and at home. John is concerned about his increasing weight and is worried that if he stops smoking, this will only add to his weight gain. This happened to several of John's friends who tried to stop smoking. John has read about ways to stop smoking and asks the nurse wheter she thinks medications, a nicotine patch, or gum make quitting easier. The nurse asks John about past attempts to stop smoking. He states that he has made many attempts over the years but was always unsuccessful. He would go without cigarettes for a short time, but if he became stressed or was around others who were smoking, he began smoking again. The best he had accomplished was to cut down on the number of cigarettes he smoked for a short while. John wonders aloud if this might be a good time to try to stop smoking again, and he asks the nurse for her opinion. After some further discussion, John tells the nurse that he will give serious thought to quitting.

Response In this case, the client has been thinking about the problem behavior that should be changed. He is open to discussing the problem with the health care provider. He is interested and has already been able to weigh the pros and con of changing or not changing the behavior. He provides insight into his motivation to change and his perception of how difficult changing his behavior has been in the past. In his past attempts to stop smoking, he has done so without a real commitment to quitting or a clear plan for change. He is seeking additional information about quitting and requesting more convincing data that this might be the ideal time and situation in which to initiate change. Some contemplation behavior is necessary for successful resolution to the problem. The client will then be ready to make a commitment to change.

Stage 2: Action

The Client with an Action Plan

Mary is a 45-year-old client with diabetes. For several years, her primary physician has been encouraging her to lose weight and to begin a regular program of exercise. He has been unsuccessful in his attempts to change Mary's behavior. Today Mary comes to the office and announces that her work place initiated a weight-loss group and that she and two of her colleagues have joined. They have been attending regularly and following the suggested dietary plan for 3 weeks. The nurse encourages Mary to discuss her efforts. Mary is eager to talk, and she reports feelings of pride and satisfaction. She states that she has always been "disgusted" at letting herself "get so heavy." She admits that she was never "really ready" to deal with the problem before. She was surprised that she was so eager to join the group when her friends made the suggestion. She is happy to have their support in making a difficult change. Mary also tells the nurse about her anxiety and doesn't want to fail because many people know that she is trying to lose weight. She has been tempted to "cheat" on the diet but has been able to "resist the urges." She also admits to being frustrated and discouraged because she did not lose the amount of weight she wanted to in the previous week. The nurse talks to Mary about weight loss, diet, exercise, and diabetes. The nurse also makes additional helpful suggestions to reduce the risk of relapse and move Mary toward long-term maintenance. Mary asks the nurse to look over the program's dietary recommendations and thanks her for the additional information. The nurse encourages Mary to report on her continued success.

Response In this case, the client has begun a set of actions intended to deal with her problem. The patient believes that her actions are achievable. She is focused on short-term gains. The patient has recognized some obstacles that might negatively affect the program. She has decided that the discomfort of diet and exercise will be worthwhile. It may be that the actual experience may become more difficult than expected. Publicizing her efforts to lose weight provides a source of support, but also a source of anxiety. By keeping the motivation for change in mind, she reinforces her commitment to change. The nurse assists the client by finding answers to questions and supporting her success. The nurse also uses strategies for establishing a positive change environment.

Stage 3: Relapse

The Client Who Relapses

Karen is a client with moderate symptoms of chronic obstructive pulmonary disease (COPD). When she was first diagnosed, she immediately entered a smoking cessation program and has been a nonsmoker for 32 months. Karen was very proud of her efforts to quit smoking.

During a follow-up appointment for an upper respiratory tract infection, Karen admits to the nurse that she is again smoking a pack of cigarettes a day. The nurse is surprised and disappointed. The nurse asks Karen to explain what happened and asks whether Karen can identify factors leading to her relapse. Karen explains about difficulties she is having with her teen-age daughter and that her husband's job was "downsized." She says that, initially, she found it relaxing to smoke a cigarette after dinner with her husband, who is also a smoker, and that she thought she could control her cravings. She did not think that she would go back to smoking a pack of cigarettes a day again. However, soon she began looking forward to a cigarette whenever she could not deal with the demands of her family. Now she has resumed her earlier smoking behaviors. The nurse reinforces the benefits to Karen of not smoking, and asks if she can help Karen find resources for dealing with her family problems. Karen makes no statements about wanting to discontinue the behavior again, so the nurse asks her directly about plans to discontinue smoking. Karen states that she would like to try again.

Response In this case, the client has an episode of problem behavior after a period of success in overcoming the problem. The client is again engaging in the undesired behavior. The client is able to describe the circumstances that led to the relapse. This is the client's first relapse, and the story of the relapse is not very complex. She does not appear to be in denial or resistance, although she does not express a plan to stop smoking. The nurse helps the client by not being judgmental or blaming. The goal is to reaffirm the health benefits to Karen of not smoking, help to find ways to deal with factors contributing to the "slip," and help the client to recommit to not smoking.

Intentional Behavior Intention is a person's beliefs about the consequences of performing a specific behavior, and how much effort the person is willing to commit to performing a targeted behavior. From this viewpoint behavior can be understood as the transmission of intention into action (Fishbein & Ajzen, 1975). This concept was first introduced in 1975 when Fishbein and Ajzen proposed that behavioral intention is a primary factor in performing targeted behaviors.

Behavioral intention, an individual's motivation to engage in a targeted behavior, is perceived as the cognitive mechanism by which attitudes influence behavior (Jennings-Dozier, 1999; Rutter, 2000). Attitudes, the overall positive or negative feelings about performing the behavior, are a function of behavioral beliefs which are perceptions about the consequences and behavior and the evaluation of those consequences. The assumption is that the harder a person is willing to try to perform a targeted behavior the more likely the targeted behavior will be performed (Werner, 2004).

Behavioral intention is also influenced by behavioral, normative and control beliefs. Behavioral beliefs are perceptions that the targeted behavior can be performed. The person must believe that he/she possesses the skills and functional capacity to carry out the targeted behavior. The performance of the targeted behavior depends not only on the decision to perform the behavior but also on skills and opportunities that may or may not be available for the performance of the targeted behavior.

Subjective norms are the person's perceptions regarding what significant others and those whose opinions are important to the person think about the targeted behavior. Decision-making whether to perform a targeted behavior does not occur in a social vacuum. This adds a social aspect to behavioral intention (Abraham, Sheeran, & Orbell, 1998). Normative beliefs reflect the person's judgment regarding significant others' preferences and support for performing or not performing the targeted behavior. If the person perceives that the targeted behavior is valued by significant others and that efforts to engage in the behavior will be supported by significant others,

the likelihood of the actual performance of the targeted behavior is greater.

Perceived behavioral control also affects behavioral intentions as well as behavior (Ajzen, 1991). Control beliefs are the perceptions regarding the extent to which the person has control to perform the targeted behavior. Perceived behavioral control is the perception regarding the extent to which performing the targeted behavior is easy or difficult.

Other factors influencing behavioral intention include: self-identity (Conner & Armitage, 1998), past behavior and habit (Norman, Conner, & Bell, 2000; Werner, Schatz, & Vered, 2001), affect (Perugini & Bagozzi, 2001), knowledge (Werner, Schatz, & Vered, 2001) and perceived susceptibility (Norman, Conner, & Bell 2000).

Self-efficacy Self-efficacy beliefs from the foundation for human motivation, well-being and personal accomplishment (Bandura, 1995; Resnick, 2004). Individuals contemplating change form perceptions regarding the outcome. Outcome expectations are the beliefs that if a specific behavior is completed there will be a certain outcome. However, outcome expectations alone are unlikely to contribute to predicting behavior (Bandura, 1995). Self-efficacy involves judgments individuals make about their capabilities to organize and execute courses of action required to attain designated types of action or performances thus meet outcome expectations. The most influential source of self-efficacy is interpretation of the result of one's prior performance. The individual's perceptions of self-efficacy influence their beliefs about mastery of outcome expectations. Individuals engage in tasks and activities, interpret the results of their actions, and use those interpretations to develop beliefs about their capability to engage in subsequent tasks or activities and act in concert with the beliefs created (Resnick, 2004). Self-efficacy aids to establish perceptions regarding outcome expectation. The outcomes an individual expects are the result of the judgments of what that person can accomplish. Vicarious experience, observing others perform tasks, are also source of information regarding self-efficacy. Although weaker than actual mastery for helping to create self-efficacy beliefs vicarious experience is a useful change strategy. People will be influenced by observation reaction when they are uncertain about their own abilities or when they have limited prior experience with a particular behavior.

Spiral Model of Change

The transtheoretical change process model proposed by Prochaska, Norcross, and DiClemente (1994) attempts to address the limitations of earlier change process frameworks. It takes into consideration the client's readiness to change and tailors the change process to meet the client's immediate needs, motivation, and commitment to change.

Prochaska, Norcross, and DiClemente's model (1994) integrates core concepts from a variety of other change process models. Two primary underlying concepts are Janis and Mann's (1977) decisional balance and Bandura's (1986) concept of self-efficacy. In the Spiral Model of Change, the phenomenon of change progresses through six stages. Progression through the stages is not linear, but cyclic. However, successful movement through one stage of change does not necessarily lead to the next stage. Clients can become impeded at any point on the spiral. Each of the stages takes place over a period of time and involves specific tasks. The six stages of the model are precontemplation, contemplation, planning and preparation, action, maintenance, and termination.

The nurse and client engage in mutual decision making and can choose one strategy or a combination of strategies to deal with complex change issues. Experiential processes are more influential than behavioral strategies for understanding client responses and predicting change progress in the early stages of change. However, behavioral strategies are more effective for understanding and predicting transitions from preparation to action and from action to maintenance (Prochaska et al., 1994). Long-term effects can be accomplished when both experiential and behavioral strategies are used in combination. Table

14-5 presents the model's six stages, with associated themes, client characteristics, and nursing interventions.

Maintenance of Change

Change is maintained best in the environment in which it is learned. A major task for maintaining behavioral change is to general ize the new or modified behavior to other situations and environments. Many factors influence change maintenance and generalization. These variables may influence cognitive, affective, or behavioral domains. Important factors that influence the maintenance of change include the following:

- Personal beliefs and attitudes that support the change
- Extent of affective and cognitive commitment to change
- Ease of incorporating change into personal lifestyles (associative learning)
- Reinforcement and rewards for engaging in changed behavior (intermittent reinforcement)
- Amount of energy involved in making a decision to change
- Personal attractiveness of actions
- Centrality of health as a value and cultural issues
- Communication of change to others (publicizing commitment to change)

Outcomes

The ultimate goal of the change process is the modification of behavior, health practices, or lifestyle, and the integration of that change into the client's lived experience. However, the nurse must assist the client at her or his level of readiness for change. Outcomes are based on the assessment of that level of readiness and the type of strategies selected for implementation in the plan for change. Assisting clients with chronic illnesses and their families involves promoting desired changes and developing skills for continuing change to reduce complication and enhance functioning, well-being, and self-actualization.

TABLE 14-5

The Spiral of Change

Stage	Theme	Characteristics/Behaviors	Interventions
Precontemplation	Resisting change	Resistive actions Rationalization Projection and displacement Denial and minimization Demoralization Argumentative Transference	Raising consciousness and insight Self-assessment Seek permission to discuss the problem with the patient Ask patient to think, talk, and read about the problem behavior or suggested change Countertransference
Contemplation	Approaching change	Wishful thinking Waiting for magic moment Weighing of pros and cons Premature action to change without a developed action plan Begins to question whether change might be beneficial Begins to make commitment to change process	Assist in the development of pros and cons for changing and development of a decisional balance scale Obtain patient's perspective of the change and its impact on life-style Create possibility frame Warmth and support Solicit feedback
Preparation	Preparing and committing to change	Accepts that the change is both essential and beneficial Commits to change process Positive view of overcoming earlier perceived obstacles Makes change plan May procrastinate about beginning date	Reinforce patient's reasons to change Stress the value of being prepared Together with the patient and significant others, develop a plan for change: Take small steps Decrease anxiety Encourage public announcement of projected change Develop a "changer's manual"
Action	Moving	Time of maximum focus and effort Following the plan for change Energetic Assertive Demonstrating commitment to change	Use change talk Stress self-authoring abilities Counter thinking Environment control Active diversion: Relaxation techniques Exercise

TABLE 14-5

Continued

Stage	Theme	Characteristics/Behaviors	Interventions
		Impulsively can lead to dropping efforts	Rewarding
		Actively attempts to prevent slips and relapse	Maintain a positive change environment
		Guilt following slips or relapses	Discuss and handle feelings of guilt
		Resolution to change can fade	Discuss difference between slips and relapse
			Discuss and support pros of change
			Reflect on short-term outcomes and benefits to the patient
			Modify plan as necessary and appropriate
Maintenance	Remaining changed	Sustained vigilance and activity are needed	Support and praise for accomplishments
		Outcome expectations achieved from concerted effort	Explore patient's positive feelings and expectation
		Levels of awareness regarding importance of vigilance of change varies	Inquire about slips and relapses
		Some ground can be lost because of slips and relapses, resulting in frustration and attack on self-esteem	Assist patient to identify danger time and danger signs
		Expresses feelings on how change has positively impacted life	Modify plan to reduce potential for slips or relapses
		Working to integrate change into life-style and preventing future slips and relapses	Assist patient to develop self-assessment skills and to know when and where to seek future professional assistance
			Support modified life-style and personal self-image
			Reflect on long-term outcomes and benefits to the patient
Termination	Exiting the cycle	New self-image with new change integrated into image and life-style	Positive regard for patient
		No temptation in any situation	Discuss positive benefits to life following change
		Solid self-efficacy	Discuss the effects of change on others
		Healthier life-style	Discuss the possibility of following the change process to deal with other problems
		Real solution to the problem, promoting change	

SOURCES: Adapted from Glanz, Rimer & Lewis, 2002; O'Connell, 1997; Prochaska, Norcross & DiClemente, 1994.

Study Questions

1. Compare and contrast planned change and drift change.
2. Discuss intentional behavior and how it can affect the change process for the client with chronic illness.
3. Why is self-efficacy an important factor for clients with a chronic illness?
4. What are potential barriers to the change process?
5. Compare and contrast the models of change addressed in this chapter. What are the pros and cons of each?
6. From your perspective, what model of change best addresses the change that may be needed in the client with chronic illness? Why?
7. What is meant by the term culturally tailored change program?
8. Describe three skills that a successful change agent must possess.

References

Abraham, C., Sheeran, P., & Orbell, S. (1998). Can social cognitive models contribute to the effectiveness of HIV-preventive behavioural interventions? A brief review of the literature and a reply to Joffe (1996, 1997), and Fife-Shaw (1997). *British Journal of Medical Psychology*, 71, 297–310.

Ajzen, I. (1991). The theory of planned behavior. *Organizational Behavior and Human Decision Processes, 50,* 179–211.

Bailey, B. (1990). Change agent. In I. Lubkin (Ed.), *Chronic illness: Impact and interventions* (2nd ed.), (pp. 262–278). Boston: Jones & Bartlett.

Bandura, A. (1986). *Social foundations of thought and action: A social cognitive theory.* Englewood Cliffs, NJ: Prentice-Hall.

Bandura, A. (1995). Exercise of personal and collective efficacy. In A. Bandura (Ed.) *Self-efficacy in changing societies*, (pp. 279–305). New York: Cambridge University Press.

Bushnell, M. (1979). Institution in transition. *Perspectives of Psychiatric Care, 12* (6), 260–265.

Caplan, G. (1964). *Principles of preventive psychiatry.* New York: Basic Books.

Chin, P., Finocchiaro, D., & Rosebrough, A. (1998). *Rehabilitation nursing practice.* New York: McGraw-Hill.

Conner, M. & Armitage, C. (1998). Extending the theory of planned behavior: A review and avenues for further research. *Journal of Applied Psychology, 28*(15), 1429–1464.

Deci, E., & Ryan, R. (1985). *Intrinsic motivation and the nursing process.* New York: Plenum Press.

Dixon, E. (1998). Change agent. In I. Lubkin & P. Larsen (Eds.), *Chronic illness: Impact and interventions* (4th ed.) (pp. 327–342). Sudbury MA: Jones & Bartlett.

Duck, J. D. (1998). Managing change: The art of balancing. In *Harvard Business Review On Change*, (pp. 55–81). Boston: Harvard Business School Publishing.

Durrant, M., & Kowalski, K. M. (1993). Enhancing views of competence. In S. Friedman (Ed.), *The new language of change constructive collaboration in psychotherapy*, (pp. 107–137). New York: Guilford Press.

Ellis, A., & Grieger, R. (1977). *Handbook of rational-emotive therapy.* New York: Springer.

Erikson, E. H. (1963). *Childhood and society.* New York: WW Norton.

Fanger, M. T. (1993). After the shift: Time-effective treatment in the possibility frame. In S. Freidman (Ed.), *The new language of change* (pp. 85–106). New York: Guilford Press.

Farley, A. M. (1992). *Nursing and the disabled across the life span.* Sudbury, MA: Jones & Bartlett.

Fishbein, M. & Ajzen, I. (1975). *Beliefs, attitudes, intention, and behavior.* New York: Wiley.

Fordyce, B. R. (1977). *Behavioral modification and the nursing process.* St. Louis: Mosby.

Friedman, S., & Fanger, M. T. (1991). *Expanding therapeutic possibilities: Getting results in brief psychotherapy.* New York: Lexington Books.

Geraci, E. (2004). Planned change. In *Middle range theories: Application to Nursing Research*, (pp. 125–147). Philadelphia: Lippincott Williams and Wilkins.

Gingerich, W., & de Shazer, S. (1991). The BRIEFER project: Using expert systems as theory construction tools. *Family Process, 30,* 241–249.

Glanz, K., Rimer, B., & Lewis, F. (2002). Theory, research, and practice in health behavior and health education. In K. Glanz, B. Rimer, & F. Lewis (Eds.), *Health behavior and health education: Theory, Research, and practice,* (pp. 22–39). San Francisco: John Wiley & Sons, Inc.

Gordon, D., & Meyers-Anderson, M. (1981). *Phoenix: Therapeutic patterns of Milton H. Erikson.* Cupertino, CA: Meta.

Greenstone, J. L., & Levitson, S. C. (1993). *Elements of crisis intervention: Crises and how to respond to them.* Pacific Grove, CA: Brooks/Cole.

Hoff, L. A. (1978). *People in crisis: Understanding and helping.* Menlo Park, CA: Addison-Wesley.

Huber, D. (2000). *Leadership and nursing case management.* (2nd ed.) Philadelphia: Saunders.

Janis, I., & Mann, L. (1977). *Decision-making: A psychological analysis of conflict, choice, and commitment.* London: Cassell & Collier Macmillan.

Jennings-Dozier, K. (1999). Predicting intentions to obtain a Pap smear among African American and Latino women: Testing the theory of planned behavior. *Nursing Research, 48* (4), 198–205.

Kubler-Ross, E. (1969). *On death and dying.* New York: Macmillan Publishing.

Kreuter, M., & Skinner, C. (2000). Tailoring: What's in a name. *Health Education Research, 15,* 1–4.

Laughlin, J. A. (1989). Rehabilitation: Unlocking the gates to change. In S. Dittmar (Ed.), *Rehabilitation nursing: Process and application,* (pp. 528–535). St. Louis: Mosby.

Lewin, K. (1947). Frontiers in group dynamics: Concept, methods, and reality in social science. *Human Relations, 5* (1), 5–42.

Lewin, K. (1951). *Field theory in social science.* New York: Harper & Brothers.

Lippitt, G. L. (1973). *Visualizing change: Model building and the change process.* La Jolla, CA: University Associates.

Lippitt, G. L., & Lippitt, R. (1978). *The counseling process in action.* San Diego, CA: University Press.

Mauksch, I. G., & Miller, M. H. (1981). *Implementing change in nursing.* St. Louis: Mosby.

Mitchell, S. (1988). *The Tao Te Ching: A new English version.* New York: Harper-Collins.

New, J. R., & Couillard, N. A. (1981). Guidelines for introducing change. *The Journal of Nursing Administration, March* (8), 7–21.

Norman, P., Conner, M. & Bell, R. (2000). The theory of planned behavior and exercise: Evidence for the moderating role of past behaviour. *British Journal of Health Psychology, 5,* 249–261.

O'Connell, D. (1997). Behavior change. In M. D. Feldman & J. F. Christensen (Eds.), *Behavioral medicine in primary care: A practical guide* (pp. 125–135). Stamford, CT: Appleton & Lange.

Pender, N. (1987). *Health promotion in nursing practice* (2nd ed.). Norwalk, CT: Appleton-Century-Crofts.

Pender, N. (1996). *Health promotion in nursing practice.* (3rd ed.) Stamford, CT: Appleton & Lange.

Perlman, D. & Takacs, G. (1990). The ten stages of change. *Nursing Management, 21* (4), 33–38.

Perugini, M. & Bagozzi, R. (2001). The role of desires and anticipated emotions in goal-directed behaviours: Broadening and deepening the theory of planned behaviour. *British Journal of Social Psychology, 40,* 79–98.

Prochaska, J. O., Norcross, J. C., & DiClemente, C. C. (1994). *Changing for good: A revolutionary six-stage program for overcoming bad habits and moving your life positively forward.* New York: Guilford Press.

Reinkemeyer, A. (1970). Nursing's need: Commitment to an ideology of change. *Nursing Forum, 9* (4), 340–350.

Resnick, B. (2004). Self-efficacy. In S. Peterson & T. Bredow (Eds.) *Middle range theories application to nursing research,* (pp. 97–124). Philadelphia: Lippincott Williams & Wilkins.

Resnicow, K. Braithwaite, R. Dilorio, C. & Glanz, K. (2002). Applying theory to culturally diverse and unique populations. In K. Glanz, B. Rimer, and F. L. Lewis (Eds.), *Health behavior and health education: Theory, research and practice,* (pp. 485–505). (3rd ed.). San Francisco: John Wiley & Sons.

Roberts, A. R., & Burgess, A. (1997). Crisis intervention. In A. Burgess (Ed.), *Psychiatric nursing promoting mental health,* (pp. 703–713). Stamford, CT: Appleton & Lange.

Rogers, C. R. (1972). Change agents, clients, and change. In G. Zultman, P. Kotlteer, & I. Kaufman (Eds.), *Creating social change,* (pp. 194–213). New York: Rinehart and Winston.

Rokeach, M. (1973). *The nature of human values.* New York: Free Press.

Rutter, D. (2000). Attendance and reattendance of breast cancer screening: A prospective 3-year test of the theory of planned behavior. *British Journal of Health Psychology, 5* (1), 1–13.

Ryan, P. (2000). Facilitating behavior change in chronically ill persons. In J. Miller (Ed.), *Coping with chronic illness Overcoming powerlessness*, (pp. 481–503). (3rd ed.). Philadelphia: Davis.

Selekman, M. D. (1993). *Pathways to change: Brief therapy solutions with difficult adolescents.* New York: Guilford Press.

Seligman, M. (1991). *Learned optimism.* New York: Alfred A. Knopf.

Shumaker, S. A., Schron, E. B., & Ockene, E. B. (Eds.). (1990). *The handbook of health behavior change.* New York: Springer.

Spector, R. S. (2000). *Cultural diversity in health and illness.* Norwalk, CT: Appleton & Lange.

Steckel, S. (1982). *Patient contracting.* New York: Appleton-Century-Crofts.

Sue, D. W. (1999). *Counseling the culturally different: Theory and practice.* New York: John Wiley & Sons.

Swansburg, R. C. & Swansburg, R. J. (2002). *Introduction to management and leadership in nurse managers* (3rd ed.). Sudbury, MA: Jones & Bartlett.

Werner, P. (2004). Reasoned action and planned behavior. In S. Peterson & T. Bredow (Eds.), *Middle range theories: Application to Nursing Research*, (pp. 125–147). Philadelphia: Lippincott Williams and Wilkins.

Werner, P., Schatz, Y. & Vered, I. (2001). Predictors of women's willingness to use dual energy x-ray: Testing the theory of planned behavior. The 17th World Conference of Gerontology, Vancouver, Canada.

Yoder-Wise, P. (2003). *Leading and managing in nursing* (3rd ed.). St. Louis: Mosby.

CHAPTER 15

Client and Family Education

Cheryl P. McCahon

Introduction

Chronic illness is a life-altering experience, but the extent of the impact is client-specific and situational. Each situation is unique, and the response of the individual (and family) to the realization of lifetime changes influences the manner, content, depth, timing, and when and how teaching should occur. What assessment parameters should be considered as the nurse determines the most appropriate teaching strategies for the client and family with a diagnosis of chronic disease? What problems can the nurse teacher anticipate? What teaching strategies will best facilitate learning? How do differences in age; disease process; physical, intellectual, and emotional status; and resources affect the teaching-learning process? Clearly, chronic illness complicates each teaching situation and challenges the nurse as teacher. This chapter presents selected findings about teaching and learning in nursing practice and provides suggestions to ensure successful learning outcomes, with the primary emphasis on the adult.

The Teaching-Learning Process

The teaching-learning process is complex, dynamic, and interactive. According to Norton (1998), teaching is a system of directed and deliberate actions that are intended to induce learning through a series of directed activities (p. 211). Specific approaches to learning as well as identification of necessary knowledge, skills, and attitudes are determined through in-depth assessment. Hogstel (2001) contends that effective teaching requires an understanding of the complex internal and external forces that shape people's lives and create barriers to successful change (p. 221).

Two theoretical perspectives of how one learns are behaviorism and cognitivism. Behaviorists concentrate on methods of strengthening or weakening new habits through the presence or absence of stimuli intended to produce a response (Hogstel, 2001). Cognitivism is based on the premise that cognition results when students apply new information to what they already know. Thus, learning is influenced by beliefs, attitudes, and the context in which the idea is taught (Hogstel, 2001, p. 224).

The Role of Teaching in Nursing

Client teaching is an essential and expected role. Both the National League for Nursing (NLN) and the American Association of Colleges of Nursing (AACN) describe competencies of teaching-learning. In the past, health education has emphasized teaching about disease processes; however, with the increased national awareness of the need for health promotion and disease prevention through work such as *Healthy People 2000* and *Healthy People 2010*, there is a new look to health education. Client education is central to professional standards of nursing care to promote the individual's empowerment (Hogstel, 2001, p. 221). Ignatavicius & Workman (2002) describe the teacher role as becoming increasingly more important as clients are discharged quicker and sicker from the hospital, subacute unit, or nursing home, or to their homes.

The Joint Commission on the Accreditation of Healthcare Organizations (JCAHO) and the Centers for Medicare and Medicaid Services (CMS) mandate client and family education for hospitals and long-term care facilities that are accredited or participating in Medicare/Medicaid programs. These mandates include the need for documentation of client teaching during hospitalization and prior to discharge and have contributed to increased accountability and leadership of nurses in client education.

JCAHO's standards for patient/family education include the following (adapted from 1998 *Comprehensive Accreditation Manual for Hospitals*: Chicago: JCAHO):

Standard PF.1: Patient/family receive education specific to patient's assessed (provided with appropriate education and training to increase knowledge of the illness and treatment) needs, abilities and readiness to learn

Standard PF.2: Patient (and family) receive education that is interactive

Standard PF.3: Any discharge instructions given to the patient/family are provided to the organization responsible for the patient's continuing care.

Standard PF.4: The organization plans and supports the provision and coordination of patient and family education activities and resources.

Fuszard (1995) contends that there isn't a practice role in the nursing profession that does not include the teaching-learning process (p. xv). This perspective is validated as all of the various roles of the professional nurse are considered: caregiver, health teacher, coordinator/collaborator, consultant, beginning researcher, advocate, and change agent. No matter what role is enacted, within each is embedded aspects of the teaching role.

Beginning with nursing students' first courses, the role of the health educator is described. Basic teaching-learning principles are identified: tenets that stem from either behaviorist or constructivist beliefs, which describe how to ensure that learning takes place. However, traditional client and family education focuses on disease information and deemphasizes the place and effect of the illness in the client's life. Nursing care plan books contain stereotypical teaching plans that address step-by-step teaching of basic knowledge or a skill.

Approaches to client education as currently taught in nursing programs are not as effective as they could be (Saarman, Daugherty & Reigel, 2000). Behavioral change does not occur simply because the client has gained the knowledge about what needs to be done. Saarman and colleagues stress that learning what needs to be done and acting on that knowledge are different processes (p. 281). They describe making a life-style change, as is often necessary in chronic illness, to be a process that includes learning about the need, becoming motivated, building resources necessary to support the change, and then making and sustaining the change.

Why do nurses believe that by addressing the knowledge component, the client will learn? How can you, as a nurse in an ever-changing health care environment, meet client and family learning needs in ways that are satisfying to all parties? What are the factors that influence learning? How does a diagnosis of chronic disease affect the teaching-learning process? How can the nurse develop teaching strategies to facilitate client and family learning as they confront the challenges posed by chronic illness? Two teaching learning theories, pedagogy and androgogy, are the basis for client and family education.

Pedagogy and Andragogy

People learn in different ways, depending on their age, developmental levels, ability to process, and individual needs. The art and science of teaching children is termed *pedagogy*. This approach is teacher-centered, with the learner assuming a passive and dependent role. The learner needs clarity and specificity. The pedagogical approach involves learners who have few life experiences and who look to the teacher to identify what, when, and how to learn, as well as evaluation of the learning (Fuszard, 1995). The teacher is responsible for providing the information and process to learn the material. Knowles (1990) describes the pedagogical approach as the teacher having full responsibility for making all decisions about what will be learned, how it will be learned, when it will be learned, and if it will be learned (p. 54).

Knowles (1990) defines *adult education,* or *andragogy,* as the art and science of helping people learn (p. 43). Knowles believes that adult learners are persons who do best when asked to use their experience and apply new knowledge to solve real-life problems. He views this self-reliant learner as one who is mature biologically, legally, socially, and psychologically. He contends that adults learn through problem solving and often have internal incentives for learning. Adults are usually goal-oriented learners, like challenging assignments that are reality based, and are willing to assume responsibility for their actions. Adult education, or andragogy, is a student-centered approach to learning, with the teacher seen as a facilitator. The emphasis is on learning, rather than teaching, with the teacher providing opportunities and activities for learning as well as encouragement to apply new knowledge and/or skills. Evaluation is done jointly by teacher and learner, and sometimes by peers (Fuszard, 1995).

It should be noted that Knowles does not believe that all learning fits exclusively into either the pedagogical or the andragogical mode. For example, the client who learns that surgery is necessary to remove a cancerous tumor in his or her intestine needs facts about the surgery, when it will occur, and what the preparation will be. At that point, the ability of the client to be a self-directed learner is not appropriate. The many challenges and needs of the client and family with a chronic disease necessitate the nurse's assessment of the appropriate theory of learning to the situation. Another example from the nurse's perspective is reflected in Reflection Exercise 1.

Phases of Learning

Another way of viewing learning is to separate learning into phases. Covey (1990) divides learning into three phases: dependence, independence, and interdependence. Within the different phases, teachers assume different roles. In the dependent phase, the teacher is responsible for all decisions. This role fits nicely with the pedagogical teaching method and is appropriate for infants and children or for adults whose learning, for a variety of reasons, cannot be independent.

In the independent phase, the learner assumes responsibility for her or his own learning. The third phase of learning—interdependence—is a decision

---

■ *Reflection Exercise 1* ■

You are an expert cardiac nurse who is taking a new position working with renal dialysis clients. You have the benefit of a good medical-surgical knowledge base; critical thinking skills; excellent communication skills, as needed to work with clients and families; and a readiness to learn. However, when you begin to work in this new setting, many of the psychomotor skills needed place you in the position of novice. What kind of teacher would you want . . . and expect? Why?

made by the individual (Covey, 1990). Interdependence is a mature, advanced concept in which, physically, the adult is self-reliant and capable; emotionally, there is a sense of self-worth with the need for loving, giving, and receiving, and there is intelligent respect for others (Musinski, 1999, p. 24).

These phases of learning can be applied to Knowles' beliefs about adult education, such as the understanding that adults recognize that they are capable of self-direction and like to plan their own learning. Brookfield (1990) describes the facilitation of learning—assisting adults to make sense and act upon the personal, social, occupational, and political environment in which they live—as an important, exhilarating, and profound activity for the facilitators and the learners. It is also a highly complex psychosocial drama in which the personalities of the individuals involved, the contextual setting for the educational transaction, and the prevailing political climate crucially affect the nature and form of teaching (p. vii).

Barriers Influencing the Teaching-Learning Process

A number of factors specific to the client, family, and the nurse influence the teaching-learning process. Addressing these factors does not guarantee learning, but these factors provide assessment parameters to consider when developing a teaching plan.

Developmental Issues

Childhood and Adolescence

Learning in children is dependent upon physical and psychological readiness. Thus, a thorough assessment of the child's developmental level, including factors such as language skills, physical ability to perform specific psychomotor tasks, intellectual ability, attention span, and memory are of paramount importance. Is the child able to communicate? Are the questions posed asked at a level that the child will understand? Does the child respond to a learning situation through verbal communication or through pictures, role playing, or a combination of instructional approaches? Children vary widely in each of the factors cited, even children within the same age range.

The child's ability to learn is influenced greatly by attention span. Often, material presented to the child necessitates concentration for a prolonged period of time. Attention span expectations should increase as the child matures. However, note that children, as well as adults, can become distracted, withdrawn, or unable to attend to the learning at hand due to physical or emotional distress. Teaching a young child, for example, a toddler or preschooler, should always be done in short 5- to 10-minute segments.

Memory is also a factor in the child's ability to learn. The nurse needs to ascertain the child's ability to retain and recall information. This ability increases as the child matures but is also influenced by illness factors. The nurse's teaching strategies should emphasize teaching methods and tools that facilitate memory, such as pictures, poems, word games, and so forth.

Physical abilities are another consideration when teaching a child. The ability of the child to carry out specific psychomotor skills that involve fine motor movements may not yet be developed in the young child. Hence, the child's ability to perform a task must be carefully assessed, not only to prevent using an inappropriate teaching method, but also to prevent frustration and promote learning.

During adolescence, the client's ability to learn can be affected by the previously identified factors, but not necessarily because of developmental reasons. Adolescence is a time of physical and psychological development that provides the child increased independence and the ability to take on new challenges. Often, the need for independence interferes with the teaching-learning process. For example, peer relationships are of extreme importance to adolescents, creating problems for the child with a chronic illness. The adolescent diabetic is torn between the expectations perceived by peer group membership and adherence to a prescribed diet, which does not include the schedule or foods of the peers. The adolescent with rheumatoid arthritis may be unable to be involved in sports or become involved in social activities, which would provide increased stressors to a body that is physically and emotionally exhausted and often in pain.

Young Adulthood

During the period of young adulthood, individuals are realizing their occupational and vocational goals and developing themselves as productive members of society. Falvo (1999) describes young adulthood as a time of building and maintaining intimate relationships and developing social responsibility. She sees the effects of limitations resulting from illness or disability as defining the young adult's ability to fulfill vocational and occupational goals (p. 12). Think of the athlete whose career plans involve a long-term contract with a professional sports team. What are the consequences of a motor vehicle accident that leaves the young person a paraplegic? What physical limitations might also result that would interfere with the individual's ability to sustain an intimate relationship? How would the injured athlete's self-image be affected?

Teaching young adults can be difficult, not only because of the multifaceted issues that must be addressed, but also because the nurse often identifies with the hopes and expectations of the individual and family. A thorough objective assessment should identify those factors that are barriers to learning. Goal setting should always include the client and spouse or significant other.

Middle and Older Age

The middle years add new dimensions and challenges to the teaching-learning process. Factors that influence learning include physical and emotional barriers that are the result of illness, past learning experiences, and new or existing client and family issues. Midlife is a time of change, when the client is continuing to develop but is also exposed to a variety of stressors. Chronic illness compounds the stressors of midlife, especially when the illness intensifies body image changes brought about by the physiological changes of aging, decreases in physical capabilities, and role changes.

With aging comes increased opportunities for chronic illness. In addition, primary aging changes, those that occur simply as the result of growing older, can also influence learning. However, simply being older does not automatically negate the individual's ability to learn, nor does a client's chronological age automatically mandate a specific approach to teaching. Older persons sustain physiological and psychosocial changes that may require adaptive teaching strategies, but application of adult learning principles to each situation is continued. A thorough assessment reveals changes with aging that may need to be addressed in the teaching situation. Smeltzer and Bare (2000) contend that older persons can learn if the material is relevant, the environment is supportive, and the pace facilitates learning (p. 42).

Changes in cognition with age include slower response time to thinking and reacting to stimuli, decreased short-term memory and concentration, and decreased ability for abstract thinking. Teaching strategies to address these changes include an environment without distractions, presenting small amounts of material that include the necessary basic information, frequent repetition and reinforcement of the learning, and a variety of alternative teaching approaches, such as written material, audiovisual aids, and additional time for practice should the desired skill be of a psychomotor nature. Stanley, Blair, and Beare (2005) have identified helpful teaching strategies to assist elders with age-associated memory decline (Table 15-1).

Sensory changes begin in midlife, are progressive, and affect an individual's ability to learn. Changes include declines in hearing, sight, pain perception, touch, taste, and smell. Has the older person not heard what is being said, is he or she ignoring you, or have you not clarified what is being taught? Teaching strategies for addressing decreased hearing includes gaining attention by facing the client, maintaining eye contact, and speaking distinctly in a clear voice. Decrease extraneous noise and do not raise your voice, as shrill or high-pitched sounds are less likely to be heard. Always provide

---

TABLE 15-1

Teaching Strategies to Offset Age-Associated Memory Decline

- Encourage association between items.
- Increase time for teaching, especially psychomotor skills.
- Eliminate environmental distractions, such as projectors, and promote physical comfort.
- Make sure that eyeglasses are clean and in place.
- Encourage verbal responses.
- Set easily achievable goals.
- Allow time for the person to respond.
- Use soft-white light to decrease glare.
- Correct wrong answers immediately and reinforce correct answers frequently.
- Sum up at the end and review all major points.
- Offer liquid nourishment and allow bathroom breaks.
- Clarify with examples that the older adult can relate to in everyday life.

SOURCE: Stanley, Blair & Beare, 2005, p. 68.

---

time for the elder to respond to you. Encourage the use of hearing aids or other adaptive devices to improve the possibility of learning and enhance the quality of life for the elder and those with whom she or he interacts.

Changes in sight result in decreased peripheral vision, decreased clarity of vision, loss of ability to see written material at close range (without corrective glasses), change in color discrimination, and an increased sensitivity to glare. Teaching strategies to address these issues include the use of large letters when providing written materials, adequate lighting in a glare-free environment, and teaching materials that have contrasting colors (e.g., white letters on a black background). Because of changes in color discrimination, assessing color perception is suggested.

Primary aging changes occur in every body system, at different times, and with varying intensity. Some changes, such as those in the musculoskeletal system, affect strength and endurance. Additional time during teaching should be allocated for changes in position or movement, and the pace and activity level should be slowed. Additionally, reaction time may be slowed, and some elders have changes in equilibrium, affecting psychomotor skill learning. Teaching should include instructions to change position slowly to prevent vertigo or loss of balance, with a resulting fall.

Changes that occur in the cardiovascular system include decreased cardiac output and stroke volume, which influence the pace of learning. Vascular changes such as decreased blood flow secondary to atherosclerosis can affect cognitive functioning, ability to concentrate, and being able to learn and process new material.

Gender

Client education is affected by historic bias in health care in regard to women and by the neglect of research on gender and sex differences in health (Redman, 1999, p. 3). Redman contends that most non-reproductive research is done on males and that the information and skills included in client education programs may not be effective for women or may be misleading. As an example, she describes the differences in male and female presenting symptoms for myocardial infarction. However, following a lengthy review of recent studies regarding gender differences, Bastable (2003) contends that the extent to which learning is affected by differences between the sexes remains open to question (p. 235).

Culture

Culture is the sum total of doing, feeling and thinking, past and present, of a social group within a given period. It is a group's design for living, a shared set of socially transmitted assumptions about the nature of the physical and social world, goals in life attitudes, roles and values . . . a complex integrated system that includes knowledge, beliefs, skills, art, morals, law, customs and any other acquired habits and capabilities (Murray & Zentner, 2001, p. 4). Individuals who live as members of an ethnic group take on the beliefs, practices, and customs of that group. Examples of these cultural and ethnic differences include issues related to health, illness, aging, death, and dying. Cultures differ in respect to basic values, the composition of the family unit, childbearing patterns, interaction with others versus privacy, time orientation, education, use of work and leisure time, and attitudes regarding change. Each of these factors needs consideration, as lack of attention to cultural norms can adversely affect learning outcomes.

Cultural factors are important because they mediate the ways in which symptoms are identified and interpreted, the appropriate modes of the expression of pain and suffering, whether the illness is stigmatized or accepted, and whether the dependency that accompanies chronic disease is devalued or considered a part of the normal life cycle (Swanson & Tripp-Reimer, 1997, p. 13). Swanson and Tripp-Reimer contend that one's ethnic affiliation strongly influences the definition, recognition, and evaluation of chronic conditions. This affiliation also influences teaching and learning. For example, if one believes that illness is God's punishment for some past indiscretion or a necessary preparation for one's eternal reward, then teaching directed at pain management in an individual who believes that the suffering is deserved may be to no avail.

When examining the reading materials provided to African American clients in an anticoagulation clinic, Wilson et al. (2003) found readability an important factor to consider when teaching clients and families. Findings revealed that the average grade completed by the clients was 12th grade, but the mean reading skills were between the seventh and eighth grade levels. At the same time, the teaching materials presented were three to four grades higher than the clients' reading abilities. Additionally, none of the educational materials were culturally sensitive (p.276). The authors contended that success of anticoagulation treatment depends upon the clients' knowledge and understanding of the risks of bleeding. However, without the ability to read the materials, the individuals may not recognize when intervention is necessary. They may also be too embarrassed about their illiteracy to question what they can't read. Also, materials that lack cultural sensitivity send signals to the client that their culture is not an important consideration.

Tripp-Reimer et al. (2001) suggest addressing cultural barriers in providing care through inversion of the problem, that is viewing the barriers from the culture of biomedicine. The researchers see barriers to care for minority groups to include ideas such as: patients who don't practice healthy behaviors don't care about their health; biomedicine is right; traditional beliefs should be changed rather than built upon; people should and will follow the directions given by health care practitioners; adherence failure is the patient's problem; everyone understands the concept "chronic illness;" science is the only appropriate basis for practice; personal health is the most important priority for each family member; patients have autonomy—except with regard to adherence; and health care is available and accessible to all (p.14). The authors believe that to address these barriers, patient education programs, including the content, teaching modalities, and the person identified to provide the information need careful consideration.

Motivation

An adult learner's motivation to learn is pragmatic, problem-centered, and internal, and that motivation arises from the learner's curiosity (Knowles, 1990). According to Wlodkowski (1985), there are six major factors that impact learner motivation: attitude, need, stimulation, affect, competence, and reinforcement. As an example, consider Mrs. Jones, a single mother newly diagnosed with multiple sclerosis in the first case study.

Readiness to Learn

Readiness to learn involves many factors. When teaching children, readiness is associated with the child's physical and psychosocial ability to learn. Physical or psychological comfort, as well as emotional disequilibria, also affects ability and motivation to learn. Unexpected emotional upheavals can impede learning, even in an individual who has requested teaching. A middle-aged client with an initial diagnosis of diverticulitis asks the nurse to help him become better informed about his diet and ways to prevent flare-ups of the disease. A teaching plan is carefully prepared and ready to present. However, upon entry into the client's room, the nurse finds the client tearful, apparently distraught, and the client tells the nurse he wants to be left alone. Concerned, she leaves the room, subsequently learning from the unit nurse that the physician had just informed the client that the biopsy had revealed numerous lesions throughout his colon, which will require surgery.

High anxiety prevents learning, even in clients who want to learn. At times, health care professionals have attempted to frighten clients into compliant behavior by raising anxiety levels, but with little success. For example, the individual in end-stage emphysema knows that his lifetime of cigarette smoking has contributed to his present condition and his present quality of life. However, telling the client that he will die soon if he doesn't quit smoking rarely makes an impression.

Communication

According to Spector (2000a), symbols of our culture, acts and sounds, form the basis of all languages (p. 80). The way in which we communicate enables us to share information through language that is verbal, nonverbal, written, through music or art, or even by silence. In some instances, what is shared is unintentional (e.g., nonverbal communication such as facial expression, gesturing, body language, noncompliant behaviors, ignoring the teacher, etc.). There are cultural differences in body language; some nonverbal communication may express similar emotions in any culture, such as fear, pain, or sadness (Murray and Zentner, (2001). A suggestion is to teach by physically moving the body of the person or showing what you want the client to learn by demonstrating, using pictures, using short sentences with easy-to-understand vocabulary, facing the client, maintaining eye contact, and speaking slowly and clearly (p. 21).

Murray and Zentner (2001), Spector (2000b), and Purnell and Paulanka (2005) describe ways that language barriers contribute to miscommunication. In many instances, nurses who are talking with clients and families from other cultures believe that they are being understood when the client nods, smiles, or provides other clues that imply that the communication is understood. In reality, the appearance to understand may be only to avoid embarrassment and save face. In some cultures, it is inappropriate to share information of a personal nature. In those situations, data gathering may be done only over a prolonged period of time. Purnell & Paulanka (2005), in a guide to culturally competent health care, have identified communication issues to consider for 28 different cultures.

Numerous authors have developed cultural assessment materials for practitioner use. Huff and Kline (1999) have developed a cultural assessment framework, and Spector, (2000) has designed a *Guide to Heritage Assessment and Health Traditions.* Purnell & Paulanka (2005) have suggested including concepts such as nutrition, health care practices, death rituals, spirituality, and high risk health behaviors as well as those identified in other assessment frameworks. In today's multicultural society a cultural assessment is necessary to ensure that the client and family receive culturally appropriate teaching.

Mrs. Jones

Mrs. Jones has recently been diagnosed with multiple sclerosis. Prior to her diagnosis, she experienced fatigue, double vision, dizziness, and "feeling clumsy," and was often "off balance," appearing unable to walk in a straight line. She is recently divorced, in part because of her symptoms, which have embarrassed her husband and led to his refusal to be seen with her in public. She has a 4-year-old who attends an all-day nursery school, and a 7-year-old who is already active in a variety of sports. Mrs. Jones is self-employed, running a mail order business from her home. She has not had any difficulty in working at her computer for periods of time. She has hired a neighbor to care for her children when they are not in school. She does, however, need to shop and cook for her family. She expresses a desire to learn all that she can about her disease and her part in dealing with the symptomatology.

Discussion: Mrs. Jones' motivation for learning can be described using Wlodkowski's factors affecting motivation. Mrs. Jones' *attitude* will influence her behavior, as will her *need* for goal-directed learning about her disease. She wants to learn about her disease so she is better able to deal with her present and future symptoms. Her need to learn is influenced by her ongoing desire to gain knowledge about her disease, so that she can provide services needed to care for her family. Mrs. Jones is *stimulated* to learn for the purpose of gaining needed knowledge and skills. Mrs. Jones' *affect* relates to her emotional experiences—how she feels about what she is learning. Her feelings will influence and motivate her behavior. If these emotions are negative and she is unable to address her behavior, then motivation will be a challenge. Mrs. Jones demonstrates *competence* by wanting to take control of her life, being empowered by her knowledge about her disease, and what she can expect. Providing positive *reinforcement* such as praise, social approval, and attention for Mrs. Jones as she problem-solves ways in which she is planning to deal with her home, her business, and her children will increase Mrs. Jones' self-concept, and will provide her with the support that she needs to achieve the outcomes she has determined for her own learning.

Abbott et al. (2002) describe a patient and education committee, within a multifaceted and multicultural health care center, that developed a survey to determine client education needs. The findings revealed a need for cultural competency. A short, user-friendly tool, Cultural Cues, was developed to increase cultural awareness. The survey also revealed additional areas needing to be addressed such as beliefs about health and illness, how health care decisions were made, and the roles of touch and modesty. Six Culture Cues have been developed and are resulting in more culturally sensitive client education.

Societal Role Considerations

One's values regarding health and health care, the meaning of illness, and the determination of treatment deemed acceptable or unacceptable are learned from one's societal group (Falvo, 1994). Deviation from values or group norms can be a source of ridicule or exclusion (p. 50). In the life of an individual with chronic illness, there are times that disease precludes an individual from fulfilling one or more expected roles, thus failing to meet either personal and/or societal expectations. Many stories have been written about an individual with end-stage disease who makes the decision to live, to be present at a wedding, to celebrate a milestone birthday, or to hold a newborn great-grandchild. Family roles will often supercede the other roles of the individual with chronic illness. The nurse needs to consider what is important to the client when developing a teaching plan. The second case study about Mrs. Smith illustrates the importance of an individual's role and its influence on client outcomes.

Physical and Functional Influences

The extent to which an individual's condition is disabling is dependent on the individual's perception of the condition, the environment, and the reaction of friends, family, and society in general (Falvo, 1999). Individual reactions to a similar illness or disability are often different. Numerous physical obstacles can interfere with or hinder learning. Pain, decreased mobility, sensory changes with aging, dizziness, nausea, and vomiting are some of the many distractions that prevent the client from concentrating on learning.

Preoccupation with bodily concerns is one of the primary needs within Maslow's hierarchy of needs framework, and thus must be satisfied before higher level issues can be addressed. A client with a new colostomy who is concerned about the odor and the leaking stool is not ready to learn about the various resources that exist in the community.

Locus of Control

Miller (2000) asserts that locus of control contributes to the way in which the client views and responds to illness. Individuals with an internal locus of control believe that their health is determined by their own actions and behaviors. Individuals with an external locus of control believe that their health is in the hands of others, beyond their control, and therefore feel powerless and helpless to address and respond to their illness. For example, the perception

that "I am in control" versus "God is in control . . . it makes no difference what I do," contributes to the way in which a client approaches and responds to teaching.

Compliance

Much has been written about noncompliance of clients to a prescribed therapeutic plan. Compliance is a factor to address when teaching individuals with chronic illness (see Chapter 10, on compliance). Reasons postulated for lack of compliance include factors related to the client, the teaching, and misperceptions set forth by the nurse educator. Uncovering the cause of noncompliance involves the nurse's skill in assessment, knowledge about the disease, the social environment, the client's beliefs and values about health and illness, and the family dynamics. There may be no clear-cut answer for failure to comply, with even the individual not certain why she or he is not acting in a certain manner. Noncompliance may relate to the need for control, to maintain independence, to show dependence, to deny the illness, or take life into one's own hands.

Nurse Factors That Influence the Teaching-Learning Process

As has been described, teaching is an expected role of the nurse. The necessary qualifications of educators in some settings are those of advanced practice nurses, such as clinical nurse specialists or nurse practitioners. However, most settings expect all staff nurses to act as educators to clients and their families. Many nurses believe that they are ill prepared for the teaching expected. Rankin and Stallings (2001, p. 126) described barriers that nurses believe limit their ability to teach clients effectively:

- ■ Time restrictions
- ■ The need for teaching skills

Mrs. Smith

Mrs. Smith is a 65-year-old woman with Type II diabetes. Three of her five grown children live nearby and bring the grandchildren to visit frequently. Mrs. Smith's self-image is that of caregiver and homemaker. She has abundant supplies of desserts and junk food on hand at all times in the event that the family drops in. Mrs. Smith still routinely cooks for large numbers of people, though the timing of visits by her children and grandchildren is sporadic. Her homemaker activities have revolved around food and the home during her entire life. A planned exercise program has never been part of her life-style, and her "matronly figure" is seen as "a consequence of cooking for my family." Her retired husband is a "meat and potatoes man" who has always expected at least one large meal daily, prepared by Mrs. Smith. Her major concern, expressed during assessment, was that she would not be a good wife and mother if she had to change her diet.

Questions:

1. What teaching method(s) would work best when teaching Mrs. Smith?
2. What assessment data are needed about Mrs. Smith in regard to her self image, her role as homemaker, and her spouse?
3. What factors need to be considered in development of a plan addressing information specific to diabetic education?

- Haphazard teaching efforts
- Patient education is neither noticed or rewarded

In many health care settings, the teaching protocols, teaching plans, and teaching materials are outdated and have not kept pace with the changes in health care. Nurses need role models and coaching to gain the skill and confidence needed to provide relevant, timely information to clients during their illness experience. Nurses tend to use medical jargon and words that are often not understood by the client, often contributing to decreased learning. It is necessary for nurse educators to transfer the needed information to clients and families in language that can be clearly understood.

Rankin and Stallings (2001) believe that the nurse should concentrate on the most critical behaviors needed by the client and family. With those priorities identified, realistic teaching plans can be created. Plans that are complex, or contain extraneous material will frustrate staff, clients, and families (p.127).

Reflection on the nurse's own culture, values, and beliefs may reveal a naiveté that can interfere with providing culturally sensitive care to clients and families. Insensitivity to dietary restrictions of the Orthodox Jew, lack of knowledge about the head-of-family role in various cultures preventing them from taking on caregiver duties, showing anger when speaking, and demonstrating poor manners are all examples of lack of knowledge related to culture, which result in teaching plans that lack cultural competence.

Spector (2000) contends that in addition to the need to consider the client's culture, health care professionals also need to realize that professional socialization into a profession teaches the student a set of beliefs, practices, habits, likes, dislikes, norms and rituals. As the student takes on the language and beliefs of the profession, care must be taken to prevent misunderstanding with the client, making certain that time is taken to listen and understand the questions and concerns set forth as treatments, discharge planning, and decision making regarding health care are discussed.

Two studies discussed the nurse as client educator. Honan and colleagues (1998) described nurses' perceptions of responsibilities in client teaching and determined factors that influenced or enhanced the nurse in fulfilling the educator role. Nurse variables influencing client teaching included knowledge level, availability of time and staff, privacy, responsibility, priority placed on role, documentation, and client teaching materials.

Trocino, Byers, & Peach (1997) examined nurses' attitudes toward client and family education to determine associated barriers and concerns. Findings included that client and family teaching was a high priority and an essential role. However, there was disagreement over who should do the teaching, with many respondents believing that teaching was the responsibility of the advanced practice nurse. Many responded that they felt uncomfortable with some topics expected to be taught and felt that additional preparation for teaching should be incorporated into all undergraduate and graduate nursing programs.

Interventions

Chronic illness affects every aspect of an individual's life. There is no cure, little predictability, and much uncertainty. During most chronic illnesses, there are different phases of the disease process. Within each phase, physical and emotional events occur that affect the adaptive abilities and the educational needs of both the client and family. Therefore, no one approach will fit each teaching-learning situation. The timing, acuity, and severity of the disease progression provide additional challenges to effective teaching.

Family reaction and perception of the chronic illness are also important influences on adaptation. It is known that family participation has an effect on the success of a client's rehabilitation program.

Thus, it is important to develop teaching plans based upon learning needs of both client and family.

The Teaching Role in Chronic Illness

The development of a teaching plan involves use of a systematic process similar to the steps in the nursing process. Although the steps of the plan are described as linear, the process itself is dynamic, relying on the nurse to constantly reflect upon the information available regarding knowledge about the disease, the resources available to the client and family, and a multitude of other factors that have an impact on the specific teaching situation. *Assessment* determines client and family needs and is the foundation upon which the teaching plan will be designed. The nurse will determine the appropriate nursing diagnoses and formulate a teaching plan.

Development of an action plan involves the nurse choosing appropriate content, with one (or more) teaching-learning strategies. This decision follows reflection upon numerous factors, including the knowledge, skills, and attitude needs of the client and family, and what is known about the illness course. Additional factors to consider include culture, environment, motivation, and readiness of the learner; physical impairments that might preclude learning; timing; age; and factors specific to the family dynamics.

Goals and outcomes identification form the basis of plan implementation. The plan will work best if the goals are mutually determined, with the client an active participant in the decision-making process. *Implementation* of the plan follows. *Evaluation* provides the nurse with information regarding client and family learning, and identifies whether there is a need for additional teaching, clarification, and support.

Developing a teaching plan for a client and family with a diagnosis of chronic illness is a challenging task. A systematic approach to assessing, planning, developing, implementing, and evaluating the teaching plan is essential. A framework to guide the teaching-learning process can be helpful. Examples of three frameworks or models—the medical model, the stress and adaptation model, and Braden's self-help model—all applicable to the chronic illness are discussed next.

Medical Model

The medical model has been widely used as the approach of choice by physicians and nurses. Using the medical model, a teaching plan is based on the signs and symptoms of a medical diagnosis. This approach addresses the needs of the known medical condition but can overlook or negate the sociocultural issues that affect the client and family's daily life.

Stress and Adaptation Model

Physical and psychosocial stressors and responses to them are described through Antonovsky's work (1979). Stressors are physical-biochemical, psychosocial, cultural, and environmental factors that evoke a certain state in an organism. Human response to stress is interpreted by nursing in relation to the behaviors exhibited by the individual. When applied to chronic illness, stressors are demands made upon an individual from the internal or external environment and that exceed the resources of the system.

Antonovsky describes the way in which the individual approaches and responds to his or her environment as a sense of coherence (p. 123). This sense of coherence provides the individual with a sense that "things will work out right." According to Antonovsky, persons with a strong sense of coherence mobilize general resistance resources (GRRs) to avoid stressors, thereby minimizing the stress response, avoiding what he terms diseases of adaptation, and maintaining the client's sense of coherence. Essentially, the GRRs overcome the stressors, allowing the client to achieve a higher level on the wellness-illness continuum.

Using this framework in developing client and family education programs in chronic illness, the nurse's assessment would include both stressors and GRR categories. Based on the findings, an individualized teaching plan could be formulated. The pa-

rameters of this model match closely with the client and family factors that influence learning, which were identified in the previous chapter.

Braden's Self-Help Model

The middle-range nursing theory—Braden's Self-Help Model: Learned Response to Chronic Illness Experience—is a framework that describes enabling factors that may enhance learning and mediate responses in chronic illness (Braden, 1990a, 1990b). According to Lefort (2000), the self-help model shows the dynamics of a learned self-management response, as opposed to a learned helplessness or passive response to the experience of chronic illness (p. 154). Braden (1993) defines *self-help* as "an informed process of facing definable, manageable adversities by maintaining control of everyday problems" (p. 38). Braden contrasts this process to individuals with a passive response who do not actively seek solutions to problems, remain uninformed, and who withdraw from definable, manageable difficulties. By understanding the dynamics of a self-help response to chronic illness stressors, nurses are better able to develop appropriate interventions, including teaching (Lefort, 2000).

Hypothesized relationships of constructs in the self-help model are found in Figure 15-1. Constructs in the model are conceptualized as antecedents (perceived severity of illness, limitation, and uncertainty), mediators (enabling skills), and outcomes (self-help and life quality). Braden (1990a) notes that perceived severity of illness can act as a stimulus to learning or result in increased exposure to the antecedents of limitation and uncertainty. Braden (1990b) conceptualized limitation as being unable to do things one wants to do and hypothesized that higher levels of severity of illness would be associated with high levels of limitations and uncertainty.

Use of either Antonovsky's stressors and GRR frame of reference or Braden's Self-Help Model will heighten the nurse's awareness of the multiple factors to consider in the teaching–learning process. Each of these models provides a rehabilitative perspective, never negating the stressors or weaknesses,

FIGURE 15-1

Hypothesized Relationships of Constructs in the Self-Help Model

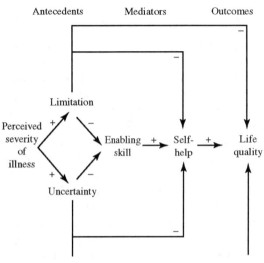

SOURCE: LeFort (2000), p. 154.

but using GRRs or enabling or managing skills to maximize quality of life for the client and family. Each model seeks to maintain optimism, with a foundation that the client is a power source.

Development of a Teaching Plan

Assessment

The accuracy of the collected assessment data depends on the interviewing and observation skills of the individual doing the assessment. Development of a systematic assessment process will improve the quality and accuracy of the teaching plan. A summary of factors to be assessed, which have been previously discussed in this chapter, include the client's values and beliefs, knowledge base, ability to learn, readiness to learn, and motivation. Additionally, there are a number of basic teaching-learning principles that need to be remembered as the nurse

completes the teaching-learning assessment and develops the teaching plan (Table 15-2).

The nursing diagnoses set the stage for determining the objectives, content, teaching strategies, expected outcomes, and evaluation methods. However, choosing the appropriate diagnosis is often difficult. Reasons for this difficulty include failure to use nursing diagnosis terminology to identify problems, problem identification using the medical model, and an inaccurate or incomplete assessment. One diagnosis that is often used incorrectly by students and practicing nurses is knowledge deficit. Carpenito (2000) states that knowledge deficit, as a nursing diagnosis, does not represent a human response, alteration, or pattern of dysfunction, but, rather, a related factor. It is when this lack of knowledge causes or could cause a problem that the nurses act on a nursing diagnosis (p. 552).

Wilkinson (2000) describes knowledge deficit as contributing to a number of problem responses, such as anxiety, altered parenting, self-care deficit, or ineffective coping, and as a result, suggests the use of knowledge deficit as an etiology of a nursing diagnoses rather than the problem itself (p. 250). Wilkinson cautions that when knowledge deficit is used as a problem, it causes the nurse to focus on providing information rather than focusing on behaviors caused by the lack of knowledge.

Once a comprehensive client and family assessment has been completed, the appropriate nursing diagnoses determined, and learner needs identified, the development of the teaching plan begins. The following checklist can help in developing a teaching plan

- What are the learner needs (client and family)?
- Are they based on a comprehensive assessment?
- Are the identified needs appropriate for the client?
- What are the priorities for teaching?
- Are the learner objectives identified? Are they clearly stated, related to the identified needs, and attainable, measurable, and realistic?
- Does the content outline address the objectives, include material to be presented, allow material

TABLE 15-2

Teaching and Learning Principles

1. The learner's biological, psychologic, sociologic, and cultural realities shape the learner's perception of the learning experience.
2. Perception is necessary for learning.
3. Conditioning is a process of learning.
4. Learning often occurs by trial and error.
5. Learning may occur through imitation.
6. Concept development is part of the learning process.
7. Motivation is necessary for learning.
8. Learner control increases learning.
9. Learning styles vary.
10. Physical and mental readiness is necessary for learning.
11. Active participation is necessary for effective learning.
12. New learning must be based on previous knowledge and experience.
13. Application of new learning in a variety of contexts broadens the generalization of that learning.
14. Learning is affected by the individual's emotional climate.
15. Repetition and reinforcement strengthen learning.
16. Success reinforces learning.
17. Accurate and prompt feedback enhances learning.
18. Good teacher-learner rapport is important in teaching.
19. Teaching requires effective communication.
20. Learning needs of clients must be determined.
21. Objectives serve as guides in planning and evaluating teaching.
22. Planning time is required for effective teaching and learning.
23. Control of the environment is an aspect of teaching.
24. Teaching skill can be acquired through practice and observation.
25. Evaluating effectiveness is a part of teaching.

SOURCE: Reprinted from Babcock & Miller, *Client Education: Theory and Practice* © 1993, Mosby, with permission from Elsevier.

to be accomplished in the allocated time, and consider the client's knowledge base?

- Are the teaching strategies appropriate to the subject, the situation, the knowledge level of the client, and realistic within the time frame?
- Are the expected outcomes realistic and attainable?
- Are the evaluation methods at the client's level, do they address the objectives identified, and are they appropriate to the situation?

Though there is no guarantee that the learning goals will be achieved, there is an increased likelihood of successful outcomes when the preceding questions are addressed.

While nursing textbooks have always advocated development of mutually determined, goal-directed teaching plans, the reality is that often the plans have been those designed by the nurse, with little input from the client or family. Miller and Capps (1997) describe a flow chart for client education that details the education process as beginning in the preadmission phase and continuing through post discharge. The chart incorporates the family throughout the process and provides a reference to the nurse in determining appropriate parameters to consider at various stages throughout the education process.

Implementing the Teaching Plan

Setting Priorities

The assessment provides data that assist the nurse in setting priorities in the teaching plan. The nurse may assume that certain topics or subjects should be discussed first, because the nurse sees them as a priority. However, the topic may not be a priority for the client for a variety of reasons. It is essential that the nurse understand what is important to the client and family. Including the client and family in the original goal setting is essential.

Instructional Strategies

The overall plan for design of a learning experience, termed an *instructional strategy,* can involve several methods of teaching (Bastable, 2003). Methods include one or more techniques or approaches used by the teacher to bring learners together with the content to be learned, and are an approach to communicate information. Examples of instructional methods include lecture, small group discussion, role modeling, role playing, gaming, simulation, computer-assisted instruction (CAI), demonstration and return demonstration, learning modules, and individual instruction techniques. Instructional tools are the mechanisms through which information is disseminated. Examples include books, videos, posters, and computer software.

Success of the designated plan depends on numerous factors, including best fit for the client, tool availability, and the learning environment. The methods should be determined following a thorough assessment and be based on learning objectives and expected client outcomes. A comprehensive summary of general characteristics of instructional methods is presented in Table 15-3.

Determination of the instructional method of choice can be determined by answering five questions:

1. Does the method help the learners achieve the stated objectives?
2. Is the learning activity accessible to the learners you have targeted?
3. Is the method efficient, given the time, energy, and resources available in relation to the number of learners you are trying to reach?
4. To what extent does the method allow for active participation to accommodate learner needs, abilities, and style of learning?
5. Is the method cost effective?

Information Technology as a Tool   Information technology has become increasingly important in the practice of nursing, and, similarly, it has become important for teaching clients and families. The American Association of Colleges of Nursing, in the *Essentials of Baccalaureate Education for Professional Nursing Practice,* state that nursing education should prepare knowledgeable workers—able to manage information and high technology on one hand and complicated clinical judgments on the other (1998, p. 13). The National Advisory Council on Nurse Education and Practice (1997) identified the need to adequately prepare the nation's nursing work force to use technology to manage information for education and practice and to help patients gain access to health care information.

One of the purposes of the new information technology is clinical data management for health care professionals. However, Lewis and Pesut (2001) see technology's influence affecting the consumer as well. They predict that clients will soon meet health care needs through e-health web sites that allow clients to receive treatment recommendations by e-mail. Through on-line decision support tools, clients will be coached in self-care and disease management. Health kiosks at malls will also provide access to health care providers, eliminating the need to go to the provider's office (Lewis & Pesut, 2001, p. 7).

Nursing education needs to incorporate competencies and skills that support a consumer health information age (Lewis & Pesut, 2001). A future expectation for nurses involved in health care educa-

TABLE 15-3

General Characteristics of Instructional Methods

Methods	Domain	Learner Role	Teacher Role	Advantages	Limitations
Lecture	Cognitive	Passive	Presents information	Cost effective Targets large groups	Not individualized
Group discussion	Affective Cognitive	Active, if learner participates	Guides and focuses discussion	Stimulates sharing ideas and emotions	Shy or dominant member
One-to-one Instruction	Cognitive Affective Psychomotor	Active	Presents information and facilitates individualized learning	Tailored to individual's needs and goals	High levels of diversity Labor intensive Isolates learner
Demonstration	Cognitive	Passive	Models skill or behavior	Preview of "exact" skill/behavior	Small groups needed to facilitate visualization
Return demonstration	Psychomotor	Active	Individualizes feedback to refine performance	Immediate individual guidance	Labor intensive to view individual performance
Gaming	Cognitive Affective	Active, if learner participates	Oversees pacing Referees Debriefs	Captures learner enthusiasm	Environment too competitive for some learners
Simulation	Cognitive Psychomotor	Active	Designs environment Facilitates process Debriefs	Practices "reality" in safe setting	Labor intensive Equipment costs
Role playing	Affective	Active	Designs format Debriefs	Develops understanding of others	Exaggeration or underdevelopment of role
Role modeling	Affective Cognitive	Passive	Models skill or behavior	Helps with socialization to role	Requires rapport
Self instruction	Cognitive Psychomotor	Active	Designs package Gives individual feedback	Self-paced Cost effective	Procrastination Requires literacy
Computer-assisted instruction	Cognitive	Active	Purchases or designs program Provides individual feedback	Consistent Immediate and continuous feedback Private Individualized	Costly to design or purchase Must have hardware
Distance learning	Cognitive	Passive	Presents information Answers questions	Targets learners who are at varying distances from expert	Lack of personal contact Accessibility

SOURCE: Bastable, S. (2003) p. 378. *Nurse as educator: Principles of teaching learning.* Sudbury, MA: Jones & Bartlett.

tion is the ability to develop technology-based education and information materials. The advent of the internet and the plethora of health-related sites available to the lay public bring informed consumers to teaching situations. These advances also afford new opportunities for nurses to aid consumers in their information-seeking and health care needs, assisting them in evaluating and judging the information obtained from the resources found.

The internet offers new teaching strategies for the nurse to use in client and family education as well. These strategies are being used by physicians (O'Conner & Johanson, 2000), by nursing professionals in community settings (Alemagno, Niles & Treiber, 2004), and are being used in specialty areas such as childbirth education (Collins, 2000). In selected nursing programs, students are helping clients and families access information on the Internet during home visits through the use of the Nightingale Tracker (Elfrink et al., 2000). Although this latter computer-based electronic communication system was developed to provide faculty access to students in the community, it has had an additional value for students teaching clients and families how to access specific health or illness information.

Technology has been used as a conduit to provide client education. Kizak & Conrad (2004) describe using technology to develop and distribute cancer education materials using storyboards. The purpose of choosing storyboards instead of posters was the ability to distribute them throughout a large health system which could then be distributed to clients, families, and the general population.

Sorrentino et al. (2002) describe use of the intranet, an internal network that operates within the larger world wide web, as an effective strategy to deliver and reinforce client education. The oncology staff created the teaching materials and found that there were significant advantages to use of the intranet. Advantages included online storage, decreased costs, easy access, real-time updates and distribution, and unlimited supply availability (p. 354).

Oermann and Wilson (2000) assessed ten websites for readability of quality care information that is available to consumers on the internet. They con-

tended that the quality of information presented was important in order for clients and families to make informed decisions and to empower them in determining if they were receiving quality care. Six of the ten documents reviewed were below recommended readability level, thus making them comprehensible to the majority of consumers.

Evaluation of Learning

Evaluation is an integral component of a teaching plan and a part of the continuous process of client education. Evaluation is dynamic, occurs throughout the teaching-learning process, and can be accomplished through a variety of methods. Evaluation is useful in determining progress toward client and family goals, the value of the plan in achieving desired outcomes, and quality of care. Evaluation also provides data to modify teaching plans.

Evaluation methods vary based on expected outcomes and involve comparing predicted outcomes with actual client and family responses. In an inpatient setting, progress toward goals can be seen or assessed by written or verbal feedback, return demonstration of a skill, or observing a change in behavior. However, the process becomes more challenging when the client is taught at discharge and is not seen again following the teaching session.

Ways in which goal accomplishment can be determined include follow-up phone calls with focused questions, client satisfaction surveys mailed to the home, return visits to the physician or nurse practitioner, and anecdotal information from family. Depending on the specific goals of the teaching plan, changes in physical abilities and evidence such as laboratory values, vital signs, and medication compliance may be seen as ways to evaluate the teaching (Bopp & Lubkin, 1998). It is important to note that behavior changes seen shortly after the teaching occurred may not be sustained over time. In evaluating teaching-learning outcomes, both the client and family are involved in the process, with their feedback providing data to ascertain the effectiveness of the teaching plan or to modify the existing plan.

Other Strategies

Development of Specially Designed Teaching Programs

Dunbar (1998) describes a client-centered teaching program for individuals with cardiac disease based on the client's specific needs. A plan was designed that focused on what the clients decided they were ready to learn before or at the time of discharge. One area that was targeted was postmyocardial infarction (MI) depression. Outcomes of the new approach have been positive, by deemphasizing the nurse's perspective of what clients want to learn. The questions posed to the client reflect more strongly the client's perception of illness rather than simply providing information about disease. Essentially, the nurse is giving the client an opportunity to provide a broader base of assessment data upon which to build a teaching plan.

Chelf et al. (2001) reviewed published results of an overview of the past decade of evaluation and research of cancer related client education. Many client educators believe that the methodology for client education research is not well developed (p. 1139). Their findings revealed that many factors previously discussed in this chapter were cited as influencing the client's ability to learn such as patient preferences, readability and literacy. They also explored computer assisted learning, telephone, audio and video use in client education, treatment education and pain and fatigue.

Jenny and Fai (2001) developed a computer-based interactive multimedia client education program on exercise and heart health for cardiac rehabilitation clients. The program used a combination of interactive teaching strategies as well as various multimedia presentations. When compared with a group who were taught with tutorial methods, the researchers found that many clients enjoyed the alternative approaches to learning, while some preferred the more traditional methods. As the internet becomes more commonplace in the lives of clients and families, the authors predict that the use of computers and interactive teaching methods for clients with chronic illness will increase.

Pierce et al. (2002) describe teaching clients using web TV as the medium to support caregivers of stroke clients. In this study, clients had 24/7 access for nurses with questions and concerns. Rationale for web interventions was to provide clients and caregivers an opportunity to ask questions of a clinical nurse specialist, to have contact via email with the nurse, caregivers and other study participants, and to provide educational information about strokes, and caregiving.

The use of automated calls with telephone nurse follow-up was a strategy used by Piette, Weinberger, and McPhee (2000) to improve mental health, self efficacy, satisfaction with care, and improved quality of life for low income diabetic clients. The study built on the model that the nurse would provide systematic monitoring and client education and targeted phone counseling. Findings included better self care and glycemic control and fewer diabetic symptoms with predictions that education for chronic illness clients in the future will frequently involve use of combination strategies such as the study described.

Teaching Plans Adapted to the Environment

Smith et al. (2000) describe a home care program by outreach nurses that includes visits to clients and families in their homes to provide support, education, and monitoring. The visits are also viewed as providing information for the physicians. In addition to the outreach nurses, some nurse practitioners also provide nursing interventions. Though the program did not result in decreased hospital admissions, the authors believe that clients with moderate COPD may have mortality and health-related quality-of-life gains from the outreach program.

Alemagno et al. (2004) described using computers to reduce medication misuse of community-based seniors. The seniors were found in senior centers across the city and were encouraged to participate in a short computer-based questionnaire which addressed questions specific to medication knowledge and compliance. The computer program also provided short educational video clips to address potential medication misuse. A two-month follow-up of clients revealed use of the medication reminder checklist, discussions of the medications with their doctors, and satisfaction with the teaching method.

Other examples of technology use in providing nursing care, specifically, telemedicine include a variety of telecommunication examples. Jenkins and Sweeney (2001) describe assessing clients with chronic congestive heart failure using a two-way telemedicine audiovisual system. Comparisons were made between real time nurse assessments and use of the telemedicine approach. Nurses and clients were favorable to the approach but felt that there continued to be a need for nurses to conduct real home visits along with the telemedicine assessments. A study by Gardner et al. (2001) was completed to determine the use of interactive video technology to assess chronic wounds being managed in the home. The rationale for the study was that the expert nurse may not be available in long term care settings or to visit clients' homes. Hence, teaching that was done using this technology was useful to assess the wound and to assist the nurse not familiar with managing chronic wounds.

Other Considerations

Caregiver Role/Education Needs

Early discharge from the hospital mandates that assistance be provided as the individual recovers from exacerbation of a chronic disease. Family members acting as caregivers, providing hands-on skills to loved ones, are being asked to learn complex skills using sophisticated technologies, and in a very short period of time. These skills are often taught in the hospital, under less than ideal circumstances, and the caregiver is expected to then apply what has been taught in a home setting. Family members who have no experience with illness must not only learn to manage difficult clinical problems, but also, at the

same time, adjust to life changes and the consequences. Caregiver stress becomes a significant factor when family members take on both new and often very difficult situations. This stress may be compounded by problematic family relationships, grieving the loss of the loved one, role changes, and a variety of factors brought about by the illness, such as financial concerns, resource availability, and fear of the unknown. Haggard (1989) suggests that deciding which family member(s) to teach deserves careful consideration. The most logical choice is the person who will be the primary caregiver. However, in some situations, more than one person will be needed. Haggard suggests that a smaller number is better and that the determination of caregiver be guided by the family, because some individuals who are thought to be most appropriate may choose not to participate. Gaining information about the caregiver initially will help determine the teaching methods as well as appropriateness of the person selected as caregiver. Realizing that the caregiver has no formal health care background prevents the nurse from bringing inflated expectations to a teaching experience. This is particularly true when dealing with elderly caregivers.

Buckwalter et al. (2002) describe a number of telehealth studies for elders and their caregivers in rural communities. The studies included the use of various technologies to provide health care either through interactive video or in conjunction with in-home nurse visits. Each of the studies described reported overall patient satisfaction.

Huber and McClelland (2003) explored client and family preferences discharge planning, piloting a tool to measure preferences. The authors found the role of the family as critical, especially when the client's dependence necessitates the need for caregiving. Findings were that caregivers and patients differed in preference leading to the recommendation that discharge planning needs to begin early and that use of a specific tool will help nurses to comprehensively develop a plan that includes needs of both the client and the caregiver. The authors found that assessing and incorporating the caregiver's needs can provide a plan that will help to keep the client from rehospitalization.

Community Resources

With the expansion of the caregiver role as health care delivery changes continue, knowledge of community resources has become an integral part of care planning. These resources can be found through places of worship, service agencies, community centers, senior centers, day care centers for children and adults, the World Wide Web, lay literature such as *Prevention Magazine,* organizations like AARP, newsletters from local hospitals, and word of mouth. Knowledge of the availability of transportation in any geographic area is also an important consideration.

Different Environments of Care

As the health care delivery system changes, nurses are expected to be able to think across settings as they teach clients and families. What are the issues that need to be considered as a skill is taught to a client who is home bound, or to a caregiver who is going to provide follow-up to your teaching? How will the equipment available to the client at home differ from that in the institutional setting? How does one teach maintaining clean or sterile technique when the environment does not provide for that option?

Time Constraints

The time required to teach a client and family will always exceed the time planned. Even with years of practice, the expert nurse realizes that unforeseen circumstances will often preclude the best laid plans. In teaching, the amount of time spent on preparation is often significant. With novice teachers, the depth and amount of material is often far greater than the client and family needs and can absorb. Most teaching within clinical settings is less than formal. In fact, teaching may be just a part of the everyday exchange that occurs between the client and nurse. If formal teaching is needed, Haggard (1989)

recommends planning a number of small sessions during a day, in contrast to presenting a major teaching plan. She also contends that nurses should use "golden" or "teachable" moments during time spent with a client. Many situations provide such moments; some are planned to appear spontaneous, but at other times, they simply happen.

Timing is important, but there is little chance that all of the necessary information will be presented to the client prior to discharge from the hospital. The use of discharge planning interventions, found to be cost-effective and improve outcomes, is being implemented around the country. These interventions provide numerous opportunities for clients and families to learn what is needed to manage their chronic illness.

End-of-Life Issues

Educational needs continue throughout the client's lifetime, even until shortly before death. Quality of life can be influenced by the client's ability to control his or her situation, and many teaching moments center upon client rights, advocacy, and issues related to control. Client and family teaching at end-of-life may be related to the physical manifestations that occur during the dying process or to ways in which to psychologically support the client and family during this time. Nurses involved in caring for clients at end-of-life have often known the individual and family for prolonged periods of time. Seeing the client's decline, even when reality dictates that the end is near, often causes role strain and a feeling of powerlessness. End-of-life education for many practicing nurses has been nonexistent, causing a sense of inadequacy in regard to the knowledge and skills necessary to provide the needed support for the client and family.

Lynn (2000) discusses the importance of professional education involving knowledge and competence in health care professionals caring for clients with chronic, eventually fatal illness. The importance of learning to communicate with, support, and care for chronically ill clients over time, in order to help them live fully within the constraints imposed by their disease, is essential.

■ Outcomes

The optimal outcome for the client and family in the teaching-learning situation is that the client either demonstrate results of the knowledge, is able to repeat the skill, or show a change in behavior that is helpful in managing the client's disease process. The specific outcomes of the teaching-learning plan dictate the client outcomes.

Study Questions

1. What factors influence learning in each of an individual's developmental stages?
2. Compare and contrast pedagogy and andragogy.
3. What specific behavioral strategies can be used to teach the individual with chronic illness?
4. What client factors affect the teaching-learning process?
5. What nurse factors affect the teaching-learning process?
6. What are the steps of the teaching-learning process? Describe each of them.
7. How is teaching an individual and family with chronic illness different from teaching those with an acute condition or disease?

References

Abbott, P., Short, E., Dodson, S., Garcia, C., et al. (2002). Improving your cultural awareness with culture cues. *Nurse Practitioner, 27* (2), 44-7, 51.

Alemagno, S. A., Niles, S. A., & Trieber, E. A. (2004). Using computers to reduce medication misuse of community–based seniors: Results of a pilot intervention program. *Geriatric Nursing, 25* (5), 281–85.

American Association of Colleges of Nursing. (1998). *Essentials of baccalaureate education for professional nursing practice.* Washington, DC: AACN.

Antonovsky, A. (1979). *Health, stress, and coping.* San Francisco: Jossey-Bass.

Babcock, D. E., & Miller, M. A. (1994). *Client education: Theory and practice.* St. Louis: C. V. Mosby.

Bastable, S. B. (2003). *Nurse as educator: principles of teaching and learning.* (2nd ed). Sudbury, MA: Jones & Bartlett.

Bopp, A., & Lubkin, I. (1998). Teaching. In I. Lubkin & P. Larsen (Eds.), *Chronic illness: Impact and interventions* (4th ed.), (pp. 343–362). Sudbury, MA: Jones & Bartlett.

Braden, C. J. (1993). Promoting a learned self help response to chronic illness. In S. Funk, E. Tornquist, M. Champagne, & R. Wiese (Eds.), *Key aspects of care for the chronically ill: Hospital and home,* (pp. 158–169). New York: Springer.

_____. (1990a). Learned self help response to chronic illness experience: A test of three alternative learning theories. *Scholarly Inquiry of Nursing Practice, 4,* 23–41.

_____. (1990b). A test of the self help model: Learned response to chronic illness experience: Self help model. *Nursing Research, 39,* 42–47.

Brookfield, S. D. (1990). *Understanding and facilitating adult education.* San Francisco: Jossey-Bass.

Buckwalter, K. C., Davis, L. L., Wakefield, B. J., Kienzle, M. G., et al. (2002). Telehealth for elders and their caregivers in rural communities. *Family Community Health, 25* (3), 31–40.

Carpenito, L. J. (2000). *Nursing diagnosis: Application to clinical practice* (8th ed.). Philadelphia: Lippincott.

Chelf, J., Agre, P., Axelrod, A., Cheney, L., et al. (2001). Cancer related patient education: An overview of the last decade of evaluation and research. *Oncology Nursing Forum, 28*(7), 1139–47.

Collins, C. (2000). Childbirth educators and the internet: Making our jobs eaiser? *International Journal of Childbirth Education, 15* (1), 11–13.

Covey, S. (1990). *The seven habits of highly effective people.* New York: Simon & Schuster.

Dunbar, C. N. (1998). Developing a teaching plan. *American Journal of Nursing, 98* (8), 16B–16D.

Elfrink, V., Davis, L. S., Fitzwater, E., Castleman, J., et al. (2000). A comparison of teaching strategies for information technology into clinical nursing education. *Nurse Educator, 25,* (3), 136–144.

Falvo, D. (1994). *Effective patient education: A guide to increased compliance.* Gaithersburg, MD: Aspen.

Fuszard, B. (1995). *Innovative teaching strategies in nursing.* Gaithersburg, MD: Aspen.

Gardner, S. E., Frantz, R. A., Specht, J. P,. Johnson-Mekota, J. L., et al. (2001). How accurate are chronic wound assessments using interactive video technology. *Journal of Gerontological Nursing, 27* (1), pp.15–20.

Haggard, A. (1989). *Handbook of patient education.* Rockville, MD: Aspen.

Hogstel, M. O. (2001). *Gerontology: Nursing care of the older adult.* Albany, NY: Delmar.

Honan, S., Krsnak, G., Petersen, D., & Torkelson, R. (1998). The nurse as patient educator: Perceived responsibilities and factors enhancing role development. *Journal of Continuing Education in Nursing, 19* (1), 33–37.

Huber, D., & McClelland, E. (2003). Patient preferences and discharge planning transitions. *Journal of Professional Nursing, 19* (3), 204–210.

Huff, R. M. & Kline, M. V. (1999). *Promoting health in multicultural populations: A handbook for practitioners.* Thousand Oaks, CA: Sage.

Ignatavicius, D. D., & Workman, M. L. (2002). *Medical-surgical nursing: Critical thinking for collaborative care.* Philadelphia: WB Saunders.

Jenkins, R. L. & McSweeney, M. (2001). Assessing Elderly patients with congestive heart failure via in-home interactive telecommunication. *Journal of Gerontological Nursing, 27* (1), pp. 21–27.

Jenny, N., & Fai, T. (2001). Evaluation the effectiveness of an interactive multimedia computer-based patient education program in cardiac rehabilitation, *Occupational Therapy Journal of Research, 21* (4), 260–74.

Joint Commission on the Accreditation of Healthcare Organizations. (1998). *Comprehensive accreditation manual for hospitals.* Chicago: Author.

Kizak, A., & Conrad, K. (2004). Using technology to develop and distribute patient education storyboards across health systems. *Oncology Nursing Forum, 31* (1), 131–135.

Knowles, M. (1990). *The adult learner: A neglected species.* Houston: Gulf Publishing.

LeFort, S. M. (2000). A test of Braden's self-help model in adults with chronic pain. *Journal of Nursing Scholarship, 32* (2), 153–160.

Lewis, D., & Pesut, D. (2001). Emergence of consumer health informatics. *Nursing Outlook, 49,* 7.

Lynn, J. (2000). Learning to care for people with chronic illness facing the end of life. *JAMA, 284* (19), 2508–2510.

Miller, B., & Capps, E. (1997). Meeting JCAHO patient-education standards. *Nursing Management, 28* (5), 55–58.

Miller, J. F. (2000). *Coping with chronic disease: Overcoming powerlessness* (3rd ed.). Philadelphia: Davis.

Murray, R. B., & Zentner, J. P. (2001). *Health promotion strategies across the life span.* Upper Saddle River, NJ: Prentice Hall.

Musinski, B. (1999). The educator as facilitator: A new kind of leadership. *Nursing Forum, 34* (1), 23–29.

National Advisory Council on Nurse Education and Practice. (Deccmber, 1997). *A national informatics agenda for nursing education and practice,* (pp. 1–32). Report to the Secretary of the Department of Health and Human Services, Health Resources and Services Administration. Washington, DC: Government Printing Office.

Norton, B. (1998). From teaching to learning. In D. Billings & J. Halstead (Eds.), *Teaching in nursing: A guide for faculty.* Philadelphia: Saunders.

O'Conner, B., & Johanson, J. (2000). Use of the web for medical information by a gastroenterology clinic population. *JAMA, 284* (15), 1962–1964.

Oermann M., & Wilson, F. (2000). Quality of care information for consumers on the internet. *Journal of Nursing Care Quality, 14* (4), 45–54.

Pierce, L., Steiner, V., & Govoni, A. (2002). In home online support for caregivers of survivors of stroke: A feasibility study. *CIN: Computer, Informatics, Nursing, 20* (4), 157–164.

Piette, J., Weinberger, M., & McPhee, S. (2000). The effect of automated calls with telephone nurse follow-up on patient centered outcomes of diabetes care. *Medical Care, 38* (2), 218–230.

Pohl, M. L. (1981). *The teaching function of the nursing practitioner* (4th ed.). Dubuque, IA: Brown.

Purnell, L.D., & Paulanka, B.J. (2005). *Guide to Culturally Competent Health Care.* Philadelphia: F.A Davis Company.

Rankin, S. H., & Stallings, K. D. (2001). *Patient education.* (4th ed). Philadelphia: Lippincott, Williams and Wilkins.

Redman, B. K. (1999). *Women's health needs in patient education.* New York: Springer.

Saarmann, L., Daugherty, J., & Reigel, B. (2000). Patient teaching to promote behavioral change. *Nursing Outlook, 48,* 281–287.

Smeltzer, S., & Bare, B. (2000). *Textbook of medical-surgical nursing.* Philadelphia: Lippincott.

Smith, B., Appleton, S., Adams, S., Southcott, A., et al. (2000). *Home care outreach nursing for COPD.* Oxford: The Cochrane Library.

Sorrentino, C., Berger, A., Wardian, S., & Pattrin, L. (Nov/Dec 2002). Using the intranet to deliver patient education materials. *Clinical Journal of Oncology Nursing,* 6(6), 354–57.

Spector, R. (2000a). *Cultural diversity in health and illness.* Upper Saddle River, N.J.: Prentice Hall Health

Spector, R. (2000b). *Cultural care: Guides to heritage assessment and health traditions.* Upper Saddle River, NJ: Prentice Hall Health.

Stanley, M., Blair, K., & Beare, P. (2005). *Gerontological nursing.* Philadelphia: FA Davis.

Swanson, E., & Tripp-Reimer, T. (1997). *Chronic illness and the older adult.* New York: Springer.

Tripp-Reimer, T, et al. (Feb 2001). Cultural barriers to care: Inverting the Problem. *Diabetes Spectrum,* 13–22.

Trocino, L., Byers, J., & Peach, A. G. (1997). Nurses' attitude toward patient and family education: Implications for clinical nurse specialists. *Clinical Nurse Specialist, 11* (2), 77–84.

Wilkinson, J. M. (2000). *Nursing diagnosis handbook.* Upper Saddle River, NJ: Prentice Hall Health.

Wilson, F., Racine, E., Tekieli, V., & Williams, B. (2003). Literacy, readability, and cultural barriers: cultural factors to consider when educating older African Americans about anticoagulation therapy. *Journal of Clinical Nursing, 12* (2), 275–283.

Wlodkowski, R. J. (1985). *Enhancing adult motivation to learn.* San Francisco: Jossey-Bass.

CHAPTER 16

Advocacy

Faye I. Hummel

Introduction

Advocacy is a core value of professional nursing and intrinsic to the practice of nursing. Advocacy is an ongoing process as opposed to a single isolated event (McGrath & Walker, 1999). Clients with chronic illnesses and their families often need information, understanding, and competent intervention to help them reformulate their lives, assimilate their losses, and adjust to the changes brought about by their illnesses (Sullivan-Bolyal, Sadler, Knafl, Gillis & Ahmann, 2003). These individuals are at risk if they are unable to represent their needs, wishes, values, and choices. Under these circumstances, others must advocate on their behalf. As a moral concept, advocacy requires the nurse to speak up for the client's rights and choices, to assist the client to clarify his or her decisions, and to protect the client's privacy and autonomy in decision making (Hamric, 2000). Nurse advocates can make a difference for clients with chronic illness in the complex health care system.

Evolution of Nursing Advocacy

The role of the nurse, as advocate, has changed as society and the health care system have evolved. Nursing advocacy can be traced to Florence Nightingale's concern for the environment she found when she went to the Crimea to provide patient care, and to Lillian Wald's concern for the social issues impacting public health. Even though nurses have always had the potential to practice advocacy, as reflected in their problem-solving skills and abilities to assess and meet human needs, the implementation of nursing advocacy as a nursing role was slow in developing. Over time, nurses have moved from a focus on coordinating hospital policy and personnel and being accountable primarily to physicians to supporting the needs and rights of clients. Table 16-1 lists the major steps in the evolution of nursing advocacy.

Military Model

Although early nurses protected the confidence of their patients, they were required to avoid criticizing the hospital, training school, fellow nurses, or physicians. Nurses obeyed physician orders without question and helped maintain patient trust in the physician-patient relationship, even if it meant overlooking errors in judgment, decisions, or violations of patient rights. During this time, nurses were torn between their desire to be loyal to the patient and their required loyalty to the physician and institution (Winslow, 1984).

375

TABLE 16-1

Major Steps in the Evolution of Nursing Advocacy

Model	Key Component
Military	Nurse as loyal soldier
	Obedience to physician
	Loyalty to institution
Rights/legal	Nurse as protector of patient rights
Advocacy	Nurse with moral and legal
	responsibility to the patient

Rights/Legal Model

In the 1960s, national social policy began to reflect the philosophy that health care was the right of every individual. This change in policy was coupled with a rise in consumer activism and loss of consumer confidence in the way medicine was practiced (Starr, 1982). Consumers of health care were no longer willing to remain dependent on their physicians for information, support, and services; they demanded an increased role in decision making that affected them and wanted to know more about their conditions as a consistent part of client care. Consequently, as a result of the patient rights movement, there was an expressed desire for nurses to become advocates. This change in philosophy and growing activism led to a dramatic change in health care delivery. Simultaneously to the changes in national policy, professional organizations, including the American Nurses' Association (ANA), began defining and securing patients' rights, including the right to information about diagnosis; the right to therapy, prognosis, and informed consent; the right to privacy and confidentiality; and the right to die.

Advocacy Model

The role of patient advocacy emerged in the nursing literature in the late 1970s, and support for the role was reflected in professional organizations and schools (Mallik & Rafferty, 2000). In the 1970s the concept of nursing advocacy was incorporated into nursing's code of ethics. The International Council of Nursing (ICN) removed language that required nurses to maintain loyalty and obedience to physicians from the code of ethics (Snowball, 1996). Similarly, the ANA code deleted rules that obligated nurses to help maintain client confidence in physicians or to obey their orders automatically (Winslow, 1984).

In 2001, the ANA adapted a revised Code of Ethics for Nurses that was responsive to the present social and health care context and contemporary ethical challenges and issues. The Code of Ethics for Nurses requires the nurse to promote, advocate for, and strive to protect the health, safety, and the rights of patients (ANA, 2001). The revised code establishes a greater foundation of patient advocacy among nurses, emphasizes the importance of patient autonomy (White, 2002) and provides a framework for nurses to use in ethical analysis and decision-making (Olson, 2001).

For nursing, the evolution of the advocate role was an important step toward recognizing and accepting the client as an active participant in health care decision making, and empowering clients as self-determining consumers of health care. Client empowerment is furthered by administrative protocols such as policies and procedures that meet individual needs.

Defining Advocacy

Advocacy is complex and multidimensional. The nursing literature presents multiple interpretations of advocacy. For some, advocacy is constructed at the macrolevel involving organizations, systems and policy (Avery & Bashir, 2003; Bassett, 2003; Grace, 2001; Milio, 2002; Smith, 2004). For other nursing scholars, advocacy focuses on empowerment (Falk-Rafael, 2001; Maliski, Clerkin, & Litwin, 2004), promoting client self-determination (Gadow, 1990) or autonomy (Breier-Mackie, 2001; Schroeter, 2000), informed decision making (Aylett & Fawcett, 2003; Kohnke, 1980), mediation (Williams & Gossett, 2001; Winslow, 1984), and humanism (Curtin, 1979). Nevertheless, what is common to all definitions and perspectives of advocacy is a primary commitment to the health care of clients.

Advocacy activities seek to redistribute power and link resources to people (individuals or groups) who demonstrate a need. While the ideal of nursing advocacy is to empower clients within the health care system, many times institutional, social, political, economic, and cultural constraints prevent clients from accessing health care. When such constraints are present, an advocate is necessary to facilitate procurement.

Self-Care Nursing Theory

To be relevant to nursing practice, advocacy must be planned within a nursing framework, and the nursing theory selected will determine which advocacy strategies will be used. This author prefers Orem's self-care theory (1995), which asserts that individuals should care for themselves unless there is a defined self-care limitation. Self-care activities are those that individuals initiate and perform on their own behalf to maintain health and well-being. Because individuals with chronic illnesses primarily care for themselves in their own environments, self-care is particularly important for them. However, many of these individuals have limited functioning— that is, self-care deficits—including limitations of knowing, limited motivation, limitations in physical ability, limitations in making judgments and decisions, and limitations in self-management (Orem, 1995). In addition, clients may lack adequate social or family support.

Orem (1995) identified the following self-care abilities:

- Gathering and using air, food, and fluid from the environment
- Excreting waste such as urine and feces in socially acceptable ways
- Providing a clean, safe environment, such as maintaining the skin as a protective barrier and maintaining a safe, comfortable temperature
- Maintaining a balance between rest and activity
- Maintaining a healthy relationship with self and with others

Often, individuals with chronic illnesses experience unrecognized requirements for assistance associated with their changed functional status. For example, new treatment regimens may not be understood by the client, who would therefore require adequate and appropriate knowledge and information. In addition, the client needs to learn about alternate courses of action that are available, including the potential consequences of each action, so an informed decision can made. The nurse is in the position to provide this information and to provide assistance, if desired by the client, once an acceptable course of action has been identified. The activities of the advocate would be determined by the limitations(s) and experience of the client, because the goal of advocacy is to promote the development of enabling capabilities—that is, power components— thus minimizing the effects of the chronic illness.

Philosophical Foundations of Advocacy in Nursing

The manner in which the nurse advocate intercedes to increase the client's power components depends on the underlying values and beliefs held by the nurse regarding the advocate role. The literature reveals a number of advocacy perspectives or models that are not mutually exclusive (Table 16-2). Elements, separate or in combination, of each of these models are evident in contemporary nursing practice.

Paternalistic Advocacy

In paternalism, the professional-client relationship is professionally dictated. Paternalism values client health above client autonomy and is guided by the principles of beneficence (protect from harm) and nonmaleficence (avoid inflicting harm). The paternalistic view centers around an authority figure, be it physician or nurse, who determines what is best

TABLE 16-2

Philosophical Foundations for Advocacy in Nursing

Type	Distinguishing Elements
Paternalistic advocacy	Beneficence "Nonmaleficence"
Consumerism advocacy	Patient autonomy
Consumercentric advocacy	Patient autonomy with nurse input
Existential advocacy	Nurse–client relationship for meaning Self-determination
Humanistic advocacy	Client autonomy within nurse–client relationship rather than client independence

for the client (Haggerty, 1985). Information is selectively distributed to or withheld from a client in order to control the decision-making process, with the caveat that the caretaker's expertise will seek the best decisions possible for the client. Paternalism uses coercion in order to provide a good outcome (in the eyes of the decision maker), but one that is not necessarily desired by the ones it is intended to benefit.

Historically, paternalism was viewed as advocacy and welcomed by both clients and communities as appropriate health care provider behavior (Haggerty, 1985). Even today, some nurses view paternalism from a positive perspective, as helpful and other-serving. In these situations, the advocate believes that decisions should be made by those most capable of knowing what actions are in the clients' best interests. Thus, they feel the client's right to the best possible care is protected.

Consumer Advocacy

Within the context of consumer advocacy, consumers are the active decision makers in the health care system. Client goals from this perspective include (1) the right to equal access to health care services, (2) the right to public education regarding health care is-

sues, and (3) the right to knowledge of alternative treatments (Bramlett, Gueldner & Sowell, 1990).

Nurses serve as consumer guides who present information to a client and then withdraw, allowing the client to make his or her decision(s) privately (Kohnke, 1980). The nurse does not assist the client in the decision-making process itself.

The actions of the consumer guide are twofold. The first is to inform clients of their rights in particular situations and ensure that they have all the necessary information and knowledge available to make informed decisions. This information must be presented so it can be understood by clients and be free of any personal biases held by the nurse. The second is to support the client in whatever decisions he or she makes, even though the nurse, other health professionals, families, or friends may not agree with this decision.

In this model, both the provision of information and withdrawal of the nurse are important, because it is assumed that the client's decisions must be made privately in order to prevent undue influence. It is possible that consumerism dehumanizes clients by assuming they require only appropriate data in order to process a decision. The model implies there is no need for any assistance beyond this point.

Consumercentric Advocacy

Consumercentric advocacy is also driven by consumer demands for access, information, and availability of alternatives; its primary aim is to mobilize resources to promote client well-being. Consumercentric advocacy is unique in its combined emphasis on the client's rights in decision making, linked with the nurse's role in promoting these rights (Bramlett et al., 1990). Components central to this model of advocacy are (1) maximum transfer of knowledge to the client, (2) client decision-making with assistance from the nurse, and (3) the nurse's support of the client's implementation of decisions.

The nurse's role in knowledge transfer serves to assure the client that all information needed is presented in understandable form. As with the consumer advocacy model, the ultimate decision rests with the client, and it is honored by the nurse, regardless of its degree of congruence with the values of others or the established norms of the health care system. Consumercentric advocacy extends consumer advocacy in that the nurse serves as an active partner of the client in the decision-making process, planning, and implementation phase to carry out the client's decision(s) if the client so wishes (Bramlett et al., 1990).

Existential Advocacy

Gadow (1990) asserts that the essence of nursing is existential advocacy, which is based on the principle that freedom of self-determination is a most fundamental and valuable human right. The model of existential advocacy focuses on the ideal "that individuals be assisted by nursing to exercise authentically their freedom of self-determination" (p. 43). In this context, *authentic* means reaching decisions that are one's own and reflective of the entire complexity of one's values.

In this model, the nurse is willing to set aside personal values and beliefs to facilitate the personal meaning of the clients' experiences. As an existential advocate, the nurse acts in the client's best interests, but the client determines what these best interests are in accordance with his or her own unique set of values. The opportunity for the nurse to assist clients in clarifying their values is enhanced because the nurse is present during the time that the client is feeling vulnerable and distressed. Nurses have sustained contact with clients, allowing the nurse to view the client as an individual rather than as a "health problem" or "diagnosis."

Existential advocacy does more than provide information; it promotes nurse interaction with clients to determine the personal, unique meaning that the experiences of health, illness, suffering, or dying have for those individuals. The ideal is for clients to be assisted by a nurse to exercise their self-determination (Gadow, 1990).

Humanistic Advocacy

Curtin (1979) believes that advocacy is "based upon our common humanity, our common needs and our common human rights" (p. 3). It is the commonality of being human that serves as the basis of any relationship between nurses and clients. As advocates, nurses must "assist patients to find meaning or purpose in their living and in their dying" (p. 7). In short, the role of the nurse advocate is to "create an atmosphere in which something intangible (human values, respect, compassion) can be realized. . . . This is not-so-simple, good nursing practice" (p. 123).

Humanistic advocacy, as the foundation of the nurse-patient relationship, requires an understanding that each client is a unique human being. In fact, the opportunity for nurses to acquire a deeper knowledge and appreciation of the client in this way is enhanced by establishing long-term relationships with clients and participating in the intimate details of their physical and emotional care.

However, how and when clients are given information is as significant as what they are told. The humanistic nurse advocate has the opportunity to provide all information relative to a situation to clients as they request it and are prepared for it. Although nurses participate in the decision-making process with clients, it is the client who determines what his or her best interests are (Curtin, 1979).

The Need for Advocacy

The role of client in and of itself calls for an advocate. Upon entry into the health care system, the client relinquishes control over his/her life, loses self-identity and initiative, and becomes distant from supportive networks. The client is in a strange environment in which institution protocols may coerce the client to adopt a subordinate role in which they agree with a powerful health care professional and feel the need to comply rather than refuse treatment (Baldwin, 2003). The client's voice may be ignored by health care professionals or quieted by dwindling energy levels that comes from the disease process itself or the side effects of treatment. Clients and their families are vulnerable and powerless in the health care power structure (Davis, Konishi, & Tashiro, 2003). Further, the reductionism tendencies of medicine in which the client is viewed in terms of a diagnosis or symptoms or treatments (Mitchell & Bournes, 2000) diminishes the individual as an active participant in health care decisions.

Client autonomy, a fundamental ethical principle within Western health care systems, embraces one's right to choose one's goals and ends and ensures that clients have the capacity and right to decide for themselves what is in their best interests (Breier-Mackie, 2001). The necessity for advocacy stems from the impact illness has on the individual's autonomy and ability to make decisions. *Individual autonomy* is commonly defined as the ability of an individual to respond, react, or develop independently without outside control—that is, the right to make independent decisions and determine individual actions. Clients face conflicts and situations that demand decision-making, yet oftentimes they are ill equipped to make such decisions. Client autonomy necessitates the empowering of clients by providing information (Breier-Mackie, 2001; Haggerty, 1985).

An antecedent to advocacy is vulnerability (Baldwin, 2003). Vulnerability is a key issue for health care professionals (de Chasnay, 2005) in that vulnerable clients have a greater probability of developing health problems (Aday, 2001) and experience compromised autonomy as they lack the ability to control the outcome. The burden of chronic illness disproportionately affects vulnerable populations (Sullivan, Weinert, & Cudney, 2003). Vulnerable clients are least able to identify and express their needs and desires beyond the completely obvious (Niven & Scott, 2003; Segesten & Fagring, 1996). Chronic conditions are a significant health care challenge, and one's vulnerability is often brought into sharp focus by illness or disease. Vulnerability is an indication that nurses need to act as advocates (Mallik, 1997).

The presence of an adversary dictates the need for an advocate. The adversary may be a disease, circumstances such as pain and suffering, or even fellow human beings, such as health care professionals. An adversary may be the difference in care priorities and autonomy perspectives between nurses and physicians. The goal of nursing emphasizes client

normality and independence as defined by clients' abilities whereas physicians emphasize beneficence through treatment provision. Advocacy is needed to ensure that the client has the opportunity to participate in health care decisions (Breier-Mackie, 2001). Advocates most frequently intercede on behalf of clients with other nursing staff to alter or modify care routines, with social welfare workers, and with family members, particularly parents, regarding decision making for children (Segesten & Fagring, 1996).

Advocate Roles

The nurse-client relationship has long served as a foundation for understanding the nature of nursing. Central to advocacy are therapeutic relationships in which the client's wishes are articulated (Roberts, 2004). Communication and listening, important components of a therapeutic relationship, are necessary for advocating (Olsen, 2001). The client's perspective is required of any advocacy work (Mitchell & Bournes, 2000). The purpose of the nurse-client relationship is to maintain and restore control to clients (Curtin, 1988) and embodies mutuality, reciprocity, and moral decision making (Gadow, 1990). As clients come to know the nature and meaning of their illnesses, their power tends to be restored and their vulnerability is reduced, which are particularly salient points for those with chronic illnesses because of the enduring nature of these illnesses.

Because nurses have a sound knowledge of health care and work closely with clients, nurses remain the most suitable profession to perform the advocacy role (O'Connell, 2000; Mallik, 1997). Despite limited nursing literature regarding the role of advocacy in the care of clients with chronic conditions, nursing advocacy is relevant to this population. As an advocate, the nurse speaks on behalf of clients who may not be able to speak for themselves and articulates their needs to those in power. The advocate may be a representative for clients, a counselor who alleviates fear, protects client rights, and restores autonomy and self-control, or a health care professional who forms the link between the client's personal values and goals and biomedical interventions. In addition, the advocate may be an information provider, a monitor of quality care, or a spokesperson. The nurse, as advocate of client autonomy, is aligned with the client rather than with physicians, families, or hospitals. The nurse does this by carrying out key functions.

Advocacy requires tact, diplomacy, specific knowledge, and skills such as effective communication, negotiation, and timing. It also requires commitment from individual nurses as well as from the profession of nursing as a whole (Black, 2004). Advocacy involves valuing client autonomy, the right to choose, as well as taking action for client self-determination (Schroeter, 2000). However, the presence of these attributes does not guarantee successful advocacy.

Professional responsibility to the health care client is a salient feature of advocacy. Four characteristics are necessary to carry out the advocacy role effectively. First, advocates need to be assertive in helping clients meet their needs. Second, the advocate must be willing to take risks for the benefit of clients. Third, the advocate must have the ability to communicate clearly and effectively, state the clients' problems in a succinct manner, and work toward problem resolution. Fourth, the advocate needs to be able to identify the power bases and work with the system in order to identify appropriate resources to facilitate change for clients (Allender & Spradley, 2005).

Decision-Making Consultant

The advocate is a consultant to the health care client who may be facing ambiguity about an illness or disease. Providing information about the illness and what services are available will enable the client to make an informed decision (Aylett & Fawcett, 2003). Nurse advocates respect clients as the primary decision makers in their own health and treatments. The goal of nursing actions, therefore, is to enhance and support the client's responsibility and self-determination to the fullest extent possible (American Nurses Association, 1985). Haggerty (1985) identified three standard conditions for rational decision-making by clients:

1. An understanding of the treatments or procedures being proposed
2. The ability to evaluate the risks and benefits of the proposed treatments or procedures, and the ability to deliberate about the pros and cons of the proposed treatments or procedures
3. The capability of making decisions regarding the proposed treatments or procedures

Others describe the Options, Outcomes, Values and Likelihood Guide (OOVL Guide), which is a decision-making guide for both professionals and consumers (Lewis, Hepburn, Corcoran-Perry, Narayan, & Lally, 1999). Nurses must provide clients all information necessary to make a decision and support the client once the decision has been made.

Translator

The nurse advocate may serve as a translator for the client with chronic illness. The advocate as translator may help clients make sense of the health care system. Frequently, health care providers use terminology or medical jargon that is not understood by the client. The advocate may need to explain and decipher the information into understandable, practical terms for the client. The client may have a conversation with the physician that s/he cannot decipher, making it necessary for the nurse to clarify patient-physician communication (Williams, & Gossett, 2001). As a translator, the advocate helps the client to transform his or her desires and wishes into a cogent treatment plan (Schwartz, 2002) and guides the health care team in the direction preferred by the client.

For those clients who are unable to communicate in English, the advocate ensures client access to linguistically appropriate services. The advocate ensures that the person used to interpret for the client is appropriate, not a family member and qualified, not a member of the ancillary staff. In settings where in-person translation is not feasible, the advocate will need to facilitate the use of other resources such as AT&T that can provide translation support via telephone. The advocate may need to provide health education materials that are written in the language of the client at a readability level that is appropriate for the client's reading abilities.

Navigator

Advocates need to protect client autonomy in a potentially overwhelming and intimidating health care system by serving as expert navigators of the system and assisting clients to do what s/he would otherwise be unable to do (Schwartz, 2002). Clients may have adequate knowledge to make informed decisions but lack the ability to navigate the complex and fragmented health care system. Nurses need to take leadership in helping clients find their way (Courts, Buchanan, & Werstlein, 2004). The advocate as a navigator promotes holistic care by ensuring the client can access the right level of care in the right setting at the right time so that all of the client's health needs are addressed. Core competencies of client navigators are client education, emotional support, scheduling, language translation and referral to other services (Curran, 2003).

Mediator

To assume the role of mediator, the advocate must know the client. It is the nurse-client relationship that empowers the nurse to represent the client to the interdisciplinary team (Breier-Mackie, 2001). To fulfill a mediating role effectively, the advocate must be reactive and sensitive to professional and societal factors that stimulate conflict. As a mediator, the nurse advocate listens, clarifies, and makes suggestions to assist parties to understand each other so as to facilitate agreement on a particular action. The nurse also mediates between the medical choice of a particular treatment and the client's personal understanding of the benefit that may exist (Gadow, 1990). Nurses mediate and clarify communications between the patient and physician and directly or indirectly influence physician-client communications (Williams & Gossett, 2001). The advocate may also intercede on behalf of others, particularly those who do not have political or economic power and those who experience barriers to access health care on their own. Nurses mediate between clients and community resources, clients and medical services, and clients and their families. The advocate needs to identify the power bases that exist and work within the system in order to find appropriate resources to facilitate change for the client (Allender & Spradley, 2005).

Information Provider

Knowledge is power, but only when that knowledge is relevant to the client. In order to provide appropriate information, the advocate must listen to the needs, wants and desires of the client. When clients feel unheard, have no voice, they feel invalidated and dismissed and feel powerless (Courts et al., 2004). Clients value knowledge about their chronic conditions and view comprehensive treatment approaches as valuable and supportive. Due to the nature of many chronic conditions, there is an ongoing need for current and specific information. Clients in health care settings need to be knowledgeable about their rights and need appropriate and adequate information to make informed decisions; that is, they need to be educated as to the nature of the intervention, treatment, care, and outcome. Advocates not only inform clients of the benefits of a specific treatment or procedure, but also of the potential risks or consequences associated with that course of action, and should be told of the "no-treatment" option, which is an important component of informed decision-making. For example, surgical intervention has inherent risks, and the outcome may not necessarily be what the client anticipated. Telling the truth requires nurses to let go of the belief that they can "fix" things for their clients (Miller, Cohen & Kagan, 2000).

Clients are increasingly knowledgeable about their chronic conditions through the Internet and mass media. Many visit their physicians with requests for specific tests or medications (Corbin & Cherry, 2001). While the nurse may not be an expert in all aspects of chronic illness, it is a nursing responsibility to seek out information through collaboration with others, such as expert clinicians. When appropriate, the advocate may refer the client to the Internet for additional information. The limitations and usefulness of the Internet as an appropriate information source for the client must be evaluated by the nurse advocate.

Anticipatory Guide

Anticipatory guidance for individuals who have chronic illnesses and their families is an important component of the nurse-advocate role. Given his or her knowledge and experience, the advocate is in a position to anticipate problems that may arise. Uncertainty of the illness trajectory suggests the need for someone to act with clients (Aylett & Fawcett, 2003). Anticipatory guidance is based on identifying expected future needs, and can begin weeks, months, or years before any actual help is required. Future needs can have a profound effect on clients' lives because major life decisions can be influenced by them. Clients need a listener, a coach, to help them chart their course throughout their chronic illness (Courts et al., 2004). For example, anticipating the need for increasing care of a spouse with Alzheimer's disease may be a factor in a wife's decision to select among respite, in-home, or institutional care. In addition, anticipating future dependency needs allows clients with progressive chronic illnesses to express their own wishes and preferences for care options. Even though informed anticipation may lack certainty, it facilitates greater rational future planning, thus avoiding potentially difficult decisions made at the last minute (Nolan, Keady & Grant, 1995).

Referral Resource

In addition, to providing information about the chronic disease itself, the advocate provides information about available, accessible, appropriate and affordable resources and services in the community to meet the client's needs. Advocacy involves linking clients with resources (Falk-Rafael, 2001). The ad-

vocate may link the client with the American Cancer Society or the American Lung Association programs that can make their lives easier. The advocate needs to maintain current information about community resources or services, which can be at the local (private or public), state, or federal level. The advocate determines the client's needs and preferences and selects available resources that are appropriate. In addition, the advocate helps the client to maximize the selected resource to its fullest potential. Finally, the advocate evaluates the effectiveness and acceptability of the resource to the client.

Spokesperson

When speaking on behalf of a client who is unable or unwilling to speak on his or her own behalf, the advocate must communicate clearly and effectively and be able to state the client's problem(s) from the client's perspective in a succinct manner. This requires that the advocate be assertive and, sometimes, outspoken. It also requires that the advocate be willing to take risks for the benefit of the client (Allender & Spradley, 2005). For example, the wife of a man with hemiplegia may tend to be overprotective and refuse to let her husband engage in many of the activities of daily living. The spokesperson can explore with the wife the benefits of allowing her husband be more independent, thus promoting the voice of the husband.

Public Relations

The advocate may also perform by providing education to community groups about particular health issues. Examples of groups with which nurse-advocates have been involved are attachment disorder groups and Alzheimer's disease groups. Another important aspect of public relations by the advocate is to help people become more aware of the availability of nurse advocacy.

In summary, the client with a chronic condition must be a full partner with the nurse in health care decision-making. This relationship must be based on an emancipatory model as opposed to the traditional authoritative relationship. When health care professionals are unable to value client expertise, their behaviors fuel a mutual alienation in chronic illness relationships (Thorne, Nyhlin & Paterson, 2000).

Problems and Issues

There are a number of potential issues linked to advocacy; awareness of these increases the possibility that they can be overcome. These issues include internal barriers, such as client and nurse factors, and external barriers, such as constraints associated with the social environment.

Client Factors Affecting Advocacy

Clients may experience alterations in their self-care capabilities that interfere with their quality of life (see Chapter 9, on quality of life). These include lack of confidence, lack of readiness, conflict with family or health care providers, functional impairments, and sociocultural influences.

Lack of Confidence

Confidence is a positive quality that enhances personal coping and success. Chronic illnesses have the potential to strip away a client's sense of self-worth and sense of confidence. Love (1995) reported that clients who lack confidence often are unable to assess their needs accurately and consequently do not protect their self-interests effectively. Such clients are at risk of being manipulated or coerced by others and may capitulate to the wishes of family members or health care professionals out of fear and guilt. Clients' confidence levels are increased when the nurse demonstrates an interest and value in the client as an individual.

For those clients who lack confidence, the advocate may need to intervene when a decision needs to be made or a treatment plan is incongruent with the client's lifestyle or personal roles. For example, a physician who orders total bed rest for a mother who has three young children in the household who require supervision and care.

Lack of Readiness

Readiness is coupled with change. When clients are no longer able to maintain status quo with their health condition, they realize a need for change. Clients with a high degree of readiness report less anger, less depression, and view their condition in a more positive light. Those who experience a low degree of readiness report feeling depressed, afraid and vulnerable in the face of change (Dalton & Gottlieb, 2003). The nurse advocate role in readiness is to trigger and support readiness by acknowledging the client's concerns, listening to his or her perspective and respecting the client's perspective about what needs to change. Imparting knowledge and information to clients is an exchange process and requires active client participation. However, there are times when clients may not desire an exchange of information due to a lack of self-esteem, fear of the information, or lack of ability to understand the information imparted by the advocate. During these times, the advocate should encourage clients to seek information at a later time, when they are ready for information.

Conflict with Family or Health Care Professionals

Chronic illness impacts the individual as well as the family and can cause major changes in family roles and functioning. The number of families caring for members who have a chronic condition is significant and growing (Sullivan-Bolyai et al., 2003). Families are increasingly replacing skilled health care workers by providing complex and ongoing care to their relatives with chronic illness (McCorkle & Pasacreta, 2001). Conflict among families can result when family members become fatigued and overwhelmed with caregiving responsibilities. In such cases, the focus of advocacy may extend beyond the individual to family caregivers who also need information and intervention strategies about physical and psychological aspects of chronic illness care (McCorkle & Pasacreta, 2001). It is important to help families consider how they will frame an issue that will be amenable to problem solving and decision-making (Walker, 2001). The advocate can relieve some caregiver anxiety and stress by providing assistance in guiding them through the health care system.

When clients make their own decisions and act on them, there may be a difference between the clients' choices and those that would be made by family members or health care professionals. Consequently, clients not only may experience disapproval from others regarding their decisions, but also may encounter resistance when attempting to implement them. In these instances, it is the responsibility of the advocate to assure clients of their rights and responsibilities to make decisions and to reassure them that they need not make changes because others may have objections to these choices (Bramlett et al., 1990).

The case study of Mr. Smith is an example of how a client and caregiver can differ regarding the course of action needed to deal with a problem. This case study generates a number of concerns for Bill Jones, who is a nurse-advocate for his clients. How much control belongs to Mr. Jones? How much to Mr. Smith? What control do family caregivers have? How do control issues affect the nurse-client rela-

tionship they have? How do control issues impact on the nurse-family relationship? How do control issues impact on the client-family relationship? What should guide Mr. Jones' approach in the care of this client?

Functional Impairments

Clients with significant physical or mental impairments may be unable to serve as their own advocates or to enlist others to be their advocates. These individuals can remain in the community if they are able to arrange for care. In some instances, the client becomes isolated and unable to access needed systems, such as home-delivered meals or transportation. It is important that the nurse-advocate determine whether the client is capable of being his or her own agent. If this is deemed unlikely, the client may need to be referred to the courts to have a conservator appointed. In these cases, the advocate's role is generally determined by the legal system.

Substituted Judgment   For clients who are incapacitated and cannot care for themselves independ-

The Problem of Pressure Ulcers—Part I

Mr. Smith is a 54-year-old man who was diagnosed with amyotrophic lateral sclerosis (ALS) eight years ago. He lives at home with his wife and their adolescent daughter and receives nursing care and support from professional and ancillary nursing staff from a local home health agency on a daily basis. His primary nurse is Bill Jones, R.N. Despite extreme muscle weakness, Mr. Smith is able to sit in his motorized wheelchair for most of the day. Although he is physically dependent on others, Mr. Smith is mentally competent and is able to continue his professional work life on a part-time basis. Mr. and Mrs. Smith are extremely knowledgeable about his disease process and prognosis.

During the last few weeks, Mr. Smith has developed pressure ulcers from sitting in his wheelchair for extended periods of time. Bill informs him that he needs to spend less time in his wheelchair to promote healing and decrease the progression of his ulcer. But Mr. Smith refuses to alter his daily routine. Additionally, he frequently stays at work late, extending the time he spends sitting in his wheelchair. When he returns home in the afternoon, he refuses to be put back into bed, stating that he wants to spend time with his family. His ulcers are becoming worse and may require extensive medical and nursing intervention to ameliorate the problem.

ently or ensure their own safety, conservatorship can be a powerful tool in the management and treatment of these individuals (Lamb & Weinberger, 1993). Under the doctrine of substituted judgment, a guardian or conservator is appointed by the courts to oversee health care or financial matters on behalf of the incapacitated person (Clark, 1997). The client may request a conservator, or others may request that one be appointed.

Conservatorship is a protective mechanism, overseen by the courts, by which a surrogate makes personal decisions on the client's behalf (Reynolds, 1997). Such protective methods require balance between maintaining the client's personal freedom or self-determination and providing protection. Even when the client (the conservatee) has relinquished his or her decision-making authority, it is imperative the decisions made by the surrogate be congruent with the desires of the client. If subjective and objective evidence is not available, the conservator is expected to make decisions deemed to be in the conservatee's best interests. Under such circumstances, the advocate may be jointly involved with the conservator in the decision-making process relative to the care of the client (Lamb & Weinberger, 1993).

The conservator not only is appointed by the courts, but also is responsible to the courts to look out for the client's interests. Among other things, the conservator plays an important role in clinical management on behalf of gravely disabled persons, such as determining the arrangements necessary to provide adequate food, clothing, shelter, and treatment, especially if the client does not have close family involvement and support (Lamb & Weinberger, 1993). In this situation, the nurse collaborates with the conservator, and possibly others, to implement the advocate role effectively.

Social and Cultural Influences

Culture is significant to the health and well being of individuals. Humans exist within culture, and culture is a universal phenomenon (Leininger, 1995). Culture is learned, shared, and dynamic (Andrews & Boyle, 2003). Leininger & McFarland

(2002) define culture care as "the subjectively and objectively learned and transmitted values, beliefs and patterned lifeways that assist, support, facilitate or enable another individual or group to maintain their health and well-being, to improve their human condition and lifeway or to deal with illness, handicaps, or death" (p. 83). Culture impacts and dictates one's responses to normal events of everyday life and is a driving force in the decisions and choices that individuals and families make about health and care (Fletcher, 2002, Salas-Provance, Erickson, & Reed, 2002). Advocates must know the cultural values, beliefs and practices of clients and act accordingly. Cultural factors are an invaluable blueprint in caring for clients with chronic illness in which care is person oriented rather than disease oriented. Culturally congruent care is care that is beneficial, satisfying and meaningful to those served by nurses (Leininger, 1995).

Critical to providing culturally appropriate care is the cultural context of the individual. Culturally appropriate care can only occur when culture care values, expressions, or patterns are known and used appropriately (Leininger, 1995). Assumptions or biased expectations cannot replace accurate assessments of clients and their families. Members of a cultural group do not necessarily fit into the textbook description of that culture's stereotypical behavior (Andrews & Boyle, 2003). Persons from some ethnic groups may seek nontraditional healers such as curendaras and shamans while others from that same ethnic group may not. Some Muslim men may not want to be touched by a female health care professional, but for others, the gender of the health care provider may not be a cultural taboo.

Advocacy which emphasizes individual autonomy may conflict with cultural customs and beliefs. Many cultural groups are group-oriented rather than individual-oriented. For group-oriented persons or families, advocacy must be modified to include all members of the family rather than just the individual. For example, Arab husbands frequently accompany their wives for health care visits limiting confidential communication with female clients. In some Native American families, health care decisions are made by the matriarch of the family rather than the individual. Failure to include her in the decision-making process significantly diminishes advocacy effectiveness. In other cultures, the oldest male is the person with whom to speak on health care matters. Japanese view individuals as embedded in social relationships (Davis, Konishi, & Tashiro, 2003). Cultural conflicts may arise when families are not consulted before an intervention or staff interferes with rituals deemed necessary by the client's family. Conversely, when a client chooses to go against a cultural norm or custom, the client has the right to do so. In situations where families are in disagreement with the person about compliance with cultural customs, the nurse advocate must support the client and give the individual the resources necessary to carry out self determination in the situation (Zoucha & Husted, 2000).

Nurse Factors Affecting Advocacy

As an advocate, the nurse must act within the context of the work situation and the possibilities available. It may, consequently, be difficult for the nurse to fulfill the responsibilities of the advocate role due to a number of barriers. Advocates are accountable for their actions and must be prepared to accept the consequences of those actions while remaining within the limits of professional codes of practice. It is not the illness that clients identify as the reason for their vulncrability but the way health care professionals relate to them (Mitchell & Bourne, 2000).

Cultural Competence

Nurses who are culturally competent serve as better advocates for health care clients (de Chesnay et al., 2005). Cultural competence is a process in which the nurse integrates cultural awareness, cultural knowledge, cultural skill, cultural encounters and cultural desire to provide care (Campinha-Bacote, 2002). This model assumes variation among persons of ethnic and cultural groups, when persons may or may not adhere to what is known about a

particular cultural or ethnic group. It is imperative for nurses to explore potential differences and similarities among clients and their beliefs to ensure culturally congruent care (Leininger & McFarland, 2002). Leininger (1995) asserts "clients who experience nursing care that fails to be reasonably congruent with the client's beliefs, values, and care lifeways will show signs of cultural conflicts, noncompliance, stresses, and ethical or moral concerns" (p. 45). Failure of advocates to acknowledge and incorporate the client's cultural perspective leads to an environment of misrepresentation and poor communication. Therefore, cultural competence is imperative for the client advocate.

Many health care professionals are not trained adequately to overcome the language and cultural barriers of clients (Thomas, Richardson, & Saleem, 2000). The advocate needs a working knowledge of cultural values, beliefs, and practices of individuals and groups to provide culturally congruent care and the ability to integrate cultural practices and beliefs into the formal health care system. When folk care and professional care are not congruent, recovery, health and well-being of the client are impacted (Leininger, 1995). Thus, it is necessary for the advocate to promote and facilitate the integration of traditional or folk health care methods such as folk healers, religious acts or ceremonies and family participation into plan of care. The role of advocate can be a cultural bridge between professional and folk care (Zoucha, 2000). While knowledge of cultural values and norms is imperative for the nurse advocate, the views held by the individual must be known as well. The desires and wishes of the individual client supersede the cultural values, beliefs and practices of the culture in which the individual and family are a part (Tang & Lee, 2004).

One's culture impacts and dictates responses to events of daily life. The advocate is also a cultural entity. Nurses come to the advocacy role with their own cultural experiences that impact their interactions. An advocate may not be conscious of his/her own cultural values and beliefs; therefore, advocates may need to examine their own values and beliefs that emanate from their personal heritage and review their own life experiences. Understanding one's own culture will enable the advocate to be more open to the world of others and advocate appropriately. Further, advocates need to examine their personal values and beliefs as they relate to the client's right to self-determination (Erlen, 2002).

Without knowledge and understanding of cultural care values, beliefs and practices of the client, nurses are more likely to impose their own values and beliefs on the client, thus failing to act as the client advocate. Further, if the nurse is unable or unwilling to honor the values of the client, advocacy will not occur.

Uncertainty

Without a consistent model of advocacy, defining the parameters of advocacy is uncertain (Hewitt, 2002). The role of nurse advocacy is poorly defined (Mallik, 1997), complex (Hewitt, 2002), and depends on knowledge of the nurse (Black, 2004).

Nurses lack the skills they need to resolve advocacy issues (Georges & Grypdonck, 2002). While some may not recognize rights violations, others lack experience and communication skills to facilitate advocacy. Problems with advocacy arise from uncertainty experienced by the nurse about what is right, legal, moral, or ethical. The development of advocacy practices is haphazard and situation-dependent as opposed to being taught in nursing education programs (Foley, Minick, & Lee, 2002). The literature provides little description of how nurses actually learn advocacy, even though advocacy is assumed to be a part of nursing education curriculum. An expected outcome of nursing education is nurses knowing how to protect clients and to be their advocate (Altun & Ersoy, 2003). Learning how to advocate involves differentiating between controlling client choices (domination and dependent) and assuring client choices (allowing freedom). Nursing education has an important responsibility for integrating ideas and concepts about client advocacy into the curriculum.

The knowledgable advocate may also experience uncertainty. If the nurse does not perceive support from the organization, that nurse may feel restricted to taking little if any action necessary for patient advocacy (Schroeter, 2000).

Role Conflict

Nurses may experience conflicting loyalties with themselves, their clients, their coworkers and their employers (Schroeter, 2002). A caveat associated with the client advocate role is a situation in which tensions among clients, employers, and professional bodies may put the nurse in a position of choosing between being an employee and the interests of clients. Under this circumstance, the nurse may be unsure as to which role comes first—advocate or employee—and therefore, must distinguish and separate the roles. If the role of employee comes first, the employer's rules and procedures take precedence; and then the nurse performs the role of advocate within those rules and procedures. Nevertheless, nurses must act to ensure safe, competent, legal and ethical care is provided to all clients (Schroeter, 2002). Nurses not only have the right but a duty to immediately report to their superiors whenever they are convinced there is an inappropriate diagnosis or treatment that will jeopardize the safety of the client. Failure of nurses to act as an advocate may result in liability for the individual nurse as well as the nurse's employer (Tammelleo, 2002).

Divergence between perspectives of nurses and physicians contributes to role conflicts. The nursing perspective is characterized by the desire to act according to client wishes while the physician perspective is characterized by the wish to act in accordance with treatment possibilities. Lack of understanding and an unwillingness to acknowledge the value of each perspective can lead to conflict (Georges & Grypdonck, 2002).

Unwillingness to Take Risks

Risk is inherent with the advocacy role. Some advocacy activities represent little if any risk to the advocate. Providing comfort measures poses little risk whereas reporting unsafe, unethical behavior by others can be of great risk to the advocate. Advocacy may require the nurse to take action on behalf of the client. Not all nurses are comfortable with conflict. Some nurses may not have the self-confidence necessary to stand up and speak out on behalf of clients. The advocate may lack empowerment due to a restrictive care environment or power hierarchies in the work environment that impact nursing autonomy (Schroeter, 2000). Nurses may be unwilling to step forward as advocates because they fear recrimination, be it loss of a job, face, status, or respect of colleagues (Martin, 1998) Those who do speak up may receive poor treatment from management. Being an advocate is a potentially difficult role for nurses to adopt (Mallik, 1997).

Nurses who refuse to enforce bad policies, to overlook poor standards of care, to hide misconduct, or to overlook the concerns of clients are frequently referred to as "whistleblowers". Nurses who report misconduct believe in client advocacy and feel they have a responsibility to clients (Ahenn & McDonald, 2002). Advocates need courage to overcome peer pressure to 'go along and get along'. Nurses need to safeguard the client when health care and safety are jeopardized by the incompetent, unethical or illegal practice of any health care professional (Mohr & Horton-Deutsch, 2001).

Appropriateness of the Advocacy Role

Mitchell and Bournes (2000) question whether advocacy may be more harmful than helpful to clients. Others question whether nurses have the autonomy, authority, and power to effectively advocate for patients within the hierarchy of the health care system (Hewitt, 2002; Hyland, 2002; Mitchell & Bournes, 2000). Some health care professionals argue that advocacy should not be the duty of the nurse and may interfere with ongoing health care. Nurses can become benevolent and believe they know what is best despite the client's independent decision (Valente, 2004).

Acting as an advocate for client rights may place the nurse in an adversarial position with the physi-

cian or institution, because there may be constraints instituted by the hierarchical systems of health care. Power imbalances between health professionals make advocacy roles difficult to fulfill. Since nurses are not the only health care professionals to perform the role of advocacy, they may need to join with other care professionals to provide a team approach to advocacy working with physicians and the health care power structure in order to maximize the benefits for all involved (Davis, Konish & Tashiro, 2003).

Time and Energy

Many nurses feel that assuming advocacy responsibilities is an additional nursing task that is time and energy consuming. Decreased personnel resources and increased client acuities are realities of health care today. Nurses may lack the time required to develop relationships with clients (Teasdale, 1998). While these and other factors may contribute to personal fatigue and perceived lack of time to advocate, it is how the nurse as an individual views humans and their illness experience that determines the advocacy. If the nurse respects clients as knowing partners, as teachers and leaders of their own illness, advocacy is not an additional role but a part of nursing practice (Mitchell & Bournes, 2000).

When advocacy is incorporated into the nursing process, advocacy does not necessarily take additional time. What may be time and energy consuming are the consequences of advocacy, which can include conferences, hearings, reports, and the time to consider, decide upon, and implement another course of action. If these changes in the plan of care are made in accordance with clients' wishes, the nurse is advocating for the clients each time he or she gives nursing care.

Undesirable Clients

The concept of undesirable exists only when an external evaluation is placed on the client by the health professional. Internal bias or prejudice held by the nurse creates visible or invisible barriers for clients. The advocate may consciously or unconsciously hold prejudices and biases toward certain groups of people. For some, it may be persons from specific ethnic groups. Some clients are viewed as having less social value than others (Glaser & Strauss, 1968). Social value is subjective and determined by such factors as age, marital status, income, living conditions, hygiene, behavior, and so forth. Other clients might be perceived as having low moral worth. The nurse might feel that the client's illness or condition is the result of behaviors chosen by the client, so the client is "getting what he or she deserves." Another group of clients who are seen as undesirable is those who do not behave within the prescribed norms of the institution or agency or are violent.

The nurse must advocate not only for the client he or she likes, but also on behalf of those who may be labeled as undesirable. This requires that nurses be aware of their own values and beliefs, and that they acknowledge their own negative feelings toward certain clients. Advocates must ensure that all persons are treated with respect and dignity.

Social Factors Affecting Advocacy

Barriers within the client's and nurse's social system may hinder or complicate advocacy. Therefore, advocacy must be considered within a broader social context.

Culture

Advocacy is practiced in a world comprised of people from many places practicing many cultures. Dramatic demographic changes are occurring in the United States with the Euro-American majority predicted to become the minority by 2050. As a result of these population shifts, nurses will be working with a greater number of clients from diverse cultural and ethnic backgrounds.

Advocacy is based upon a Western concept of individualism, a society consisting of autonomous individuals. Western societies promote the realization of the individual self as the goal, yet other cultures do not. The Western principle of autonomy is

self-determination, whereas the East Asian principle of autonomy is family-determination. Family is viewed as an autonomous social unit in which the entire family, not the client alone, has real authority in decision-making (Takemura, 2005). Culture is the context and driving force in the health care decisions individuals, families, and groups make.

Stratification

A number of competing forces operate within society that perpetuate inequities in the distribution of wealth and resources. The health care system in the United States is enormously costly and is characterized by both a poor distribution of resources and significant inequities of access (see Chapter 27, on financial impact). There is a correlation between poverty and illness (Bezruchka, 2000; 2001). Those persons who experience a marginalized sociocultural status and have limited access to economic resources have a greater than average risk of developing health problems (Aday, 2001). Advocacy activities are aimed at the macrolevel in which organizations and systems are modified and policy initiated to address the redistribution of power and resources to individuals or aggregates with an identified need. At the personal level, the advocate may connect clients to resources that are available and accessible to them in the community.

Stigma

There is evidence in the literature that negative attitudes about persons with chronic illnesses are held by society (see Chapter 3, on stigma). Stereotypes and misconceptions about chronic illnesses lead to a lack of inclusion.

Stereotypes are a set of inaccurate, simplistic generalizations about a group of individuals, based on unjustified preconceptions, allowing them to be treated adversely. Stigma is a response to any physical or social attribute or characteristic that devalues a person's social identity and disqualifies him or her from full social acceptance (Goffman, 1963). For the individual with an invisible stigma, this may not be a problem. For example, the person who has diabetes is in a better position to manage his or her illness without any adverse response from others. If the attribute is visible, such as being wheelchair-bound, others may indeed stigmatize the person.

For individuals with chronic illness, it may be necessary for the advocate to overcome his or her own preconceived notions and focus on identifying the client's needs. In addition, the advocate may focus attention on the stereotypes held by the general public and provide community education about children and adults with chronic conditions.

Health Care Policy

In general, contemporary health care policy focuses on reducing health care costs. Managed care systems have been implemented in a growing number of private and public health care programs for cost savings as well as control of future cost increases (see Chapters 27 and 26, on financial impact and politics and policy, respectively). Under a capitated reimbursement system, insurers may refuse to pay for costly rehabilitative services, may institute financial incentives to abbreviate care, or may cite lack of empirical data to deny rehabilitation as "medically necessary" (Banja, 1999). For example, many HMOs restrict access to needed hospitalization and other costly health care services for both children and adults. Individuals who experience an exacerbation of their mental illnesses may be denied needed hospitalization because of cost containment. Saving money frequently takes precedence over quality care. As another example, managed care programs may channel persons with diabetes to a general practitioner who lacks adequate training or experience with state-of-the-art diabetes treatment. Because diabetes is a complex chronic illness, a special level of expertise and experience is required to maintain an optimal level of wellness for clients.

Health Care System

The health care system perpetuates client vulnerability. The health care system has the potential to restrict the autonomy of people, and to disable and dominate them by virtue of its bureaucracy, scientific expertise and technology. Clients surrender their independence to the health care system where the physician is omniscient and the client begins the process of learned helplessness and an inability to speak for themselves (Hewitt, 2002). The focus of the contemporary health care system is cost containment and managed care. Private medical practice is being replaced with clinical conglomerates. Fee-for-service is being replaced by salaried and capitated payments. Hospitals have merged into investor-owned corporations wherein the bottom line is fiscal responsibility rather than quality care. Decisions in the health care system are made by power brokers who are neither providers nor consumers of health care, but insurance companies, Wall Street firms, think tanks, consultants, and pharmaceutical companies (Sheridan-Gonzalez, 2000). Many HMOs offering a comprehensive scope of services control utilization by means of a primary physician "gatekeeper" for diagnostic tests and procedures, specialist referrals, and tertiary care. Private insurance companies and publicly funded insurance programs have incorporated managed care by requiring preauthorization for testing, consultation, or hospital admission. Control of health care costs is achieved by regulating physician activities and client care; these acts are, in essence, managed care.

Since the 1970s individualism has extended into the health care system. Advanced directives, health care proxies, durable power of attorney and other mechanisms have been developed to ensure individual determination in health care decisions. Client empowerment has led to a population not only aware of their rights, but one that seeks remedy for perceived violation of those rights. The litigious nature of the health care system impacts advocacy. Advocates need to balance the humanistic values of nursing with the highly technological and specialized health care delivery system.

Paternalism

Health care professionals who impose their own values and beliefs on the client limit clients' possibilities and create situations of domination and dependence (Mitchell & Bournes, 2000). Professional dominance creates and exacerbates social differences between physicians and clients. The physician is assumed to be the knowledgeable expert, while clients are considered only recipients of the physician's professional services. Because knowledge is power, one way to retain professional power is to control the flow of information to clients.

The imbalance of power is characteristic of the physician-client relationship. Clients may not feel comfortable asking their physicians questions, so they often turn to the nurse to clarify communications. For example, elderly clients frequently do not question their physicians when they feel that treatment is inappropriate or needs to be modified but may feel comfortable in telling their nurse with whom they have developed a trusting relationship. Clients may be unable to verbalize their needs to their physicians either because they are intimidated by the physicians' perceived power or because the physicians lack the time to listen to the client's concerns. Nurses are ideally positioned to assist clients and their families to clarify their needs and wishes (Breier-Mackie, 2001).

Clients may see nurses as paternalistic based on two underlying assumptions: (1) the nurse has superior knowledge to decide what is best for clients, and (2) the nurse has the authority to make decisions on behalf of the clients (Haggerty, 1985). Even though the nurse may have the education and experience to make many decisions on behalf of clients, when the nurse does so without considering client consent, the nurse strips away a basic human right—the right to self-determination.

Paternalism can be harmful to clients and self-serving to health care professionals as paternalism fails to respect the individual and the right to participate in the decision-making process (Mitchell & Bournes, 2000). Persons living with chronic illness are particularly vulnerable to the harmful effects of paternalism. McCurdy (1997), an individual who lives with muscular dystrophy, reports vulnerability stems not only from his illness but the way health care professionals relate to him, specifically, the dehumanizing, controlling, punitive, judgmental practices of health care professionals.

Irresolvable Problems

When conflict develops between clients and the physician, the nurse advocate seeks to uncover and clarify the client's and physician's perspectives. The nurse may not be able to address all advocacy problems and issues because some issues are beyond the scope of the nurse. There are problems of distortion when the individual's perception of a situation differs from reality, that is, when there is a belief that the problem has no solution or that the problem does not exist. Under these circumstances, the problem may need to be redefined in solvable terms. There may also be problems beyond the grasp of the advocate, such as legislation, regulations, or policy (Chafey et al., 1998).

■ Interventions

The essence of advocacy is to empower the client for independence in the health care system. The client may need information or guidance in services and resources to meet their specific needs. The advocate may need to focus on the system itself to make the system more responsive and relevant to the needs of clients. By calling attention to inadequate, inaccessible, or unjust care, the nurse can influence change on behalf of the client. An advocacy situation can be triggered in any of the following ways (Segesten & Fagring, 1996):

- A verbalized request from the client. For example, "Would you ask the doctor for me?"
- A stated problem from the client. For example, "This medication is making me feel sicker and I've stopped taking it."
- An independent decision by the nurse who may act on behalf of, and in the best interest of, the client, particularly when the client is very ill.

Each advocacy situation and every nurse who performs the advocate role is unique, making the advocacy process complex. Four advocacy models are presented to assist the nurse in adjusting the advocate role to the client situation. Each of these models reflects the same goal—promoting the clients' right to autonomy and self-determination—yet they differ somewhat in nursing strategies and approaches.

Advocacy within any of the models involves a process similar to the nursing process. The nurse-advocate needs to assess both the client's need for advocacy and any barriers that may prevent clients from acting on their own behalf. Barriers include such factors as the type of chronic condition and nature of symptoms, the presence or absence of resources (knowledge and information, social support, time, money), client confidence and readiness, social and cultural influences, the setting where advocacy will occur (home or facility), and the political and economic climate that affect health-related legislation. In addition, it is important to obtain a detailed chronological account of events and validating support that a problem exists and that action is needed; having all available facts about a situation contributes to effective advocacy. Should the advocate be unable to intervene independently, he or she may need to present the client case to the appropriate decision makers, a task that requires tact and interpersonal skills in order to promote a collaborative relationship.

The advocate then determines the point at which advocacy will be most effective. It is important to remember that the activities of the advocate are carried out collaboratively between the nurse and client. The timing of advocacy is based on knowledge of past efforts and prior actions that address the issue. Effort should be made to coincide with the activities of local regulatory agencies and with state or federal legislative bodies if that is appropriate.

Effective advocacy of the nurse results in self-advocacy by clients. Clients need to learn to speak on their own behalf for the future without nursing intervention. Feedback of the entire process allows the nurse and client to determine how effective the intervention has been. If the problem continues, the client and nurse-advocate can then decide whether new goals are necessary and/or whether certain aspects of the intervention need to be changed.

Advocacy Models

The four advocacy models presented are: 1) *the advocacy process* (Brower, 1982); 2) *the decision-making process based on self-determination* (Gadow, 1980); 3) *the decision-making process* advocated by Haggerty (1985); and 4) *self-advocacy* (Brashers et al., 2000) (Table 16-3). As mentioned, the nursing process serves as a foundation for each of these models. These four models are useful tools for the nurse in promoting the clients' abilities to make informed, self-determined choices in their health care.

The Advocacy Process

The advocacy process model consists of six steps (Brower, 1982). The first step requires building a relationship between the client and advocate that reflects openness and mutual understanding of realistic expectations. Also included in this step is the identification of norms of particular clients or groups to honor their cultural values and beliefs. The nurse needs to evaluate the client's understanding of the situation, provide information appropriate to the client's literacy level, and discuss other factors that would have an impact on decisions, such as financial or legal matters. Clients would be informed about the nature of their choices and the content and consequences of those choices.

The second step in the advocacy process is problem diagnosis. The underlying causes of the problem need to be identified. Alternatives and consequences relative to the problem are then generated. The advocate would explore pertinent resources relative to the identified problem. Resources at the micro level (self-care agency) and macro level (societal) would be considered.

The identification of a specific aspect of the larger problem is the third step in the advocacy process. Long-term and short-term goals are negotiated and established. The fourth step is decision making or choosing a solution derived in part from prior experience and research of the client-advocate. The fifth step is to agree on the goals and objectives in order to build interest and identification with the

TABLE 16-3

Nursing Process Advocacy Models

Nursing Process	Self-Advocacy (Brashers et al., 2000)	Advocacy Process (Brower, 1982)	Decision-Making Process Based on Self-Determination (Gadow, 1980)	Decision-Making Process (Haggerty, 1985)
Assessment/diagnosis	• Evaluate client expertise, including: —Knowledge of personal responses —Outcome preferences —Knowledge of personal, social, financial resources	• Build relationship • Diagnose problem	• Patient self-determination • Nurse–patient relationship • The nurse's values • The patient's values	• Evaluate situation • Determine client knowledge regarding situation • Determine benefits/risks • Determine goals of client and nurse
Planning/outcome	• Explore client-provider relationship • Identify possible treatment options goals	• Delineate problem: —Set long-term goals —Set short-term goals • Choose solution	• Patient individuality	• Explore situation with client • Negotiate common goals • Identify responsibilities of client and nurse relative to
Implementation	• Negotiate treatment plan	• Gain acceptance of solution		• Carry out proposed plan
Evaluation	• Evaluate treatment plan	• Evaluate advocacy project		• Client perspective • Nurse perspective

specified problem. The advocate would support the clients' rights to make choices and act on those choices and affirm the client's decisions.

The last step is the evaluation of the successes and failures of the advocacy project. During this process, the exchange of information between the advocate and client may occur so that the client's choices remain viable. Affirmation advances the process of reevaluation and commitment to promote self-determination.

Decision Making Based on Self-Determination

Based on the client's right to self-determination, this advocacy model focuses on assisting clients to achieve self-determination concerning health alternatives (Gadow, 1980). The model outlines five steps for promoting client decision making. While each element requires consideration by the nurse and client, the steps of the process have no predetermined sequence. This model assumes that the appropriate amount and type of information cannot be determined without client participation.

1. Provide relevant, adequate, and sufficient types and amounts of information to the client so that he or she understands and can respond to situations. With more information, clients are more likely to exercise self-determination in decision making.
2. Let the relationship between nurse and client evolve so that the nurse can ascertain whether the client needs more information. Nurses should not wait for clients to request information, but should offer assistance in this process. The nurse can ask questions such as, "Would more information help you make a decision?" Or the nurse can be less direct by saying something like, "Some people are helped in making a decision when they have more information. Would this be helpful for you?"
3. The nurse's views should be disclosed as part of the relevant information given to the client so that the client can understand the nurse's behavior. The purpose of such disclosure is not to persuade the client, but merely to inform and affirm the importance of articulation of values in the decision-making process.
4. The client should be helped to determine his or her own values. Clarification of the client's values is enhanced with the disclosure of the nurse's values. However, it is the values of the client concerning the quality-of-life and treatment decisions that are decisive.
5. The client should be assisted in determining freely the meaning that health, illness, or dying will have to him or her. It is important to remember that individuals are a composite of their unique understanding of themselves and their bodies. When the client makes such determinations, the nurse can then attend to considerations other than values. The nursing task involved in this step is to assist clients in determining the meanings their illnesses have to them.

The Decision-Making Process

The steps in the decision-making process proposed by Haggerty (1985) parallel the steps of the nursing process. This model is useful to the nurse as he or she seeks to help the client make informed, self-determined choices in health care.

Assessment/Problem Diagnosis   The advocate initially evaluates the situation and determines to what extent clients are informed of their conditions. Then the advocate decides how much the client is willing to change behaviors that impact his or her health or whether the client intends to continue the same behaviors. The advocate would determine the extent to which the chronic illness has altered the client's sense of control over his or her health.

The advocate also determines the client's knowledge regarding the chronic disease, the client's awareness of important components of the treatment plan, and the client's ability to make choices regarding management of the chronic illness.

Planning   The advocate examines the situation with the client, and together they discuss possible options of managing the chronic illness and the benefits and risks associated with a specific decision. The goals of the client and nurse are determined along with the degree of congruence between them. This action is followed by the negotiation of mutual goals emphasizing the responsibilities and obligations of both the nurse and the client. A contract or agreement is written that clearly sets forth the responsibilities of both parties to enhance the understanding of and commitment to the established goals.

Implementation   Implementation of the proposed plan is carried out. Both parties would perform their responsibilities relative to the goals stated in the contract.

Evaluation   Evaluation from the client's perspective allows a determination of the extent to which his or her responsibilities were fulfilled. The client can also determine how much control he or she had in the decision-making process and whether identified needs were met.

Evaluation from the nurse's perspective would determine whether the nurse's actions supported and enhanced client autonomy. The nurse would also evaluate the extent to which the client had opportunities to take control of the decision-making process relative to care and whether the problem was resolved, at least in part. Part II of the case study about Mr. Smith's pressure ulcers demonstrates how the decision-making model can be used.

Self-Advocacy

Self-advocacy assists clients to recognize and adapt to the uncertainty that goes hand in hand with chronic conditions (Gould, 2001). Brashers, Haas, and Heidig (1999) provide a description of client self-advocacy. Self-advocacy is described as persuasive efforts and behaviors of an individual that are in the individual's interest. Self-advocacy behaviors frequently have an impact on encounters with health care personnel. Following are components that are central to self-advocacy at the collective and individual levels:

1. Information Acquisition: Information is an important component of self-advocacy. The level of understanding the client has about a particular chronic illness is an important part of negotiating his or her health care. Increased knowledge about treatment options is important and leads to an awareness of the broader range of options, giving clients the ability to critique the quality of their care and to challenge the expertise of the health care provider.
2. Assertive Stance toward Health Care: Assertiveness allows the client to confront the paternalistic or authoritarian interactional styles frequently found in health care relationships and settings. Even though clients may begin a health care relationship as passive, they develop more assertive behaviors as they become more accustomed to the health care setting and their health care providers.
3. Mindful Nonadherence: Mindful nonadherence is a form of reasoned, rational decision making in which the suggested treatment is declined in favor of another alternative. Mindful nonadherence allows clients to decide what treatment options are best for them, to reject treatment recommendations, and offer reasons for doing so.

Self-advocacy is the process in which individuals are enabled to gain the confidence and skills to make choices and speak for themselves. Persons with chronic conditions are able to challenge their position of relative powerlessness, and self-advocacy is viewed as a helpful strategy within the process of empowerment. The client develops knowledge and skills needed to exercise control over their own lives. Self-advocacy is the most empowering form of advocacy and is the preferable strategy within health care settings as it minimizes the risks involved (Teasdale, 1998). While some health care professionals may have difficulty accepting an active client

The Problem of Pressure Ulcers—Part II

Bill Jones, the primary nurse, uses the *decision-making process* in working with the identified problem of Mr. Smith's pressure ulcers.

Problem Identification

Bill determines that Mr. Smith's most pressing desire is to remain up and that he is willing to risk further skin breakdown. Because they have a positive rapport, Mr. Smith is able to discuss this situation at great length with Bill and to articulate his awareness of what additional skin breakdown might mean. Given his deteriorating physical status, Mr. Smith feels that staying in the wheelchair improves the quality of his life at home.

Planning

Together they explore options that would promote healing of Mr. Smith's ulcer while still honoring his wish to remain in control of the situation. They establish a goal to initiate activities that might stop the progression of the ulcer and still allow him to spend time with his family. They establish a contract whereby the responsibilities of both are clearly delineated. The schedule they agree on requires that Mr. Smith be put to bed for a period of time after he returns home from work to get weight off of his sacral area. During this time, Mrs. Smith will apply continuous moist compresses to the area. Mr. Smith would then return to his wheelchair for dinner and socializing with his family.

Implementation

Bill teaches Mrs. Smith how to apply moist compresses correctly, and Mr. Smith goes to bed after his return home every afternoon.

Evaluation

After a couple of weeks, Bill and Mr. Smith discuss the schedule and progress of the ulcer. Mr. Smith voices that he feels he has control in the decision-making process and that he is willing to adhere to the schedule despite the inconvenience of returning to bed during the day.

Bill notes that although the ulcer has not gotten any better, it has not progressed. Although he would like Mr. Smith to spend more time off his sacral area, he is encouraged that the ulcer has not worsened. He feels that his advocacy action has allowed Mr. Smith to retain his self-determination and the quality of life he wishes to have.

---

model, increased participation by clients leads to higher quality decisions and commitment to those decisions as well as increased satisfaction with health care. In this model, the role of the nurse advocate is to ensure that the barriers such as attitudinal, practical and financial, to self-advocacy are reduced.

Regardless of the model used, the role of the advocate is to empower clients to make the best decisions from their own perspectives. Client decision-making is enhanced by the use of the information exchanged, the nursing process, written techniques such as contracts, lists and advanced directives, and reflective listening and role playing to explore the different options and potential consequences. Informed decision-making is a powerful tool to increase clients' self-confidence and build skills that can strengthen their autonomy and confidence for future decision making.

Summary and Conclusions

Advocacy is creating environments that foster care and healing for all clients. Human worth does not rest exclusively on bodily functions or abilities. It is when we come to recognize this that we will become more enlightened and empowered to act as advocates for justice for all (Gold, 2002). Advocacy is a role that must be learned and developed, valued and practiced. Advocacy is central to professional nursing.

Advocacy requires scientific knowledge, expert communication, facilitation skills, problem-solving abilities, and affirmation techniques. It may be as informal as acknowledging a human condition or as formal as employing an advocacy process for the unmet needs of clients. Advocacy issues that affect persons with chronic illnesses are broad, ranging from public considerations, such as health policy, to private concerns, such as threats to clients' well-being.

Advocacy may involve the nurse in political action to activate change, or it may be a quiet, private function of support and intuition, allowing clients to put meaning into their situations. The advocate acknowledges the personal values and hopes of clients and shapes an atmosphere of caring. In some circumstances, advocacy may be the only intervention that can make a difference for a client within the health care system.

Given that knowledge is power, advocacy empowers clients to make informed decisions affecting both health and the satisfaction of their needs. Empowered caring creates for clients the possibility for choice and control (Zerwekh, 2000). The client not only is the recipient of care, but also becomes an active participant in defining both health needs and the appropriate use of resources. Using a holistic approach, advocates respond not only to biologic needs, but also to socioeconomic circumstances that affect the well-being of clients.

Study Questions

1. In what ways have historical events had an impact on the advocate role in nursing?
2. What is your definition of *advocacy*?
3. Discuss the three self-care deficits in relation to chronic illnesses. How do the power components as set forth by Orem (1995) affect these limitations?
4. What are the similarities and differences among "existential advocacy," "consumerism advocacy," and "paternalism"? What are the strengths and limitations of each approach?
5. Are nurses ever justified in acting paternalistically? Why? If so, when and under what circumstances?
6. Can the nurse assist a client in the decision-making process without imposing undue influence on the process? What factors facilitate or obstruct this process?
7. How do the values and beliefs of the nurse influence the manner in which the nurse implements the advocate role?
8. Discuss the client and nurse factors that have an impact on advocacy.
9. Identify the social-structural factors affecting advocacy. How are these factors similar or different from the nurse and client factors?
10. Discuss the interrelationships between culture and advocacy.
11. Compare and contrast the models of advocacy in Table 16-3.
12. Given a client situation, how would you implement advocacy using one of the models in Table 16-3?
13. In what ways do you anticipate the advocacy role in the nursing profession changing and evolving in the future?

References

Aday, L. (2001). *At risk in America.* San Francisco, CA: Jossey-Bass.

Ahern, K., & McDonald, S. (2002). The beliefs of nurses who were involved in a whistleblowing event. *Journal of Advanced Nursing, 38* (3), 303–309

Allender, J. A., & Spradley, B. W. (2005). *Community health nursing: Promoting and protecting the public's health* (6th ed.). Philadelphia: Lippincott.

Altun, I., & Ersoy, N. (2003). Undertaking the role of patient advocate: A longitudinal study of nursing students. *Nursing Ethics, 10* (5), 462–471.

American Nurses Association (2001). *Code of ethics for nurses with interpretive statements.* Washington, D.C.: American Nurses Publishing.

Andrews, M. M., & Boyle, J. S. (2003). *Transcultural concepts in nursing care* (4th ed.). Philadelphia: Lippincott.

Avery, B., & Bashir, S. (2003). The road to advocacy—searching for the rainbow. *American Journal of Public Health, 93* (8), 1207–1211.

Aylett, E., & Fawcett, T. N. (2003). Chronic fatigue syndrome: The nurse's role. *Nursing Standard, 17* (35), 33–37.

Banja, J. (1999). Patient advocacy at risk: Ethical, legal and political dimensions of adverse reimbursement practices in brain injury rehabilitation in the US. *Brain Injury, 13* (10), 745–58.

Bassett, M. T. (2003). Public health advocacy. *American Journal of Public Health, 93* (8), 1204.

Bezruchka, S. (2000). Culture and medicine: Is globalization dangerous to our health? *Western Journal of Medicine, 172,* 332–334.

Bezruchka, S. (2001). Societal hierarchy and the health Olympics. *Canadian Medical Association Journal, 164,* 1701–1703.

Black, J. M. (2004). Blind obedience or plain stupidity? *Plastic Surgical Nursing, 24* (2), 37.

Bramlett, M. H., Gueldner, S. H., & Sowell, R. L. (1990). Consumer-centric advocacy: Its connection to nursing frameworks. *Nursing Science Quarterly, 3* (4), 156–161.

Brashers, D. E., Haas, S. M., & Neidig, J. L. (1999). The patient self-advocacy scale: Measuring patient involvement in health care decision-making interactions. *Health Communication, 11* (2), 97.

Brashers, D. E., Haas, S. M., Klingle, R. S., & Neidig, J. L. (2000). Collective AIDS activism and individuals' perceived self-advocacy in physician-patient communication. *Human Communication Research, 26* (3), 372–402.

Breier-Mackie, S. (2001). Patient autonomy and medical paternity: Can nurses help doctors to listen to patients? *Nursing Ethics, 8* (6), 510–521.

Brower, H. T. (1982). Advocacy: What it is? *Journal of Gerontological Nursing, 8* (3), 141–143.

Campinha-Bacote, J. (2002). The process of cultural competence in the delivery of health care services: A model of care. *Journal of Transcultural Nursing, 13* (3), 180–184.

Chafey, K., Rhea, M., Shannon, A. M., & Spencer, S. (1998). Characterizations of advocacy by practicing nurses. *Journal of Professional Nursing, 14* (1), 43–52.

Clark, E. G. (1997). Substituted judgment: Medical and financial decisions by guardians. *Estate Planning, 24* (2), 66–73.

Corbin, J. M. & Cherry, J. C. (2001). Epilogue: A proactive model of health care. In R. B. Hyman and J. M. Corbin (Eds.). *Chronic illness research and theory for nursing practice.* New York: Springer.

Courts, N. F., Buchanan, E. M., & Werstlein, P. O. (2004). Focus groups: The lived experience of participants with multiple sclerosis. *Journal of Neuroscience Nursing, 36* (1), 42–47.

Curran, C. R. (2003). Navigation the chaotic health care system. *Nursing Economics, 21* (6), 261.

Curtin, L. (1988). Ethics in nursing practice. *Nursing Management, 19* (5), 7–9.

Curtin, L. (1979). The nurse as advocate: A philosophical foundation for nursing. *Advances in Nursing Science, 1,* 1–10.

Dalton, C. C., & Gottlieb, L. N. (2003). The concept of readiness to change. *Journal of Advanced Nursing, 42*(2), 108–117.

Davis, A. J., Konishi, E., & Tashiro, M. (2003). A pilot study of selected Japanese nurses' ideas on patient advocacy. *Nursing Ethics, 10* (4), 404–413.

de Chesnay, M. (2005). Vulnerable populations: Vulnerable people. In M. de Chesnay (Ed.). *Caring for the vulnerable: Perspectives in nursing theory, practice, and research.* Sudbury, MA: Jones & Bartlett.

de Chesnay, M., Wharton, R., & Pamp, C. (2005). Cultural competence, resilience, and advocacy. In M. de Chesnay (Ed.). *Caring for the vulnerable: Perspectives in nursing theory, practice, and research.* Sudbury, MA: Jones & Bartlett.

Erlen, J. A. (2002). Adherence revisited: The patient's choice. *Orthopaedic Nursing, 21* (2), 79–82.

Falk-Rafael, A. R., (2001). Empowerment as a process of evolving consciousness: a model of empowered caring. *Advances in Nursing Science, 24* (1), 1–16.

Fletcher, S. N. E. (2002). Cultural implications in the management of grief and loss. *Journal of Cultural Diversity, 9* (3), 86–90.

Foley, B. J., Minick, M. P., & Kee, C. C. (2002). How nurses learn advocacy. *Journal of Nursing Scholarship, 34* (2), 181–186.

Gadow, S. (1980). A model for ethical decision making. *Oncology Nursing Forum, 7* (4), 44–47.

_____. (1990). Existential advocacy: Philosophical foundations of nursing. In R. Pence & J. Cantrall (Eds.), *Ethics in nursing: An anthology.* New York: National League for Nursing.

Georges, J. J., & Grypdonck, M. (2002). Moral problems experienced by nurses when caring for terminally ill people: A literature review. *Nursing Ethics, 9* (2), 155–178.

Glaser, B. G., & Strauss, A. L. (1968). *Time for dying.* Chicago: Aldine.

Goffman, E. (1963). *Notes on management of spoiled identity.* Englewood Cliffs, NJ: Prentice-Hall.

Gold, S. (2002). Beyond pity and paternalism: Even progressive persons committed to social justice are unable to embrace the disability rights movement. Are we afraid of something? *The Other Side, 38* (5), 16–21.

Gould, M. A. (2001). Too many patients, too few registered nurses: Developing an advocacy plan. *Nephrology Nursing Journal, 28* (4), 381.

Grace, P. J. (2001). Professional advocacy: Widening the scope of accountability. *Nursing Philosophy, 2* (2), 151–161.

Haggerty, M. C. (1985). Ethics: Nurse patron or nurse advocate. *Nursing Management, 16* (5), 340–347.

Hamric, A. B. (2000). What is happening to advocacy? *Nursing Outlook, 48* (3), 103–104.

Hewitt, J. (2002). A critical review of the arguments debating the role of the nurse advocate. *Journal of Advanced Nursing, 37* (5), 439–445.

Hyland, D. (2002). An exploration of the relationship between patient autonomy and patient advocacy: Implications for nursing practice. *Nursing Ethics, 9* (5), 472–482.

Kohnke, M. F. (1980). The nurse as advocate. *American Journal of Nursing, 80,* 2038–2040.

Lamb, H. R., & Weinberger, L. E. (1993). Therapeutic use of conservatorship in the treatment of gravely disabled psychiatric patients. *Hospital and Community Psychiatry, 44* (2), 147–150.

Leininger, M. (1995). *Transcultural nursing: Concepts, theories, research and practices* (2nd ed.). New York: McGraw-Hill.

Leininger, M., & McFarland, M. R. (2002). *Transcultural nursing concepts, theories, research and practice* (3rd ed.). New York: McGraw-Hill.

Lewis, M., Hepburn, K., Corcoran-Perry, S., Narayan, S., et al. (1999). Options, outcomes, values, likelihoods decision-making guide for patients and their families. *Journal of Gerontological Nursing, 25* (12), 19–25.

Love, M. B. (1995). Patient advocacy at the end of life. *Nursing Ethics, 2* (1), 3–9.

Maliski, S. L., Clerkin, B., & Litwin, M. S. (2004). Describing a nurse case manager intervention to empower low-income men with prostate cancer. *Oncology Nursing Forum, 31* (1), 57–64.

Mallik, M., & Rafferty, A. M. (2000). Diffusion of the concept of patient advocacy. *Journal of Nursing Scholarship, 32* (4), 399–404.

Mallik, M. (1997). Advocacy in nursing—A review of the literature. *Journal of Advanced Nursing, 25* (1), 130–138.

Martin, G. W. (1998). Communication breakdown or ideal speech situation: The problem of nurse advocacy. *Nursing Ethics, 5* (2), 147–157.

McCurdy, A. H. (1997). Mastery of life. In J. Young-Mason (Ed.). *The patient's voice: Experiences of illness.* Philadelphia: F. A. Davis.

McCorkle, R., & Pasacreta, J. V. (2001). Enhancing caregiver outcomes in palliative care. *Cancer Control, 8* (1), 36–45.

McGrath, A., & Walker, A. (1999). Nurses' perception and experience of advocacy. *Contemporary Nurse, 8* (3), 72–78.

Milio, N. (2002). A new leadership role for nursing in a globalized world. *Topics in Advanced Practice Nursing eJournal, 2* (1).

Miller, S. H., Cohen, M. Z., & Kagan, S. H. (2000). The measure of advocacy. *American Journal of Nursing, 100* (1), 61–64.

Mitchell, G. J., & Bournes, D. A. (2000). Nurse as patient advocate? In search of straight thinking. *Nursing Science Quarterly, 13* (3), 204–209.

Mohr, W. K., & Horton-Deutsch, S. (2001). Malfeasance and regaining nursing's moral voice and integrity. *Nursing Ethics, 8* (1), 19–35.

Niven, C. A., & Scott, P. A. (2003). The need for accurate perception and informed judgement in determining the appropriate use of the nursing resource: Hearing the patient's voice. *Nursing Philosophy, 4,* 201–210.

Nolan, M., Keady, J., & Grant, G. (1995). Developing a typology of family care: Implications for nurses and other service providers. *Journal of Advanced Nursing, 21* (2), 256–265.

Olsen, D. P. (2001). Protection and advocacy: An ethics practice in mental health. *Journal of Psychiatric and Mental Health Nursing, 8,* 121–128.

Olson, L. L. (2001). Nursing's new code of ethics: A collaborative process. *Chart, 98* (5), 8.

Orem, D. E. (1995). *Nursing concepts of practice* (5th ed.). St. Louis: Mosby.

Reynolds, S. L. (1997). Protected or neglected: An examination of negative versus compassionate ageism in public conservatorship. *Research on Aging, 19* (1), 3–25.

Roberts, D. (2004). Patient advocacy: The *real* restraint-reduction strategy. *MEDSURG Nursing, 13* (1), 7.

Salas-Provance, M. B., Erickson, J. G., & Reed, J. (2002). Disabilities as viewed by four generations of one Hispanic family. *American Journal of Speech-Language Pathology, 11,* 151–162.

Schroeter, K. (2000). Advocacy in perioperative nursing practice. *AORN Journal, 71* (6), 1207–1222.

Schroeter, K. (2002). Ethics in perioperative practice—patient advocacy. *AORN Journal, 75* (5), 941–946.

Schwartz, L. (2002). Is there an advocate in the house? The role of health care professionals in patient advocacy. *Journal of Medical Ethics, 28* (1), 37–40.

Segesten, K., & Fagring, A. (1996). Patient advocacy—An essential part of quality nursing care. *International Nursing Review, 43* (5), 142–144.

Sheridan-Gonzalez, J. (2000). It's not my patient. *American Journal of Nursing, 100* (1), 13.

Smith, A. P. (2004). Patient advocacy: Roles for nurses and leaders. *Nursing Economics, 22* (2), 88–90.

Snowball, J. (1996). Asking nurses about advocating for patients: 'reactive' and 'proactive' accounts. *Journal of Advanced Nursing, 24,* 67–75.

Starr, P. (1982). *The social transformation of American medicine.* New York: Basic Books.

Sullivan-Bolyai, S., Sadler, L., Knafl, K. A., Gilliss, C. L., et al. (2003). Great expectations: A position description

for parents as caregivers: Part 1. *Pediatric Nursing, 29* (6), 457–461.

Sullivan, T., Weinert, C., & Cudney, S. (2003). Management of chronic illness: Voices of rural women. *Journal of Advanced Nursing, 44* (6), 566–574.

Takemura, Y. (2005). Cultural traits and nursing care particular to Japan. In M. de Chesnay (Ed.). *Caring for the vulnerable. Perspectives in nursing theory, practice, and research.* Sudbury, MA: Jones & Bartlett.

Tammelleo, A. D. (2002). Nurses failed to 'advocate' for their patient. *Nursing Law's Regan Report, 42* (8), 2.

Tang, S. T., & Lee, S. C. (2004). Cancer diagnosis and prognosis in Taiwan: Patient preferences versus experiences. *Psycho-Oncology, 13,* 1–13.

Teasdale, K. (1998). *Advocacy in healthcare.* Oxford, UK: Blackwell.

Thomas, V., Richardson, A., & Saleem, T. (2000). The efficacy of bilingual health advocacy in ethnic minority patients with cancer. *Nursing Standard, 14* (26), 32–33.

Thorne, S. E., Nyhlin, K. T., & Paterson, B. L. (2000). Attitudes toward patient expertise in chronic illness. *International Journal of Nursing Studies, 37* (4), 303–311.

Valente, S. M. (2004). End-of-life challenges: Honoring autonomy. *Cancer Nursing, 27* (4), 314–319.

Walker, E. (2001). How do we facilitate caregivers' involvement in decision-making? *Journal of Advanced Nursing, 34,* 329–337.

White, G. (2002). The code of ethics for nurses: responding to new challenges in a new century. *Nevada RNformation, 11* (1), 21.

Williams, C. A., & Gossett, M. T. (2001). Nursing communication: Advocacy for the patient or physician? *Clinical Nursing Research, 10* (3), 332–340.

Winslow, G. R. (1984). From loyalty to advocacy: A new metaphor for nursing. *The Hastings Center Report, 14,* 32–40.

Zerwekh, J. V. (2000). Caring on the ragged edge: Nursing persons who are disenfranchised. *Advances in Nursing Science, 22* (4), 47–61.

Zoucha, R. (2000). The significance of culture in caring for Mexican Americans in a home health setting. *Home Health Care Management Practice, 12* (6), 46–52.

Zoucha, R., & Husted, G. L. (2000). The ethical dimensions of delivering culturally congruent nursing and health care. *Issues in Mental Health Nursing, 21,* 325–340.

CHAPTER 17

Research in Chronic Illness

Barbara B. Germino

Introduction

As the population ages, chronic illness, more than ever before, presents imposing challenges to professionals in all arenas of health care. Those in nursing and other clinical fields seek to assist individuals, families, and communities not only in the prevention of chronic illness and managing the day-to-day work of chronic illness, but also in maintaining optimal functioning and quality of life over time. Many risk factors, preventive strategies, and suggested management approaches are based on evidence generated by research. However, there are still significant unanswered questions in all areas. Continuing research is clearly needed to strengthen the scientific knowledge base for practice in the prevention of chronic illness and the care of clients with chronic illness. Although this chapter focuses on research for clinical practice, there are other areas of research that are equally important if evidence-based care is to be delivered effectively. Other areas include research on the quality of chronic illness care, chronic illness care delivery costs, and studies of health policy, which impact morbidity and mortality at the national and international levels. Such work serves as part of the foundation for changing the shape of healthcare delivery in chronic illness

and is crucial to address, but is beyond the scope of this chapter.

Types of Research in Chronic Illness

Research about chronic illness may be categorized as focusing on either prevention or management. Within each of these broad domains, studies using a variety of designs and methodologies may be grouped into descriptive and intervention-focused research. Descriptive research provides data on risk factors; the natural history of illness and responses to it; factors that predict or modify health promotion behavior; factors that moderate or mediate the incidence or impact of chronic illness on clients and their families, as well as on communities; relationships among aspects of illness processes; and predictors of specific illness outcomes.

Intervention research in chronic illness focuses on evaluating the efficacy of specific strategies targeted to individuals, groups, populations, and communities. Outcomes may relate to chronic illness prevention, for example, changing life-style behaviors in children to prevent later development of cardiovascular disease (Gittelsohn et al., 1998; Gortmaker et al., 1999; Harrell et al., 1999; McMurray et al., 2000,

2002; McMurray, Bauman & Harrell, 2000; Nader et al., 1999). Other studies may focus on outcomes related to management of chronic illness, for example, self-help interventions for persons with arthritis (Braden, 1993). Still others focus on preventing chronic conditions, maintaining optimal functioning, and maximizing quality of life over time. An example of the latter is a study of exercise with frail rural elderly clients (Hogue & Cullinan, 1993).

This chapter is organized into research on prevention of and management of chronic illness—and, within each of these domains, categorized as descriptive or intervention research. Because this body of work is so large, research cited exemplifies but in no way serves as a complete representation of work in any of these areas, on any particular age group, or on any particular chronic disease. Conceptual and methodological issues in each area are identified and discussed and, finally, future directions for research in chronic illness are proposed.

Theoretical Support for Chronic Illness Research

Much research in chronic illness has been theoretically based and/or has contributed to the growing body of mid-range theory available to guide the study of a variety of questions. Prevention research in nursing has been guided by a number of nursing and other theories: Wellness Motivation theory (Fleury, 1996); the Health Belief Model (Becker, 1974); The Health Promotion Model (Pender, 1987); the Theory of Reasoned Action (Ajzen & Fishbein, 1980); the Theory of Planned Behavior (Ajzen, 1985; Ajzen & Timko, 1983); Social Cognitive and Self-Efficacy Theory (Bandura, 1986; Baranowski, Perry & Parcel, 2002); and the Transtheoretical Model (Prochaska, Reding & Evers, 2002).

Theories of management of chronic illness that have been useful in generating research include Illness Trajectory theory (Corbin & Strauss, 1991), Self-help and Self-care theories (Braden, 1990), Cognitive Behavioral theory (Fishel, 1999; Gelder, 1997), Stress and Coping theories (Tennen et al., 2000), Uncertainty theory (Mishel, 1990), and Social

Support theories (Hupcey, 1998). In addition, models and theories generated inductively from qualitative research, specifically Normalization (Charmaz, 1990) and Quality of Life (Nuamah et al., 1999; Padilla, 1993), have been developed and refined by research on a variety of management and quality-of-life issues.

Theory development in chronic illness has not moved forward at the same pace as chronic illness research but recent work on theories that have been used for some time is exciting and reminds us that this kind of scholarly work is as essential to evidence-based practice as research. Paterson, Russell, & Thorne (2001) have questioned assumptions underlying self-care theory, particularly in the area of everyday self-care decision-making. This work has raised questions about some of the assumptions that have shaped much of the self-care research and pointed out their flaws and limitations. Burton (2000) has written about re-thinking stroke rehabilitation using the Corbin and Strauss chronic illness trajectory framework, noting that nursing interventions for those who have had strokes have often focused on the progression of the client through the health care system, rather than on future recovery. Paterson (2000) has criticized the three main constructions of chronic illness that have persisted over time in spite of research evidence to the contrary. Alternative or additional theoretical perspectives have been discussed in the recent literature on medically fragile children (Mentro & Steward, 2002); in linking HIV/AIDS clients' self-care with outcomes (Chou & Holzemer, 2004); using a developmental science perspective to enhance nursing research with children and families (Miles & Holditch-Davis, 2003); including positive outcomes in stress and coping research (Folkman & Moskowitz, 2000); refining a mid-range theory of comfort for outcomes research (Kolcaba, 2001); combining a stigma and a normalization perspective to capture the dynamic and evolving experiences of chronic illness (Joachim & Acorn, 2000); using a life-span development perspective in research with individuals and families to integrate biological, sociohistorical and non-normative aspects of chronic illness (Rankin, 2000);

and testing a new theory of chronic pain (Tsai, Tak, Moore & Palencia, 2003).

Research on the Prevention of Chronic Illness

Research about the prevention of chronic illness takes a number of different forms. Basic descriptive work in this area includes studies to determine how biological (including genetic), biobehavioral, environmental, psychosocial, behavioral, and contextual factors influence the development and progression of specific chronic illnesses (Harrell et al., 2001; McMurray, Harrell & Brown, 2000). Case studies presented and published by clinicians may generate initial questions about such factors. Such dialogue may lead to highly focused basic research to replicate observations in other than human models and to explore mechanisms by which outcomes such as chronic disease occur. Large epidemiological studies assist scientists in identifying risk factors for chronic disease by verifying associations between predictors and outcomes. These studies raise questions about but do not clarify the mechanisms by which predictive factors are associated with certain outcomes. Research studies that attempt to establish cause need to be based on theory and carefully designed to control for possible confounding factors. In nursing, exemplars of areas of prevention research include risk and vulnerability of people of varying ages to chronic illnesses or other negative health or developmental outcomes, and the enhancement of knowledge and attitudes that motivate people to positive health promoting behaviors or to screening for chronic illnesses.

Descriptive Research on the Prevention of Chronic Illness

The risk and vulnerability of infants and children have been areas of concern in relation to short- and long-term developmental outcomes of these children. The programmatic research of Barnard, Snyder and Spietz (1991) and Diane Holditch-Davis (1987; 1994; 2003a, 2003b) serves to exemplify nursing research contributions in which the investigators have identified factors predictive of long-term developmental problems, including such predictors as parent–infant interactions, sleep–wake states, and breathing patterns. Barnard's work has been based on an ecological model of development in which the child and his or her environment are in ongoing interaction and affect each other in reciprocal ways (Barnard, 1978). The parents are seen as part of the child's environment, making parent–infant interaction one of the key foci for study. One proposition of the conceptual model is that interventions targeting the environment or the interaction between the infant and environments would affect the child's development both in the short and long term. Barnard's team has followed a cohort of high-risk children from birth well into school age to examine long-term effects of intervening with parent–infant interactions in feeding, playing, and other daily activities (Barnard, Snyder & Spietz, 1991).

Since the eradication of many acute infectious diseases, the long-term health of children has become a concern. The concept of a "new morbidity" in children, a shift in their health profile to biological, psychological, and social factors that can have a significant impact on the potential of children, was first used in the mid-1980s (Haggerty, 1984). Examples of more recently recognized factors included poverty, lack of prenatal care, a dysfunctional home life, child abuse, and neglect (Simeonsson & Gray, 1994). The focus on infancy and early childhood expanded to concerns about school-age children—a developmental period when children begin to make choices about life-style behaviors that will have lifelong impact on their health and well-being (Simeonsson & Gray, 1994). As life-threatening infectious diseases were eliminated, it became clear that life-style–related risk factors such as smoking, alcohol, and other substance abuse, sedentary life-styles, high-fat diets, and obesity were factors that needed to be targeted in school-age children. Physical health was redefined as researchers linked life-style behaviors with increased risk for cardiovascular disease. The discovery of atherosclerotic fatty streaks in the arteries of children as young as 3 years old and in 45 to 77 percent of those under age 22 (Jopling, 1992) precipitated the development of national guidelines on risk factors and nutrition (NIH Consensus Conference, 1985) and continue as part of a national agenda for fostering the health and well-being of children in the United States (Healthy People 2000, 1991; Healthy People 2010, U.S. DHHS, 1999). Recently, there has been national concern about what is seen as an epidemic of childhood obesity with health care providers reporting premature chronic illness such as Type II diabetes in obese children.

Other investigators have focused on poverty as a health risk (Nelson, 1994) and the cost burden of low birth weight (Gennaro et al., 1993). Essentially, these studies are based on the assumption that inadequate resources—physiological or biobehavioral and environmental/interpersonal—have the potential of affecting child health. Childhood indicators of cardiovascular disease risk factors, their interaction with genetic susceptibility, and factors contributing to their progression continue to be heavily studied in a number of disciplines (Gittelsohn et al., 1998; Gortmaker et al., 1999; Harrell et al., 1996, 1999; Nader et al., 1999). In particular, nursing can contribute research on factors in the child's environment that are tied to risk factors including family health behaviors, peer behavior, values for and availability of exercise, smoking rules and nutritious school lunches (Lee & Cubbin, 2002; Miles & Holditch-Davis, 2003). There is a growing need for examination of how children at various socioeconomic levels, with different cultural backgrounds, and living in rural or urban locations, adapt to acute or chronic illness; the intergenerational aspects of health including family medical history and the influence of parental illness; and the factors that influence child health behaviors (Miles & Holditch-Davis, 2003; Vohr et al., 2000).

In the decades since the AIDS epidemic began, there have been a number of studies describing knowledge, attitudes, and behaviors of adolescents in relation to risk and exposure to HIV/AIDS. Substantial misinformation has been described in surveys of primary grade teachers and students (Glenister et al., 1990). Studies of teenagers, espe-

cially African Americans, indicated that in spite of knowledge about AIDS, children of this age group frequently participated in risky sexual behaviors (Walker, 1992; Koniak-Griffin & Brecht, 1995).

Descriptive research on chronic illness prevention in adults over the past two decades also focused first on the identification of risk factors for major chronic illnesses (particularly for cancer and cardiovascular diseases). The Framingham Heart Study and the Nurses' Health Study were major longitudinal epidemiological studies that verified and clarified the impact of life-style factors on the risk of major life-threatening chronic illnesses. In particular, the role of smoking, alcohol, diet, exercise, obesity, hypertension, family history, and occupational risks emerged as key in planning future intervention research. Recent research literature contains a variety of examples of studies of determinants and predictors on health-related behaviors, targeting previously understudied groups including women and ethnic minorities (Blue & Marston-Scott, 2001; Carter & Kulbok, 2002; Lucas, Orshan & Cook, 2000; Rockwell & Riegel, 2001).

In addition to learning about risk factors of major chronic illnesses, studies on the effects of such knowledge on participation in chronic disease screening (Weinrich et al., 1998b) are another component of descriptive prevention research. Initial identification of risk factors lead to a major investment in public education throughout school curricula and focused on adults using the most up to date marketing and media strategies. Studies on the knowledge people have gained from these efforts, the effect of public education programs on life-style behaviors, and screening participation demonstrate equivocal or conflicting results.

Questions have been raised about the impact of long-standing racial discrimination on the willingness of some minority groups, particularly African Americans, to participate in screening for major chronic illnesses like cancer, even when their ethnicity puts them at particularly high risk (Underwood, 1995, 1999). Others have questioned whether prolonged life in poverty circumstances, with the physical, physiological, psychological, and educational deprivation that such experience brings, can, in subtle cumulative ways, increase risk for some diseases. Whether cultural proscription, lack of knowledge, perceived discrimination and distrust, or cumulative biological or immunological factors are involved in the willingness of minorities to be screened, to seek follow-up care, to persist in treatment, remain issues for future research. Progress is beginning to be evident in recent research that takes cultural factors into account as potentially powerful behaviors. Recent work focuses on underserved groups, particularly ethnic minorities, and their knowledge and information needs, as well as beliefs and attitudes toward the specific chronic illness (e.g. cancer) and toward screening, screening behaviors, and risk appraisal (Frank, Swedmark & Grubbs, 2004; Grindel, Brown, Caplan & Blumenthal, 2004; Lee et al., 2004; Radosevich et al., 2004; Reynolds, 2004; Sheridan, Felix, Pignone & Lewis, 2004; Thomas, 2004; Watts, Merrell, Murphy & Williams, 2004). Just focusing on underserved minorities in such studies is an important albeit small step in moving forward our understanding of the influences that may be linked to culture and ethnicity, religious beliefs, and social experiences such as racism and sexism.

Intervention Research on Prevention of Chronic Illness

Population Studies Interventions for preventing chronic illness target either the entire population or those at high risk. Population-focused interventions are more effective in reducing a particular disease problem for the population as a whole (Harrell et al., 1999; Rose, 1980). An example of this is the expanding number of school-based studies designed to test interventions for improving cardiovascular health. These studies are based on the fact that cardiovascular diseases are the number one health problem in the United States today, that descriptive research has documented the beginning of atherosclerosis in childhood, that progression of disease is linked to risk factors, and that one-fourth to one-

third of children entering school have at least one elevated risk factor (Williams & Wynder, 1993). Knowing that the majority of children up to age 16 in this country are in school and assuming that health behaviors can be influenced through the school, nurse investigators and others have conducted trials of interventions to prevent or reduce smoking and obesity, favorably influence lipid profiles, lower body fat, lower blood pressure, and increase physical activity (McMurray et al., 2002). In a recent review of ten such studies that linked cognitive and behavioral interventions with physiologic outcomes, Meininger (2000) notes "there were no consistent effects of school-based interventions on the risk factor profiles of children and adolescents" (p. 239). Earlier studies had more significant effects on blood pressure and lipids than did later studies. More recent studies used behavioral and cognitive strategies and addressed the environment—school, family, and/or community—but changes in physiological risk factors were infrequent. There were, however, some changes in knowledge and health behaviors with these studies (Meininger, 2000).

Although a wide range of ethnic groups was represented across the studies in Meininger's review, there was little information on differential effects. Changes in risk factors were inconsistent by gender and ethnicity, indicating that theoretical models guiding the studies must be reexamined and/or that interventions must be more gender- and culture-sensitive (Meininger, 2000).

It was clear that population-focused studies achieved better results in cardiovascular health, and this supports earlier literature (Harrell et al., 1999; Meininger, 2000). Additionally, dealing with the school environment and including families proved to be ineffective in changing key outcomes. Meininger recommended that broader public health components to school-based interventions, including mass media campaigns, education and screening programs for adults, and policy changes to reinforce interventions at all levels, be part of future preventive interventions (Meininger, 2000). Other recent school-based intervention research has resulted in important changes in outcomes such as reducing body fat and blood pressure in young adolescents (McMurray et al., 2002).

In spite of the greater efficacy of population-based interventions, targeting groups known to be at high risk may be a first step in testing an intervention or may be the best use of available resources. An exemplar of this approach is the work of Weinrich et al. (1998a, 1998b), who have focused on interventions to enhance participation of African Americans in screening for cancers for which they are at high risk. Using cultural knowledge and prior intervention experience, this group of investigators included peer educator and client navigator interventions that incorporated phone calls aimed at overcoming screening barriers and provided reminders for screening. The men who received these tailored interventions were significantly more likely to participate in screening (Weinrich et al., 1998b). In addition, the study indicated that low-income African American men were more likely to be recruited for screenings if work sites and churches were used as community screening sites (Weinrich et al., 1998a). Recent work by Powe, Ntekop, & Barron (2004) evaluated the effectiveness of a culturally relevant intervention on colorectal cancer knowledge and screening behaviors in community elders. Other research has tested the efficacy of a brief decision aid on information needs of men about prostate cancer screening (Sheridan, Felix, Pignone & Lewis, 2004).

Family Studies   The growing problem of substance abuse in adolescents, part of the "new morbidity" mentioned earlier in this chapter, leads to subsequent chronic addictions and risk factors for a number of chronic conditions, including cancer and cardiovascular disease, and disability from violence or accidents. Because the majority of adolescents are living in a family environment and families are seen as responsible for their health and development, interventions to prevent substance abuse have often been family-based. Family prevention strategies in substance abuse have been categorized as universal, selective, or indicated. Universal prevention programs target populations; selective, interventions

focus on high-risk individuals and families; and indicated programs are designed for those who already demonstrate problem-related behavior (Loveland-Cherry, 2000). Family interventions may be embedded in broader school and community programs or may be exclusively family based. Loveland-Cherry (2000) critically reviewed intervention programs of each type, as well as exclusive family interventions, comparing conceptual approaches, format and content, populations, level of intervention, adequacy of design, and magnitude and duration of effects. Short-term effectiveness was more often documented than were long-term outcomes. The costs of these interventions or feasibility of implementing them outside of the research project have not been well studied. Unlike the research on primary prevention of cardiovascular health problems, there has been more support in this body of work for targeting interventions to specific at-risk groups, although experts in this area continue to debate where the emphasis should be along the continuum from primary to tertiary prevention. Some argue that all adolescents are at risk and that intervening at the universal level is most cost effective (Loveland-Cherry, 2000). Loveland-Cherry (2000) argued that the evidence is equivocal and will require many controlled studies to adequately support a clear conclusion.

Efficacy or empowerment concepts are important influences on health and health behaviors across the life span. Evidence in support of this may be found in a number of successful intervention studies (LeFort, 2000; Lorig, Ritter & Gonzalez, 2003; Luepker et al., 1996; Stone et al., 1994). The importance of nursing's perspective to the interdisciplinary collaboration on optimal approaches to health promotion is clear.

Research on the Management of Chronic Illness

Descriptive research on the management of chronic illness in adults and their families includes studies of the experience and impact of the illness on the client and family and their responses to coping with that illness. Part of response to illness, to use the language of trajectory theory (Corbin & Strauss, 1991), is learning to do the work associated with the particular illness trajectory—both the management work of balancing the demands of illness and having some semblance of a normal life; and the biographical work of shaping and dealing with a changed identity as the illness affects the person. Management of chronic illness involves dealing with the meaning of the illness for the self, the family, and the future. This includes living with uncertainty and dealing with many transitions as the illness trajectory unfolds over time. Transitions occur not only in working with health care professionals, but also in managing uncertainty, and symptoms, dealing with changes in functional status, maintaining or adapting roles and relationships, dealing with fears of recurrence or worsening of the illness, and developing effective coping strategies.

For children with chronic illness and their families, research has also focused on child and family responses, with emphasis on alterations in parenting roles, quality of life and family relationships, and the negotiation of caregiving roles. As technology has kept preterm, low-birth-weight babies alive, the literature reflects that their immaturity may put them at risk for future development of chronic problems. In addition, those chronic illnesses most common in young children and most threatening and intrusive to the child and family's life have created needs for understanding that have been addressed in descriptive work and intervention studies that may enhance management of asthma, diabetes, epilepsy, cystic fibrosis, and other chronic diseases of childhood.

Descriptive Research on Management of Chronic Illness

Qualitative Research　One of the richest resources in the management of chronic illness is the qualitative work being done by nurse investigators over the past two decades. In the *Annual Review of Nursing Research*, Thorne and Paterson (2000) discuss studies of the experience of chronic illness from the perspective of the ill person—the "insider"

perspective. The proliferation of qualitative studies describing the chronic illness experience and its management have enlarged our view from strictly an "outsider" perspective to one that incorporates both the outsider and insider views of the complexities of living with chronic illness (Conrad, 1990; Gerhardt, 1990; Kralik, 2002; Soanes & Timmons, 2004; Sullivan, Weinert & Cudney, 2003; & Thorne & Paterson, 1998).

In the process of inquiry that has resulted in an insider perspective, nurse investigators have contributed greatly to our understanding of chronic illness. But, at the same time, the results of this inquiry have "complicated our theoretical understanding of what it is like to live with a chronic disease" (Thorne & Paterson, 2000, p. 3).

In studying the experience of chronic illness, researchers have either focused on a specific chronic disease or looked for commonalities and differences in a wide variety of chronic diseases within the same study. The investigator who looks for themes of living with chronic illness across disease types assumes there is an overriding concept of chronicity and that crosses disease-specific boundaries. In fact, there are a number of studies documenting that fatigue, pain, and suffering are examples of powerful factors in living with a variety of chronic illnesses. On the other hand, findings about chronic illness derived from studies of particular chronic diseases indicate that some diseases create unique impingements, demands, or experiences that are particular to those diseases and more salient than those features that are common to other chronic problems. Neither approach by itself allows a model of what it is like to live with a chronic illness that is comprehensive enough to guide clinical practice or health policy (Thorne & Paterson, 2000).

Political and social trends change the way that people view, discuss, and label chronic illnesses. These trends can have significant effects on how and what information is exchanged and presented to clients and families, how it is perceived by both the health care professional and the person and family who have to deal with it. The meaning of the chronic illness and the relationship of mind and body in the particular illness may affect the extent to which family members and others react (May, Doyle & Chew-Graham, 1998; Wilde, 2003). An illness like cancer, once stigmatized strongly as a "death sentence" and a disease that was seen as unclean, evoked responses such as pseudonyms for the disease (e.g., "the big C"), whispers or lack of any discussion of the illness, and the assumption that the person with the illness was as good as dead.

Compliance or adherence is another example of a chronic illness experience that has evolved over time but is still strongly influenced by a paternalistic medical model. In spite of evidence that many chronically ill persons become quite expert at self-management and know their bodies better than their health care providers, there is still the notion among health care providers that what is prescribed as treatment and management by them should be followed without question or challenge, and to not do so is to risk being labeled as "noncompliant" or "non-adherent"— not doing what is best for him or her (Wellard, 1998) (see Chapter 10, on compliance).

There has been an increase in the nursing research describing specific problems of living with chronic illness and self-care strategies is noticeable in recent nursing research literature. In particular, studies of self-care including strategies for symptom management (Bennett et al., 2000); complementary/alternative medicine as informed self-care decision-making (Thorne et al., 2002); spiritual coping mechanisms (Narayanasamy, 2004); and special populations and their management strategies e.g. rural women (Sullivan, Weinert & Cudney, 2003); and midlife women (Kralik, 2002) lead nursing knowledge in very practical directions, providing evidence to guide the design and testing of self-care interventions.

As children and adults with chronic illness live longer, developmental and other transitions will influence the reshaping of the chronic illness experience and self-management strategies. A recent study focusing on the transition from adolescent to adult care exemplifies attention to this important consideration (Soanes & Timmons, 2004). Miles & Holditch-Davis (2003) argue that nursing research

with children and families, because of the complexity of interactions of the biological, behavioral and psychological systems of the person and family, and the complexity of their ongoing interactions with multiple aspects of the environment, requires a developmental science perspective that is systems-oriented, developmentally-focused, holistic and integrated.

As discussed, the theory generated by qualitative methods, will have been influenced by those who have not participated in qualitative research, past and current discourse shaping the meaning of particular chronic illness, and by the notion of compliance with prescription by a powerful other, rather than a partnership in management of the disease. The insider view has also raised questions about how gender and age shape responses to chronic illness. Other study factors not addressed to date include the chronic illness experiences of those who are poor, poorly educated, and marginalized by virtue of ethnicity, poverty, or lack of education (Thorne & Paterson, 2000). In addition, we need to reexamine factors such as compliance in light of the findings of such studies—to understand whether noncompliance may have more to do with the complexity of gender, culture, and other factors, than we have thought previously. Thorne and Paterson (2000) point out that findings of these types exemplify the kind of complexity that may be uncovered when we use research methods that allow examination of factors "in interaction rather than in isolation."

Quantitative Research on Children with Chronic Illness and Their Families

Quantitative descriptive research on management of chronic illness reveals a significant body of work focused on both chronically ill children and their families. In the descriptive literature on children with chronic illness, certain themes are common in specific diseases (e.g., epilepsy) or in chronicity itself. The attributes of the chronically ill child include characteristics of the chronic condition and the child's condition, health behaviors, child psychosocial adjustment, the child's perceptions of self, coping, and social support, and affect (Austin & Sims, 1998; D'Auria, Christian, Henderson & Haynes, 2000;). As part of, or in addition to, studies of child characteristics, there are a number of instrument development studies, because developmentally appropriate measures of many concepts in the area have not been available.

The literature on chronically ill children, unlike that of adults, often includes the idea of family as context if not a variable for study. A content analysis of family assessments in 13 studies revealed a focus on family concepts, including family stressors, family functioning, family resources and coping, and family member involvement and adjustment (Austin & Sims, 1998). In most studies, *family* was operationalized as a parent or parents, but a number of studies included siblings as well as the ill child. The impact of chronic illness of infants and children on parental caregiving (Miles, 2003) as well as parental caregiving by chronically ill parents (Holditch-Davis, Miles, et al., 2001) have become important issues for study, especially in relation to developmental outcomes for children and adolescents (Christian, 2003) and responses of siblings (VanRiper, 2003).

As technology becomes more available to chronically ill children and their families outside the hospital, issues of care for technology-dependent children at home have been a focus of more research. In a recent review of this literature, the authors conclude there is a need for ongoing research in pediatric home care, to address changes in the meaning of home to these families; how family dynamics may be impacted by the care of a technology-dependent child in the home; social isolation of these families; costs; and parent-professional relationships (Wang & Barnard, 2004)

Quantitative Research on Adults with Chronic Illness

Much of the descriptive research on adults with chronic illness over the past decade has focused on psychosocial factors characterizing or influencing

the course of chronic illness. Some of this work has focused on the notion of chronicity and characteristics of chronic illness as overriding the specifics of particular chronic diseases. Other research has focused on specific chronic diseases and the factors that accompany them. Both approaches have contributed to our understanding of what it is like to live with chronic illness, of predictors of quality of life and adjustment outcomes, and, increasingly, of the physiological and biobehavioral outcomes of self-care behaviors over time.

Uncertainty has been described as a universal experience of chronic illness for adults (Mast, 1995). Some of the causes of uncertainty in chronic illness are related to the severity of the illness, the erratic nature of symptomatology, and the ambiguity of symptoms as well as uncertainty about the outcomes of serious illness and the personal and social aspects of life (Bailey & Nielsen, 1993; Braden, 1990; Brashers et al., 2003; Cochrane, 2003; Janson-Bjerklie, Ferketich & Benner, 1993; Mishel, 1999; Wineman et al., 1996).

Uncertainty also arises from concerns about an unknown future (Brown & Powell-Cope, 1991; Smeltzer, 1994; Pelusi, 1997; Nelson, 1996). The impact of chronic illness on daily routines has been described as initiating changes in the person's concept of self and a questioning of one's identity, another source of uncertainty (Mishel, 1999; Charmaz, 1994; Brown & Powell-Cope, 1991; Fleury, Kimbrell & Kruszewski, 1995; Mishel & Murdaugh, 1987). Chronic illness demands lifelong management by the person experiencing it, and adequate knowledge and understanding of the illness and effective management strategies do not come quickly or easily to many. Lack of information is a major source of uncertainty at various points in the illness trajectory—with a new diagnosis, as the trajectory changes; with initiation of new treatment or new complications; and with the possibility or recurrence or exacerbations (Beach, 2001; Mishel, 1999; Small & Graydon, 1992; Nyhlin, 1990; Moser et al., 1993; Hilton, 1988).

In spite of the uncertainties accompanying chronic illness, the work involved in managing treatment and self-care regimens has been well described since the early research of Strauss et al. (1984). Some research has focused on the relationship of clients' health beliefs to regimen adherence (Roberson, 1992). The role and importance of social supports (Morgan et al., 2004; Primomo, Yates & Woods, 1990), and coping variables (Dodd, Dibble & Thomas, 1993; Raleigh, 1992) in the client's success in management have been addressed in a few studies. In addition to studies of how chronically ill persons successfully manage their illnesses (Kralik, Koch, Price & Howard, 2004), predictors of self-care behaviors across a variety of chronic illnesses have been a recent focus of attention in research (Rockwell & Riegel, 2001); self-care is also being linked to outcomes (Chou & Holzemer, 2004).

Another important area of descriptive research on chronic illness is the impact of the illness on clients and families. Studies on the trajectory of chronic illness (Corbin & Strauss, 1991; Fagerhaugh et al., 1987; Jablonski, 2004; Corbin & Strauss, 1991; Wiener & Dodd, 1993) focus on disease consequences and work done by clients and others to manage the illness. The illness trajectory model has generated rich theory for nursing practice and has led to studies of illness management and coping in many diseases, such as cancer, cardiac disease, HIV, mental illness, multiple sclerosis, diabetes, and epilepsy (Morse & Fife, 1998; Roe, 2000; Robinson et al., 1993; Smeltzer, 1991). Studies on the natural history of chronic disease-related or treatment-related symptoms, and predictors of these symptoms have grown exponentially in the nursing research literature. In particular, studies have focused on pain and fatigue which are common symptoms across many chronic diseases and are particularly intrusive symptoms that can affect the quality of life of chronically ill persons in many domains. Studies describing risk factors for particular symptoms, associations of particular symptoms with specific treatment(s), clusters of symptoms, and the ways in which people learn to manage their symptoms over time provide an important foundation for the development of effective interventions to predict, prevent, minimize, alleviate and manage symptoms of chronic illness (Armer, Radina, Porock & Culbertson, 2003). The symptom

experiences of under-studied populations with chronic illness are exemplified by a review of 32 studies of the symptom experiences of women with chronic illness (O'Neill & Morrow, 2001).

Stimulated by new technology and the aggressive treatment of life-threatening illness that cannot be cured, there is a large and growing body of research literature on the quality of life in adults (Breitmeyer et al., 1992; Brostrom, Stromberg, Dahlstrom & Fridlund, 2004; Burckhardt et al., 1989; Ferrell et al, 1998a, 1998b; Franks, McCullagh & Moffatt, 2003; McSweeny & Labuhn, 1990; Widar, Ahlstrom & Ek, 2004) as well as in children. Quality of life has evolved from a global conceptualization of the ability to function in several domains to complex models that reflect the complexity of life quality in multiple domains, such as physical/functional well being, psychological well-being, social well-being, and spiritual well-being. Unfortunately, although there seems to be agreement within nursing and other disciplines about the first three domains, there is little agreement about measurement of the domain. A variety of global and disease-specific quality of life instruments have created a fragmented literature that is difficult to synthesize. What has become clear, however, is that neither a global nor a disease-specific measure alone can capture the complexity of quality of life, so the current gold standard for measurement has become to combine the two. This addresses one of the issues mentioned earlier in this chapter—the notion of whether chronicity overrides specific chronic disease demands or whether the specific demands provide a more accurate picture. In essence, it is only in the combination of the two that we begin to capture the complexity of quality of life in chronic illness (see chapter 9, on quality of life).

As chronic illness increases in our aging population, and as families or others are the primary caregivers for chronically ill adults as well as children, the literature on caregiving in chronic illness has grown tremendously. Findings from caregiving studies provide useful information about specific caregiving tasks, the burdens and satisfactions of caregiving, the risks of prolonged caregiving to the caregiver, the characteristics of caregiver/care receiver relationships, and the social and economic costs of caregiving (Acton & Wright, 2000: Barer & Johnson, 1990; Cartwright et al., 1994; da Cruz, Pimenta, Kurita & de Oliveira, 2004; Given et al., 1997; Kuhlman et al., 1991; Reinhard & Horvitz, 1995; Strand & Haughey, 1998; and Winslow, 1997). Most studies on caregiving focus on spouse or family caregivers of chronically ill individuals or elders. However, caregiving acts of clients for each other also have been studied by nurse researchers (Hutchinson & Bahr, 1991) (see Chapter 11, on family caregivers).

Intervention Studies in the Management of Chronic Illness and Outcomes

Intervention studies related to the management of chronic illnesses comprise the recent and most rapidly growing aspect of the chronic illness literature. The majority of these studies in nursing have been conducted within the past ten to 15 years. The proliferation of clinical intervention studies may be attributed to increased nursing research funding with an emphasis on funding agencies' preferences for this type of research. This shift in emphasis was based on the belief that an adequate body of descriptive work had been developed and, while there were still clearly gaps in that work, the time had come to develop and test clinical interventions that would directly influence practice and outcomes. The shift to intervention work may also have been given some impetus by the movement in nursing research to address the problem of research dissemination—a highly funded national effort during which a number of groups of investigators described barriers to dissemination of research in nursing and attempted to address those barriers in innovative dissemination models (Cronenwett, 1990; CURN Project, 1983; Funk, Tornquist & Champagne, 1995; Rutledge & Donaldson, 1995). At any rate, intervention research with both chronically ill children and adults, clearly took a giant leap in the decade of the 1990s. The link between chronic illness problems, the efficacy and cost effectiveness of interventions to address those prob-

lems, and outcomes to document efficacy became the focus of much nursing research.

Unlike intervention studies in chronic illness prevention, intervention trials in the management domain are targeted to a sample of the population deemed to be most in need and therefore likely to be most responsive to the intervention. The design of such intervention trials, to be valid tests of efficacy, must have some or all of the following components: a treatment (or treatments) group and a control or comparison group, random assignment to one or the other, a clearly defined treatment or intervention with a clearly defined "dose." The intervention is preferably theory-driven and has been tested in pilot studies. The design of the intervention trial should include pre- and post-test measurement of outcomes. More than one post-test measure—for example, a short-term post-intervention and a longer-term post-intervention measure, provides better estimates of the intervention's effects over time.

Intervention Research with Children with Chronic Illness and Their Families

Prior to the 1990s, some of the best-known intervention research with children and families focused on parent–infant interaction in the perinatal period that addressed the potential developmental outcomes for babies at high social risk (Barnard, 1972, 1978; Barnard & Neal, 1977; Barnard & Bee, 1983). Results from these studies determined that interventions were most effective if tailored to the characteristics of the caregivers. In addition, timing of the intervention was found to be crucial. At the other end of the trajectory, early intervention studies focused on the setting and nature of care for terminally ill children who were dying at home and in the hospital (Martinson et al., 1978). Outcomes included not only social and psychological variables, but also economic factors. Research over a period of 20 years that tested the empowerment of children to participate in their own illness-related care concluded that, to be successful, interventions must also include families and health care professionals (Lewis & Lewis, 1989, 1990).

Finally, a study by the U.S. General Accounting Office (1990) reviewed home visiting in the United States and Europe to describe its effectiveness as an early intervention strategy for low-birth weight infants, socially disadvantaged first-time mothers, and others. These researchers found that home visiting was important as a nursing intervention with high-risk populations, in that it was related to better outcomes at birth and improved child health and development (Brooten et al., 1986; Olds et al., 1986).

In an integrative review of intervention research with chronically ill children and their families, Deatrick (1998) addressed the question of what intervention strategies had been effectively used with this group, and what interventions had not been successful, and analyzed the methodological adequacy of the studies as well as the psychometric properties of the outcome measures. Of the nine studies that met the criteria for review, most did not identify conceptual or theoretical frameworks. Two, however, did use ecological systems frameworks (Black et al., 1994; Pless et al., 1994), and two used social psychological theories (Heiney et al., 1990; Hills & Lutkenhoff, 1993); the frameworks in all cases were consistent with study purposes. Most of the interventions were clearly educational or psychoeducational; one was a series of seven sessions of group therapy, the goal of which was to increase social adjustment of siblings of children with cancer (Heiney et al., 1990). The one individual intervention was a series of 12 contacts between child and parent and a BSN-prepared nurse over one year; it was designed to optimize family and parent functioning to increase psychosocial adjustment (Pless et al., 1994). Perhaps because of the lack of theoretical perspectives for many of the interventions, none of the studies described their rationale for the timing of their interventions (Walker, 1992).

Interventions in these studies were targeted to the ill children, their siblings, or the family, although outcomes were sometimes measured for other than the target sample. Family-focused interventions appeared more successful than child-focused interventions. Outcomes for child-focused interventions

included increased problem-focused coping strategies, decreased detachment strategies, and enhanced self-care abilities and range of motion (Brandt & Magyary, 1993; Hills & Lutenhoff, 1993; Lewis & Lewis, 1990; Pless et al., 1994; Smith et al., 1991). Sibling outcomes included social adjustment and qualitative reports of trust, sadness, anger, and uncertainty (Heiney et al., 1990).

More recently, intervention research in chronically ill children and adolescents has focused on improving a variety of outcomes including such examples as resilience and quality of life in children and adolescents with cancer (Nelson et al., 2004); activity outcomes for adolescents who have corrective surgery for scoliosis (LaMontagne, Hepworth, Cohen & Salisbury, 2004): self-management in diabetes (Gage et al., 2004); and management of feelings through poetry in mentally ill children and adolescents (Raingruber, 2004).

Intervention studies aimed at promoting health and preventing chronic illness in children and adolescents comprise what is probably the fastest growing area of research in the last few years. Studies targeting health behaviors in order to decrease the morbidity and mortality of children and adolescents have included a focus on overall health from a holistic perspective and using holistic interventions (Rew, Johnson, Jenkins & Torres, 2004); using culturally and developmentally appropriate interventions to prevent or change behaviors that put children and adolescents at risk for HIV/AIDS (DeMarco & Norris, 2004); preventing osteoporosis by intervention during adolescence (Brown & Schoenly, 2004); preventing sexually transmitted infections in high incidence minority groups (Steenbeek, 2004); promoting self-efficacy for healthy eating (Long & Stevens, 2004); and testing strategies for successful adolescent smoking cessation (Hamilton, O'Connell & Cross, 2004).

Intervention Research with Adults with Chronic Illness

It is not surprising that cancer and heart disease, as the number one and two causes of death for middle-aged and older adults in the United States, have been the chronic illnesses in which, more often, a variety of interventions have been studied. In cardiovascular diseases, exercise interventions, stress management, and life-style changes to reduce risks after an acute event have been the focus of a number of intervention studies (Allen, 1996; Barnason, Zimmerman & Nieveen, 1995; Blumenthal et al., 1997; Fletcher & Vassallo, 1993) as have multidisciplinary team and advanced practice nursing models for care delivery to those with intermittent congestive heart failure, with the goal of managing the illness and preventing episodes of failure requiring treatment and care resources (Cline et al., 1998; Martens & Mellor, 1997; Venner & Seelbinder, 1996).

Psychosocial interventions, both outpatient and home-based, have been tested to enhance recovery from myocardial infarction as well as from cardiac surgery, particularly coronary artery bypass graft surgery, with varying effects (Buselli & Stuart, 1999; Frasure-Smith et al., 1997; Gilliss et al., 1993; Hill, Kelleher & Shumaker, 1992; Moore, 1997). Specific goals of psychosocial interventions have been to decrease physiological arousal and response, including subsequent disease progression; to improve the individual's ability to identify stressors and appraise them in a realistic manner; and to promote a sense of connection with self and others and a sense of meaning and purpose in life (Buselli & Stuart, 1999; Lunsford & Fleury, 2000).

As the medical management of cardiovascular problems has become more successful in allowing people to live longer at home in spite of these problems, nursing interventions have been developed and tested to enhance not only the management of symptoms but the optimization of function and quality of life, and the prevention or at least delay of more severe problems. Psychoeducational interventions for the management of chronic stable angina have recently been reviewed for methodological rigor (McGillion, Watt-Watson, Kim & Yamada, 2004). In spite of positive report of their effectiveness, the authors critiqued the studies' methodological problems and concluded that these intervention trial results are really inconclusive. Preventing re-hospitalizations and emergency room visits has been a focus of interventions for cardio-

vascular problems, as an example, a home based intervention to prevent hospitalization for chronic atrial fibrillation has been developed (Inglis et al., 2004). In addition, recent attention to intervention trials in under-studied, often high-risk populations is a welcome trend in nursing research (Lorig, Ritter & Gonzalez, 2003; Miles et al., 2003).

Significantly more intervention studies have been conducted in men with cardiovascular disease than in women. Rarely have subjects been compared by gender in any intervention study, generally because subsamples of women are so small and because investigators have not addressed the potential importance of gender. Preliminary research indicates that interventions need to be based in part on clients' individual perceptions of illness and of themselves in response (Fleury et al., 1995; Hill, Kelleher & Stuart, 1992). Gender, as a factor in shaping illness perceptions and perceptions of responses, has not been included in many intervention studies, but there does seem to be a trend to target under-studied populations with major chronic illnesses, including women as well as ethnic minorities.

The findings across psychosocial intervention studies in cardiovascular disease have been inconsistent (Lunsford & Fleury, 2000; Moore, 1997). Some studies have indicated that the addition of psychosocial treatments to standard rehabilitation regimens reduced morbidity and mortality, psychological distress, and some biological risk factors, while many other studies show little effect of interventions. Many interventions were multifaceted, making it difficult to identify the differential benefits of any single strategy. Lunsford and Fleury (2000) suggest that developing interventions around an organizing theory would assist in elucidating the pathways to improvement and the benefits of specific interventions, the dose and timing of which derive from the theory.

In cancer care, many of the intervention studies of the past decade and a half, both group and individual, have focused predominantly on helping people with cancer learn more about the disease and treatment, deal more effectively with treatment decisions and choices to be made, and manage the emotional responses to the illness trajectory (Scura,

Budin & Garfing, 2004). Additional studies have examined sharing concerns with others, maintaining or enhancing their social support systems, managing the side effects and sequellae of treatment, increasing satisfaction with sexual relations, and enhancing satisfaction with and quality of life (Anderson, 1992; Devine, 2003; Devine & Westlake, 1995; Fawzy et al., 1995; Forester et al., 1993; Mishel et al., 2002; Molenaar et al., 2001; Trijsburg, van Knippenberg & Rijpma, 1992). Most intervention studies have used a combination of educational, psychological, or combined psycho-educational interventions to enhance cancer clients' knowledge about their illness, improve their communications with health care professionals, enhance their assertiveness when dealing with the health care system, solve problems, and deal with feelings (Anderson, 1992; Devine & Westlake, 1995; Fawzy et al., 1995; Forester et al., 1993; Germino et al., 1998; Mishel et al., 2002; Trijsburg, van Knippenberg & Rijpma, 1992). Increasingly however, exercise interventions have been tested and found to be useful in certain kinds of cancer (Blanchard, Courneya & Laing, 2001; Kolden, Strauman & Ward, 2002; Schwartz, 2000); and cognitive behavioral strategies are being adapted to manage the stresses of serious illness and treatment (Antonu, Lehman & Kilbourn, 2001).

Intervention Research Targeted to Cancer Caregivers In addition to interventions for clients with cancer, there is a growing, however slowly, body of intervention studies that have targeted caregivers of clients with cancer. In a review of interventions on caregiver outcomes in cancer, Pasacreta & McCorkle (2000) reviewed studies that examined educational interventions, support, counseling and psychotherapy interventions, and hospice and palliative home care services. Models to facilitate family caregivers in obtaining needed information included linking of specific nurses with families. This intervention was received well by families, but the outcomes of the study were not described well enough for subsequent research or replication (Carmody, Hickey & Bookbinder, 1991). In a more standardized test of a psycho-educational curriculum designed specifically for cancer caregivers (Barg et al., 1998), the investigators included clearly measurable and appropriate outcomes but found that many caregivers were unwilling to attend a strictly group-organized intervention. The researchers raised the question about whether those caregivers who attended group interventions may actually be a self-selected sample least in need of intervention because they may be able to garner and use social support (Pasacreta & McCorkle, 2000). Ferrell and colleagues, focusing on an intervention related to cancer pain management for caregivers, demonstrated the intervention's effectiveness in improving caregiver knowledge and quality of life (Ferrell et al., 1995).

Support, counseling, and psychotherapy interventions targeting family care providers are still limited in number. Houts et al. (1996) described a prescriptive problem-solving model for training family caregivers. The acronym COPE (creativity, optimism, planning, and expert information) is used to describe the program that teaches caregivers how to plan and implement responses to or in anticipation of problems, both psychosocial and medical. The program is reported as being empowering and can help to moderate stress, but no outcomes are used in the research design that documents the program's effectiveness. Another problem-solving intervention, this one individualized for problems identified by spouses of cancer clients, comprised six sessions. At the six-month follow-up, spouses who received the intervention showed no improvement in their distress, although the clients of those spouses showed decreased depression (Blanchard, Toseland & McCallion, 1997). The authors do not have an explanation for this finding but suggest that the client-spouse dyad may be a more appropriate focus for study. A recent pilot study tested a cognitive behavioral intervention to enhance the quality of interpersonal relationships between mothers with breast cancer and their school-age children (Davis Kirsch, Brandt & Lewis, 2003). This intervention was reflective of prior research that demonstrated problems in parenting by mothers with breast cancer who are depressed (Zahlis & Lewis, 1998).

With cost-effectiveness of family caregiver interventions in cancer being a critical issue, creative use of strategies other than face to face contacts are being increasingly tested. Telephone support interventions for family caregivers have recently targeted caregivers of seriously ill cancer clients (Walsh, Estrada & Hogan, 2004) and caregivers of cancer clients at the end of life (Walsh & Schmidt, 2003). A combination of telephone and in person contacts structured an intervention designed to improve depressive symptoms among cancer caregivers; this intervention targeted caregivers of those with newly diagnosed cancer, providing information on symptom monitoring and management, education about cancer, emotional support, coordination of services and caregiver preparation to care (Kozachik et al., 2001). The intervention appeared to be effective in slowing the rate of depressive symptoms, but not in decreasing levels of depression. Sampling bias was an issue since more severely depressed caregivers tended to withdraw from the study.

In the larger field of oncology, increasing openness to complementary and alternative interventions is beginning to be reflected in nursing intervention research with family caregivers. A recent pilot study of art intervention with family caregivers serves as an interesting example (Walsh & Weiss, 2003).

With more individuals with cancer being cared for at home by family, several intervention studies have focused on palliative home care models. These models emphasize support and education of family care providers and the stress they experience. Some of the important findings of these studies included that caregivers of cancer clients who have physical problems of their own are at risk for psychological morbidity as they assume the caregiving role (Jepson et al., 1999). A number of recent descriptive studies validate this finding (Kurtz, Kurtz, Given & Given, 2004; Nijboer et al., 2001; and Rossi Ferrario et al., 2004). The length of time caregivers were involved with hospice has been positively related to the number of communication tasks reported and consistent with the hospice approach to management of the terminally ill. There were no significant results for the effect of duration of caregiving and length of time in hospice on caregivers' outcomes (Yang & Kirschling, 1992; McMillan & Mahon, 1994; McMillan, 1996). Other findings related to bereavement outcomes indicate that bereaved caregivers have special needs that, when managed by those with appropriate training, result in positive outcomes (Fakhoury, McCarthy & Addington-Hall, 1997). The spousal relationship, older age, and perception of substantial emotional burden have been related to difficulties with bereavement (Rossi Ferrario et al., 2004).

Intervention Research on Other Chronic Illness

As the population has aged, there has been increasing interest in some of the chronic conditions of aging, including urinary incontinence. The management of urinary incontinence in ambulatory, otherwise functional populations has been of increasing interest to nurse investigators because of its prevalence, costs, and impact on quality of life (Wyman, 2000). Research identifying risk factors and information from the physical medicine and rehabilitation literature on bladder training in those with neurological impairments has been foundational to the current generation of intervention studies. In spite of poor understanding of how bladder training achieves its effects, bladder training interventions for both women and men have been successful in decreasing the severity of incontinence, decreasing the number of incontinence episodes, reducing stress or urge incontinence, and subjective improvement (Columbo et al., 1995; Fantl et al., 1991; Wiseman, Malone-Lee & Rail, 1991; Wyman et al., 1997, 1998).

Pelvic floor muscle exercises, with a variety of adjuvant and supportive devices, such as audiocassette practice tapes, biofeedback, vaginal weight training, electrical stimulation, and drug therapy, have been shown, as has bladder training, to have short-term effectiveness, although long-term treatment maintenance tends to be lower (Wyman, 2000). Adherence rates tend to drop over time, and some have suggested that the physiological and psychological theories on which these interventions are based are at least part of the problem because they do not take knowledge about health behavior change into account (Wyman, 2000). There has been little or no research on long-term prevention of incontinence, even with knowledge of the risk factors.

Nursing interventions targeting clients with chronic pain (deWit & van Dam, 2001) chronic wounds or ulcers (Orsted et al., 2001); and depression (Smith, Leenerts & Fajewski, 2003; Zust, 2000) are also of increasing interest as are complementary and alternative strategies including, as examples, meditation (Bonadonna, 2003) and journaling for emotional disclosure and benefit finding (Stanton et al., 2002).

Issues in Chronic Illness Research

Issues of Descriptive Research in Prevention of Chronic Illness

In this area of research, there are a number of issues. First, the research is largely interdisciplinary, and while there are more nurse investigators with programmatic research than in prior decades, some of the work consists of only one or two studies. Nurses who increasingly work with interdisciplinary research teams, particularly in school-based research, bring a variety of valuable perspectives to complex problems. The theories and models guiding the research reflect the balance of nursing and interdisciplinary work. The majority of the work in this area is quantitative, and there seems to be some consensus on priorities across disciplines over time. Recent emphasis on children's risk factors for cardiovascular disease, especially childhood obesity and early onset of Type II diabetes as well as HIV/AIDS is clear.

Issues in Intervention Research in the Prevention of Chronic Illness

A few years ago, in an integrative review of intervention models for health promotion of children and families, Hayman and colleagues (1995) discussed a common theme in chronic illness literature, the cross-disciplinary nature of the research and few programmatic efforts in this area. Given the relative recency of descriptive work in chronic illness, Hayman et al. noted that it is not surprising that theory-based intervention research is just beginning to emerge. Today, the gold standard for nursing interventions on the prevention of chronic illness includes a basis in theory, attention to the clinical realities of intervention delivery, evaluation of costs, and clear, salient outcomes. In the area of chronic illness prevention, there are some programmatic intervention studies led by nurse principal investigators—most notably Harrell (Harrell et al., 1995; 1996; 1999; 2001) and Jemmott (Jemmott & Jemmott, 1992). The theoretical base for this area of chronic illness research is more complex because, in children and families, contextual and developmental factors vary over time, and studies demand models that can reflect change at the individual and family levels, and that can target a variety of outcomes and account for multiple contexts (Hayman, Meininger, Coates & Gallagher, 1995).

Issues in Descriptive Research on Chronic Illness Management

In a literature review of children with chronic illness and their families, Austin and Sims (1998) note several areas of concern. Many studies up to that time had focused on the child's general psychosocial adjustment rather than on adjustment to the illness—the domain for nursing care. Without more attention to illness adjustment, and factors that may influence it at various points in time, it will be difficult for nurses to design appropriate and effective interventions. The source and type of assessment data continue to be a concern, because many investigators still use only one source and do not make appropriate use of other techniques, such as observational methods. The use of multiple sources and methods for measurement of the same concept is one strategy for addressing method variance bias and needs to be used more consistently by nurse investigators (Lorenz & Melby, 1994). Many of the instruments used in these studies were developed for the general population and may not be valid measures for children with chronic health conditions. In addition, inadequate attention has been given to the developmental level of the child, with age often the only developmental variable measured. In a recent chapter of the *Annual Review of Nursing Research*, Miles and Holditch-Davis (2003) call for a developmental science perspective to guide this research because this perspective allows an integrative view of systems both internal and external to the child and family and with which they interact, having mutual influence.

In the descriptive research on adults with chronic illness, there are a number of issues for consideration in future work. Early work was rarely theory-driven, but there have emerged a number of mid-range theories in nursing and adaptation of theories from other disciplines that have enhanced this literature and given it direction and substance. New models continue to be developed and adapted, and modern statistical techniques have enhanced our ability to test complex models in a meaningful way. At this point in time, qualitative theory development work and quantitative theory testing research are both considered crucial to the development of chronic illness knowledge. As we learn more about the complexities of chronic illness prevention and management in our progress to intervention studies, it is essential that we find better ways for the results of these two kinds of research to "speak" to each other.

Measurement issues continue to abound in this, as in many other areas. The development and testing of measures that fit emerging conceptualizations continue as ongoing issues.

The search for commonalities across models of childhood and adult chronic illness is revealing, and adult-oriented investigators can learn from the data on the inclusion of family that are evident in much of the work on chronically ill children. The need to address developmental and timing issues in terms of assessing risk in disease management continues to be unaddressed. A recent article points out a limitation in most chronic illness research, the discrepancy between the "temporal patterning of chronic illness as it is played out slowly and the majority of research that is undertaken and funded in one-, two-, or three-year cycles with an eye to achieving statistical significance" (Russell & Gregory, 2000, p. 100). The need for longitudinal designs remains an issue that must be balanced against funding constraints, attrition problems, and other issues.

Finally, we need to attend to the gaps in our knowledge—about the relationship of gender, culture, age/development, marginality, poverty, and other circumstances—in regard to responses to and ability to manage chronic illness. Non-mainstream populations of chronically ill people have not often been studied, but inquiry in the area of HIV/AIDS has provided us with some important lessons that need wider application. Gender differences remain an issue in many chronic illnesses.

Issues in Intervention Studies in Chronic Illness Management

Intervention studies disproportionately test efficacy with Caucasian, middle-class people, and many intervention subjects, depending on the illness, have been one gender or the other, with few comparisons by gender. Particular illness populations are not representative of all chronic illness; for instance, with cancer, interventions have, for a long time, come out of studies of those with breast cancer (Devine & Westlake, 1995). Fortunately, that has changed in recent years as high risk, underserved groups and more studies of men with prostate cancer and other specific kinds of cancers for both men and women have been targeted in interventions (Germino, 2001). For many years women were excluded from studies or present in very small numbers in cardiovascular disease and incorporated in the samples of men. Management interventions targeting caregivers need theory-based, pilot-tested, standardized group and individual interventions. This area of information would benefit greatly, too, from some consistency in outcomes and consistency in measurement of those outcomes.

Summary and Conclusions

Research about prevention and management of chronic illness crosses many categories of illness and chronic problems, of which only a few are represented here. The literature on children tends to include families, a strength that the adult literature does not necessarily include. However, there is growing attention to families of adults in terms of the caregiving role, as well as interventions to alleviate the risks of and enhance the positive aspects of giving care to a family member. A diverse foundation of descriptive research, a changing health care system, and a focus on cost effectiveness have all contributed to a growing body of intervention research in chronic illness, both prevention and management interventions. Lack of consistency in theory being tested and applied, variability in outcomes, gaps in measurement, and sampling bias are the key issues

that pervade this body of knowledge. Future work requires a focus on these issues and on methodological rigor that will produce findings on which effective practice can be based.

Across all areas of chronic illness research in nursing, there is a need for more mid-range theory specific to aspects of chronic illness. More research that systematically tests and provides data for refinement of such theory would move nursing knowledge forward. Chronic illness focused, multidisciplinary journals or other venues, in which the literature, rather than being disease-specific, can be related to each other, develop a better view of common phenomena. Also, combining biological and behavioral methods better fits nursing's holistic perspective of the many aspects of people's lives that are affected by chronic illness. Finally, dissemination of research findings into practice will help the development of evidence-based practice.

Study Questions

1. What are the barriers that face researchers in chronic illness research in general?
2. What are the issues in designing an intervention study on the management of chronic illness?
3. What issues are apparent with research in children and chronic illness?
4. What has been the major impetus for doing intervention studies in chronic illness?

5. Describe the pros and the cons of doing descriptive research from a disease-specific perspective versus a study examining individuals' commonalities across several different diseases.
6. What does the future hold in regard to chronic illness research?

References

Acton, G. J., & Wright, K. B. (2000). Self-transcendence and family caregivers of adults with dementia. *Journal of Holistic Nursing, 18* (2), 143–158.

Ajzen, I. (1985). From intentions to actions: A theory of planned behavior. In J. Kuhl & J. Beckman (Eds.), *Action control: From cognition to behavior,* (pp. 11–39). New York: Springer.

Ajzen, I., & Fishbein, M. (1980). *Understanding attitudes and predicting social behavior.* Englewood Cliffs, NJ: Prentice-Hall.

Ajzen, I., & Timko, C. (1983). Attitudes, perceived control and the prediction of health behavior. Unpublished manuscript. University of Massachusetts, Amherst.

Allen, J. K. (1996). Coronary risk factor modification in women after coronary artery bypass surgery. *Nursing Research, 45* (5), 260–265.

Anderson, B. L. (1992). Psychological interventions for cancer patients to enhance quality of life. *Journal of Consulting and Clinical Psychology, 60*, 552–568.

Antonu, M. H., Lehman, J. M., & Kilbourn, K. M. (2001). Cognitive behavior stress management intervention decreases the prevalence of depression and enhances benefit finding among women under treatment for early-stage breast cancer. *Health Psychology, 20* (1), 20–32.

Armer, J. M., Radina, M. E., Porock, D. & Culbertson, S. D. (2003). Predicting breast cancer-related lymphedema using self-reported symptoms. *Nursing Research, 52* (6), 370–379.

Austin, J., & Sims, S. (1998). Integrative view of assessment models for examining children's and families' responses to chronic illness. In M. Broome, K. Knafl, K. Pridham, and S. Feetham (Eds.), *Children and families in health and illness*, (pp. 196–220). Thousand Oaks: Sage.

Bailey, J. M., & Nielsen, B. I. (1993). Uncertainty and appraisal of uncertainty in women with rheumatoid arthritis. *Orthopaedic Nursing, 12* (2), 63–67.

Bandura, A. (1986). *Social foundations of thought and action: A social cognitive theory.* Englewood Cliffs, NJ: Prentice-Hall.

Baranowski, T., Perry, C. K. & Parcel, G. S. (2002). How individuals, environments and health behavior interact: Social Cognitive Theory. In Glanz, K., Rimer, B. K., & Lewis, F. M. (Eds.). *Health behavior and health education: Theory, research and practice* (3rd ed.) (pp. 165–184). San Francisco: Jossey-Bass Publishers.

Barer, B. M., & Johnson, C. L. (1990). A critique of the caregiving literature. *The Gerontologist, 30* (1), 26–29.

Barg, F. K., Pasacreta, J. V., Nuamah, I. F., Robinson, K. D., et al. (1998). A description of a psychoeducational intervention for family caregivers of cancer patients. *Journal of Family Nursing, 4*, 394–413.

Barnard, K. E., & Neal, M. V. (1977). Maternal-child nursing research: Review of the past and strategies for the future. *Nursing Research, 26*, 193–200.

Barnard, K. E. (1972). The effect of stimulation on the duration and amount of sleep and wakefulness in the premature infant (doctoral dissertation, University of Washington, 1968). *Dissertation Abstracts International, 33*, 2167b.

———. (1978). *Nursing child assessment training project learning resource manual.* Seattle: University of Washington School of Nursing.

Barnard, K. E., & Bee, H. L. (1983). The impact of temporally patterned stimulation on the development of preterm infants. *Child Development, 54*, 1156–1167.

Barnard, K. E., Snyder, C., & Spietz, A. (1991). Supportive measures for high-risk infants and families. In A. L. Whall & J. Fawcett (Eds.), *Family theory development in nursing: State of the science and the art.* Philadelphia: FA Davis.

Barnason, S., Zimmerman, L., & Nieveen J. (1995). The effects of music interventions on anxiety in the patient after coronary artery bypass grafting. *Heart and Lung, 24*, 124–132.

Beach, W.A. (2001). Stability and ambiguity: Managing uncertain moments when updating news about mom's cancer. *Text, 21* (1/2), 221–250.

Becker, M. J. (Ed.). (1974). *The health belief model and personal health behavior.* Thorofare, NJ: Charles B. Slack.

Bennett, S. J., Cordes, D. K., Westmoreland, G., Castro, R. et al. (2000). Self-care strategies for symptom management in patients with chronic heart failure. *Nursing Research, 49* (3), 139–145.

Black, M., Nair, P., Knight, C., Awachtel, R., et al. (1994). Parenting and early development among children of drug-using women: Effects of home intervention. *Pediatrics, 94*, 440–448.

Blanchard, C. G., Toseland, R. W., & McCallion P. (1997). The effects of a problem solving intervention with spouses of cancer patients. *Journal of Psychosocial Oncology, 14*, 1–21.

Blanchard, C. M., Courneya, K. S. & Laing, D. (2001). Effects of acute exercise on state anxiety in breast cancer survivors. *Oncology Nursing Forum, 28* (10), 1617–1621.

Blue, C., Wilbur, J. & Marston-Scott, M. (2001). Exercise among blue collar workers: Application of the theory of planned behavior. *Research in Nursing and Health, 24*, 481–493.

Blumenthal, J., Jiang, W., Babyak, M., Krantz, D., et al. (1997). Stress management and exercise training in cardiac patients with myocardial ischemia. *Archives of Internal Medicine, 157*, 2213–2223.

Bonadonna, R. (2003). Meditation's impact on chronic illness. *Holistic Nursing Practice, 17* (6), 309–319.

Braden, C. J. (1990). A test of the self-help model: Learned response to chronic illness experience. *Nursing Research, 39*, 42–47.

_____. (1993). Promoting a learned self-help response to chronic illness. In S. G. Funk, E. M. Tornquist, M. T. Champagne, & R. A. Wiese (Eds.), *Key aspects of caring for the chronically ill: Hospital and home*, (pp. 158–169). New York: Springer.

Brandt, P. A., & Magyary, D. L. (1993). The impact of a diabetes education program on children and mothers. *Journal of Pediatric Nursing, 8*, 31–40.

Brashers, D. E., Neidig, J. L., Russell, J. A., Cardillo, L. W., et al. (2003). The medical, personal and social causes of uncertainty in HIV illness. *Issues in Mental Health Nursing, 24* (5), 497–522.

Breitmayer, B. J., Gallo, A. M., Knafl, K. A., & Zoeller, L. H. (1992). Social competence of school-age children with chronic illnesses. *Journal of Pediatric Nursing, 7*, 181–188.

Brooten, D., Kumar, S., Brown, L., Butts, P., et al. (1986). A randomized clinical trial of early hospital discharge and home follow-up of very low birthweight infants. *New England Journal of Medicine, 315*, 934–939.

Brostrom, A., Stromberg, A., Dahlstrom, U. & Fridlund, B. (2004). Sleep difficulties, daytime sleepiness and health-related quality of life in patients with chronic heart failure. *Journal of Cardiovascular Nursing, 19* (4), 234–242.

Brown, M. A., & Powell-Cope, G. M. (1991). AIDS family caregiving: Transitions through uncertainty. *Nursing Research, 40*, 338–345.

Brown, S. J., & Schoenly, L. (2004). Test of an educational intevention for osteoporosis prevention with U.S. adolescents. *Orthopedic Nursing, 23* (4), 245–251.

Burckhardt, C. S., Woods, S. L., Schultz, A. A., & Ziebarth, D. M. (1989). Quality of life of adults with chronic illness: A psychometric study. *Research in Nursing and Health, 12*, 347–354.

Burton, C. R. (2000). Re-thinking stroke rehabilitation: The Corbin and Strauss chronic illness trajectory framework. *Journal of Advanced Nursing, 32* (3), 595–602.

Buselli, E., & Stuart, E. (1999). Influence of psychosocial factors and biopsychosocial interventions on outcomes after myocardial infarction. *Journal of Cardiovascular Nursing, 13* (3), 60–72.

Carmody, S., Hickey, P., & Bookbinder, M. (1991). Preoperative needs of families. *Association of Operating Room Nurses Journal, 54*, 561–567.

Carter, K., & Kulbok, P. (2002). Motivation for health behaviors: A systematic review of the nursing literature. *Journal of Advanced Nursing, 40* (3), 316–330.

Cartwright, J. C., Archbold, P. G., Stewart, B. J., & Limandri, B. (1994). Enrichment processes in family caregiving to frail elders. *Advances in Nursing Science, 17* (1), 31–43.

Charmaz, K. (1990). Discovering chronic illness: Using grounded theory. *Social Science and Medicine, 30* (11), 1161–1172.

_____. (1994). Identity dilemmas of chronically ill men. *The Sociological Quarterly, 35* (2), 269–288.

Chou, F.Y., & Holzemer, W.L. (2004). Linking HIV/AIDS clients' self-care with outcomes. *Journal of the Association of Nurses in AIDS Care, 15* (4), 58–67.

Christian, B. (2003). Growing up with chronic illness: Psychosocial adjustment of children and adolescents with cystic fibrosis. *Annual Review of Nursing Research, 21*, 151–172.

Cline, C. M. J., Israelsson, B. Y. A., Willenheimer, R. B., Broms, K., et al. (1998). Cost effective management program for heart failure reduces rehospitalization. *Heart, 80*, 442–446.

Cochrane, J. (2003). The experience of uncertainty for individuals with HIV/AIDS and the palliative care paradigm. *International Journal of Palliative Nursing, 9* (9), 382–388.

Columbo, M., Zanetta, G., Scalambrino, S., & Milani, R. (1995). Oxybutynin and bladder training in the management of female urinary urge incontinence: A randomized study. *International Urogynecology Journal, 6*, 63–67.

Conrad, P. (1990). Qualitative research on chronic illness: A commentary on method and conceptual development. *Social Science and Medicine, 30*, 1257–1263.

Corbin, J., & Strauss, A. (1991). A nursing model for chronic illness management based upon the trajectory framework. *Scholarly Inquiry for Nursing Practice, 5* (3), 155–174.

Cronenwett, L. (1990). Improving practice through research utilization. In S. Funk, E. Tornquist, M. Champagne, L. Copp, & R. Wiese (Eds.), *Key aspects of recovery: Improving nutrition, rest and mobility*, (pp. 7–22). New York: Springer.

CURN Project (Horsley, J. A., Crane, J., Crabtree, M. K. & Wood, D. J.) (1983). *Using research to improve nursing practice: A guide*. New York: Grune & Stratton.

D'Auria, J. P., Christian, B. J., Henderson, Z. G. & Haynes, B. (2000). The company they keep: The influence of peer relationships on adjustment to cystic fibrosis during adolescence. *Journal of Pediatric Nursing, 15*, 175–182.

daCruz, Dde A., Pimenta, C. A., Kurita, G. P., & de Oliveira, A. C. (2004). Caregivers of patients with chronic pain: Responses to care. *International Journal of Nursing Terminology and Classification, 15* (1), 5–14.

Davis Kirsch, S. E., Brandt, P. A., & Lewis, F. M. (2003). Making the most of the moment: When a child's mother has breast cancer. *Cancer Nursing, 26* (1), 47–54.

Deatrick, J. A. (1998). Integrative review of intervention research with children who have chronic conditions and their families. In M. E. Broome, K. Knafl, K. Pridham, & S. Feetham (Eds.), *Children and families in health and illness*, (pp. 221–235). Thousand Oaks, CA: Sage.

DeMarco, R., & Norris, A. E. (2004). Culturally relevant HIV interventions: Transcending ethnicity. *Journal of Cultural Diversity, 11* (2), 65–68.

Devine, E. C. (2003). Meta-analysis of the effects of psychoeducational interventions on pain in adults with cancer. *Oncology Nursing Forum, 30* (1), 75–89.

Devine E. C., & Westlake, S. K. (1995). The effects of psychoeducational care provided to adults with cancer: Meta-analysis of 116 studies. *Oncology Nursing Forum, 22* (9), 1369–1381.

DeWit, R., & van Dam, F. (2001). From hospital to home care: A randomized controlled trial of a pain education programme for cancer patients with chronic pain. *Journal of Advanced Nursing, 36* (6), 742–754.

Dodd, M. J., Dibble, S. L., & Thomas, M. L. (1993). Predictors of concerns and coping strategies of cancer chemotherapy outpatients. *Applied Nursing Research, 6* (1), 2–7.

Fagerhaugh, S., Strauss, A., Suczek, B., & Wiener, C. (1987). *Hazards in hospital care.* San Francisco: Jossey-Bass.

Fakhoury, W. K. H., McCarthy, M., & Addington-Hall, J. (1997). Carers' health status: Is it associated with their evaluation of the quality of palliative care? *Scandinavian University Press, 25,* 297–301.

Fantl, J. A., Wyman, J. F., McClish D. K., Harkins, S. W., et al. (1991). Efficacy of bladder training in older women with urinary incontinence. *Journal of the American Medical Association, 265,* 609–613.

Fawzy, F. I., Fawzy, N. W., Arndt, L. A., & Pasnau, R. O. (1995). Critical review of psychosocial interventions in cancer care. *Archives of General Psychiatry, 52,* 100–113.

Ferrell, B. R., Grant, M., Chan, J., Ahn, C., et al. (1995). The impact of cancer pain education on family caregivers of elderly patients. *Oncology Nursing Forum, 22,* 1211–1218.

Ferrell, B. R., Grant, M., Funk, B., Otis-Green, S., et al. (1998a). Quality of life in breast cancer Part I: Physical and social well-being. *Cancer Nursing, 20* (6), 398–408.

Ferrell, B. R., Grant, M., Funk, B., Otis-Green, S., et al. (1998b). Quality of life in breast cancer Part II: Psychological and spiritual well-being. *Cancer Nursing, 21* (10), 1–9.

Fishel, A. (1999). Psychosocial and behavioral health care. In C. Shea, L. Pelletier, E. Poster, G. Stuart, & M. Verhey (Eds.), *Advanced practice nursing in psychiatric and mental health care*, (pp. 190–202). St. Louis: Mosby.

Fletcher, B. J., & Vassallo, L. M. (1993). Exercise testing and training in physically disabled subjects with coronary artery disease. In S. G. Funk, E. M. Tornquist, M. T. Champagne, & R. A. Wiese (Eds.), *Key aspects of caring for the chronically ill: Hospital and home,* (pp. 189–201). New York: Springer.

Fleury, J. (1996). Wellness motivation theory: An exploration of theoretical relevance. *Nursing Research, 45* (5), 277–283.

Fleury, J., Kimbrell, C., & Kruszewski, M. A. (1995). Life after a cardiac event: Women's experience in healing. *Heart and Lung, 24,* 474–482.

Folkman, S., & Moskowitz, J.T. (2000). Positive affect and the other side of coping. *American Psychologist, 55* (6), 647–654.

Forester, B., Kornfeld, D. S., Fleiss, J. L., & Thompson, S. (1993). Group psychotherapy during radiotherapy: Effects on emotional and physical distress. *American Journal of Psychiatry, 150,* 1700–1706.

Frank, D., Swedmark, J. & Grubbs, L. (2004) Colon cancer screening in African-American women. *ABNF Journal, 15* (4), 67–70.

Franks, P. J., McCullagh, L., & Moffatt, C. J. (2003). Assessing quality of life in patients with chronic leg ulceration using the Medical Outcomes Short Form-36 questionnaire. *Ostomy and Wound Management, 49* (2), 26–37.

Frasure-Smith, N., Lesperance, F., Prince, R., Verrier, P., et al. (1997). The scientific foundations of cognitive behaviour therapy. In D. Clark & C. Fairburn (Eds.), *Science and practice of cognitive behaviour therapy*, (pp. 27–46). Oxford: Oxford University Press.

Funk, S. G., Tornquist, E. M., & Champagne, M. T. (1995). Barriers and facilitators of research utilization. *Nursing Clinics of North America, 30* (3), 395–407.

Gage, H., Hampson, S., Skinner, T. C., Hart, J., et al. (2004). Educational and psychosocial programmes for adolescents with diabetes: Approaches, outcomes and cost-effectiveness. *Patient Education and Counseling, 53* (3), 333–346.

Gelder, M. (1997). The future at behavior therapy. *Journal of Psychotherapy Practice and Research, 6* (4), 285–293.

Gennaro, S., Brooten, D., Klein, A., Stringer, M., et al. (1993). Cost burden of low birthweight. In S. G. Funk, E. M. Tornquist, M. T. Champagne, & R. A. Wiese (Eds.), *Key aspects of caring for the chronically ill: Hospital and home,* (pp. 271–280). New York: Springer.

Gerhardt, U. (1990). Qualitative research on chronic illness; the issue and the story. *Social Science and Medicine, 30,* 1149–1159.

Germino, B. B. (2001). Educational and Psychosocial Intervention Trials in Prostate Cancer. *Seminars in Oncology Nursing, 17* (2), 129–137.

Germino, B. B., Mishel, M. H., Belyea, M., Harris, L., et al. (1998). Uncertainty in prostate cancer: Ethnic and family patterns. *Cancer Practice, 6* (2), 107–113.

Gilliss, C., Gortner, S., Hauck, W., Shinn, J., et al. (1993). A randomized clinical trial of nursing care for recovery from cardiac surgery. *Heart and Lung, 22,* 125–133.

Gittelsohn, J., Evans, M., Helitzer, D., Anlikeer, J., et al. (1998). Formative research in as school-based obesity prevention program for Native American school children (Pathways). *Health Education Research, 13* (2), 251–265.

Given, B. A., Given, C. W., Helms, E., Stommel, M., et al. (1997). Determinants of family caregiver reaction: New and recurrent cancer. *Cancer Practice, 5* (1), 17–24.

Glenister, A. M., Castiglia, P., Kanski, G., & Haughey, B. (1990). AIDS knowledge and attitudes of primary grade teachers and student. *Journal of Pediatric Health Care, 4,* 77–85.

Gortmaker, S. L., Peterson, K., Wiecha, J., Sobol, A. M., et al. (1999). Reducing obesity via a school-based interdisciplinary intervention among youth. *Archives of Pediatric and Adolescent Medicine, 153,* 409–418.

Grindel, C. G., Brown, L., Caplan, L., & Blumenthal, D. (2004). The effect of breast cancer screening messages on knowledge, attitudes, perceived risk and mammography screening of African American women in the rural South. *Oncology Nursing Forum, 31* (4), 801–808.

Haggerty, R. J. (1984). The changing role of the pediatrician in child health care. *American Journal of Diseases of Children, 127,* 545–549.

Hamilton, G., O'Connell, M. & Cross, D. (2004). Adolescent smoking cessation: Development of a school nurse intervention. *Journal of School Nursing, 20* (3), 169–174.

Harrell, J. S., Bomar, P., McMurray, R., Brown, S. A., et al. (2001). Leptin and obesity in biracial mother-child pairs. *Biologic Research in Nursing, 3* (2), 55–64.

Harrell, J. S., Gansky, S. A., McMurray, R. G., Bangdiwala, S. I., et al. (2001). School-based interventions to improve the health of children with multiple cardiovascular risk factors. In S. G. Funk, E. M. Tornquist, J. Leeman, M. S. Miles & J. S. Harrell (Eds.), *Key aspects of preventing and managing chronic illness* (pp. 71–83). New York: Springer.

Harrell, J. S., McMurray, R. G., Bangdiwala, S. J., Frauman, A. C., et al. (1996). The effects of a school-based intervention to reduce cardiovascular disease risk factors in elementary school children: The Cardiovascular Health in Children (CHIC) study. *Journal of Pediatrics, 128,* 797–805.

Harrell, J. S., McMurray R. G., Gansky, S. A., Bangdiwala, S. I., et al. (1999). A public health vs. a risk-base intervention to improve cardiovascular health in elementary school children: The Cardiovascular Health in Children Study. *American Journal of Public Health, 89* (10), 1529–1535.

Hayman, L. L., Meininger, J. C., Coates, P. M., & Gallagher, P. R. (1995). Nongenetic influences of obesity on risk factors for cardiovascular disease during two phases of development. *Nursing Research, 44,* 277–283.

Healthy People 2000: National health promotion and disease prevention objectives. (1991). Washington, DC: Public Health Service, U.S. Department of Health and Human Services.

Heiney, S., Goon-Johnson, K., Ettinger, R. S., & Ettinger, S. (1990). The effects of group therapy on siblings of pediatric oncology patients. *Journal of Pediatric Oncology Nursing, 7* (3), 95–100.

Hill, D., Kelleher, K., & Shumaker, S. (1992). Psychosocial interventions in adult patients with coronary heart disease and cancer. *General Hospital Psychiatry, 14S,* 28S–42S.

Hills, R. G., & Lutkenhoff, M. L. (1993). Social skills group for physically challenged school age children. *Pediatric Nursing, 19*, 573–577.

Hilton, B. A. (1988). The phenomenon of uncertainty in women with breast cancer. *Issues in Mental Health Nursing, 9*, 217–238.

Hogue, C., & Cullinan, S. M. (1993). Exercise training for frail rural elderly: A pilot study. In S. G. Funk, E. M. Tornquist, M. T. Champagne, & R. A. Wiese (Eds.), *Key aspects of caring for the chronically ill: Hospital and home*, (pp. 202–211). New York: Springer.

Holditch-Davis, D., Bartlett, T. R., Blickman, A., & Miles, M. S. (2003b). Post-traumatic stress symptoms in mothers of premature infants. *Journal of Obstetric, Gynecological & Neonatal Nursing, 32*, 161–171.

Holditch-Davis, D., & Black, B. (2003a). Care of preterm infants: Programs of research and their relationship to developmental science In J.J. Fitzpatrick (Series Ed.); M. Miles and D. Holditch-Davis (Vol. Eds.). *Annual Review of Nursing Research Vol. 21*. Research on child health and pediatric issues (pp. 23–60). New York: Springer.

Holditch-Davis, D., Edwards, L. J., & Wigger, M. C. (1994). Pathologic apnea and brief respiratory pauses in preterm infants: A pilot study. *Pediatrics, 56*, 361–367.

Holditch-Davis, D., Miles, M.S., Burchinal, M., O'Donnell, K., et al. (2001). Parental caregiving and developmental outcomes of infants of mothers with HIV. *Nursing Research, 50* (1), 5–14.

Holditch-Davis, D., & Thoman, E. B. (1987). Behavioral states of premature infants: Implications for neural and behavioral development. *Developmental Psychbiology, 20*, 25–38.

Houts, P. S., Nezu, A. M., Nezu, C. M., & Bucher, J. A. (1996). The prepared family caregiver: A problem-solving approach to family caregiver education. *Patient Education and Counseling, 27* (1), 63–73.

Hupcey, J. (1998). Clarifying the social support theory-research linkage. *Journal of Advanced Nursing, 24*, 1231–1241.

Hutchinson, C., & Bahr, R. (1991). Types and meanings of caring behaviors among elderly nursing home residents. *Image, 23* (2), 85–88.

Inglis, S., McLennan, S., Dawson, A., Birchmore, L., et al. (2004). A new solution for an old problem? Effects of a nurse-led, multidisciplinary, home-based intervention on readmission and mortality in patients with chronic atrial fibrillation. *Journal of Cardiovascular Nursing, 19* (2), 118–127.

Jablonski, A. (2004). The illness trajectory of end-stage renal disease dialysis patients. *Research, Theory and Nursing Practice, 18* (1), 51–72.

Janson-Bjerklie, S., Ferketich, S., & Benner, P. (1993). Predicting the outcomes of living with asthma. *Research in Nursing and Health, 16*, 241–250.

Jemmott, L. S., & Jemmott, J. B. III. (1992). Increasing condom-use intentions among sexually active Black adolescent women. *Nursing Research, 41*, 273–279.

Jepson, C., McCorkle, R., Adler, D., Nuamah, I. O., et al. (1999). Effects of home care on caregivers' psychosocial status. *Image: Journal of Nursing Scholarship, 31*, 115–120.

Joachim, G. & Acorn, S. (2000). Living with chronic illness: The interface of stigma and normalization. *Canadian Journal of Nursing Research, 32* (3), 37–48.

Jopling, R. J. (1992). Physical fitness in children. In S. B. Friedman, R. A. Hoekelman, N. M. Nelson, & H. M. Seidel (Eds.), *Primary pediatric care* (2nd ed.). (pp. 246–256). St. Louis: Mosby.

Kolcaba, K. (2001). Evolution of the mid range theory of comfort for outcomes research *Nursing Outlook, 49* (2), 86–92.

Kolden, G. G., Strauman, T. J., & Ward, S. A. (2002). A pilot study of group exercise training for women with primary breast cancer. *Psycho-Oncology, 11*, 447–456.

Koniak-Griffin, D., & Brecht, M. (1995). Linkages between sexual risk taking, substance use and AIDS knowledge among pregnant adolescents and young mothers. *Nursing Research, 44*, 334–346.

Kozachik, S. L., Given, C. W., Given, B. A., Pierce, S. J., et al. (2001). *Oncology Nursing Forum, 28* (7), 1149–1157.

Kralik, D. (2002). The quest for ordinariness: Transition experienced by midlife women living with breast cancer. *Journal of Advanced Nursing, 39* (2), 146–154.

Kralik, D., Koch, T., Price, K. & Howard, N. (2004). Chronic illness self-management: Taking action to create order. *Journal of Clinical Nursing, 13* (2), 259–267.

Kuhlman, G. J., Wilson, H. S., Hutchinson, S. A., & Wallhagen, M. (1991). Alzheimer's disease and family caregiving: Critical synthesis of the literature and research agenda. *Nursing Research, 40* (6), 331–337.

Kurtz, M. E., Kurtz, J. C., Given, C. W. & Given, B. A. (2004). Depression and physical health among family caregivers of geriatric patients with cancer—a longitudinal view. *Medical Science Monitor, 10* (8), CCR447–456.

LaMontagne, L. L., Hepworth, J. T., Cohen, F., & Salisbury, M. H. (2004). Adolescent scoliosis: Effects of corrective surgery, cognitive-behavioral interventions and age on activity outcomes. *Applied Nursing Research, 17* (3), 168–177.

Lee, C. Y., Ko, I. S., Kim, H. S., Lee, et al. (2004). Development and validation study of the breast cancer risk appraisal for Korean women. *Nursing and Health Sciences, 6* (3), 201–207.

Lee, R. E., & Cubbin, C. (2002). Neighborhood context and youth cardiovascular health behaviors. *American Journal of Public Health, 92,* 428–436.

LeFort, S. M. (2000). A test of Braden's Self-Help Model in adults with chronic pain. *Journal of Nursing Scholarship, 32* (2), 153–160.

Lewis, C. E., & Lewis, M. A. (1989). Educational outcomes and illness behaviors of participants in a child-initiated care system: A 12-year follow-up study. *Pediatrics, 84,* 845–850.

_____. (1990). Consequences of empowering children to care for themselves. *Pediatrician, 17,* 63–67.

Long, J. D., & Stevens, K. R. (2004). Using technology to promote self-efficacy for healthy eating in adolescents. *Journal of Nursing Scholarship, 36* (2), 134–139.

Lorenz, F. O., & Melby, J. N. (1994). Analyzing family stress and adaptation: Methods of study. In R. D. Conger & G. H. Elder (Eds.), *Families in troubled times: Adapting to change in rural America,* (pp. 21–54). New York: Aldine de Gruyter.

Lorig, K. R., Ritter, P. L. & Gonzalez, V. M. (2003). Hispanic chronic disease self-management: A randomized community-based outcome trial. *Nursing Research, 52* (6), 361–369.

Loveland-Cherry, C. J. (2000). Family interventions to prevent substance abuse: Children and adolescents. *Annual Review of Nursing Research, 18,* 195–218.

Lucas, J., Orshan, S. & Cook, F. (2000). Determinants of health-promoting behavior among women ages 65 and above living in the community . *Scholarly Inquiry for Nursing Practice: An International Journal, 14* (1), 77–92).

Luepker, R. V., Perry, C. L., McKinlay, S. M., Nader, P. R., et al. (1996). Outcomes of a field trial to improve children's dietary patterns and physical activity: The child and adolescent trial for cardiovascular health (CATCH). *JAMA, 275,* 768–776.

Lunsford, V., & Fleury, J. (2000). Interventions to promote psychosocial recovery in women with coronary heart disease: An integrated literature review, (unpublished).

Martens, K. H., & Mellor, S. D. (1997). A study of the relationship between home care services and hospital readmission of patients with congestive heart failure. *Home Healthcare Nurse, 15,* 123–129.

Martinson, I., Armstrong G. D., Geis, D., Anglim, M. A., et al. (1978). Home care for children dying of cancer. *Pediatrics, 62,* 106–113.

Mast, M. E. (1995). Adult uncertainty in illness: A critical review of research. *Scholarly Inquiry for Nursing Practice: An International Journal, 9,* 3–24.

May, C., Doyle, H., & Chew-Graham, C. (1998). Medical knowledge and the intractable patient: The case of chronic low back pain. *Social Science and Medicine, 48,* 523–534.

McGillion, M., Watt-Watson, J., Kim, J., & Yamada, J. (2004). A systematic review of psychoeducational intervention trials for the management of chronic stable angina. *Journal of Nursing Management, 12* (3), 174–182.

McMillan, S. C. (1996). Quality of life of primary caregivers of hospice patients with cancer. *Cancer Practice, 4,* 191–198.

McMillan, S. C., & Mahon, J. (1994). The impact of hospice services on the quality of life of primary caregivers. *Oncology Nursing Forum, 21,* 1189–1195.

McMurray, R. G., Bauman, M. J., Harrell, J. S., & Bangdiwala, S. I. (2000). Effects of improvement in aerobic power on resing insulin and glucaose concentrations in youth. *European Journal of Applied Physiology, 81* (1–2), 132–139.

McMurray, R. G., Harrell, J. S., Bangdiwala, S. I., Bradley, C. B., et al. (2002). A school-based intervention can reduce body fat and blood pressure in young adolescents. *Journal of Adolescent Health, 31,* 125–132.

McMurray, R. G., Harrell, J. S. & Brown, S. (2000). Circulating leptin concentrations are not related to physical activity levels in youth. *Clinical Exercise Physiology, 2* (3), 159–164.

McSweeney, A. J., & Labuhn, K. T. (1990). Chronic obstructive pulmonary disease. In B. Spilker (Ed.), *Quality of life assessments in clinical trials,* (pp. 391–418). New York: Raven Press.

Meininger, J. C. (2000). School-based interventions for primary prevention of cardiovascular disease: Evidence of effects for minority populations. *Annual Review of Nursing Research, 18,* 219–246.

Mentro, A. M. & Steward, D. K. (2002). Caring for medically fragile children in the home: An alternative theoretical approach. *Research and Theory in Nursing Practice, 16* (3), 161–177.

Miles, M. S. (2003). Parents of children with chronic health problems: Programs of nursing research and their relationship to developmental science. *Annual Review of Nursing Research, 21*, 247–277.

Miles, M. S., & Holditch-Davis, D. (2003). Enhancing nursing research with children and families using a developmental science perspective. In J. J. Fitzpatrick (Ed.). *Annual Review of Nursing Research, 21*, 203–243.

Miles, M. S., Holditch-Davis, D., Eron, J., Black, B. P., et al. (2003). An HIV self-care symptom management intervention for African American mothers. *Nursing Research, 52* (6), 350–360.

Mishel, M. H. (1990). Reconceptualization of the Uncertainty in Illness Theory. *Image: Journal of Nursing Scholarship, 22*, 256–262.

Mishel, M. H. (1999). Uncertainty in chronic illness. *Annual Review of Nursing Research, 17*, 269–294.

Mishel, M. H., Belyea, M., Germino, B., Stewart, J., et al. (2002). Helping patients with localized prostate carcinoma manage uncertainty and treatment side effects. *Cancer, 94* (6), 1854–1866.

Mishel, M. H., & Murdaugh, C. L. (1987). Family adjustment to heart transplantation: Redesigning the dream. *Nursing Research, 36* (6), 332–338.

Molenaar, S., Sprangers, M. A. G., Rutgers, E. J., Luiten, E. J., et al. (2001). Decision support for patients with early-stage breast cancer: Effects of an interactive breast cancer CDROM on treatment decision, satisfaction and quality of life. *Journal of Clinical Oncology, 19* (6), 1676–1687.

Moore, S. (1997). Effects of interventions to promote recovery in coronary artery bypass surgical patients. *Journal of Cardiovascular Nursing, 12* (1), 59–70.

Morgan, P. A., Franks, P. J., Moffatt, C. J., Doherty, D. C., et al. (2004). Illness behavior and social support in patients with chronic venous ulcers. *Ostomy and Wound Management, 50* (1), 25–32.

Morse, J. R., & Fife, B. (1998). Coping with a partner's cancer: Adjustment at four stages of the illness trajectory. *Oncology Nursing Forum, 25* (4), 751–760.

Moser, D. K., Clements, P. J., Brecht, M. L., & Weiner, S. R. (1993). Predictors of psychosocial adjustment in systemic sclerosis: The influence of formal education level, functional ability hardiness, uncertainty and social support. *Arthritis and Rheumatism, 36*, 1398–1405.

Nader, P. R., Stone, E. J., Lytle, L. A., Perry, C. L., et al. (1999). Three-year maintenance of improved diet and physical activity: The CATCH cohort. *Archives of Pediatric and Adolescent Medicine, 153*, 695–704.

Narayanasamy, A. (2004). Spiritual coping mechanisms in chronic illness: A qualitative study. *Journal of Clinical Nursing, 13* (1), 116–117.

National Institutes of Health Consensus Conference. (1985). Lowering blood cholesterol to prevent heart disease. *Journal of the American Medical Association, 253*, 2080–2086.

Nelson, A. E., Haase, J., Kupst, M. J., Clarke-Steffen, L.et al. (2004). Consensus statements: Interventions to enhance resilience and quality of life in adolescents with cancer. *Journal of Pediatric Oncology Nursing, 21* (5), 305–307.

Nelson, J. P. (1996). Struggling to gain meaning: Living with the uncertainty of breast cancer. *Advances in Nursing Science, 18* (3), 59–76.

Nelson, M. A. (1994). Economic impoverishment as a health risk: Methodologic and conceptual issues. *Advances in Nursing Science, 16*, 1–12.

Nijboer, C., Tempelaar, R., Triemstra, M., van den Bos, G. A., et al. (2001). The role of social and psychologic resources in caregiving of cancer patients. *Cancer, 91* (5), 1029–1039.

Nuamah, I. F., Cooley, M. E., Fawcett, J., & McCorkle, R. (1999). Testing a theory for health-related quality of life in cancer patients: A structural equation approach. *Research in Nursing and Health, 22* (3), 231–242.

Nyhlin, K. T. (1990). Diabetic patients facing long-term complications: Coping with uncertainty. *Journal of Advanced Nursing, 15*, 1021–1029.

Olds, D. L., Henderson, C., Tatelbaum, R., & Chamberlin, R. (1986). Improving the delivery of prenatal care and outcomes of pregnancy: A randomized trial of nurse home visitation. *Pediatrics, 77*, 16–28.

O'Neill, E. S., & Morrow, L. L. (2001). The symptom experience of women with chronic illness. *Journal of Advanced Nursing, 33* (2), 257–268.

Orsted, H. L., Campbell, K. E., Keast, D. H., Coutts, P., & Sterling, W. (2001). Chronic wound caring—a long journey toward healing. *Ostomy and Wound Management, 47* (10), 26–36.

Padilla, G. V. (1993). State of the art in quality of life research. *Communicating Nursing Research, 26* (1), 71–80.

Pasacreta, J. V., & McCorkle, R. (2000). Cancer care: Impact of interventions on caregiver outcomes. *Annual Review of Nursing Research, 18*, 127–148.

Paterson, B. L. (2000). "Are we in Kansas yet, Toto?" The construction of chronic illness in research. *Canadian Journal of Nursing Research, 32* (3), 11–17.

Paterson, B. L., Russell, C., & Thorne, S. (2001) Critical analysis of everyday self-care decision making in chronic illness. *Journal of Advanced Nursing, 35* (3), 335–341.

Pelusi, J. (1997). The lived experience of surviving breast cancer. *Oncology Nursing Forum, 24,* 1343–1353.

Pender, N. J. (1987). *Health promotion in nursing practice* (2nd ed.). Norwalk, CT: Appleton-Century-Crofts.

Pless, I. B., Feeley, N., Gottlieb, L., Rowat, K., et al. (1994). A randomized trial of a nursing intervention to promote the adjustment of children with chronic physical disorders. *Pediatrics, 94,* 70–75.

Powe, B. D., Ntekop, E. & Barron, M. (2004). An intervention study to increase colorectal cancer knowledge and screening among community elders. *Public Health Nursing, 21* (5), 435–442.

Primomo, J., Yeates, B., & Woods, M. F. (1990). Social support for women during chronic illness: The relationship among sources and types to adjustment. *Research in Nursing and Health, 13,* 153–161.

Prochaska, J. O., Redding, C. A., & Evers, K. E. (2002). The Transtheoretical Model and Stages of Change. In K. Glanz, B. K. Rimer, & F. M. Lewis (Eds.), *Health behavior and health education: Theory, research and practice (3rd ed.),* (pp. 99–120). San Francisco: Jossey Bass Publishers.

Radosevich, D. M., Partin, M. R., Nugent, S., Nelson, D., et al. (2004). Measuring patient knowledge of the risks and benefits of prostate cancer screening. *Patient Education and Counseling, 54* (2), 143–152.

Raingruber, B. (2004). Using poetry to discover and share significant meanings in child and adolescent mental health nursing. *Journal of Child and Adolescent Psychiatric Nursing, 17* (1), 13–20.

Raleigh E. D. (1992). Sources of hope in chronic illness. *Oncology Nursing Forum, 19* (3), 443–448.

Rankin, S. H. (2000). Life-span development: Refreshing a theoretical and practice perspective. *Scholarly Inquiry in Nursing Practice, 14* (4), 379.

Reinhard, S. C., & Horwitz, A. V. (1995). Caregiver burden: Differentiating the content and consequences of family caregiving. *Journal of Marriage and the Family, 57,* 741–750.

Rew, L., Johnson, R. J., Jenkins, S. K., & Torres, R. (2004). Developing holistic nursing interventions to improve adolescent health. *Journal of Holistic Nursing, 22* (4), 298–319.

Reynolds, D. (2004). Cervical cancer in Hispanic/Latino women. *Clinical Journal of Oncology Nursing, 8* (2), 146–150.

Roberson M. H. (1992). The meaning of compliance: Patient perspectives. *Qualitative Health Research, 2,* 7–26.

Robinson, L. A., Bevil, C., Arcangelo, V., Reifsnyder, J., Rothman, N., & Smeltzer, S. (1993). Operationalizing the Corbin & Strauss Trajectory Model for elderly clients with chronic illness. *Scholarly Inquiry for Nursing Practice, 7* (4), 253–268.

Rockwell, J. M., & Riegel, B. (2001). Predictors of self-care in persons with heart failure. *Heart and Lung, 30* (1), 18–25.

Roe, B. (2000). Effective and ineffective management of incontinence: Issues around illness trajectory and health care. *Qualitative Health Research, 10* (5), 677–690.

Rose, G. (1980). Relative merits of intervening on whole populations versus high-risk individuals only. In R. M. Llauer & R. B. Shekelle (Eds.), *Childhood prevention of atherosclerosis and hypertension,* (pp. 351–566). New York: Raven Press.

Rossi Ferrario, S., Cardillo, V., Vicario, F., Balzarini, E., & Zotti, A.M. (2004). Advanced cancer at home: Caregiving and bereavement. *Palliative Medicine, 18* (2), 129–136.

Russell, C. K., & Gregory, D. M. (2000). Capturing day-to-day aspects of living with chronic illness: The need for longitudinal designs. *Canadian Journal of Nursing Research, 32* (3), 99–102.

Rutledge, D. N., & Donaldson, N. E. (1995). Building organizational capacity to engage in research utilization. *Journal of Nursing Administration, 25* (10), 12–16.

Schwartz, A. (2000). Daily fatigue patterns and effect of exercise in women with breast cancer. *Cancer Practice, 8* (1), 16–24.

Scura, K. W. E., Budin, W., & Garfing, E. (2004). Telephone social support and education for adaptation to prostate cancer: A pilot study. *Oncology Nursing Forum, 31* (2), 335–338.

Sheridan, S. L., Felix, K., Pignone, M. P. & Lewis, C. L. (2004). Information needs of men regarding prostate cancer screening an the effect of a brief decision aid. *Patient Education and Counseling, 54* (3), 345–351.

Simeonsson, N. W., & Gray, J. N. (1994). Healthy children: Primary prevention of disease. In R. J. Simeonsson (Ed.), *Risk, resilience and prevention: Promoting the well-being of all children,* (pp. 77–102). Baltimore: Paul H. Brookes.

Small, S. P., & Graydon, J. E. (1992). Perceived uncertainty, physical symptoms and negative mood in hospitalized patients with chronic obstructive pulmonary disease. *Heart and Lung, 21,* 568–574.

Smeltzer, S. C. (1991). Use of the trajectory model of nursing in multiple sclerosis. *Scholarly Inquiry for Nursing Practice, 5* (3), 219–234.

_____. (1994). The concerns of pregnant women with multiple sclerosis. *Qualitative Health Research, 4,* 497–501.

Smith, C. E., Leenerts, M. H., & Gajewski, B. J. (2003). A systematically tested intervention for managing reactive depression. *Nursing Research, 52* (6),401–409.

Smith, K., Schreiner, B. J., Brouhard, B., & Travis, L. (1991). Impact of a camp experience on choice of coping strategies by adolescents with insulin-dependent diabetes mellitus. *Diabetes Educator, 17,* 49–53.

Soanes, C., & Timmons, S. (2004). Improving transition: A qualitative study examining the attitudes of young people with chronic illness transferring to adult care. *Journal of Child Health Care, 8* (2), 102–112.

Stanton, A. L., Danoff-Burg, S., Sworowski, C. A., Collins, A. D., et al. (2002). Randomized controlled trial of written emotional expression and benefit finding in breast cancer patients. *Journal of Clinical Oncology, 20,* 4160–4168.

Steenbeek, A. (2004). Empowering health promotion: A holistic approach in preventing sexually transmitted infection among First nations and intuit adolescents in Canada. *Journal of Holistic Nursing, 22* (3), 254–266.

Stone, E. J., McGraw, S. A., Osganian, S. K., & Elder, J. P. (1994). Process evaluation in the Multicenter Child and Adolescent Trial for Cardiovascular Health (CATCH). *Health Education Quarterly, 16,* 155–168.

Strand, V. R., & Haughey, M. (1998). Factors influencing the caregiver's ability to experience respite. *Journal of Family Nursing, 4* (3), 231–254.

Strauss, A. L., Corbin, J., Fagerhaugh, S., Glaser, B., et al. (1984). *Chronic illness and the quality of life.* St. Louis: Mosby.

Sullivan, T., Weinert, C., & Cudney, S. (2003). Management of chronic illness: Voices of rural women. *Journal of Advanced Nursing, 44* (6), 566–574.

Tennen, H., Affleck, G., Sarmeli, S., & Carney, M. A. (2000). A daily process approach to coping: Linking theory, research and practice. *American Psychologist, 55* (6), 626–636.

Thomas, E. C. (2004). African American women's breast memories, cancer beliefs and screening behaviors. *Cancer Nursing, 27* (4), 295–302.

Thorne, S., & Paterson, B. (1998). Shifting images of chronic illness. *Image: Journal for Nursing Scholarship, 30,* 173–178.

Thorne, S., & Paterson, B. (2000). Two decades of insider research: What we know and don't know about the chronic illness experience. *Annual Review of Nursing Research, 18,* 3–25.

Thorne, S., Paterson, B., Russell, C., & Schultz, A. (2002). Complementary/alternative medicine in chronic illness as informed self-care decision making. *International Journal of Nursing Studies, 39,* 671–683.

Trijsburg, R. W., Van Knippenberg, F. G., & Rijpma, S. E. (1992). Effects of psychosocial treatment on cancer patients: A critical review. *Psychosomatic Medicine, 54,* 489–517.

Tsai, P. F., Tak, S., Moore, C., & Palencia, I. (2003). Testing a theory of chronic pain. *Journal of Advanced Nursing, 43* (2), 158–169.

Underwood, S. (1995). Enhancing the delivery of cancer care to the disadvantaged. *Cancer Practice, 3* (1), 31–36.

_____. (1999). Breast cancer screening among African American women: Addressing the needs of African American women with known and no known risk factors. *Journal of the National Black Nurses Association, 10* (1), 46–55.

U.S. Department of Health and Human Services. (January 2000). *Healthy People 2010* (Conference edition, in two volumes). Washington, DC: Government Printing Office.

U.S. General Accounting Office. (1990). *Home visiting: A promising early intervention strategy for at-risk families.* Gaithersburg, MD.

Van Riper, M. (2003). The sibling experience of living with childhood chronic illness and disability. *Annual Review of Nursing Research, 21,* 279–302.

Venner, G. H., & Seelbinder, J. S. (1996). Team management of congestive heart failure across the continuum. *Journal of Cardiovascular Nursing, 10,* 71–84.

Vohr, B. R., Wright, L.LO., Dusick, A.M., Mele, L., et al. (2000). Neurodevelopmental and functional outcomes of extremely low birth weight infants in the National Institute of Child Health and Development Neonatal Research Network, 1993–1994. *Pediatrics, 105,* 1216–1226.

Walker, L. O. (1992). *Parent–infant nursing science: Paradigms, phenomena, methods.* Philadelphia: FA Davis.

Walsh, S. M., Estrada, G. B., & Hogan, N. (2004). Individual telephone support for family caregivers of seriously ill cancer patients. *Medical Surgical Nursing, 13*(3), 181–189.

Walsh, S. M., & Schmidt, L. A. (2003). Telephone support for caregivers of patients with cancer. *Cancer Nursing, 26* (6), 448–453.

Walsh, S. M., & Weiss, S. (2003). Online exclusive: Art intervention with family caregivers and patients with cancer. *Oncology Nursing Forum, 30* (6), E115–20.

Wang, K. W., & Barnard, A. (2004). Technology-dependent children and their families: A review. *Journal of Advanced Nursing, 45* (1), 36–46.

Watts, T., Merrell, J., Murphy, F., & Williams, A. (2004). Breast health information needs of women from minority ethnic groups. *Journal of Advanced Nursing, 47* (5), 526–535.

Weinrich, S. P., Atwood, J., Cobb, M. D., Ellison, G., et al. (1998a). Cost for prostate cancer educational programs in work and church sites. *American Journal of Health Behavior, 22* (6), 421–433.

Weinrich S. P., Boyd, M. D., Weinrich, M., Green, F., et al. (1998b). Increasing prostate cancer screening in African American men with peer-educator and client-navigator interventions. *Journal of Cancer Education, 13* (4), 213–219.

Wiener, C. L., & Dodd, M. J. (1993). Coping amid uncertainty: An illness trajectory perspective. *Scholarly Inquiry for Nursing Practice: An International Journal, 7,* 17–31.

Widar, M. , Ahlstrom, G., & Ed, A. C. (2004). Health-related quality of life in persons with long-term pain after a stroke. *Journal of Clinical Nursing, 13* (4), 497–505.

Wellard, S. (1998). Constructions of chronic illness. *International Journal of Nursing Studies, 35,* 49–55.

Wilde, M. H. (2003). Embodied knowledge in chronic illness and injury. *Nursing Inquiry, 10* (3), 170–176.

Williams, C., & Wynder, E. (1993). A child health report card 1992. *Preventive Medicine, 22* (4), 604–628.

Wineman, N. M., Schwetz, K. M., Goodkin, D. E., & Rudick, R. A. (1996). Relationships among illness uncertainty, stress, coping and emotional well-being at entry into a clinical drug trial. *Applied Nursing Research, 9,* 53–60.

Winslow, B. W. (1997). Effects of formal supports on stress outcomes in family caregivers of Alzheimer's patients. *Research in Nursing and Health, 20* (1), 27–37.

Wiseman, P. A., Malone-Lee, J., & Rai, G. S. (1991). Terodiline with bladder retraining for detrusor instability in elderly people. *British Medical Journal, 302,* 994–996.

Wyman, J. (2000). Management of urinary incontinence in adult ambulatory care populations. *Annual Review of Nursing Research, 18,* 171–194.

Wyman, J., Fantl, J. A., McClish, D. K., Bump, R. C., et al. (1998). Comparative efficacy of behavioral interventions in the management of female urinary incontinence. *American Journal of Obstetrics and Gynecology, 179,* 999–1007.

Wyman, J. F., Fantl, J. A., McClish, D. K, Harkins, S. W., et al. (1997). Effect of bladder training on quality of life of older women with urinary incontinence. *International Urogynecology Journal and Pelvic Floor Dysfunction, 8,* 223–229.

Yang, C. T., & Kirschling, J. M. (1992). Exploration of factors related to direct care and outcomes of caregiving: Caregiving of terminally ill older persons. *Cancer Nursing, 15,* 173–181.

Zahlis, E. H., & Lewis, F. M. (1998). Mothers' stories of the school-age child's experience with the mother's breast cancer. *Journal of Psychosocial Oncology, 16* (2), 25–43.

Zust, B. L. (2000). Effect of cognitive therapy on depression in rural, battered women. *Archives of Psychiatric Nursing, XIV* (2), 51–63.

CHAPTER 18

Ethics in Chronic Illness

Judith A. Erlen

Introduction

Advances in health care technology continue to make new treatment options available for individuals with chronic illness. The result is that more health conditions are now managed as chronic disorders. These advances in technology address some of the technical questions of care and make additional therapies possible for clients; however, *can* does not become *ought*. There is a considerable difference between being able to do an intervention and saying that the intervention should be used in a particular client situation. Clients, families, health care professionals, and society must make hard choices regarding when, how, and with whom to use these therapies. Consequently, ethics has a more prominent role in client management decisions than ever before.

Incorporating ethical considerations into health care decision making is not new. In the 1960s, an anonymous selection committee used social worth criteria to make decisions for the Seattle Artificial Kidney Center at the University of Washington concerning which clients with end-stage renal disease were to receive a limited supply of kidney dialysis (Sanders & Dukeminier, 1968). At that time, hemodialysis machines were not readily available for all of the individuals diagnosed with this chronic condition. Committee members had to decide who was to be given a chance to live.

Similar ethical questions arise today when one considers individuals living with chronic illnesses. Although the ethical concerns, such as allocation of scarce resources, quality of life, discrimination and stigma, and powerlessness, may not be new, the context and/or the circumstances surrounding the ethical issues have changed, thereby increasing the complexity of the decision-making. The facts and the technical aspects of care are important considerations when making ethical decisions; however, new knowledge, values, beliefs, and the context of the situation are also necessary components. The challenge for nurses is to think "outside the box." This chapter describes basic concepts in ethics, discusses selected ethical issues that may arise when caring for clients with chronic illness, and offers strategies that nurses can use to understand and address these issues, as well as see ethical questions from another perspective.

Living with a Chronic Illness

Focusing on the experience of living with a chronic illness helps one identify relevant ethical issues. As clients and their families tell their ongoing stories, they provide rich descriptions of the meaning of the illness both for the individual and others (Toombs, 1995). Their narratives express the troubling situations and suffering that occur in their lives and tell of their vulnerability and their dependence on others. When individuals recount their stories, they help others to recognize the similarities and differences of the experience of living with chronic disorders. Telling the stories provides the context for identifying and understanding the ethical concerns. Often, the experiences are unique to the specific disorder (Gillick, 1995).

Chronic illnesses are relentless, progressive, and deteriorating, and create disruptions in the lives of individuals. Living with the disorder often becomes burdensome to those with the condition and to their families. Over time, these individuals need not only more, but also different health care services. Some people also have to confront the question of "how long."

Understanding the ebb and flow of daily life helps one to recognize the ethical questions that arise from living with a chronic illness. Agich (1995) states, "With the chronically ill patient, managing the illness is coincident with managing one's life. . . . In chronic illness, one undergoes the illness not as an intrusion into one's life, but as a way of life" (pp. 138–139). Unlike the transient nature of acute illnesses, chronic illnesses are pervasive and persistent.

Ethics

Ethics is the branch of philosophy that focuses on the study of the moral life. Ethics addresses the important questions of human conduct and whether actions are right or wrong. Thus, ethics directs one's attention to what it means to do good and to not harm (Beauchamp & Childress, 2001). However, determining what is good, what is right, or what is harmful can be difficult and requires conscious reflection on one's moral values and beliefs (Volbrecht, 2002).

Ethics is an integral part of the everyday experience of nursing and is reflected in the conversa-

tions that nurses have with their clients (Skott, 2003). The involvement with and understanding that nurses have about their clients provides an important perspective that needs to be incorporated into identifying ethical dilemmas and making ethical decisions. "The essence of nursing ethics is not what patients do or what nurses do but the way the dynamic of the healing relationship unfolds . . ." (Thomasma, 1994, p. 94).

Ethics is central to nursing practice because of the special relationships nurses have with clients and their families (Lucke, 1998). Nurses focus on clients who have an illness or health problem, rather than only on the disorder or condition. Clients seek out nurses because they believe nurses understand how the illness experience affects them and their families. Nurses are with clients when they are in the valleys of despair and when they have mountaintop experiences.

Curtin (1979), a seminal nurse ethicist, states "nursing is a moral art" (p. 2) because its goal is the welfare of clients. In nursing, as in other health disciplines, science and morality are joined together so that the health professional can be responsive to the needs of clients. Nurses are concerned with the human response within the context of the illness experience. Thus, they need to have an understanding of science, the use of technologies, and ethics, and value the human experience.

Ethical Practice in Nursing

Historical Perspectives

Ethical practice has always been at the heart of modern nursing. Through the years, there have been continuing efforts to develop codes of nursing ethics, position statements on ethical issues, and ethics textbooks. Research on ethics continues to expand, giving practitioners scientific data to use in their practice.

Examining the literature of the past century demonstrates how nursing and the nurse–client relationship have been affected by the changes in health care and its technology. Isabel Hampton

Robb's (1900) pioneering book, *Nursing Ethics: For Hospital and Private Use*, portrayed both ethics and etiquette. This work provided guidance and direction for novices in nursing in terms of appropriate moral behavior. The expectation was that if nurses possessed the right character, they would act accordingly. Thus, the early emphasis in nursing was on virtues. Personal behavior was indistinguishable from professional behavior.

The Florence Nightingale Pledge written by Lystra Gretter in 1893 affirmed nursing's commitment to society (Davis et al., 1997). This oath, first taken by the graduate nurses at the Farrand Training School for Nurses in Detroit, Michigan, preceded the development of an official code of ethics for nurses. This pledge reflected the moral ideals of nursing at the end of the nineteenth century. Although originally written for the graduates of the Farrand Training School, other schools of nursing in the United States soon began to have their graduates recite this pledge.

In 1896, the Nurses' Associated Alumnae of the United States and Canada (the forerunner of the American Nurses Association and the Canadian Nurses Association) was formed. One purpose of this organization was to develop a code of ethics. Yet, developing a distinct code of ethics did not occur until the 1920s. Despite earlier drafts, the American Nurses Association (ANA) only adopted its first code of ethics in 1950 (Viens, 1989). Because a code of ethics needs to reflect the changing values of both the profession and the society, nurses have continued to refine their code of ethics. Thus, for example, revisions to the code of ethics occurred in 1960, 1968, 1976, 1985, and 2001. The latter revisions of the code of ethics included interpretive statements for each tenet of the code.

Current Practice

Because a professional code of ethics guides nurses in meeting the ethical challenges in everyday practice, the ANA modified its *Code for Nurses and Interpretive Statements* (ANA, 1985) to assure that it reflects current thinking about ethical issues. The revised document was presented to and approved by the ANA House of Delegates in June 2001. Rather than have an approach based primarily on ethical principles, the *Code of Ethics for Nurses* (ANA, 2001) has a broader base in ethical theory, incorporating such perspectives as feminist, virtue, and communitarian ethics. The code includes nine general tenets with interpretive statements designed to help nurses with the new and ongoing ethical challenges inherent in nursing practice (ANA, 2001).

Nursing's code of ethics is a public statement demonstrating to society the profession's values, commitment, and acceptance of the responsibility invested in it by society. The standards set forth in the code frequently go beyond those required by the law. This code of ethics serves as a standard for self-regulation of professional conduct, provides a framework for discerning and analyzing ethical issues, and offers guidelines for ethical practice so that nurses can choose the right action rather than just acting rightly (Scanlon, 2000). The code does not provide nurses with specific answers to ethically troubling situations; however, the code does provide a starting point for examining ethical dilemmas, because its content reflects the collective moral thinking of nursing.

The International Council of Nurses (ICN) was organized in 1899, and like the Nurses' Associated Alumnae of the United States and Canada, also recognized the importance of ethics and began to develop a code in 1923 (Oulton, 2000). However, the first code of ethics of the ICN was not adopted by the membership until 1953; this code was revised in 1968 and 1973. The ICN code has sections addressing nurses' responsibilities to people (clients), practice, society, the profession, and co-workers, and provides a framework for nurses' ethical conduct (Oulton, 2000).

Ethical Principles

Ethical principles offer guidance and direction for one's decisions and actions. Most ethicists within Western society identify three predominant principles: respect for persons, beneficence, and justice.

Understanding these principles is important for identifying ethical options or choices. The concepts of veracity (truthtelling), confidentiality, privacy, and fidelity are inherent within the primary ethical principles (Table 18-1).

Respect for Persons

Respect for persons refers to recognizing and honoring the inherent dignity and the uniqueness of the individual. This principle is broader than respect for autonomy. Individuals have a personal set of values that govern their choices (Beauchamp & Childress, 2001). Respect for persons claims that each individual is free to make choices, is in control of self, is equal to another person, and has rights. These rights include privacy, confidentiality, nondeception, and noncoercion.

While the principle of respect for persons focuses on the individual, this principle also recognizes that individuals are a part of a larger community (Davis et al., 1997). Each person interacts with and affects others. Likewise others interact with and affect the individual. Connections and relationships form through these interactions. Individuals have rights and responsibilities because of their role in the community and are thereby a part of, rather than separate from, the whole.

TABLE 18-1

Ethical Principles

Principle	Definition
Respect for persons	Respecting another's autonomy or their ability to be self-determining
Beneficence	Promoting good or well-being
Nonmaleficence	Doing no harm
Justice	Fairness
Veracity	Truthtelling, honesty
Fidelity	Faithfulness, loyalty
Privacy	Noninvasiveness
Confidentiality	Nondisclosure

The principle of respect for persons also includes protecting the rights of those individuals who are not fully autonomous according to legal or ethical criteria. Each individual has value. Surrogate decision makers are asked to make decisions when individuals lack decision-making capacity (Beauchamp & Childress, 2001; Bosek, Savage, Shaw, & Renella, 2001).

Adults who become incapacitated because of illness or other circumstances that limit their ability to make choices need to be protected, when there are important decisions to make. The amount of protection by others that the individual will need varies according to the balance of harms and benefits. As one's condition(s) changes, so might the client's ability for decision making; therefore, determinations about whether or not one is able to decide for self need to be examined periodically.

Beneficence

Beneficence is the ethical principle stating that one "ought do good and to prevent or avoid doing harm" (Frankena, 1973, p. 45). A person is to take positive action and do good, to promote the well-being of another person, or to provide benefits. The person is not to do harm, to intend harm, or to place another at risk of harm. Frankena (1973) views this principle as a continuum from not harming (nonmaleficence) to doing good (beneficence). The latter maximizes benefits and is usually considered to be the action that requires more from the individual, because one has to actually do something so that the other benefits.

Beauchamp and Childress (2001) discuss nonmaleficence and beneficence separately, noting that distinctions have to be made, even when beneficence is considered to be an all-encompassing principle. Nonmaleficence focuses on not intending or causing harm; one does not take particular actions in which another person will be injured, wronged, or placed at risk for harm. On the other hand, beneficence centers on taking actions that benefit others or promotes their significant and legitimate interests (Beauchamp & Childress, 2001). Thus, the person is required to prevent or remove harm and to promote good; one makes a contribution to the other person's well-being. To determine the appropriate ethical action, the decision maker may have to balance the harms and benefits, often doing this balancing in the midst of uncertainty.

Justice

The ethical principle of *justice* is called into question to address issues related to inequalities within society. Distributive justice addresses the fair allocation of limited resources (Beauchamp & Childress, 2001). Some persons within the society will not receive these goods. How does one distribute benefits so that there is equitable treatment of each person? What constitutes a fair distribution of burdens within society? How does a society distribute goods so that the action is not considered to be unjust by those who will be left out?

Ahronheim and colleagues (2000) point out that according to Aristotelian thinking, likes are to be treated in a like manner, and unlikes in an unlike manner. However, this concept of justice provides no direction regarding the criteria to use to make these distributions. Also, what about situations of special need? What is the morally relevant feature to use? The philosopher John Rawls (1971) focuses on justice as fairness. He uses this approach to justify the distribution of social goods and giving more to those who have less (Ahronheim, Moreno & Zuckerman, 2000; Rawls, 1971).

Because all will not receive the good or service to be distributed, there is a need to make some comparisons. Making such comparisons requires that there be some relevant criteria for making particular distinctions among people when distributing a good or service. These criteria are often labeled as *material principles of justice*. These principles identify the particular characteristics that can be used when making macroallocation (societal level) or microallocation (individual level) decisions. For example, the basis for allocation decisions can be an equal distribution of the resources or individual need, merit, or contribution

to society. However, problems can arise when applying these criteria, as they may conflict with each other. Addressing such conflicts requires that there be specificity and some balancing of the criteria (Beauchamp & Childress, 2001).

Veracity

Veracity refers to being honest with others or telling the truth. The client–provider relationship is built on a foundation of trust, respect, and promise keeping (Beauchamp & Childress, 2001). Thus, one has an obligation to be open with the other and not conceal information. The material that is provided to the client is in accord with the facts. Health care providers need to acknowledge whenever information is unknown, incomplete, or uncertain (Jonsen, Siegler & Winslade, 1998). One does not lie, deceive, or manipulate the other. Instead, one corrects untruths, factual errors, and mistaken beliefs. A lack of respect is shown and trust relationships are eroded when information is intentionally withheld or deception occurs.

For individuals to make informed decisions about their health care, there needs to be both disclosure and understanding of information. To enable a person to be self-determining requires that the individual have adequate, reliable, and relevant information. Frequently, disclosing information about health matters to clients and their families occurs over time in small segments. This ongoing dialogue provides an opportunity for questions and better assimilation of the material, so that clients remain in control of decisions being made.

Fidelity

Loyalty, or *fidelity*, is another important component of the trust relationship (Beauchamp & Childress, 2001). Fidelity expresses the commitment that exists between health professionals and society, and thus encompasses promise keeping. This means that one honors an agreement. The expectation is that health care professionals will provide care to their clients and will not abandon them. Nurses' primary professional obligation is to their clients; there is a commitment to faithfulness.

Privacy

Privacy focuses on noninvasion and nonintrusiveness. Clients have a right to privacy and can expect that others will acknowledge and respect this right. Respecting one's privacy means that a person has authorized access to the other individual. One does not enter into another's space without permission. The Health Insurance Portability and Accountability Act (HIPAA) implemented in 2003 underscores the importance of the privacy rights of clients and their control over sharing of personal information (www.hhs.gov/ocr/hipaa/privacy.html). Privacy is one aspect of the respect that we owe others and is related to confidentiality.

Confidentiality

Confidentiality refers to nondisclosure of information about another without that person's consent (Beauchamp & Childress, 2001). Codes of ethics make explicit the promise that health professionals will protect client confidences. Because clients expect that information will be held in confidence, they are willing to disclose sensitive information about themselves and their health to health care providers (Jonsen, Siegler & Winslade, 1998). Like veracity, confidentiality is necessary for the trust relationship to exist between clients and providers. Breaching confidentiality makes the other person increasingly vulnerable. A client expects that the health care professional will not divulge information that has been shared unless that person is authorized to do so by the client (www.hhs.gov/ocr/hipaa/privacy. html). Thus, maintaining confidentiality is a demonstration of the respect one owes another.

Challenges to preserving confidentiality and privacy exist. The current information age raises new questions about access to, storage of, and retrieval of information and may require increased security in order to limit access to confidential information (www.hhs.gov/ocr/hipaa/privacy.html).

There may be a need to release confidential information, because the interests of others may be threatened. For example, disclosure to the health department is necessary to prevent the spread of communicable diseases or to the appropriate authorities when child abuse is suspected.

Ethical Perspectives

There are various perspectives that assist health care professionals in understanding and making ethical choices. Two traditional Western approaches are grounded in teleological and deontological thinking. More recently, the ethic of care, virtue ethics, and casuistry have taken on greater importance in nursing. Each of these perspectives provides a different approach to reasoning in ethical situations and may lead to different ethically justified actions (Table 18-2).

The *teleological approach* focuses on goals, outcomes, and consequences. Utilitarianism, as described by John Stuart Mill (1806–1873) and Jeremy Bentham (1748–1832), is probably the best known teleological theory. This philosophy has the principle of utility as its central tenet. According to this principle, one chooses to act according to what will yield the most happiness or pleasure for the majority (Beauchamp & Childress, 2001). Right actions are those that produce the best outcomes or the greatest amount of good for the most people. Thus, individuals need to calculate a happiness value for the possible outcomes and then select the outcome that provides the most utility. Intuitively, utilitarian thinking is very appealing.

Utilitarianism is a consequence-based theory. To use this approach requires information in order to predict which decision and action will result in the best outcomes. Obtaining this information in the clinical setting takes time, and some of the information may not be available. One has to consider anticipated consequences and weigh those consequences to determine the likelihood that an action will produce a particular outcome. However, uncertainty exists when calculating and predicting consequences.

In contrast, the *deontological approach* of Immanuel Kant (1724–1804) focuses on a person's duties, obligations, or responsibilities. One decides

TABLE 18-2

Ethical Perspectives

Perspective	Key Figures	Focus
Utilitarian	John Stuart Mill Jeremy Bentham	• Principle of utility • Consequences, goals, or ends
Kantian	Immanuel Kant	• Duties or obligations • Right reasons for decision
Ethic of Care	Nel Noddings Carol Gilligan	• Connections • Trust • Context
Virtue	Plato Aristotle	• Character • Motivation
Casuistry	Al Jonsen Stephen Toulmin	• Paradigm cases • Similarities and dissimilarities of cases

what action to take according to a set of principles or rules that can be generalized to similar individuals or situations. According to Kant, for a decision to be morally correct, it must be done for the right reasons. The motives and the chosen action need to coincide for this approach to be a morally worthy act. Kant's categorical imperative also states that an individual should be treated as an end rather than exclusively as a means to another's end (Beauchamp & Childress, 2001).

Using a deontological approach makes ethical reasoning seem straightforward. One needs only to follow the duties that are derived from the principles. This view, however, is too simplistic, as duties will conflict and one has to decide which competing duty takes precedence, as well as determine the basis or rationale for the ordering of principles. Additionally, the deontologic approach does not consider the context or circumstances surrounding the ethical decision.

The feminist movement has influenced nursing and refocused nursing's attention on an ethic of care. Making and justifying ethical decisions based on the best consequences or following particular moral principles addresses more the outcome or product (the decision) that results when a person engages in ethical reasoning. The *care ethic* centers on process or the communication and relationship, rather than on the outcomes or moral rules (Volbrecht, 2002).

Late twentieth century nurse leaders described caring as the moral ideal of nursing (Benner & Wrubel, 1989; Carper, 1979; Gastman, 1999; Watson, 1988). In many respects, the caring component of nursing remains hidden because of the current medical focus on curing and technology. Yet, in situations involving chronic disorders, caring is more prominent because of the vulnerability, isolation, and suffering of these clients.

Caring is relational. Because of the connection that exists between individuals, there is a concern about the well-being of the other. One focuses on what matters to the other (Benner & Wrubel, 1989). The care ethic means that one becomes a part of, rather than removed from, the situation. Context is important, as the emphasis is on this particular set of circumstances. There is an exchange—a reciprocity. Within the care ethic, there is subjectivity rather than impartiality. There is a sense of presence, involvement, emotion, understanding, and action. Caring is increasing nurses' sensitivity to the need to restructure existing relationships and institutions within health care, recognize the diversity of both client and provider populations, and focus on dialogue inclusiveness, and empowerment (Volbrecht, 2002).

The focus of *virtue ethics* is on the person who is making the ethical choices and "asks what sort of person ought I be" (Davis et al., 1997, p. 2). Good character is primary. The moral fiber of the person influences whether the individual will identify ethical issues, how the person will respond to the ethical question, and what behaviors will characterize the person.

Virtues are qualities, attributes, or character traits that a person possesses that have moral value. Examples of virtues include integrity, discernment, compassion, and trustworthiness (Beauchamp & Childress, 2001). Virtue ethics is concerned with motivation and focuses on a way of being. One's behavior is congruent with one's virtues; there is a pattern to how one behaves. Thus, the compassionate nurse does not treat a client with indifference, but is caring, tolerant, and respectful. Yet, acting according to one's virtues has its own set of problems. One also must make appropriate judgments and have an understanding of what actions are right and/or good. Volbrecht (2002) points out that there isn't a common understanding of the desirable virtues or meaning and purpose of life because of the pluralism within society.

In contrast to the theories that focus on principles and rules, *casuistry* contends that cases provide the basis for moral judgments (Jonsen & Toulmin, 1989). Casuists argue that there are paradigm or standard cases about which ethicists can agree. Cases that are similar are compared with each other. The casuist examines analogous cases and appeals to experience, wisdom, and tradition in order to justify whether an action in the new case is ethically appropriate (Beauchamp & Childress, 2001). Thus, a more inductive approach to ethical reasoning emerges.

Casuists gradually move from simple to more complex cases. The simple cases are more readily resolved, and their resolutions provide the basis for discerning the right action in the more difficult cases. Paradigm cases emerge that can be used to support or refute ethical positions when examining future cases (O'Keefe, 2001). Where there are no paradigm cases to follow, ethicists have to develop new solutions to the ethical dilemma that they have identified.

Influencing Factors

Religion, culture, and law are important factors influencing the process of ethical analysis and rea-

soning. Pluralism abounds as there are many diverse religious traditions and cultural and ethnic groups coexisting in our society. The different values and beliefs held by individuals who follow these traditions and are members of these groups strike at the heart of many ethical dilemmas. These different perspectives are becoming more pronounced and present a challenge for health care providers attempting to resolve ethical dilemmas in health care.

Religion, culture, and the law shape a person's values and views on a particular ethical issue. These factors affect one's perspective about life and death, suffering, disease, and health. The interpretations that people place on their religious and cultural values and beliefs and society's legal framework influence the ethical decisions that they make.

Religion

Our society espouses the separation of church and state; however, can one's religion be separated from one's ethics? Since religion affords insights into morals, beliefs and ethics, clients confronting an ethical dilemma may seek the position of their religious tradition on that particular question. The individual may look to religious beliefs to support the ethical decision. Many of the dominant religions have developed position statements on important ethical questions, such as abortion and euthanasia. However, the individual may not be aware of their religion's particular views, even though such statements exist. Thus, they may seek guidance for their ethical decisions from their religious advisors so that their decisions are congruent with the tenets of their faith.

In keeping with the principle of respect for persons, health care providers should respect the religious views of competent adult clients (Ahronheim, Moreno & Zuckerman, 2000). Yet, a conflict can arise whenever the client makes a decision based on religious beliefs with which the health care provider does not agree. This is often more problematic for the health care provider whenever a parent is making a decision for a child and is basing that decision on religious beliefs.

What, then, is the role of religion in ethical decision making, particularly within a pluralistic society? Religion can enrich dialogue about ethical issues, and alternative perspectives can be shared. Alternatively, religion can limit dialogue when one claims that his or her deeply held religious values are the right ones, and there can be no discussion (Volbrecht, 2002).

Likewise, spiritual values may play an important role in making ethical decisions (Ahronheim, Moreno & Zuckerman, 2000). All persons do not ascribe to a particular religion; however, they may espouse deeply held spiritual values. When caring for persons with chronic illnesses, nurses need to consider how spiritual values may influence their clients' ideas about the meaning of life and death and their perception of quality of life. Recognizing the relevance of these values and beliefs is inherent in the principle of respect for persons.

Culture

Increasingly, health care professionals are reminded of the need to respect the diversity of their clients and their co-workers. One's cultural and ethnic background helps to shape one's values and beliefs. However, like religious beliefs, all persons from a particular culture may not espouse the same values and beliefs. Even though the nurse may have an understanding of the values of a particular culture, the nurse cannot make assumptions about the decisions that a person from that culture may make, as each person is a unique individual deserving of respect (Ahronheim, Moreno & Zuckerman, 2000).

Cultural differences can lead to ethical dilemmas in the client-provider relationship (Doswell & Erlen, 1998). In particular, the belief system of the client may be discredited because it does not fit with the provider's belief system. Cultures have their own beliefs and values regarding such matters as health and illness, pain and suffering, and death and dying. If one is unaware of another's cultural beliefs, there is the distinct possibility that there will be a clash related to the treatment decision of the client and what the health care provider sees as an appropriate option.

Law

Laws limit the flexibility of one's decision-making because laws do not include exceptions. Laws identify what a society has determined to be acceptable behavior based on that society's definition of right and wrong. These laws are often the result of considerable compromise. Laws are enforceable rules (O'Keefe, 2001). Although laws are sometimes used to resolve an ethical dilemma, they provide a minimalist or an insufficient justification for one's course of action when resolving ethical issues. Thus, although laws may be an appropriate starting point for discussing ethical issues, laws are not the end point of deliberations (Ahronheim, Moreno & Zuckerman, 2000).

Laws do not address all of the complexities that surround an ethical question (O'Keefe, 2001). By appealing to the law, one only knows what to do to uphold the law. However, the most appropriate ethical action may require going beyond the law. Ethics holds one to a higher standard of behavior, because what is legal may not be ethical.

Ethical Dilemmas

Ethical dilemmas involve moral claims that are in conflict with each other (Davis et al., 1997). There are no clear solutions, because the available choices may present equally unsatisfying alternatives. Individuals who are involved in making ethical decisions may place different values on the possible alternatives. The decision makers have to address several questions. These questions include who should decide, what ought to be done, and what is the right choice.

When faced with an ethical dilemma, individuals may feel as if they are lost in a wilderness, with its tangled undergrowth. In this unknown territory, there seems to be no clearly discernible single path. Paths lead in various directions. Which path should one choose? How does one make that choice? To whom does one turn for help? What questions need to be asked and answered in order to determine the best course of action?

The Ethical Decision-Making Process

Resolving an ethical dilemma requires the use of critical thinking skills. One draws conclusions, rather than jumps to conclusions, and engages in a dynamic process of deliberation rather than inserting predetermined actions. The person needs to discern the facts—what is known? Having the facts is essential to ethical decision-making; however, the facts alone are not sufficient to determine the ethically appropriate choice. One needs to also identify the values that are related to the question—what is important? There is a need to examine the context of the situation—what is happening? Who is involved? How are they involved? Examining the facts, values, and context will help to determine what is of concern or troubling about the situation and will help one to bring the ethical issue(s) into clearer focus Table 18-3).

One needs to also consider the alternatives. Why are some alternatives more appealing? Analyzing the situation and reasoning about the possible choices will help a person to determine the right action, justify it, and defend it when others question this decision (Ahronheim, Moreno &

TABLE 18-3

The Process of Resolving an Ethical Dilemma

Examine the evidence (facts, values, context).
    Be inquisitive.
    Be open to various ideas and perspectives.
Determine the focus of the ethical dilemma.
    Make distinctions.
Identify alternatives.
    Brainstorm about the alternatives.
    Consider creative resolutions.
Analyze alternatives for their fit.
    Examine alternatives against personal and
    professional values.
Select the most ethically appropriate alternative.
Justify the choice of that alternative.
Act on the chosen alternative.
Evaluate the decision making process and the results.
Use this evaluation as feedback.

Zuckerman, 2000; Volbrecht, 2002). Once one makes her or his ethical choice, then one needs to do the right thing.

Deliberating about a case and determining the right action is very different from acting on that ethical choice. There is some risk involved and some uncertainty. Making and acting on ethical decisions requires courage. One may not be able to predict the outcome. After the ethical dilemma is resolved, one needs to critically evaluate the results and the process that led to the outcome. This evaluation will provide important feedback for future ethical deliberations.

■ Ethical Challenges and Concerns

As advances in health care technology increase the available therapeutic options, individuals with chronic illness have the potential to live longer. The result is that numerous ethical challenges are occurring for persons living with a chronic disorder and/or for those individuals providing their care. Three fundamental ethical concerns affecting people with a chronic illness are lack of control, suffering, and access to services. These issues are not meant to be, nor can they be, all encompassing, because situations change over time.

Lack of Control

Individuals with a chronic condition often feel they are being controlled by their illness. They need to adhere to medication protocols and dietary and exercise regimens. Following these complex regimens continually reminds the client of their illness (Erlen & Mellors, 1999). Clients are also vulnerable to other health-related assaults. In diseases that include exacerbations and remissions, individuals often wonder when the next exacerbation will occur. Lacking control increases their dependency on others, and often individuals feel powerless (see Chapter 13, on powerlessness).

An underlying reason for this lack of control is the uncertainty about one's future health and the quality of that life. The person begins to question.

How long will I live? How will I know when it is time to stop treatment? Will there be financial resources for my family's needs? Are there facilities to provide the necessary care that I will need? These questions have no clear answers, lack predictability, and present ethical challenges for clients and their caregivers.

Individuals with chronic illness may feel limited in their ability to affect health-related decisions. They may be unable to effectively influence the outcome that they are seeking because they lack information or understanding of what they have been told. They may be confused by or be unclear about the situation. Because they lack control over other aspects of their lives, they often believe that they have no control over health-related decisions. However, because one is bedfast or wheelchair bound does not mean that the person cannot make decisions.

Lack of control also occurs when there are imbalances in the relationship between the client and the care provider. Persons with chronic disorders are vulnerable, and there is the potential for others to exploit them. Consequently, these clients may experience anger and frustration because they feel their rights are not being respected. They may be neither partners nor consultants in the decision-making, even though decisions are being made about them. They may not be presented with treatment options and/or the related risks and benefits. The person's values may not be considered, and, thus, their voice is not heard. Decisions are, in fact, being made for them. Yet the complex nature of current treatment decisions requires that the client's perspective be included (Erlen, 1998).

The health care professional may develop a treatment regimen and then tell the client to follow the plan as prescribed. What the provider may not have considered when planning the regimen was the uniqueness of the client's situation: The health care provider took control rather than including the client. Yet, to follow the prescribed plan may require significant life-style changes for the client. Only clients know what is important to them, what they are willing to risk, and how much burden or suffering they are willing to bear. Thus, clients and health-care providers must mutually establish the goals, strategies, and treatment regimen. Shared decision making increases personal control and trust and decreases the power imbalance (see Chapter 10, on compliance).

For example, often there is a need for life-style changes when clients living with HIV infection are prescribed combination antiretroviral therapy. Clients in one study reported that their level of adherence to a regimen of antiretroviral medications was closely aligned with their participation in the treatment decision (Erlen & Mellors, 1999). When the clients were involved, they felt as if they mattered and their opinion counted.

On the other hand, the person with a chronic illness may not be included in the treatment decision making because there is a concern that the ill person lacks the capacity to make these decisions. Another reason may be that the person is too "sick" and therefore should not be burdened with decision-making. These others (family or professional caregivers) decide on behalf of, rather than at the behest of, the client and act to protect the client's best interests as perceived by the decision maker(s) (Beauchamp & Childress, 2001). The caregiver's choice is substituted for the client's wishes, and respect for client autonomy is thwarted.

Competent adult clients should participate in the decision-making of their care. However, individuals do not always make rational choices; irrational choices may cause others to question the competence of the decision maker. "*Decision-making capacity* signifies the ability to make a particular decision and is not considered a legal standard" (Council on Ethical and Judicial Affairs, 1992, p. 2229). Rather than making assumptions about whether particular clients can make decisions, health care providers need to assess the client's ability to understand, reason, and communicate (Bosek, Savage, Shaw, & Renella, 2001; Volbrecht, 2002). Family members and health care providers need to realize that clients do not necessarily lack decision-making capacity when they make decisions with which others do not agree.

Making informed decisions about their care requires that clients have knowledge and understanding of the situation. Ingelfinger's (1972) classic article called for health care professionals to do more than provide information; they need to educate clients about possible treatment options and the risks and the benefits (Once they inform a client, providers need to assess how well the person understands that information).

Assessing understanding requires that providers consider both the level of completed education and the level of functional health literacy. Persons with functional health illiteracy have trouble reading, understanding, and making decisions (Williams et al., 1995). The silent nature of this problem makes it difficult to detect as individuals have learned ways to cover their inability to understand. Clients who are functionally health illiterate are impaired and may make inappropriate decisions (Blacksher, 2002).

Treatment decisions require that clients and providers consider the technical aspects, the contextual factors, and the values and beliefs that influence decision-making. Values and beliefs are particular to and are an inherent part of the person. Because all persons do not share the same values, clients need to disclose their values and their plans to family or friends who will then use that information to make health-related decisions with them. However, making decisions based on the client's values can be troubling for others. Using the client's values and goals for the future may lead the surrogate decision makers to make very different decisions than they would make under the same circumstances.

Because clients may become incapacitated and others may need to make decisions for them, there is now greater emphasis on the importance of having advance directives. The 1990 Patient Self-Determination Act (Omnibus Budget Reconciliation Act, 1990) requires that health care agencies that receive Medicare and Medicaid funding ask clients on admission whether they have advance directives and, if not, provide them with this information. Advance directives provide instructions for others about the medical care which individuals want or do not want in regard to end-of-life care when they are unable to speak for themselves (Mezey et al., 2000). These directives are used at the time when persons are no longer able to direct their own care. Advance direc-

tives afford clients the opportunity to remain in charge of their care to the extent that this is possible. Living wills are one example of an advance directive. Another example is the health care power of attorney. In this instance, the person documents who is to be responsible for making health care decisions when the client becomes unable to make these decisions.

People mistakenly believe that their family members will know what to do at the time these health care decisions need to be made, and that there is no need to prepare directives in advance. Problems arise when there is a lack of clarity about the person's wishes. While advance directives may not answer every question that arises, they do provide a guide for decision-making that helps to protect the interests of the client. To help assure that all understand the health care wishes of the person with the chronic illness, a discussion of the advance directive needs to occur among the client, family members and health care providers. These conversations will help to clarify the person's living will, because it cannot include every possible health situation and type of treatment. A copy of the advance directive document needs to be kept in a prominent location and given to others so that it is available when the need arises. Additionally, individuals need to review their advance directives periodically, because their wishes and treatment options may change as their life situation changes.

Competence, knowledge, and understanding provide the basis for making informed decisions. These decisions are also congruent with the person's values. In other words, the choice fits with that person. To do otherwise would compromise the individual's integrity. Therefore, clients with chronic illnesses will not always opt for an available treatment, and they may decide to refuse treatment (President's Commission, 1983). Health care providers and family may have difficulty accepting this fact. However, respect for persons admonishes others to respect the client's decision to refuse whenever that decision is an informed one and the person is capable of making a decision.

Suffering

A second set of ethical challenges for persons with chronic conditions focuses on suffering. Cassell

(1991) defines *suffering* as "the state of severe distress associated with events that threaten the intactness of the person" (p. 33). These events can be physical, psychosocial, financial, and/or spiritual in nature. They create demands and generate conflicts for the person who is trying to reconcile and respond to them.

Currently, increasing emphasis is being placed on pain management and palliative care. When pain medication is used correctly, clients with chronic illness can have improved quality of life and be more productive. Pain control is necessary for people to manage other aspects of their lives. Even though there are medications available to alleviate most pain, they are not being used to their fullest extent. Frequently, pain is mismanaged because of the lack of a standardized method and protocol for pain assessment. Many health care providers have limited knowledge in this area or continue to believe the myths about pain and drug addiction. They mistakenly believe that the client will become addicted if large doses of narcotics are prescribed. Thus, the client suffers needlessly.

Health care professionals also lack knowledge of the law (Sieger, 1997). Legislative barriers prohibit physicians from prescribing large doses of narcotic medications; physicians' prescribing practices may be monitored. Further, clients may be unable to get the prescriptions filled because they cannot afford the medication or the physician writing the prescription is in a different state (Pain Undertreatment, 1999). As a result, the clients' pain is not managed appropriately or effectively. This mismanagement of pain presents an ethical dilemma for nurses. The client, rather than being helped, is being harmed.

Another harm that clients can experience is created by the stigma associated with particular diseases. Stigma is seen through the social interactions of people. Therefore, the sociological meaning of chronic illness provides a means for understanding the stigmatization that occurs. Within this framework, health is valued and illness is devalued. Individuals with chronic illness may have physically defining characteristics of their illness, or they may have varying degrees of disability that affect their ability to function. The ill individual may experience stigma because of these discrediting attributes that can spoil their social identity (Goffman, 1963) (see Chapter 3, on stigma).

Thus, those who have a chronic illness may be discredited by society. Because of their differences, they may be set apart from others. The chronically ill may be stigmatized, labeled, and avoided. Consequently, to avoid the destructive effect that stigma may have on one's social ties, individuals may try to mask their differences; they may not disclose their diagnoses as they try to fit into society. A potential problem can arise, as others can be placed at risk as a result. For example, clients with HIV infection may not disclose their diagnosis because of the potentially devastating effects that this might have on their job, their health insurance, their children, and their relationships with others.

The client's diagnosis is a label and a means of classifying the person. Labels can have both negative and positive effects. The negative effect of labels is that they stereotype behavior and may result in prejudicial or biased judgments. Labeling someone can lead to shunning behavior toward that person by others. The person with the label may be avoided, set apart, and isolated. This shunning behavior may occur because those who are "normal" do not understand the problems faced by those that are "different." The result is a lack of respect and discrimination toward the person with the label. The individual seemingly has neither rights nor status within the society. In effect, their freedom may be limited.

On the other hand, labels can have a positive effect. Even though labels set the person apart, it is this setting apart and being different that makes a person eligible for, or becomes the reason others lobby for, some specialized services. The label becomes the relevant reason for, or the condition upon which one is granted, access to particular services.

The degree of discrimination or stigma one experiences can affect quality of life. *Quality of life* is defined in terms of how satisfying or important particular aspects of one's life are to the person (Ferrans, 1990). People living with a chronic illness may not seek longevity. Instead, they may be more interested in the quality of their lives (Cella, 1992). Just being alive may be a burden that some find difficult to bear. Thus, the definition of *quality of life* is subjective and highly individualized and reflects an evaluation of the current situation. There is no agreed upon definition (Frytak, 2000). What is "good" quality of life for one person is not necessarily true for another individual with the same chronic illness. The person's life circumstances, the amount of support from family and others, and the person's values affect what matters to the individual. Therefore, quality of life becomes one's "subjective assessment of an amalgamation of possible life domains. . . ." (Frytak, 2000, p. 202) (see Chapter 9, on quality of life).

Technology can benefit many individuals with chronic illnesses and improve their quality of life. However, to what degree do people receive benefit? Is the benefit one that enables individuals to express themselves in their unique way and to continue to make a contribution to their family or society? Or, is the benefit the fact that they are able to be alive but require care from others? Does the use of technology prolong living or prolong dying? These are ques-

tions that need to be considered as one examines the ethical challenges inherent in quality of life. Clients' definitions of quality of life will guide their decision making as they consider the question, "Do I want to live like this?" Health care providers need to treat the illness experience affects the life of to the person.

Curing and managing the illness are important goals in health care. The potential exists for these goals to direct the care that the client receives. These goals focus on the notion of preserving life. For some, preserving life is the most important goal. However, for others, quality of life is the most important goal. Focusing only on the body or on preserving life exclusively threatens the humanity of the individual, can increase suffering, and can decrease the person's quality of life (Erlen, 2003a).

Accessing Services

The third ethical challenge for persons living with a chronic illness is access to services. These individuals have a greater need for health care re-

---

Decisions in Continuing Treatment

Mr. Brown, 72 years old, was diagnosed with multiple myeloma 15 months ago. He has had several recent hospitalizations, and each time he is discharged from the hospital, he is somewhat weaker. The time between his blood transfusions is decreasing as well. After his last hospitalization, he and his wife of 51 years decide that nursing home placement would probably be best for him because of the care he requires. One evening, Mr. Brown asks the nurse whether or not he should continue with the blood transfusions. He now needs to have these blood transfusions two times each week. He has to go to the hospital for the transfusion, which takes, at minimum, 8 to 10 hours. He tells the nurse, "I know I am not getting better. All that the blood transfusions are doing is prolonging the inevitable." Mrs. Brown is visiting her husband at the time. She quickly responds, "Don't say that. Look how much stronger you were after you came back from the hospital today."

Questions:

■ What are the facts/context/values in this case?
■ Given what is known from the case, what is the ethical dilemma?
■ What are possible alternatives?
■ What is the most appropriate alternative? Why?

sources, because they experience exacerbations in their illness and may have existing comorbidities. However, this potential need for health care resources raises many questions. Is society willing to provide these health services? Are the resources available to all or to only those who can pay? How much of a gap exists between the demand for services and the commitment to provide services? How do the principle of justice and the value that society places on health inform these questions?

Within society all persons are not the same nor do they have the same opportunities. Health disparities exist because of such factors as age, ethnicity, educational level, employment status. Those experiencing health disparities are particularly vulnerable, have increased morbidity and mortality, and bear heavier burdens when accessing and paying for needed health services (Thomson, 1997). The issues that are raised by health disparities as society attempts to address the goal of "health for all" by 2010 (U.S. Department of Health and Human Services, 2000) requires a reconsideration of the distribution of benefits and burdens within a society (Erlen, 2003b).

Persons with chronic illnesses have variable levels of health, depending on their disorders. Thus, the amount of health care that they need is also variable. Frequently, the problem for these clients is accessing and paying for the health care that they need. There are some ethicists and policy makers who argue that health care is a consumer good. When people need health care, they can go out and purchase it. The cost becomes what the market will bear, which is similar when purchasing any other consumer good. However, health care is not a commodity like a television or a computer that one can purchase for a specified price. Without health, people are unable to compete for the same opportunities as others in society. Without health, they cannot live meaningful lives. To maximize their health potential, persons with chronic conditions need to be able to access health care services. However, how much health care needs to be allocated to each person?

Some ethicists argue that there should be equal access to services, regardless of one's ability to pay. This approach is theoretically appealing and results in a benefit for all. Yet, the costs of providing all or even some services for all may be prohibitive. Society does not have an infinite budget to spend on health care. Inevitably, equal access means that society will need to make allocation decisions.

Others argue that basing access to services on one's ability to pay means that the quality of the services may be better, and more specialized services may be available. The premise of this approach is that those who can afford services are able to access more services. However, some societal groups will be excluded because they do not have the financial resources to access the services. These people know that they need the services and that having access to these services would help them manage their health problems. However, if they cannot afford the services, in effect, the services are being rationed. Only those who can afford to pay for the services have access to them (Erlen, 2002).

Another perspective is that equal access should occur only in relation to basic health services. This viewpoint serves as a basis for Charles Fried's (1976) historic call for providing a "decent minimum." The decent minimum is a standard benefit or a basic health care package. Beyond this basic plan, people have to pay for health services that they need.

Despite the availability of more health care services and advancing technologies, there continues to be an increasing demand for even more. People seem to have an almost insatiable demand for these services. Health care wants far exceed needs. These health care wants increase the demand for and the cost of services; they also limit the availability and accessibility of services.

Because limited health care resources exist, which services should be provided? How are these decisions made? To provide these necessary services at a cost that people can afford and to have quality care require intricate balancing. This balancing has to be based on reasons of fairness. The goal is to develop a system that even those who are denied particular services view as being fair.

Having health care services available says nothing about where those services are located. Accessibility is closely tied to availability. Individuals living outside major urban areas may find that travel costs and travel time become prohibitive as they try to access services. When one has a chronic illness, time and cost factors increase rapidly, because the need to access services may occur frequently.

Individuals who have chronic lung, heart, liver, or kidney conditions are acutely aware of accessibility, availability, and cost issues. These clients may need to move closer to a transplant center. They sit and wait, not knowing when an organ may become available or whether there will be a match.

However, making services available does not address the issue of the quality of those services. When costs are contained, quality may decrease (Emanuel, 2000). One way to decrease costs is to hire less educated personnel to perform services that more highly qualified people have been providing. When the focus is on the "bottom line" and whether or not the budget balances, client care may be compromised.

With managed care now pervasive across the United States, other issues about accessing care arise. Managed care is a system that purports to organize health care providers and facilities in order to maximize efficiency. Managed care integrates finances and the delivery of health care in order to control costs and to improve quality. However, the focus is on efficiency and effectiveness rather than client care.

An ethical problem associated with managed care and chronic illness is conflict of interest (Emanuel, 2000; Loewy, 2001). Health care providers may advocate for more services for clients or for more frequent follow-up care, yet the managed care plan may not permit this. The health care provider in trying to serve the employer and the client finds that each has different goals, which are in direct conflict with the other.

Long-term client–provider relationships are important when managing clients with chronic illnesses. These relationships promote trust and confidence. However, with the advent of managed care, this trust can be eroded, because clients may no longer feel that their interests or their rights are important. If they try to access a specialist without a referral from their primary care provider, they may be denied access. If they obtain this referral, clients may have to wait extended periods for an appointment.

This controlled access to specialists reduces client autonomy and compromises one's rights. There may also be threats to informed consent. Health care providers may have less time to explain treatment options to clients, and clients may feel that there is no time to ask questions. Clients may

Disclosure

Jerry is a 35-year-old White gay male who has been highly successful as a loan officer in a large bank in an East Coast city. He does not deny the fact that he is gay; however, he does not openly disclose the fact to others. Jerry was diagnosed with HIV almost three years ago. He has not disclosed his diagnosis to his family or to anyone at the bank. He always plans his appointments with his doctor for evenings or Saturdays. Recently, he was placed on antiretroviral therapy. He has to take some of his medications while he is at work. Jerry is wondering how he will be able to unobtrusively take his medications. He is concerned that people will begin to ask him questions. He is also concerned about his family and what they will say, as there is a good chance that he will have to take medications whenever he visits them. He knows that his family will learn of his illness sooner or later, but he is afraid of how they will react. Jerry discloses his situation to the nurse in the doctor's office and asks her what he should do.

find that their choices are also limited in regard to accessible treatments and medications.

Despite managed care, the cost of health care services continues to rise. One area with the greatest increases is the cost of prescription drugs. As people are living longer, they are more likely to develop more than one chronic disorder and need medications to manage their illnesses. But how expensive are the medications? Does the person's health care insurance cover the cost of prescriptions? Does the individual even have health insurance? Does the person have to make decisions about which prescription(s) to have filled or whether to take the medication as directed in order to reduce their health care costs?

Genetic testing and counseling is a service that individuals with chronic illness may want to access, yet this service may not be available to them. The Human Genome Project is unraveling information about the genetics of various chronic conditions. Of particular interest to many is the genetics related to Alzheimer's disease, breast cancer, and Huntingdon's chorea. How does knowledge of one's risk for a disorder affect the health-related decisions that they make? Who does one tell? What information needs to be kept confidential? If one carries the gene for a disorder, should that person have children? What is the individual's responsibility? If clients want to obtain answers to these questions, they need to have access to genetic services. To gain knowledge of risk for a genetic disorder, genetic testing and counseling services need to be available.

A related issue affecting health care costs is nonadherence to treatment regimen. Nonadherence can lead to a worsening of the chronic illness, causing the person to be hospitalized, with the ensuing additional expenses (see Chapter 10, on compliance).

Interventions for Creating an Ethical Climate

Interventions are needed to address the ethical challenges of chronic illness. The purposes of these interventions are to enable clients to have control and to participate in decision-making, to decrease suffering, and to increase accessibility to and affordability of services. The specific interventions depend on the situation. This section describes three broad categories of actions that promote an ethical health care environment for individuals with chronic conditions and their caregivers and uphold the standards of professional practice as set forth in the *Code of Ethics for Nurses* (ANA, 2001). These strategies are increasing the nurse's understanding of ethics, being an advocate for persons with chronic disorders, and engaging in effective communication. When nurses are practicing within an ethical environment, they have opportunities to learn and to dialogue. They are supported and encouraged to be client advocates. Nurses will "have the necessary freedom to act in a morally autonomous fashion for promoting the well-being of their clients" (Maier-Lorentz, 2000, p. 25). Additionally, there is a cross-disciplinary exchange of ideas.

Increasing the Nurse's Understanding of Ethics

To create and sustain an ethical environment, to be proactive, and to recognize and effectively address ethical issues, nurses must have knowledge of ethics. A strong foundation in ethics helps nurses to practice ethically. Because nurses often find themselves "caught in the middle," it is important that they be able to recognize and analyze ethical dilemmas in order to identify an ethically justified action. When ethical dilemmas occur, nurses can be assertive and request ethics consultations. To feel confident about the ethical action one is taking requires knowledge and experience. As nurses become more "expert" in the practice of nursing, they will use this knowledge and experience and take the necessary risks to address ethical dilemmas in their practice.

Nursing education programs need to include specific ethics content within their curricula. This content may be taught through a separate course or may be integrated throughout the curriculum. The national nursing accrediting bodies, the Commission on Collegiate Nursing Education and the National

League for Nursing Accrediting Commission, have criteria specifying ethics and values content in the curriculum at all levels of nursing education. Likewise, the American Nurses Association's standards for clinical nursing practice incorporate ethics in their document as well.

Nursing curricula need to provide opportunities for students at all educational levels to identify ethical dilemmas and to analyze actual and/or hypothetical ethical cases (Holland, 1999). Nurses need to experience analyzing typical cases. One format that can effectively facilitate ethical analysis and reasoning is problem-based learning. Small groups of students identify what they need to know in order to address the hypotheses and learning issues that they generate when reviewing the case. This process enables students to identify various ethical perspectives, to clarify their personal and professional values, and to understand the complexity of cases. Students are able to recognize that all persons, and likewise all nurses, do not view situations similarly. They are able to gain an understanding of the many ways that religion and law, and cultural and family backgrounds exert a strong influence on how people

understand ethical dilemmas and develop possible resolutions.

Ethics education needs to be included in staff development and continuing education programs. An effective means of increasing understanding and knowledge is the use of ethics case conferences or ethics rounds. These opportunities are situation-specific and provide insight into the ethical challenges within the nurse–client–family relationship. Focusing on actual cases provides an opportunity for nurses to clarify and examine the issues and various options. These interactive methods become a means for nurses to challenge their own thinking about their ethical choices and whether they were the most ethically appropriate.

Another possible educational strategy is the invitational conference. Kupperschmidt (2000) discussed the use of this method to explore the ethical issues related to the use of unlicensed assistive personnel. A few highly selected participants are provided with reading material prior to the conference in order to prepare themselves for the discussion that will occur. There is a highly skilled facilitator who keeps the selected participants and the discus-

Access to Care

The changes in health care reimbursement are forcing home health nursing services to alter their practices. The reimbursement policy allows clients to have a set number of visits from the nurse. At the end of that time, the client has to be discharged. The nurses in the agency, however, are concerned that clients still require care, because they are unable to adequately care for themselves. Some clients have very limited support from family and friends. The nurses in Generic Home Health Care Agency are concerned that these clients will need to be hospitalized or, worse, may die because of the lack of care. Thus, the nurses try to include visits whenever they

are in the neighborhood even though there is no scheduled visit or payment to be collected. They realize that these visits are only providing a "Band-Aid;" the basic problem is not getting better. In fact, there are increasing numbers of clients who are being seen by the nurses, for which they receive no reimbursement. The supervisor of Generic Home Health Care Agency meets with the nurses and praises them for their devotion to their clients, but tells them that they are going to have to stop this practice. The nurses ask, "What are the clients to do? How can we just ignore their needs? Don't we have a moral obligation to these clients?"

sion centered on the topic. A theater-in-the-round setting helps to focus the audience's attention on the discussion. This educational strategy requires that participants expend effort, be willing to take risks when there are conflicting ideas, and engage in thoughtful dialogue.

Nurses can also increase their knowledge of ethics by participating in journal clubs that focus on ethical issues. The readings that are selected direct participants to consider different ethical perspectives and to discuss research related to ethics in health care. Often, journal clubs have a leader whose purpose is to facilitate the discussion rather than reiterate the content of the selected article(s). The leader engages the participants in a meaningful conversation that is triggered by the article(s) in order to increase their knowledge of ethics.

Additionally, nurses can review research findings on nursing ethics or become involved with a research project examining current ethical challenges. Research contributes to the nursing profession's body of knowledge and provides the evidence for nursing practice. Within the past 25 years, there has been a significant increase in research on nursing ethics. Many of the early studies focused on the decision-making process (DeWolf, 1989; Smith, 1996). The emphasis of current research has turned to examining ethical issues (Douglas & Brown, 2002; Houtepen & Hendrikx, 2003). Nurses in clinical practice need to become aware of these findings and to use this knowledge as they care for clients.

Additionally, the novice nurse needs to identify a mentor who has experience with analyzing ethical dilemmas. Mentors model ethical behavior and help young nurses identify ethical conflicts within their caseload of clients. Mentors need to encourage ethical practice. Less experienced nurses need to discuss troubling cases and receive feedback from an individual they trust and respect. Mentors can help young nurses deliberate about these ethical dilemmas and identity possible resolutions and their consequences. Mentors can provide support for less experienced nurses as they implement their ethical actions. Mentors can also help these novice nurses to evaluate the results of their ethical choices and provide feedback that nurses can use when confronted by ethical dilemmas in the future.

When there are no opportunities available that address the ongoing educational needs of nurses, they need to "seize the moment" and create the forums that will support their learning. Nurses need to be proactive and initiate educational programs for nurses. This action on their part is more likely to meet their educational needs and to make others aware of a need for an ethical environment in which to practice nursing.

Advocacy

A nursing intervention clearly identified in the *Code of Ethics for Nurses* (ANA, 2001) is advocacy. Nurses are not to keep silent when there are unethical practices affecting their clients. To advocate for another means that one represents that person and, in so doing, protects that person's interests and rights. The advocate promotes the well-being of another (Woods, 1999). Because of the ethical issues surrounding chronically ill persons, advocacy is an important intervention. Nurses, however, are not the only health care providers who serve as advocates for clients. Because nurses establish ongoing relationships with clients and their families, nurses are often uniquely aware of the clients' values and interests. Thus, nurses can advocate for clients because they generally know what their clients want. The shared human experience that nurses have with their clients provides the foundation of their relationship one with the other. As a result, nurses can support and sustain the difficult ethical decisions that clients make. Nurses can serve as liaisons among the client, family, and other members of the health care team (see Chapter 16, on advocacy).

Advocacy may mean taking cases to the institutional ethics committee (IEC) or seeking ethics consultations. Because of their unique position in providing care to clients, nurses need to be key participants on these IECs. An ethical environment has an IEC available to provide support when difficult ethical situations arise. Persons with chronic illness may not be residing in institutions that have ethics committees. Home care and long-term care facilities are only beginning to establish IECs. Given their pivotal role in the care of clients, nurses can be instrumental in developing these committees. When no such committee exists, a neutral third party, such as a member of the clergy, a social worker, or an ethicist from a nearby college or university, may be available to serve as an ethics consultant.

Advocacy involves risk taking. As nurses advocate for clients, they may experience a conflict between fulfilling their role to clients and their role to the health care organization (Riley & Fry, 2000). Nurses may find themselves at risk of losing their jobs when they push the limits of the health care system. There is also risk when being an advocate results in nurse–physician conflict. Nurses may find that they cannot disclose information to clients that will help them make decisions. Nurses feel "caught in the middle" and powerless and may experience moral distress.

Moral distress occurs when nurses cannot act on their moral choices (Erlen, 2001; Volbrecht, 2002). Nurses are angry and frustrated; they feel powerless and may want to leave nursing. Situational constraints make it difficult for nurses to engage in what they consider to be professional and ethical practice.

To help decrease the feeling of being "caught in the middle" and experiencing moral distress, nurses can facilitate the development of policies and the promotion of high professional standards that will help to create an ethical climate. Nurses are in an ideal position to alter the ethical climate within the institution to make it more responsive to the client. Developing policies that clearly promote the client's role in making ethical decisions will help nurses as they advocate for client involvement. These policies will specify the procedures to follow and provide direction for nurses as they negotiate the health care system for their clients. Such policies demonstrate that the institution values and supports advocacy and professional practice (Maier-Lorentz, 2000).

Nurses can advocate for persons with chronic disorders and help them to advocate for themselves so that they are included in any decision making. Nurses can provide educational sessions or work with public and medical libraries to identify consumer resources that will help clients be their own advocates and provide information on various ethical issues. When individuals are informed about their medical conditions, others are less likely to diminish their rights.

Nurses need to become sensitized to the human side of persons with chronic illness, and recognize their clients' pain, anguish, suffering, and uncertainty. Although it is important to understand the technical aspects of care, it is imperative that nurses realize the personal side. Nurses are taught to be objective and to discern the facts as they assess their clients; yet, this information alone will not tell nurses enough about their clients. To provide ethical care, nurses need to understand their clients as people, to respond to them as people, and to be less calloused in their interactions.

Communicating Effectively

Ethical deliberation requires effective and open communication. There needs to be ongoing dialogue between and among the various persons involved in the case. Time is not always one's ally when making ethical decisions; thus, time needs to be used wisely. Calling on the IEC or an ethics consultant may provide the most expeditious means of addressing a troubling issue. Using the available expertise helps focus the discussion about the case. Ethics committees and consultants can serve various functions; however, their role is not to take the decision making away from the bedside or to interfere with client decision making. These committees are not the primary decision makers; rather, they facilitate decision making.

The ethics committee can conduct reviews of current client cases raising ethical concerns, as well as retrospective reviews of troubling cases, and thereby provide advice about ways to resolve the issues. They can educate and inform health care workers about ethical concerns. The committee can also examine existing and proposed legislative action in order to determine the impact that such decisions may have on residents, their families, and health care providers within the institution. Likewise, this group can initiate or advise on institutional policy that has ethical implications.

To advance their clients' interests, nurses need to lobby effectively in the public policy arena. Health policies are the result of the political process. Inherent in these policies are the values of various key players. Nurses and clients are two of these vital groups. Nurses have the knowledge that is needed to shape health policy and must be included in these discussions. They need to inform legislators about the special needs of clients with chronic illness. Frequently, lawmakers have little or no understanding of the issues that confront their constituents with chronic illness. Because nurses are with these clients on a regular basis, nurses have unique knowledge of these issues.

Laws and policies need to be established that will protect the rights of persons with chronic illness and provide them with opportunities to be contributing members of society. Establishing these laws and policies is not the only way to address these ethical issues; however, without laws there can be no enforcement of laws aimed at increasing accessibility and availability of health care services for those with chronic conditions. Because lawmakers may have limited understanding of the health and/or everyday living problems that persons with chronic disorders confront, nurses need to keep the explanations at a less sophisticated level and not use jargon.

Through their professional associations, nurses can help to define health policy issues and identify potential strategies to address the problems (Olson, 2004). Working through professional nursing organizations to further the interests of persons with chronic illnesses is important; however, nursing's efforts can be multiplied by joining forces with organizations that have legislative agendas already in place.

Nurses can talk with reporters about issues and encourage newspapers to include human interest stories that demonstrate the ethical issues that persons with chronic illness address regularly. These stories and accompanying pictures can vividly portray the issues, bring them to the attention of society, and help to engage the public. These stories can identify the ethical dilemmas regarding access to care and obtaining medications for adequate pain relief. Nurses are in a unique position to raise society's level of consciousness concerning the ethical issues of persons with chronic disorders. Likewise, because of the trust the public has in nurses, they can work together to identify solutions to these complex ethical questions.

Outcomes

When nurses engage in ethical practice, they serve as advocates for persons with chronic conditions. Upholding the well-being of the client becomes the primary goal. Clients gain control rather than relinquish it to others. The result is that the clients' voices are heard. Clients and their values become central when health care decisions are made, and their quality of life improves. Attention becomes focused on making health care resources accessible and affordable to meet the needs of those with chronic disorders.

Study Questions

1. Discuss the influences that should be considered in ethical decision making in the care of the client with chronic illness.
2. What are the key concepts within nursing ethics?
3. Identify a situation from your clinical practice that has ethical overtones. Using interventions discussed in this chapter, how would you create an ethical climate to deal with the situation?
4. Differentiate between the utilitarian and Kantian ethical perspectives. Provide an example of how each could be applied to a clinical situation.

5. How does the nursing code of ethics guide practice?

6. Most ethicists identify three predominant principles: respect for persons, beneficence, and justice. Describe each of those principles and give an example of how the principle can be applied to an actual client situation.

7. How does the care ethic provide direction for nurses caring for clients with chronic disorders?

8. Describe the difference between law and ethics.

9. Suffering is an ethical challenge for health care professionals caring for individuals with chronic disease. Explain that statement.

10. Technology is both a boon and a bane to health care. Using an ethical decision-making framework, how would one make a decision to prolong the life of a 70-year-old individual with end stage renal disease, diabetes mellitus, and osteoarthritis?

11. What is an ethical dilemma?

12. Casuistry is a newer model of viewing ethical dilemmas. How does one use that ethical perspective in a clinical situation?

References

Agich, G. J. (1995). Chronic illness and freedom. In S. K. Toombs, D. Barnard, R. A. Carson (Eds.), *Chronic illness: From experience to policy*, (pp. 129–153). Bloomington: Indiana University Press.

Ahronheim, J. C., Moreno, J. D., & Zuckerman, C. (2000). *Ethics in clinical practice* (2nd ed.). Gaithersburg, MD: Aspen Publishers.

American Nurses Association (1985). *Code for nurses with interpretive statements.* Washington, DC: Author.

American Nurses Association (2001). *Code of ethics for nurses.* Washington, DC: Author.

Beauchamp, T. L., & Childress, J. F. (2001). *Principles of biomedical ethics* (5th ed.). New York: Oxford University Press.

Benner, P., & Wrubel, J. (1989). *The primacy of caring: Stress and coping in health and illness.* Menlo Park, CA: Addison-Wesley.

Blacksher, E. A. (2002). On being poor and feeling poor: Low socioeconomic status and the moral self. *Theoretical Medicine, 23,* 455–470.

Bosek, M. S. D., Savage, T., Shaw, L. A., & Renella, C. (2001). When surrogate decision-making is not straightforward: Guidelines for nurse administrators. *JONA's Healthcare,Law, Ethics, and Regulation, 3*(2), 47–57.

Carper, B. A. (1979). The ethics of caring. *Advances in Nursing Science, 1* (3), 11–19.

Cassell, E. J. (1991). *The nature of suffering.* New York: Oxford University Press.

Cella, D. F. (1992). Quality of life: The concept. *Journal of Palliative Care, 8* (3), 8–13.

Council on Ethical and Judicial Affairs, American Medical Association (1992). Decisions near the end of life. *Journal of the American Medical Association, 267* (16), 2229–2233.

Curtin, L. L. (1979). The nurse as advocate: A philosophical foundation for nursing. *Advances in Nursing Science, 1* (3), 1–10.

Davis, A. J., Aroskar, M. A., Liaschenko, J., & Drought, T. S. (1997). *Ethical dilemmas and nursing practice* (4th ed.). Stamford, CT: Appleton & Lange.

DeWolf, M. S. (1989). Ethical decision making. *Seminars in Oncology Nursing, 5* (2), 77–81.

Doswell, W. M., & Erlen, J. A. (1998). Multicultural issues and ethical concerns in the delivery of nursing care interventions. *Nursing Clinics of North America, 30* (2), 353–361.

Douglas, R., & Brown, H. N. (2002). Patients' attitudes toward advance directives. *Journal of Nursing Scholarship, 34* (1), 61–65.

Emanuel, E. J. (2000). Justice and managed care: Four principles for the just allocation of health care resources. *Hastings Center Report, 30* (3), 8–16.

Erlen, J. A. (1998). Treatment decision making: Who should decide? *Orthopedic Nursing, 17* (4), 60–64.

_____. (2001). Moral distress: A pervasive problem. *Orthopaedic Nursing, 20* (2), 76–80.

_____. (2002). When there are limits on health care resources. *Orthopedic Nursing, 21* (2), 69–73.

_____. (2003a). Caring doesn't end. *Orthopedic Nursing, 22* (6), 446–449.

_____. (2003b). When all do not have the same: Health disparities. *Orthopedic Nursing, 22* (2), 151–154.

Erlen, J. A., & Mellors, M. P. (1999). Adherence to combination therapy in persons living with HIV: Balancing the hardships and the blessings. *Journal of the Association of Nurses in AIDS Care, 10* (4), 75–84.

Ferrans, C. E. (1990). Quality of life: Conceptual issues. *Seminars in Oncology Nursing, 6*, 248–254.

Frankena, W. K. (1973). *Ethics* (2nd ed.). Englewood Cliffs, NJ: Prentice-Hall.

Fried, C. (1976). Equality and rights in medical care. *Hastings Center Report, 6*, 29–34.

Frytak, J. R. (2000). Assessment of quality of life in older adults. In R. L. Kane & R. A. Kane (Eds.), *Assessing older adults: Measures, meaning, and practical applications,* (pp. 200–236). New York: Oxford.

Gastman, C. (1999). Care as a moral attitude in nursing. *Nursing Ethics, 6* (3), 214–223.

Gillick, M. R. (1995). The role of the rules: The impact of the bureaucratization of long term care. In S. K. Toombs, D. Barnard, & R. A. Carson (Eds.), *Chronic illness: From experience to policy*, (pp. 189–211). Bloomington: Indiana University Press.

Goffman, E. (1963). *Stigma: Notes on the management of a spoiled identity*. Englewood Cliffs, NJ: Prentice-Hall.

Holland, S. (1999). Teaching nursing ethics by cases: A personal perspective. *Nursing Ethics, 6* (5), 434–436.

Houtepen, R., & Hendrikx, D. (2003). Nurses and the virtues of dealing with existential questions in terminal palliative care. *Nursing Ethics, 10* (4), 377–387.

Ingelfinger, F. J. (1972). Informed (but uneducated) consent. *New England Journal of Medicine, 287*, 465–466.

Jonsen, A. R., Siegler, M., & Winslade, W. (1998). *Clinical ethics: A practical guide to ethical decisions in clinical medicine* (4th ed.). New York: McGraw-Hill.

Jonsen, A. R., & Toulmin, S. (1989). *The abuse of casuistry: A history of moral reasoning*. Berkeley: University of California Press.

Kupperschmidt, B. (2000). The invitational conference: A strategy for exploring ethical issues. *Nursing Forum, 35* (2), 25–31.

Loewy, E. H. (2001). Health care systems and ethics. In E. H. Loewy & R. S. Loewy (Eds.), *Changing health care systems from ethical, economic, and cross-cultural perspectives* (pp. 1–14). New York: Kluwer Academic/Plenum.

Lucke, K. T. (1998). Ethical implications of caring in rehabilitation. *Nursing Clinics of North America, 33* (2), 253–264.

Maier-Lorentz, M. M. (2000). Invest in yourself: Creating your own ethical environment. *Nursing Forum, 35* (3), 25–28.

Mezey, M. D., Leitman, R., Mitty, E. L., Bottrell, M. M., et al. (2000). Why hospital patients do and do not execute advance directives. *Nursing Outlook, 48*, 165–171.

Office for Civil Rights, (2003, May). *Summary of the HIPAA Privacy Rule*. Retrieved September 7, 2004 from the U. S. Department of Health and Human Services Office for Civil Rights. Access: http://www.hhs.gov/ocr/hipaa/privacy.html

O'Keefe, M. E. (2001). *Nursing practice and the law: Avoiding malpractice and other legal risks*. Philadelphia: FA Davis.

Olson, L. L. (2004). Politics, health policy, and ethics: Is there a relationship? *Chart, Journal of Illinois Nursing, 100* (7), 9–10.

Omnibus Reconciliation Act of 1990, Section 4206: Medicare provider agreements assuring the implementation of a patient's right to participate in and direct health care decisions affecting the patient and Section 4751: Requirements for advance directives under state plans for medical assistance. *Statutes at Large*, November 5, 1990.

Oulton, J. A. (2000). ICN's *Code of Ethics for Nurses*: Serving nurses and nursing care world-wide. *International Nursing Review, 47*, 137–141.

President's Commission for the Study of Ethical Problems in Medicine and Biomedical and Behavioral Research. (1983). *Deciding to forego life-sustaining treatment: Ethical, medical, and legal issues in treatment decisions*. Washington, DC: U.S. Government Printing Office.

Rawls, J. (1971). *A theory of justice*. Cambridge, MA: Harvard University Press.

Riley, J. M., & Fry, S. T. (2000). Troubled advocacy: Nurses report widespread ethical conflicts. *Reflections on Nursing Leadership, 26* (2), 35–36.

Robb, I. H. (1900). *Nursing ethics: For hospital and private use*. Cleveland, OH: C. Koeckert Publishers.

Sanders, D., & Dukeminier, J. Jr. (1968). Medical advance and legal lag: Hemodialysis and kidney transplantation. *UCLA Law Review, 15*, 366–380.

Scanlon, C. (2000). A professional code of ethics provides guidance for genetic nursing practice. *Nursing Ethics, 7* (3), 262–268.

Sieger, C. (Winter, 1997). Pain management: The role of the law. *Choices: The Newsletter of Choice in Dying, 6* (4), 1, 4–5.

Skott. C. (2003). Storied ethics: Conversations in nursing care. *Nursing Ethics, 10* (4), 368–376.

Smith, K. V. (1996). Ethical decision-making by staff nurses. *Nursing Ethics, 3* (1), 17–25.

State Initiatives in End-of-Life Care. (April, 1999). Pain undertreatment: A strikingly large problem. *4,* 2–8.

Thomasma, D. C. (1994). Toward a new medical ethics: Implications for ethics in nursing. In P. Benner (Ed.), *Interpretive phenomenology: Embodiment, caring, and ethics in health and illness,* (pp. 85–98). Thousand Oaks, CA: Sage.

Thomson, G. E. (1997). Discrimination in health care. *Annals of Internal Medicine, 126* (11), 910–912.

Toombs, S. K. (1995). Sufficient unto the day: A life with multiple sclerosis. In S. K. Toombs, D. Barnard, & R. A. Carson (Eds.), *Chronic illness: From experience to policy,* (pp. 3–23). Bloomington: Indiana University Press.

Viens, D. C. (1989). A history of nursing's code of ethics. *Nursing Outlook, 37* (1), 45–49.

Volbrecht, R. M. (2002). *Nursing ethics: Communities in dialogue.* Upper Saddle River, NJ: Prentice Hall.

Watson, J. (1988). *Nursing: Human science and human care: A theory of nursing.* New York: National League for Nursing.

Williams, M. V., Parker, R. M., Baker, D. W., Parikh, N. S., et al. (1995). Inadequate functional health literacy among patients at two public health hospitals. *Journal of the American Medical Association, 274,* 1677–1682.

Woods, M. (1999). A nursing ethic: The moral voice of experienced nurses. *Nursing Ethics, 6* (5), 423–433.

U.S. Department of Health and Human Services (1998). *Healthy people 2010: Understanding and improving health.* Washington, DC: Author.

CHAPTER 19

Nurse Case Management

Patricia A. Chin ▪ Judith Papenhausen ▪ Connie Burgess

Introduction

One of the many challenges facing nursing professionals in today's reactive economical climate continues to be the development and promotion of proactive, innovative clinical nursing interventions that are cost sensitive, theoretically dependable, and outcome efficacious. Pivotal driving forces in the delivery of health care today are cost containment, technology, access, and increasingly restrictive private and federal reimbursement policies.

The impact of present cost-effectiveness strategies under the rubric of managed care, such as restraints on length of stay and restrictions on reimbursement for health care services, continues to be controversial. Some cost-containment methods, accepted without benefit of published research, have altered the distribution of health care and negatively influenced individuals who are least likely to afford private payment (Cohen & Cesta, 2005; Rossi, 2003). These methods have been implemented with little concern for their effect on the elderly or individuals with chronic illness (Miller, 2000; Ware et al., 1996). These clients are often discharged from acute care facilities early in the recuperative and restorative phases of their illnesses. It is the labile health care status of these vulnerable groups that requires frequent monitoring and periodic interventions to decrease future hospital admissions.

Increasingly, lower cost alternatives include early transfer to extended care facilities or returning home with or without the support of informal caregivers or home health care. The employment of these alternatives often occurs before the formulation of a comprehensive health care plan that includes a support network of multidisciplinary health professionals and services to meet health care needs (Powell, 2000; Rossi, 2003; Zander, 1990a). Cost containment has fostered the development of managed care and case management delivery systems.

The intrusion of a chronic illness is a significant life crisis posing major challenges for individuals and their support systems. The long-term nature of chronic illness, the uncertainty, expense, efforts at palliation, symptom control, prevention and management of medical crises and physical deterioration present issues that cannot be effectively dealt with in the traditional curative medical model. Because of the diversity of client needs and the complexity of the existing health care delivery system, clients with chronic illness and their families require professional guidance in coordinating, implementing, and evaluating their health care plans. This situation has created the opportunity for the evolution of the role of the nurse case manager (NCM) and the development of nursing case management models to serve selected client populations (Bower, 1992; Burgess, 1999; DeBack & Cohen, 1996; Kostlan, 2003; Stuart, 2003; Rossi, 2003; Zrelak, 2003).

Differentiating Managed Care and Case Management

Managed care and *case management* became buzz words in the delivery of acute care services during the 1980s and 1990s (Cesta, 2002; Faherty, 1990; Lewenson, 2003; Powell, 2000; Rossi, 2003). The interchangeable usage of these terms has created confusion in the literature because both have the common goal of cost effectiveness and both are guided by client outcomes. Their operational characteristics, however, are distinctly different.

Managed Care

Since the 1990s, managed care has been the number one force that has most transformed health care delivery in the United States. Managed care evolved as a process in the effort to deflate the everexpanding health care cost bubble. The transition to managed care was necessary to grapple with the unaffordable excesses produced by earlier forces that expanded health care services and the costs to provide those services (Shi & Singh, 2004).

There is no single, universal definition of *managed care* because various organizational forms and models are still evolving. The term broadly refers to a health care delivery system in which a predetermined amount of money is available to deliver necessary and indicated health care to a group of individuals and/or organizations. Chang, Price and Pfoutz (2001) define managed care as "a health-care system willing to be held accountable both clinically and financially for the health outcomes of an enrolled population for a capitated (fixed) payment" (p. 299).

Managed care has become deeply entrenched in the United States health care system. It combines both the delivery and the financing of health care

into a single system that emphasizes coordinated delivery of services across a continuum of care with incentives for cost effectiveness (Chang, Price & Pfoutz, 2001; Shi & Singh, 2004). Managed care systems include preferred provider organizations (PPOs) and health maintenance organizations (HMOs). The fee-for-service (FFS) reimbursement system, dominant in the 1960s and 1970s, now comprises approximately 5% of health care plans, while HMOs (26%), PPOs (51%) and point-of service plans (POS) 18% represent the bulk of the market share (Shi & Singh, 2004).

The PPO serves medium to large private businesses who arrange health care for their employees through a health care plan derived from a network of hospitals, physicians, and other health care professionals for a negotiated fee. The PPO model does not assume financial risk for health services but provides these services at a discounted rate.

Point-of-Service plans were generated by HMOs. The POS plans combine features of the HMO, tight utilization management, with less restrictive patient choice. Enrollees pay extra for the privilege of using nonparticipating providers who charge for service at fee-for-service rates. This option reached a peak in popularity in 1999; however, enrollment in POS plans has gradually declined (Hoffman, 2002; Shi & Singh, 2004).

An HMO is a type of managed care plan that either assumes or shares financial risk for care. HMOs may administer health care directly, arrange for care with specific contracted providers, or both. HMOs have progressively focused on prevention as well as care and are viewed in the United States as the most cost-effective type of plan. Capitation is the predominant payment mechanism (Chang, Price & Pfoutz, 2001; Shi & Singh, 2004).

Irrespective of the specific model, managed care is a strategy that can be implemented within a variety of settings and is usually based on collaboration between different disciplines, resulting in a cost-effective, quality-oriented health plan (Cohen & Cesta, 1993; Powell, 2000; Rossi, 2003, Shi & Singh, 2004). Within a managed care system, the average patterns of cost and care outcomes for a specific case type (e.g., acute myocardial infarction or coronary artery bypass) are identified with an expected length of stay (LOS). This information becomes the basis for developing clinical approaches that stipulate cost data and clinical parameters that are used to monitor the client's progress. A critical pathway or care map is a clinical tool that is developed to manage and monitor a client's course of care. These clinical approaches are increasingly evidence-based and are generated by a multidisciplinary team and function as a "standardized plan of care which addresses the usual needs of a defined client population" (Bower & Falk, 1996, p. 163).

Managed care is provided either directly or through a contract with an outside provider at an agreed upon, usually discounted rate for every subscriber (Redman, 2005; Shi & Singh 2004). This process, called *capitation*, shifts the financial risk associated with health care from the health plans to the providers and is a major influence in transforming compartmentalized, but comprehensive, care into care continuum systems. Care continuums range from health promotion and disease prevention in homes and neighborhood community health centers to primary, acute, and long-term care. To be financially feasible, capitation mandates the need for early identification of health care needs and management of health risk. If care continuums are to be successful, all providers across the network must agree on the same interventions, particularly support of self-care strategies essential to well-being and early recognition of illness (Chang, Price & Pfoutz, 2001).

Impact of Managed Care   Many acute care services, formerly provided in inpatient settings, have shifted to outpatient settings and challenge providers to achieve at least the same quality outcomes while containing costs. Robinson (1996) reported a decline in inpatient acute care utilization of services and a rise in outpatient and subacute care services, especially in areas with a high managed care presence. Robinson concluded that "care must be taken to distinguish conceptually between the role of the hospital as a facility for in patient services and the role of the hospital as a social and economic institution" (p. 1063).

The laws of economics, which serve as the basis of managed care, suggest that to be most effective in ensuring the financial viability for managed care, there needs to be a decrease in client expectations, demands, and needs and an increase in society's awareness of the limitations of health care. Such change would contribute to a sound national economy (Riggs, 1996; Shi & Singh, 2004). It is precisely this dichotomy between individuals' health needs and the nation's economy that presents the greatest challenge to today's health care professional.

Challenges   Managed care has changed the way individuals' health care needs are taken care of. Consumers have been accustomed to a health care system that is individually oriented. However, managed care and capitation demand a shift in focus from individuals to populations. These health plans increasingly limit choice in order to manage costs. They do so by changing covered benefits, clinic locations, and out-of-pocket premiums without consideration of access, quality, or consumers' loyalty to specific providers (Christianson et al., 1995). Showstack and associates (1996) assert that the system not only should be able to provide individual care to its members, but should also consider programs and activities that address broader populations. In other words, although consumers continue to schedule appointments with a designated primary care provider, they will need substantially more services that are oriented toward prevention, identification, and risk reduction.

Managed care systems of today, and in the future, have the potential to correct the imbalances between individuals and populations in our health care system. Collaborative community relationships with key constituencies (public health officials, physicians, hospitals, employers, and consumers) enable managed care systems to act as catalysts or change agents in the community (Showstack et al., 1996).

Case Management

Case management is a care strategy frequently found within a managed care plan. In case management, an individual health care professional consistently follows an individual or a specific client population (e.g., individuals with chronic obstructive pulmonary disease) across health care settings, collaborates with other health care team members to determine outcome goals, and provides access to and monitors utilization of resources. The case manager works with the client, identifies specific needs, and interfaces with all providers across a continuum, with the goal of facilitating access to quality, cost-effective care (Weydt, 1997; Zerull, 1997). The American Nurses Association (ANA) offers the following definition of *case management:*

> A dynamic and systematic collaborative approach to providing and coordinating health care services to a defined population. It is a participative process to identify and facilitate options and services for meeting individuals' health needs, while decreasing fragmentation and duplication of care and enhancing quality, cost-effective clinical outcomes. The framework for nursing care management includes five components: assessment, planning, implementation, evaluation, and interaction (ANA, 1999, p. 3).

When an illness is chronic, case management is ongoing across clinical settings to increase self-care or family care capacity to avoid or minimize exacerbations and more costly hospitalization. *Service management, care coordination,* and *care management* are alternate terms for *case management* (Cohen & Cesta, 2005).

Nursing Case Management Most definitions of nursing case management include (1) the use of a nurse case manager to identify high-risk/high-cost clients; (2) health assessment; (3) health care planning to improve quality and efficacy; (4) procurement, delivery, and coordination of services; and (5) monitoring of the client's total care to ensure optimum outcomes (ANA, 1999; Bower, 1992; Cohen & Cesta, 2005). Nursing case management

models have the premise of service brokerage as a central theme.

Nurse case management has been defined as "a system, a role, a technology, a process and a service" (Bower, 1992, p. 4). Faherty (1990) states that "case management is the nursing process expanded in scope and made operational" (p. 20), and this view is supported by Zander (1990a), who sees the formal nursing process as "directly analogous to the process of case management" (p. 201). Zander (1988b) states that "nursing case management is both a model and a technology for restructuring the clinical production process and a role that facilitate cost/quality outcomes. It builds on the concept of managed care and the accountability practiced in primary nursing" (p. 503). Cesta (1997) defined nursing case management as an approach that focuses on the coordination, integration, and direct delivery of patient services and places internal control on the resources used for care. "It is a nursing care delivery system that supports cost-effective, patient outcomes oriented care" (Powell & Ignatavicius, 2001).

The driving forces in the evolution of the nurse case manager role within the managed care environment are financially based. Most influential has been the continued escalating cost of care. These escalating health care costs are attributed to:

■ Fragmentation and duplication of services
■ Acute care hospitals are the primary setting for care
■ Provider-forced delivery systems
■ A complex health care delivery system
■ Lack of knowledge and understanding of the administrative processes required in the managed care environment (Powell, 2000; Shi & Singh, 2004)

Goals of Nursing Case Management In nursing case management models, the professional nurse serves clients in acute care institutions and home settings and provides transitional and long-term care. The following are important goals of all nursing case management models. Adapted from ANA

(1999), Bower (1992), Cohen & Cesta (2005), and Blank (2005).

1. Optimize the client's self-care capability and increase the client's self-care abilities.
2. Enhance the client's quality of life, sense of autonomy, and self-determination.
3. Help the client to adjust to and manage his or her altered health state and manage his or her symptoms.
4. Enable the client and family to implement a complex health care plan through the development of an interactive relationship with a nurse case manager who serves in an educational and supportive role.
5. Prevent inappropriate hospitalizations and contain health care costs.
6. Provide quality health care along a continuum, with decreased fragmentation of services across many settings.

Nurse Case Management and Chronic Illness
Chronic illness care has become the most costly area of health care today. Both the traditional delivery models of public health and the traditional medical care model have been ineffective in dealing with the complexity of chronic illness and addressing the issues of cost and access to care. It is estimated that by the year 2010 as many as 141 million Americans will have a chronic condition. The cost of chronic illness care is expensive, incurring more than 75% of the total medical expenditure ($1 trillion annually) (The Robert Wood Johnson Foundation, 1996; Shi & Singh, 2004; US Department of Health and Human Services and Centers for Disease Control and Prevention, 1998).

However, our current health care delivery system emphasizes the acute illness model, which seeks cure as the ultimate outcome. In this type of health care delivery model, health care professionals assume responsibility for management of the client's care and practice primarily in acute care institutions. The acute illness model is expensive and less effective for clients with chronic illness. Increasingly, professional nurses are performing the case manager role with selected client populations. The target populations for nursing case management interventions are persons who are designated as high risk for the development of complex, continuous health care problems that require high-volume and diverse health care services (ANA, 1999; Bower, 1992).

Despite the availability of community-based and institutional care services many individuals are not getting the assistance needed for basic personal care. Unmet needs lead to increased health problems, costly treatment, and unnecessary pain and suffering (The Robert Wood Johnson Foundation, 1996; Shi & Singh, 2004). There is a serious need to implement health care delivery that is efficient and accessible for these high-risk populations. The traditional curative medical model is not effective for individuals with disease that cannot be cured. The goals of chronic care management must be quality oriented, and focused on symptom relief and the prevention of further functional decline (Cesta, 2002; Krentzman, 2002; Powell, 2000; Rossi, 2003). Meeting these goals requires consideration for services that are not usually characteristic of medical care.

A Harris national interactive survey released by Partnership for Solutions of Americans living with chronic illness identified the challenges both adults and children face (Rossi, 2003, p. 436–437).

■ 45% report that the cost of care is a financial burden,
■ 89% report difficulty in obtaining adequate health insurance,
■ 14% report that different doctors diagnosed them with various medical problems for the same set of symptoms,
■ 22% with insurance reported that not all types of needed care were covered,
■ 17% report that they received contradictory information from health care providers,
■ 72% of those living with chronic illness report having difficulty getting necessary care from health care providers,
■ 74% report difficulty obtaining prescriptive medications,

■ 78% report difficulty in obtaining help from their family or significant others.

How much longer managed care and case management strategies can continue to hold down cost increases in health care is unclear. Future cost reductions may have to come from decreased utilization of new technology and the introduction of unpopular explicit rationing strategies into the health care delivery system. It may also be difficult to contain cost without increasing tensions regarding access and quality of care. There is likely to be an increase in the use of deductibles and co-payments to reduce the demand for services (Shi & Singh, 2004). For now, though, managed care and the case management strategies are effective in holding costs, increasing access and improving the quality of care for those with chronic illnesses.

Characteristics of Nurse Case Managers   The legitimacy of the role of the NCM is strongly supported by the literature. The Nursing Social Policy Statement (ANA, 2003) notes that an outcome of a nursing intervention is the creation of a physiological, psychological, and sociocultural environment, allowing the client to gain or maintain health. Because the processes of case management and nursing are similar (Cesta, 2002; Rossi, 2003; Zander, 1990a) suggests that nurses are ideally suited for this role. In addition, Zander notes that nurses can provide case management because they have intimate access to clients and families over extended periods of time. With nurses in this role, case management is provided by an expert clinician with advanced educational preparation, who is with a client throughout the entire episode of care (Cesta, 2002; Rossi, 2003; Zander, 1990a).

Many authorities support the view that nurses are the logical candidates to become case managers because professional nurses have a generalist background. Practicing nurses have experience in assessment, diagnosis, and treatment of client responses to disease and disability, and, historically, they have participated in the implementation and monitoring of medical protocols in acute care and community health settings (Bower, 1992; Leclair, 1991; Zander, 1990b).

Characteristics of a Successful Nurse Case Manager:

■ Effective as a change agent
■ Effective in a consultant role
■ Effective as a collaborator
■ Effective as an educator of client, family, and other health team members
■ Abreast of current advances in clinical care, disease management and resources
■ Effective as a guide in multi-/interdisciplinary team processes
■ Effective in facilitating client care services and coordinating resources
■ Effectives as a manager of client care and allocating resources
■ Effective as a client and family advocate
■ Effective as a quality improvement facilitator
■ Effective in gathering date to assess clinical outcomes, quality improvement and process modification

Goals of Case Management for Individuals with Chronic Illness   Case management for those with chronic illness is evolving in both its technology and longevity. Those caring for individuals with a chronic illness will deal with chronic illness along a trajectory of care requiring systematic support of self-management skills and care coordination rather than a series of events. Improvement of self-management skills and development of a therapeutic nurse-client relationship is essential for meeting case management outcomes. Nursing case management supports the individual with chronic illness to:

■ Maintain self-management skills
■ Increase the coordination of care
■ Decrease the fragmentation of care
■ Decrease the consumption of health care dollars and

■ Improve the quality of life for the individual and family members.

Educating Nurse Case Managers The qualifications and training needs of case managers have been defined by several authors. Case managers require knowledge and skill in three general areas: (1) clinical expertise relative to the client's health care needs, (2) an ability to determine client resources and to negotiate for health care services, and (3) an ability to implement the steps in the process of case management. It is generally agreed that this process includes client assessment, care planning, and monitoring (Chin & Papenhausen, 2003; Leclair, 1991).

NCMs should have advanced academic preparation and previous experience in clinical practice (Fondiller, 1991; Rogers, Riordan & Swindle, 1991). The shift from acute care to community-based care is "more than a change in location . . . it [requires] new ways of thinking, different preparation of the professional, enhanced structures for collaboration, and more comprehensive attention to how all parts of [the] system work together" (Lamb, 1995, p. 19). There has been continued growth in baccalaureate and graduate programs offering curricula of advanced concepts in community health, case management, medical–surgical nursing, client–family assessment, health teaching, and coordination of health care services.

As case management has evolved from being a trend in managed care to a common practice, nurse educators have recognized the need for the incorporation of managed care and case management concepts and experiences into nursing curricula (Chin & Papenhausen, 2002). The case management process helps promote a client-centered approach to care. This requires a broad knowledge base and sound reasoning skills. The nurse involved in case management just also develop competencies in negotiating, coordinating, and procuring services and resources. The baccalaureate degree curriculum prepares nurses to provide care for individuals and families with complex diagnoses and unpredictable illness and trajectories. Graduates of these programs have a greater understanding and appreciation of the interdisciplinary nature of planning and caring for individuals and a broader perspective of client care.

Nursing Case Management Models

Historical Development of Case Management Models

There is lack of agreement regarding the origin of the case management concept, with the disciplines of mental health and social work claiming credit for its development (Applebaum & Wilson, 1988). In the early 1980s, federally mandated cost containment led to the emergence of case management models in community and acute care settings (Simpson, 1982). Additionally, the implementation of the prospective Medicare reimbursement system, diagnostic related groups (DRGs), imposed limitations on the length of hospitalization and stimulated growth in the home health care market (see Chapter 22, on home health care). Since the implementation of DRGs, home health clients have been more ill and have had more complex nursing needs after discharge from acute care settings (Graham, 1989), so the focus of case management has been on providing services that are economically efficient (Giuliano & Poirier, 1991).

During this same time period, the Health Care Financing Administration (HCFA) and state agencies funded demonstration projects to provide community-based case management services for the elderly (Capitman, Haskins & Bernstein, 1986; Grau, 1984). Later in that decade, the National Long-Term Care Channeling Project Study was funded to evaluate the ability of community-based case management models to provide home services to elderly clients in a cost-effective manner and prevent institutionalization (Carcagano & Kemper, 1988). These early projects represented the first use of nurses in the specific role of case manager (Grau, 1984; Shipp & Jay, 1988). However, Knollmueller (1989) and others (ANA, 1999) argue that the basic tenets of case management have been practiced by community health nurses for years.

The development and use of nurse case management proliferated by the late 1980s, with several emerging models to guide practice in a variety of settings and involving many client populations (Del Bueno & Leblanc, 1989; Knollmueller, 1989; Stillwaggon, 1989). Some were primarily community health models, such as the nursing center model for the provision of long-term eldercare (ANA, 1999; Bower, 1992; Dolson & Richards, 1990; DuBois, 1990; Igou et al., 1989; Miller, 1990), and the home health care model (Jones et al., 1990), which utilizes existing home health and visiting nurse services to provide continuity of discharge planning. Others, such as HMOs (Abrahams, 1990; ANA, 1999; Bower, 1992) and insurance-based models (Bower, 1992; Henderson, Souder & Bergman, 1987; Henderson & Wallack, 1987; Knollmueller, 1989), provide case management to high-cost clients who have catastrophic illness or injury and require permanent or transitional home care. Institutional long-term case management models are also used with the elderly in nursing home settings (Putney et al., 1990) and in rehabilitation and extended care settings (Blake, 1991; Loveridge, Cummings, & O'Malley 1988).

Some acute care models were developed for specific client populations, such as low-birth-weight infants (Brooten et al., 1988; Mazoway, 1987), high-risk pregnant teenagers (Combs & Rusch, 1990; Korenbrot et al., 1989), and persons with acquired immune deficiency syndrome (AIDS) (ANA, 1999; Bower, 1992; Littman & Siemsen, 1989). Other acute care models have a general application for a broader range of clients (Bower, 1992; Ethridge & Lamb, 1989; Zander, 1988a, 1988b).

The goals of all models of nurse case management are sensitive to both cost and quality, and these models hold great promise for cost containment. The facilitating and gate-keeping functions of the NCM have decreased the fragmentation of services across multiple settings, improved the coordination of the treatment plans across health care professionals, and prevented inappropriate hospitalizations (ANA, 1999; Bower, 1992; Ethridge, 1991; Ethridge & Lamb, 1989; McKenzie, Torkelson & Holt, 1989; Papenhausen, 1995, 1996; Rogers, Riordan & Swindle, 1991; Zander, 1988b).

Community-Based Case Management Models

Of all the case management programs, community-based models for long-term clients received the earliest and most rigorous evaluation. These models were developed for a variety of high-risk populations, and their major focus was to broker and monitor health care services delivered in the home environment or in long-term care settings. In general, clients who require community-based case management services are the elderly or those with chronic or terminal illnesses. Some community-based models focus only on long-term care service for the elderly. Medicare beneficiaries over age 65 voluntarily enroll and receive all services covered under Medicare, as well as an extended long-term care package that includes skilled nursing home and home health care services. Case managers in this type of program are either nurses or social workers (Abrahams, 1990; Scott & Boyd, 2005).

Other community-based models provide private case management on an FFS basis (Miller, 1990; Bower, 1992). FFS groups provide multidimensional assessment, client and family consultation, community resource referral and coordination, and care planning services. NCMs often have a master's degree and advanced preparation in gerontology (Bower, 1992). The client may be either an elderly client or, more commonly, the primary caregiver. Fees are charged on an hourly basis (Miller, 1990).

Some community-based models provide case management services to target populations, including clients who are technology-dependent and receive supportive care in their home; retirement community residents who receive direct personal care; and informal caregivers who receive respite care (Scott & Boyd, 2005). There are also specialized community-based models that work exclusively with children who have special health needs and potentially chronic conditions. In such models, the case manager is a public health nurse with clinical experience in pediatrics (Rossi, 2003). Community-based care models using nurse case managers have striven to be key enablers of care for those with chronic illness. Community-based nurse case management has demonstrated successful outcomes in enabling care and access with more cost-effective health care utilization (Scott & Boyd, 2005, p. 131).

Insurance-Based Case Management Models

Most major private insurance carriers in the United States have implemented some form of case management primarily as a cost-control measure. Initial use of these programs was focused at medical management in workers' compensation cases. However, as group health insurance companies reviewed claims data of their insured clients, it was noted that approximately 80 percent of the total health care costs could be attributed to 20 percent of those clients (Bower, 1992). Further analysis of data identified that those with chronic and catastrophic diagnoses resulted in high-cost, long-term care. These catastrophic and chronic conditions were (1) high-risk neonatal, (2) severe head trauma, (3) spinal cord injury, (4) ventilator dependency, (5) coma, (6) multiple fractures, (7) AIDS, (8) severe burns, (9) cerebral vascular accidents, (10) amputations, (11) terminal illnesses, and (12) substance abuse (Bower, 1992).

In private insurance–based case management, the coordination function of the case manager is critical to controlling cost and avoiding duplication and fragmentation of services. A case manager in this model begins with case identification and referral through screening activities that are often initiated by the insurance company. For a client with a high-risk profile, the case manager sets up a network of communication among health care providers, health care professionals, and the client so that alternatives can be explored and a plan of care determined. The case manager then monitors the plan regularly, contacting the involved parties until goals are reached, the client dies, or insurance coverage is depleted. Most of the case managers in this model

are registered nurses with five years or more of clinical experience, although some companies utilize rehabilitation counselors or social workers for this role (Bower, 1992).

Within-the-Walls (Hospital-Based) Nursing Case Management Models

The origins of the hospital-based nurse case management model are usually attributed to the New England Medical Center (NEMC) Hospitals, following a 13-year history of primary nursing and the investigation of nursing and physician practice patterns. This model entails the collaboration of physicians and staff nurses who formulate a case management plan and develop a critical pathway that indicates time-ordered client outcomes to be achieved during the acute care hospitalization (Etheredge, 1989; Zander, 1988a, 1988b, 1990a). With this model, the relationship between the NCM and the client is limited and usually ends with the client's discharge from the hospital (Cohen & Cesta, 1993).

Since its initial introduction, this model's case management plans and critical pathways have been linked to quality improvement practices and the development of care maps for specific client groups or case types. These care maps provide for the monitoring of resource allocation, cost-reimbursement systems, variances in the delivery of care, and client care outcomes (Cohen & Cesta, 1993). Many versions of within-the-walls case management models are currently being used in acute health care facilities to lower costs, improve effective use of resources, and maintain quality of care (Cohen & Cesta, 2005; Owens, 2003; Rossi, 2003).

Within this model, the role and qualifications of the NCM varies. NCMs may practice as the clients' primary caregivers and participate in the coordinating and monitoring of services throughout hospitalization, irrespective of the client's location (Cohen & Cesta, 2005). Other within-the-walls models use a differentiated practice model based on the educational preparation of the case manager. In these models, direct client care is provided by staff nurses, and the NCM is responsible for coordinating, monitoring, and evaluating care delivery (Cohen & Cesta, 2005). The qualifications of NCMs in these models are typically based on clinical competency and leadership qualities, and a bachelor's or master's degree may be required.

Continuum-Based Nursing Case Management Models

Originally called "beyond-the-walls nurse case management," this title was changed to "continuum-based nursing case management" to reflect case management across the continuum of all health services. Unlike the within-the-walls models that serve clients in acute care settings, the continuum-based model generally serves clients in other settings, such as their homes, their neighborhoods, and subacute institutions.

Because clients with chronic illness often need services in more than one setting, it is common for health care professionals to frequently pass care coordination responsibilities back and forth between themselves and discharge planners or clinical specialists, depending on the client's location in the health care system. This process can lead to duplication and fragmentation of services as well as greater health care costs. In addition, a change of case manager requires the development of new professional–client relationships.

The continuum-based model, in which health care services are provided by nurses in a professional group practice (the professional nurse case management model, or PNCM model), differs from other case management models in that it provides continuity of case management from the acute care setting to the home setting (Bower, 1992; Ethridge, 1991; Michaels, 1992). Consequently, the PNCM model holds great promise in alleviating the problems seen with other models, and may be the most advantageous for the client with chronic illness. The PCNM model strives for high quality, improved access to care, and risk identification and provides clients with the tools and skills necessary to effectively deal with long-term disease management. This model functions best in a health care delivery system that provides a broad range of services across acute care and community settings; provides preventive, acute, and restorative health care; allows for flexible movement of nurse case management personnel across settings; and has a financial incentive to reduce acute care admissions and recidivism.

The continuum-based model is based on the belief that high-risk clients with chronic illness can be identified early, such as at enrollment in the health care plan or after the first exacerbation of their illness. The continuum-based NCM can, therefore, establish an ongoing nurse–client–family therapeutic relationship and coordinate the entire spectrum of care for an extended and indefinite period of time.

Other goals of the model include improved cost and quality outcomes (including reduced recidivism), more appropriate service utilization, improved chronic illness management, and increased client satisfaction. This model blends the elements of both hospital and community models by allowing a single nurse case manager to design a multidisciplinary plan of care that is initiated on enrollment or during the client's hospitalization. The care manager can then follow the client into the home setting and continue to execute and monitor the plan of care (Bower, 1992; Ethridge, 1991; Michaels, 1992).

The role of the NCM within the continuum-based model includes the following (Cohen & Cesta, 2005):

1. Identifying high-risk clients, such as those who are chronically ill and those who have limited social and financial support
2. Assessing the client and family and developing a comprehensive plan of care
3. Coordinating and brokering community and agency resources
4. Collaborating with interdisciplinary health care team members and serving as the client's advocate
5. Making home visits to provide direct nursing care interventions such as emotional support, counseling, and education, designed to increase

the client's self-care and symptom management abilities

6. Monitoring and evaluating client outcomes
7. Serving as the health care liaison in the event of readmission to the hospital

Client Care Outcomes

The experience of working with NCMs has been explored from the client's perspective (Lamb & Stempel, 1994). Using grounded theory to explore the social process of the NCM–client relationship, interviews of subjects were tape-recorded and verbatim responses coded and analyzed. The subjects identified three distinctive stages or phases of the process: *bonding, working together,* and *changing*. The bonding phase consisted of establishing a nurse–client relationship (Lamb & Stempel, 1994). Early in this phase, the NCM was viewed as an expert who could assist in the assessment and stabilization of physiological problems related to disease exacerbation, and could, therefore, facilitate access to needed health care services. As the client became more physically stable, the relationship became progressively more holistic and focused on emotional and spiritual concerns. The NCM moved from being an "expert outsider" to an "insider expert," a notion coined by Lamb and Stempel (1994) based on clients' phrases describing their relationship with NCMs.

In the working together and changing phases of the process, clients' attitudes, reactions, and behaviors that contribute to exacerbation of their illnesses or prevent them from using the health care system effectively are identified (Lamb & Stempel, 1994). Clients note that the case manager makes them feel worthwhile, improves their outlook, and provides a sense of being highly supported (Lamb & Stempel, 1994). Changes in client behaviors occur in two major areas: learning improved self-care activities and mastering the ability to more appropriately access health care services.

Clients also reported an improved ability to recognize the signs of exacerbation of their symptoms and responded by seeking early assistance. They also reported improved medication adherence and other health-related regimens. At the termination of nurse case management services, several clients reached a level of independence at which they acted as their own insider expert, characterized by the ability to recognize the symptoms of exacerbation and access the health care system in a timely and appropriate way (Lamb & Stempel, 1994).

■ Nurse Case Management Interventions

One of the most difficult challenges NCMs face is identifying an appropriate framework for both long-term care planning and cost management. Multiple strategies for case management have been developed, but not all fit each situation and some only deal with specific populations. The NCM often has to modify interventions according to the changing health care environment and the setting in which the case management is being implemented. Consequently, it is important to continually reevaluate or determine what is most effective and what may require modification.

Although chronic conditions, like acute disorders, are traditionally considered in terms of pathological phenomena and subsequent physiological impairment, this perspective is actually unrelated to individuals who have chronic conditions. "By isolating thoughts of disease from consideration of the sufferer, the consequences tend to be neglected. These consequences—responses by the individual himself and by those to whom he relates or upon whom he depends—assume greater importance as the burden of illness alters" (World Health Organization, 1980, p. 23).

The most important feature in planning the care of an individual with chronic illness and his or her family is a comprehensive, individualized assessment of needs. In addition, the demands of any health care environment dictate that there are multiple plans to manage both costs and care. Rehabilitation, for example, requires the need to manage costs while delivering effective care. Unlike the current medical model, rehabilitation's goal is to reduce or eliminate the consequences of the injury or illness rather than cure (see Chapter 25, on rehabilitation). Care planning that is based on acute care models lacks the sensitivity to address the chronic long-term consequences to the individual. When evaluating the individual's quality of life after a catastrophic event, these predetermined plans of care often consume enormous amounts of resources without producing commensurate outcomes. To develop the best possible cost-effective plan for a client, appropriate strategies must be selected.

Selecting Appropriate Case Management Strategies

The notion that "one size fits all" has no more application in health care than in the clothing industry. NCMs and other clinicians have a responsibility for the economic welfare of their company or institution while providing quality care to their clients. However, regional and individual client factors may influence the care planning process and strategies to be used. Following are some of these factors:

■ Forces influencing health care delivery are frequently local, not national: adoption of Los Angeles-based strategies by a hospital in New York could well bankrupt the New York institution.

■ Resources available in one community may vary from those found in another.

■ Consequences to individuals with the same diagnosis may range from insignificant to major, depending on their individual responses.

■ The type of reimbursement mechanisms and managed care contracts differ dramatically from one community to the next.

■ Hospitals within the same corporation but located in different cities must compete in their community and must use local, not corporate-wide strategies, to do so.

In other words, different populations may require different strategies. While predetermined clinical pathways can be used in a number of un-complicated client situations, their use for all individuals suggests that individual plans of care are not required. This "cookie cutter" approach to care planning wastes valuable fiscal resources on those people who do not need them and limits resources for those who do.

Salient Factors Framework

The salient factors model is a framework for client care planning and also a specific strategy for care delivery. It is a philosophy of care that reinforces client-driven care and shifts goal determination away from professional staff exclusively and into a shared decision-making process with the client. This framework takes a broad view of all factors influencing the individual's life over time and builds an interdisciplinary plan of care, with the client, based on those agreed-upon needs. It identifies client needs at the beginning of the hospital stay and establishes the best clinical, cost-effective means to achieve specific outcomes. The Salient Factors Framework is the most appropriate framework for working clients with chronic illness and complex care needs.

About Salient Factors

Simply stated, salient factors are the key issues generated from specific, individual client needs. Instead of treating the client by diagnosis and placing him or her on a predetermined clinical pathway, or framing outcomes from physician orders, a long-term, individualistic plan of care and outcomes is developed based on the individual client. Before development of the plan, the client is asked, "Where are you going, who will be there, what must you be able to do to function in the environment, and what do you think will work best for you?"

Additional parameters include the client's functional abilities, human and fiscal resources, available benefits, and clinical services offered in the client's community. Starting with the desired outcomes, the clinical team begins working backward to determine the appropriate resources necessary for success.

Under the umbrella of the salient factors framework, each NCM has a number of strategies available from anything such as "fast track" acute care hospital stays to care provision for complex and/or chronic long-term disabilities or conditions. For some clients, a clinical pathway may be all that is needed. Other clients with higher social risks and medical needs may require a combination of clinical strategies and a significant amount of case management. By assessing individual client needs, resources are focused only on the interventions that are required.

Salient Factors: Multiple Clinical Strategies

Within the client care planning process, a combination of clinical and cost strategies are selected because they address specific needs. Four specific strategies have been identified as treatment options for simple to complex clients within the salient factors framework. The NCM may use one or all of these strategies depending on the client's needs:

■ *Process Pathway:* This strategy involves the sequencing and timing of care-related events. The process is *anticipatory* and reflects the early need for information, education, and family interaction to prevent delays in the client progressing through the program. It establishes timely and efficient communication and promotes activities such as early discharge planning. The process pathway includes the following:

1. *Timing of clinical events* to determine the best time to initiate a process or intervention, such as scheduling a family conference on the first day instead of the third day of hospitalization
2. *Flexibility* based on when the client requires an intervention, not when the intervention is dictated by a predetermined criteria or template
3. *Increased staff efficiency* and *real-time decision making* that can move care along faster if the client's readiness is evident

■ *Clinical/Critical Pathways:* These strategies are used when clients require highly predictable, routine, recurring care. Pathways are:

1. *Patternable,* physical care for a particular procedure or diagnosis. There is an expectation that the same treatments will be required for similar noncomplicated clients.
2. *Based on diagnosis,* such as a client with a hip replacement with no complications.
3. *Few, if any, long-term residual limitations;* a client with a hip replacement who, upon walking again, will not need long-term treatment, adaptations, or adjustments in their previous lifestyle.
4. *No comorbidities;* A single diagnosis can be addressed by a single pathway.

■ *Protocols:* This strategy uses procedures that were specifically developed to focus treatment on a syndrome or function. Examples may include chemotherapy, bladder training, pain management, and skin protocols. Protocols can be used if the outcomes have a high degree of predictability or are based on consistency in treatment methodology. They are also useful if they are imbedded in pathways or salient factor plans of care.

■ *Salient Factors:* As a clinical strategy, this methodology identifies the issues specific to the individual client. Each client's needs determine the issues and goals for the client. The goals are then prioritized and the team establishes which interventions are to be delivered at which level of care across the continuum. This strategy reflects long-term care needs of the client, encourages early discharge planning, and is particularly useful for chronic and catastrophic conditions.

Salient Factors: The Clinical Strategy

The salient factors strategy is used to identify the key physical, social, and resource needs most important to each client. The strategy includes the following:

- Constructing a single plan of care at the beginning of an illness episode and projecting care needs through an entire continuum
- Focusing interventions for the specific needs of each individual that are client rather than professionally driven
- Prioritizing care and costs and allowing the team to predict and plan for appropriate interventions in the right setting at the right time for the right cost
- Predicting and managing cost and outcomes of care in real time rather than retrospectively
- Identifying functional requirements for advancement through the continuum to discharge and return to the community
- Identifying barriers to discharge at each level of care and supporting staff to take steps toward effective action

The Salient Factors strategy prioritizes care and distributes available fiscal resources across services. It requires the identification of an individual client's needs at the beginning of the institutional stay and establishes the best and most cost-effective clinical strategies for achieving specific outcomes. The assessment process addresses long- and short-term needs at the point of entry into the formal system.

Categories of the Salient Factors Strategy

Five salient factor categories have been identified to guide the care-planning process and to assist the clinical team in addressing each person's complete set of needs at the beginning of the stay: (1) the physical, psychological, and behavioral consequences of the injury or illness; (2) discharge planning; (3) clinical services; (4) resources; and (5) health benefits.

Physical, Psychological, and Behavioral Consequences of the Injury or Illness This impact should consider both specific consequences to the

client and the changes that have occurred in the following areas:

- *Physical:* Is this a life-altering event, such as a traumatic brain injury, or is it a temporary impairment that will be resolved in a short, or relatively short, time with no residual impairments? What are the clinical interventions to restore the client to health or accommodate for the resulting loss of function (Burgess, 2002)?
- *Psychological:* Are there, or will there be, short- or long-term psychological effects for this individual, as may be present, for example, with cancer or a stroke?
- *Behavioral:* Has the condition altered the individual's behavior, requiring specific interventions, such as cognitive retraining or safety measures?

What must be determined is what will be necessary for the client to reach an acceptable level of functioning (Burgess, 2002).

Discharge Planning Home is a destination not a discharge plan. Because discharge planning includes management through the care continuum and back into the community, the clinician should ask the following:

- Where is the client going (home, to an assisted living or long-term care nursing home, or other place), and will they need assistance? Answers to these questions will drive care planning and client education. In addition, these questions focus on both appropriate discharge interventions and the distribution of fiscal resources.
- What will the client need so that he or she can function in the discharge setting? Decisions of this kind should be made collaboratively with the client and family.

From the perspective of case management, discharge planning occurs before treatment or at the initial point of hospitalization or initial interaction with the health care professional.

Sara: Undergoing an Uncomplicated Total Hip Replacement

Sara is a 66-year-old woman who is scheduled for a total left hip replacement. She lives at home with her able-bodied husband and has a daughter who lives ten minutes away. Although her left hip has had increased pain and reduced function over the past six months, Sara has remained active and independent in her daily activities and is expected to return home without any long-term problems.

Table 19-1 indicates use of the salient factors framework in planning Sara's care.

Clinical Services The clinician must be knowledgeable about services offered in each part of the care continuum, the location of services, and which services are included in the client's benefit package. The clinician should also know whether recommended home health or outpatient services exist where the client lives and if such services are accessible.

TABLE 19-1

Total Hip Replacement: Planning Sara's Care

Key Issues	Clinical Strategy	Continuum Location	Reasoning
▶ Physiologic/Functional What are the consequences? • No long-term deficits • No complicating factors	Clinical pathway	Acute care	No complicating or long-term residual effects that require special interventions. This patient will benefit from a "fast track" approach.
▶ Emotional/Behavioral • Anxious • Cognitively intact			Anxiety most likely will be short-lived, with interventions at the time of surgery.
What are the discharge planning needs?	Clinical pathway	Acute care/Home health	Discharge planning is included in the pathway and, in most cases, will require little or nothing more.
What are the treatment services (continuum sites) needed? • Acute care • Home health therapy • Outpatient (optional)	Clinical pathway	Acute care Home health	Postop care and follow-up included in pathway; routine course of care. In many cases, outpatient therapy will not be needed.
What are the available human resources? • Husband at home • Daughter in community	Salient factors	Home Home health	Will ambulate with walker in home. Husband and daughter will assist with ADLs.
What are the benefits/fiscal resources available? • PPO Contract with MD/Hospital	Critical pathway	Continuum	All costs covered by insurance based on PPO contracted case rate. Straightforward and known prior to surgery.

Jim: A 47-Year-Old with a Stroke

Jim is a 47-year-old contractor who has suffered a stroke. His condition has stabilized, and he is now ready for discharge to his home. He lives with his wife in a two-story house. His wife works from 8 A.M. to 5 P.M. Monday through Friday. There are no family members or close friends who can be at home with Jim on a regular basis during the day.

When this case is analyzed, it becomes obvious that more extensive thought and planning will need to occur for adequate and safe discharge home. Because of the individual differences in his home situation, predetermined clinical pathways will not accommodate his needs. Through this logical approach, the situation becomes manageable in a short period of time.

Table 19-2 indicates use of the salient factors framework in planning Jim's care.

Resources It is important for the health care professional to know what health care benefits the client has access to as well as the level of treatment systems and continuum of care covered by the client's health benefits plan. It is equally important that the clinician be knowledgeable about the human, community, and fiscal resources that are available. For instance, the clinician needs to know whether family and friends are available and to what degree they plan to participate in this person's life; whether there are community resources in place (churches, Meals on Wheels, transportation, social clubs, and so forth); or whether there are fiscal resources over and above the client's available health benefits.

Health Benefits All case managers and clinicians assess clients. However, the clinical information is kept separate from fiscal information, if, in fact, appropriate fiscal information can be obtained at all. There seems to be a prevailing attitude that clinical staff does not need to know specific contract information in order to deliver care. This factor alone may be a major contributor to the high cost of care. Today's case manager and health care team can contribute to cost savings if they have the fiscal information needed to plan care within the available resources. The clinician must have knowledge of the benefits that are available to the client and the specific care settings that are fully covered. The clini-

---

TABLE 19-2

Right CVA/Left Hemiplegia: Planning Jim's Care

Key Issue	Functional Consequence	Clinical Strategy	Continuum Location	Reasoning
▶ Physiological impact • Left hemiplegia • Difficulty swallowing	Unable to feed self (left-handed) or swallow	Salient factors	Acute care Rehab SNF rehab	Priorities on achieving specific short-term goals of feeding self and swallowing. Focus on learning to eat with right hand and not choking on food.
• Neurogenic bladder	Bladder incontinence			Timed voiding program for bladder control
• Hemianopsia/visual field disturbance	Walking into walls	Protocols		Compensatory strategies for seeing all fields of view

TABLE 19-2

Right CVA/Left Hemiplegia: Planning Jim's Care

Key Issue	Functional Consequence	Clinical Strategy	Continuum Location	Reasoning
▶ Cognitive/behavioral				
• Impulsive	Judgment and	Salient factor		Team approach for consistent
• Confused	safety in environment	and protocol Salient factors		interventions and reinforcement of decision making
▶Discharge planning				
• Where is he going?	Home	Salient factors	Acute care Rehab and SNF rehab	Discharge needs and reprioritized in each care setting as gains toward DC goals are made
• Who will be there?	Alone 8 A.M. to 5 P.M. M–F. Wife home at night.			
• What must he be able to do for himself when alone?	Feed self, transfer, toilet Be mobile, get help			The team must uniquely equip Jim to function in his own environment.
• Will he be able to function?	Yes, if above goals met before DC			Can Jim meet the minimum requirements to be home? His wife will participate in the decision of what is safe.
▶ Treatment services				
• Acute care	NA	Salient	NA	Move to the least costly level of
• Rehab		factors		care at the earliest possible
• SNF rehab				moment
• Home health				*Rehab/SNF rehab:* Bladder, bowel,
• Outpatient				skin, feeding, and swallow
• Transportation				*Home health:* Bathing, dressing, grooming, ambulation *Outpatient:* Endurance
▶ Resources				
• Human	Wife and friends			Care needs must be planned around these people. No money to hire additional help.
• Community	Community transportation			Can teach Jim to access transportation to get to outpatient care.
• Fiscal	Limited for out-of-pocket expenses			Loss of income and limited resources tell team to weigh costs of each decision.
▶ Benefits				
• Maximum coverage 100K/year	Have met inpatient capitation. HH/OP offer 5 visits each	Salient factors	Home health Outpatient	Education model of care to be carried out by family can deliver necessary services within available benefits.

cian also needs to know whether there will be any out-of-pocket dollars required for the client.

Application of the Salient Factors Framework and Strategies

When the previously mentioned questions are applied to an uncomplicated case, the result is a care planning process in which the clinical team can project probable outcomes. When there are more complex issues or comorbidities present, the process requires a more in-depth, individualized plan of care. The previous two case studies present clients with chronic conditions. Each case study has an accompanying table that demonstrates how the salient factors framework could be used with the client.

Outcomes

Evaluation of achieving case management goals and client well-being should be measured in terms of:

■ client functionality,
■ stabilization of physical symptoms,
■ extent of self-management ability,
■ client and family knowledge of the illness,
■ system, and client satisfaction.

The outcomes of all nurse case management are reduced costs, provision of quality care, and client satisfaction.

Summary and Conclusions

The growing challenge during the current economic climate involves developing cost-sensitive and outcome-efficacious interventions for individuals with unique chronic illness trajectories requiring complex care, ongoing monitoring and periodic interventions. Lower cost alternatives have evolved so that holistic nursing care can be provided. Case management that provides a consistent individual health care professional working across health care settings can help clients achieve desired outcomes. Nurse case management continues to evolve to help the client deal with the psychosocial impact of chronic illness and to adapt to an altered state of health. This role is well served by nurses, who possess both acute and chronic health care experience and knowledge of the physiological and psychosocial ramifications of specific health conditions. Nurses have a generalist background in assessment, diagnosis, and treatment of diseases, and experience in implementing and monitoring medical protocols.

Study Questions

1. Discuss the relationship between managed care and case management.
2. State four goals or objectives of nurse case management.
3. Why is nursing case management an effective strategy for planning care for clients with chronic illnesses?
4. What are the characteristics of an effective nurse case manager?
5. Discuss the limitation of the tradition medical model in providing care for clients with chronic illnesses?

6. What are the major differences between within-the-walls and continuum-based models of nurse case management? What are the advantages of each?
7. What are the steps in the salient factors strategies? How does this differ from the nursing process?
8. Select a client with whom you have worked and identify the advantages and disadvantages of applying each of the nurse case management models discussed in this chapter.

References

Abrahams, R. (1990). The Social HMO: Case management in an integrated acute and long-term care system. *Caring, 9* (8), 30–39.

American Nurses' Association. (1999). *Modular certification examination catalog.* Washington, D.C.: American Nurses Credentialing Center.

_____. (2003). *Nursing: A social policy statement.* Washington, DC: American Nurses' Publishing.

_____. (1995). *Nursing: A social policy statement.* Washington, DC: American Nurses' Publishing.

Applebaum, R. A., & Wilson, N. L. (1988). Training needs for providing case management for the long-term care client: Lessons from the national channeling demonstration. *The Gerontologist, 28* (2), 172–176.

Blake, K. (1991). Rehabilitation nursing program management. *Nursing Management, 22* (1), 42–44.

Blank, A. (2005). Linking the restructuring of nursing care with outcomes: Conceptualizing the effect of nursing case management using measurement and logic models. In E. L. Cohen & T. Cesta (Eds.), *Nursing case management: From essential to advanced practice applications,* (pp. 548–559). St Louis: Elsevier Mosby.

Bower, K., & Falk, C. (1996). Case management as a response to quality, cost and access imperatives. In E. Cohen (Ed.). *Nurse case management in the 21st century,* (pp. 161–167). St. Louis: Mosby.

Bower, K. A. (1988). Managed care: Controlling costs, guaranteeing outcomes. *Definition, 3* (3), 1–3.

_____. (1992). *Case management by nurses.* Kansas City, MO: American Nurses' Publishing.

Brooten, D., Brown, L., Munro, B., York, R., et al. (1988). Early discharge and specialist transitional care. *Image: The Journal of Nursing Scholarship, 20* (2), 64–68.

Burgess, C. (1999). Managed care: The driving force for case management. In E. L. Cohen & V. DeBeack (Eds.). *The outcomes mandate: Case management in health care today,* (pp. 12–19). St. Louis: Mosby.

Burgess, C. (2002). Managed care: What next? In T. Cesta (Ed.) *Survival strategies for nurses in managed care,* (pp. 105-117). St. Louis: Mosby.

Capitman, J. A., Haskins, B., & Bernstein, J. (1986). Case management approaches in coordinated community-oriented long-term care demonstrations. *The Gerontologist, 26* (4), 398–404.

Carcagano, G. J., & Kemper, P. (1988). An overview of the channeling demonstration and its evaluation. *Health Services Research, 23* (1), 1–22.

Cesta, T. (2002). *Survival strategies for nurses in managed care.* St. Louis: Mosby.

Chang, C. F., Price, S. A., & Pfoutz, S. K. (2001). *Economics and Nursing.* Philadelphia: F. A. Davis.

Chin, P., & Papenhausen, J. (2002). Integrating concepts of managed care and nursing case management into academic curricula. In T. Cesta (Ed.) *Survival strategies for nurses in managed care,* (pp. 196–217). St. Louis: Mosby.

Christianson, J., Dowd, B., Dralewski, J., Hayes, S., et al. (Summer, 1995). Managed care in the Twin Cities: What can we learn? *Health Affairs, 14* (2), 114–130.

Cohen, E. L., & Cesta, T. G. (1993). *Nursing case management: From concept to evaluation.* St. Louis: Mosby.

Cohen, E. L., & Cesta, T. (2005). *Nursing case management: From essential to advanced practice application.* St. Louis: Elsevier Mosby.

Combs, J. A., & Rusch, S. C. (1990). Creating a healing environment. *Health Progress, 71* (4), 38–41.

Curtin, M., & Lubkin, I. (1998). What is chronicity? In I. Lubkin & P. Larsen (Eds.), *Chronic illness: Impact and Interventions* (4th ed.), (pp. 3–25). Sudbury, MA: Jones & Bartlett.

DeBack, V., & Cohen, E. (1996). The new practice environment. In E. L. Cohen (Ed.), *Nursing case management in the 21st century,* (pp. 3–9). St. Louis: Mosby.

Del Bueno, D. J., & Leblanc, D. (1989). Nurse managed care: One approach. *Journal of Nursing Administration, 19* (11), 24–25.

Dolson, R., & Richards, L. (1990). Area agencies on aging: The community care connection. *Caring, 9* (8), 18–23.

DuBois, M. M. (1990). Community-based homecare programs are not for everyone—yet. *Caring, 9* (7), 24–27.

Ethridge, P. (1991). A nursing HMO: Carondelet St. Mary's experience. *Nursing Management, 22* (7), 22–27.

Ethridge, P., & Lamb, G. (1989). Professional nursing case management improves quality, access and costs. *Nursing Management, 20* (3), 30–35.

Faherty, B. (1990). Case management, the latest buzzword: What it is, and what it isn't. *Caring, 9* (7), 20–22.

Fondiller, S. H. (1991). How case management is changing the picture. *American Journal of Nursing, 91* (1), 64–80.

Giuliano, K. K., & Poirier, C. E. (1991). Nursing case management: Critical pathways to desirable outcomes. *Nursing Management, 22* (3), 52–55.

Graham, B. (1989). Preparing case managers. *Caring, 7* (2), 22–23.

Grau, L. (1984). Case management and the nurse. *Geriatric Nursing, 5* (6), 372–375.

Grinnell, S. K. (1989). Post conference reflections: Autonomy and independence for health professionals? *Journal of Allied Health, 18* (1), 115–121.

Harris, M., & Bergman, H. (1988). Capitation financing for the chronic mentally ill: A case management approach. *Hospital and Community Psychiatry, 39* (1), 68–72.

Health Care Financing Administration. (1999). *The 1998 Medicare chart book.* Baltimore, MD: Author.

Henderson, M. G., Souder, B. A., & Bergman, A. (1987). Measuring the efficiencies of managed care. *Business and Health, 4* (12), 43–46.

Henderson, M. G., & Wallack, S. S. (1987). Evaluating case management for catastrophic illness. *Business and Health, 4* (3), 7–11.

Igou, J. F., Hawkins, J. W., Johnson, E. E., & Utley, Q. E. (1989). Nurse-managed approach to care. *Geriatric Nursing, 10* (1), 32–34.

Jones, K., Kopjo, R., Goodneer-Laff, L., & Weber, C. (1990). Gaining control in a changing environment. *Caring, 9* (7), 38–42.

Knollmueller, R. (1989). Case management: What's in a name? *Nursing Management, 20* (10), 38–42.

Korenbrot, C. C., Showstack, J., Loomis, A., & Brindis, C. (1989). Birth weight outcomes in a teenage pregnancy case management project. *Journal of Adolescent Health Care, 10* (2), 97–104.

Kostlan, M. (2003). Geriatric Considerations. In P. Rossi (Ed.), *Case management in health care,* (pp. 585–596). Philadelphia: Saunders.

Krentzman, M. (2002). Community-based health programs in a managed care environment. In T. Cesta (Ed.), *Survival Strategies for nurses in managed care,* (pp. 290–303). St. Louis: Mosby.

Lamb, G. S. (1995). Early lessons form a capitated community-based nursing model. *Nursing Administration Quarterly, 19* (3), 18–25.

Lamb, G. S., & Stempel, J. E. (1994). Nursing case management from the client's view: growing as insider-expert. *Nursing Outlook, 42* (1), 7–13.

Leclair, C. L. (1991). Introducing and accounting for RN case management. *Nursing Management, 22* (3), 44–49.

Lewenson, S. B. (2003). Historical perspectives on managed care. In T. Cesta (Ed.). *Survival strategies for nurses in managed care,* (pp. 24–36). St Louis: Mosby.

Littman, E., & Siemsen, J. (1989). AIDS case management: A model for smaller communities. *Caring, 7* (11), 26–31.

Lorig, K., (2001). Self-management in chronic illness. In S. Funk, E. Tornquist, J. Leeman, M. Miles, & J. Harrell (Eds.), *Key aspects of preventing and managing chronic illness,* (pp. 35–42). New York: Springer.

Loveridge, C. E., Cummings, S. H., & O'Malley, J. (1988). Developing case management in a primary nursing system. *Journal of Nursing Administration, 18* (10), 36–39.

Mazoway, J. M. (1987). Early intervention in high cost care. *Business and Health, 4* (3), 12–16.

Mazzuca, S. (1982). Does patient education in chronic disease have a therapeutic value? *Journal of Chronic Disease, 35* (9), 521–529.

Michaels, C. (1992). Carondelet St. Mary's experience. *Nursing Clinics of North America, 27* (1), 77–85.

Miller, J. (2000). *Coping with chronic illness: Overcoming powerlessness* (3rd ed.). Philadelphia: F. A. Davis.

Miller, K. (1990). Fee-for-service case management. *Caring, 9* (8), 46–49.

National Center for Health Statistics. (1999). *Employer-sponsored health insurance.* Hyattsville, MD: Author.

Owens, M. S. (2003). Changes in case management. In P. Rossi (Ed). *Case management in health care,* (pp. 19–32). Philadelphia: Saunders.

Papenhausen, J. (1995). The effects of nursing case management intervention on perceived severity of illness, enabling skill, self-help, and life quality in chronically ill older adults. Unpublished dissertation, University of Texas at Austin.

_____. (1996). *Discovering and achieving client outcomes.* In E. L. Cohen (Ed.), *Nursing case management in the 21st century,* (pp. 257–268). St. Louis: Mosby.

Powell. S. K. (2000). *Case management: A practical guide to success in managed care.* Philadelphia: Lippincott Williams Wilkins.

Powell, S., & Ignatavicius, D. (2001). *Core curriculum for case management.* Philadelphia: Lippincott.

Putney, K. A., Hauner, J., Hall, T., & Kobb, R. (1990). Case management in long-term care: New directions for professional nursing. *Journal of Gerontological Nursing, 16* (12), 30–33.

Redman, R. (2005). Financing health care in the United States: Economic and policy implication. In E. L. Cohen & T. Cesta (Eds.), *Nursing case management: From essential to advanced practice applications,* (pp. 219–226). St Louis: Elsevier Mosby.

Riggs, J. E. (September 1996). Managed care and economic dynamics. *Archives of Neurology, 53* (9), 856–858.

Robinson, J. C. (1996). Decline in hospital utilization and cost inflation under managed care in California. *Journal of the American Medical Association, 276* (13), 1060–1064.

Rogers, M., Riordan, J., & Swindle, D. (1991). Community-based nursing case management pays off. *Nursing Management, 22* (3), 30–34.

Rossi, P. (2003). Introduction to complex care. In P. Rossi (Ed.) *Case management in health care,* (pp. 343–510). Philadelphia: Saunders

Scott. J., & Boyd, M. (2005). Outcomes of community-based nurse care management programs. In E. L. Cohen & T. Cesta (Eds.), *Nursing case management: From essential to advanced practice applications,* (pp. 129–140). St Louis: Elsevier Mosby.

Shi, L. & Singh, D. (2004). *Delivering health care in America: A systems approach.* Sudbury, MA : Jones & Bartlett.

Showstack, J., Lurie, N., Leatherman, S., Fisher, E., et al. (1996). Health of the public: The private-sector challenge. *Journal of the American Medical Association, 276* (13), 1971–1974.

Simpson, D. F. (1982). *Case management in long-term programs.* Washington, DC: The Center for the Study of Social Policy.

Sinnenn, M. T., & Schifalacqua, M. M. (1991). Coordinated care in a community hospital. *Nursing Management, 22* (3), 38–42.

Stillwaggon, C. A. (1989). The impact of nurse managed care on the cost of nurse practice and nurse satisfaction. *Journal of Nursing Administration, 19* (11), 21–27.

Stuart, B. (2003). Hospice and the transition to end-of-life-care. In P. Rossi (Ed.), *Case management in health care,* (pp. 687–700). Philadelphia: Saunders.

The Robert Wood Johnson Foundation, (1996) (November). Chronic care in America: A 21st century challenge. http://www.rwif.org/library

US Department of Health and Human Services and Centers for Disease Control and Prevention. (1998) (May). *Chronic diseases and their risk factors: The nation's leading causes of death: A report with expanded state-by-state information.* vii, 3.

Walstedt, P., & Blaser, W. (1986). Nurse case management for the frail elderly: A curriculum to prepare nurses for that role. *Home Healthcare Nurse, 4* (2), 30–35.

Ware, J. E., Bayliss, M. S., Roger, W. H., Kosinsik, M., et al. (1996). Differences in 4-year health outcomes for elderly and poor, chronically ill patients treated in HMO and fee-for-service systems: Results from the medical outcomes study. *Journal of the American Medical Association, 276* (13), 1039–1047.

Weil, M. (1985). Professional and educational issues in case management practice. In M. Weil & J. Karl (Eds.), *Case management in human service practice,* (pp. 357–390). San Francisco: Jossey-Bass.

Weydt, A. (1997). Unpublished interview/survey. Emmanuel-St Joseph's, Mankato, MN.

World Health Organization. (1980). International classification of impairments, disabilities, and handicaps: A manual of classifications relating to the consequences of disease. Geneva, Switzerland: WHO Publications.

Zander, K. (1988a). Nursing case management: Strategic management of cost and quality outcomes. *Journal of Nursing Administration, 18* (5), 23–29.

_____. (1988b). Nursing case management: Resolving the DRG paradox. *Nursing Clinics of North America, 23* (3), 503–520.

_____. (1990a). Case management a golden opportunity for whom? In J. C. McCloskey & H. K. Grace (Eds.), *Current issues in nursing* (3rd ed.), (pp. 199–204). St. Louis: Mosby.

_____. (1990b). Differentiating managed care and case management. *Definition, 5* (2), 1–2.

Zerull, L. (1997). Unpublished interview/survey. Winchester Medical, Winchester, Virginia.

Zrelak, P.A. (2003). Case management of the transplant patient. In P. Rossi (Ed.). *Case management in health care,* (pp. 524–565). Philadelphia: Saunders.

CHAPTER 20

The Advanced Practice Nurse in Chronic Illness

Sue E. Meiner

Introduction

Over the past decade, there has been a growing need for advanced practice nurses (APNs). The management of chronic diseases has become the practice for many APNs across North America. Besides the benefits of having a professional nurse provide care that accentuates support for human response to changes in health, that care also emphasizes client and family education that prevents recurrence of easily controlled health conditions.

Two primary issues emerged that prompted the need for APNs. Those factors included an increasing demand to provide better care to underserved populations and the changing demographics of the United States. While major cities have an abundance of physicians to serve their population, many rural areas of the United States and other areas have not been as fortunate. The need for practitioners in those areas is great, and the ability to attract a physician to those areas is poor. Additionally, the demographic changes in the United States, with the increasing number of older adults, and many of those individuals with more than one chronic illness, have further increased the need for a mid-level practitioner who can manage health care in a cost-effective manner.

An APN has many skills that benefit individuals with chronic illness, such as conducting health histories, physical examinations, diagnosing and treating common acute illness and injuries, and providing supportive, ongoing care of the client. An APN may order and interpret laboratory tests and counsel clients and their families on health promotion as well as health care options (AACN, 1994). APNs may also practice in hospitals or rehabilitation facilities to assist staff nurses in providing the most effective bedside care during an inpatient stay.

The care that individuals with chronic illness need can be provided by APNs because of their knowledge of the health care system, community resources, when and how to make referrals, and how to work collaboratively with other health professionals. As the number of older adults rises steadily and advances in treatment options for chronic illnesses continue, APNs will become the primary health care professionals to many persons across the United States and Canada.

Advanced Practice Nursing Education

Advanced practice nursing includes education and skills that are additions to the basic nursing education of the registered nurse (RN). The additional education is at the graduate degree level, with concentration in an advanced nursing practice specialty. Education includes clinical components appropriate to the specialty and didactic studies in advanced knowledge of nursing theory, physical and psychosocial assessment, interventions based on that advanced assessment, and client health care management (American Nurses Association, 2004).

A statement of the essentials of masters education for APNs was developed by the American Association of Colleges of Nursing (AACN) in 1994. The statement lists three components that should be included in all programs providing APN education:

1. A generic graduate core basic to all master's of nursing degree programs.
2. An advanced practice generic core.
3. A specialty role core specific to the selected APN role.

The generic graduate core may include nursing theory, health policy, multicultural issues of care, ethical/legal issues, nursing research, and health care delivery systems. The advanced practice generic core usually includes theories of individuals, families, and communities; physiology and pathophysiology; advanced health assessment; health promotion; advanced pharmacology; clinical decision making; advanced nursing interventions and therapeutics; and role differentiation.

The specialty core specific to the selected concentration includes the nurse practitioner (NP) role, the clinical nurse specialist role (CNS), the certified registered nurse anesthetist (CRNA), and the certified nurse midwife (CNM) role. These roles have components that have expansion and specialization of skills and knowledge. The issue of expansion refers to adding new practice skills and knowledge that prepare the APN for autonomy within the specific practice area. This autonomy may overlap boundaries that have been thought of as traditional medical practice. Specialization is the concentration of focus in practice to a more limited practice field (American Nurses Association, 2003). Examples of

specialization are pain management, psychiatric/mental health, palliative care, or hospice nursing.

The CRNA is a graduate of a nurse anesthesia educational program accredited by the Council on Accreditation of Nurse Anesthesia Educational Programs (COA) or its predecessor, and has passed the certification examination administered by the Council on Certification of Nurse Anesthetists. The CRNA provides significant care pre- and postoperatively to persons requiring procedures under anesthesia. Working with anesthesiologists (either MD or DO), the CRNA administers a variety of sedatives and anesthesia and facilitates the safety of the client undergoing invasive procedures or surgery. Other areas that are within the skills of the CRNA include pain management, respiratory care and emergency resuscitation (American Nurses Association, 2004).

The CNM is educated in both nursing and midwifery. Certification is gained through the American College of Nurse-Midwives. The CNM usually provides independent management of women's health care, including prescriptive needs. Many CNMs practice in collaboration with family practice physicians or with obstetricians serving maternity clients. The CNM role is directed primarily toward the women's reproductive health specialty. However, childbearing is only one component of this role. Care also includes care of the newborn. Family planning, diagnosis, and treatment of diseases of the reproductive system are a major component of this specialty practice. The CNM will refer those clients that are indicated by their health status (American Nurses Association, 2003). The APN specialties of the CRNA and the CNM are not discussed further in this chapter, as their roles generally do not include long-term involvement with individuals with chronic illness.

Regulation of advanced study is controlled by internal and external means. The quality of graduates from APN programs is regulated internally by the nursing faculties of each program. This continuous self-assessment process analyzes the multiple components of the educational process and the outcomes of the graduates. External evaluation of APN programs is provided by accrediting organizations. These organizations include the National League for Nursing Accrediting Commission (NLNAC), the Commission on Collegiate Nursing Education (CCNE), the American Academy of Nurse Practitioners, the American Nurses Credentialing Center, and specialty groups that focus on specific practice orientation (e.g., oncology nursing, perioperative nursing, maternal–newborn nursing). Organizations that provide accreditation serve as an external check and balance for programs (Craven, 1998).

Roles

Clinical Nurse Specialist

Advanced practice nursing in the United States began with the development of the nurse clinician role in 1943 by Frances Reiter. This role set the precedent of APNs having additional education and training past basic nursing education preparation. By the 1960s, the term *nurse clinician* had evolved to *clinical nurse specialist*. The roles of the CNS include those of advanced direct patient care provider, educator (staff, client, and community), consultant, and researcher.

The CNS works or consults with various members of the health care team to attain optimum quality of care for clients. This consultative effort requires multidisciplinary management skills. Often the CNS's work may include indirect care as she or he consults with staff nurses on care issues. When client education is needed, the CNS prepares individualized learning materials for the client and/or family members.

The CNS serves as an advocate for the client, family, or community through involvement in legislative activities aimed at health promotion and screening programs. The goals of these actions are to decrease the cost of health care and increase clients' quality of life.

Interpreting and/or conducting nursing research is an integral component of the CNS role. As new breakthroughs occur in care options for clients with chronic illness, the CNS may interpret and apply the research data to the practice setting. Often, application of research findings may include inservice education to staff as well. When areas of high

volume, high cost, and high risk are identified, the CNS can establish research protocols to ensure that quality standards are maintained.

The majority of CNS graduates complete educational programs that award a master's degree in nursing. Specialty areas include pediatric, adult, family, or geriatric practice areas. Other CNS programs may be more general, such as a medical–surgical CNS.

Nurse Practitioner Role

The first NP demonstration project was initiated in 1965 at the University of Colorado under the direction of Dr. Loretta Ford. The project developed a new role of nursing practice specifically designed to improve the overall health care of children and families. The NP project was the outcome of a physician–nurse collaborative effort based on the medical model. The physician was instrumental in all facets of the NPs' education and skills training.

During this development of the NP role, certificate NP programs proliferated, and produced the majority of the original practicing NPs. These programs were generally nine to 12 months in length (certainly short compared with current graduate programs preparing NPs) (Snyder et al., 1999).

In 1979, the National League for Nursing (NLN) stated their position regarding this advanced education for nurses. NLN's position was that NP education should be in a graduate program that awarded a master's degree in the nursing specialty. This action was taken to protect the public and to ensure that practitioner competence and quality of client/family care were cornerstones of each program (Luggen, Travis & Meiner, 1998).

A current trend emerging in graduate programs preparing APNs is combining the two roles, CNS and NP, into a single program. A student graduating from a master's program would be educated as both a CNS and an NP (a blended role) and be eligible to take the appropriate certification examinations associated with each. Because the blending of the CNS and NP into one role is new, and data documenting and evaluating outcomes do not currently exist.

Theory-Based Practice

The practice of APNs is guided by knowledge, skills, and clinical experience acquired throughout basic and advanced nursing education. Nursing theories have been a component of the majority of APN educational programs accredited by national organizations since the 1960s. Models and theories from nursing and other disciplines provide the intellectual framework that guides professional practice.

While many APNs use models or theories to guide their clinical practice, others are reluctant to do so. These individuals may be unclear how to apply a theory to their practice or lack general knowledge about theories in advanced practice settings. Others use the medical model versus a nursing framework for their practice. The medical model is comfortable and predictable. Other reasons to use the medical model might include insufficient information to select a practice model and distrust in self-selection of an applicable theory.

The inability to use a nursing or related theory in clinical practice has been referred to as the "theory–practice gap" (Kenney, 1999). Some question the value of nursing theories in practice because a number of the profession's theories have evolved from other disciplines. However, the richness of nursing theory and concepts from other disciplines support the APN in collaborating with others; listening to the client; educating client, family, and staff; initiating research; and consulting with others on a regular basis.

Research has identified seven criteria for selecting theories that can be applied to nursing practice (Table 20-1). These criteria include identifying the type of client, the health care setting, the realistic nature of the theory, having an understanding of the premises, and other areas pertinent to use in a practice setting (McKenna, 1997).

Debate continues regarding the use of one or more theories in clinical practice. Nursing, like many professions, has multiple theories that represent different and unique perspectives about the phenomena in its practice. Nursing models or theories include grand theories, mid-range theories, broad conceptual models, and specific practice theories. Some are more appropriate than others for use in advanced practice.

Early nursing theories primarily identified the recipients of nursing care as passive and nondimensional. Contemporary nursing models view humans as continuously changing, with reciprocal interactions with their environment. As a result, an individuals' reactions to nursing care are not predictable,

---

TABLE 20-1

Seven Criteria for Selecting Models and Theories for Clinical Practice

1. *Type of client:* The client's needs should direct the choice because the theory provides guidelines to achieve the client's goals.
2. *Health care setting:* The type of clinical setting and nursing practice are contextual factors that affect selection of theories.
3. *Parsimony/simplicity:* Simple and realistic theories are more likely to be understood and applied in practice.
4. *Understanding:* Nurses must understand a theory if they are expected to use it.
5. *Origins of the theory:* The credibility, prior use, and testing of the theory should also be considered.
6. *Paradigms as a basis for choice:* Nurses must decide between the totality or simultaneity paradigm, as each provides a different view of clients and nursing actions.
7. *Personal values and beliefs:* The theory must be congruent with the nurse's own views about humans, health, and nursing.

SOURCE: From McKenna, H. (1997). Choosing a theory for practice. In H. McKenna (Ed.), *Nursing theories and models*, (pp. 127–157). New York: Rutledge. Reprinted with permission of Thomson Publishing Services on behalf of Taylor & Francis Books.

nor can they be controlled. While the earlier theories provided specific nursing guidelines, contemporary models are more abstract and do not provide specific direction for care.

A well-defined decision-making model as well as a code of ethics provides the APN with the foundation to perform appropriately in ethical dilemmas, which are bound to occur from time to time. The PRACTICE Model was developed to help with resolution of essential ethical issues for APNs. This Model has eight defining words.

- Patient—facts that are pertinent;
- Relationships—connections with significant others;
- Advocacy—decision-making ability;
- Conflicts—involving ethics, family members;
- Treatment—risks and benefits of treatment modalities;
- Interests—advance directives, living will, motives of interested parties;
- Consequences—short and long term responses to actions; and
- Ethical Principles—identify the principles that are at stake (Robinson & Kish, 2001).

Selecting and using one or more models or theories in clinical practice depends on the nurse having a broad knowledge base and understanding of the interrelationship of various models and theories. When a model or theory is used in a practice setting, the APN is demonstrating accountability for decisions and actions related to the plan of care established for each client (Kenney, 1999).

American Nurses Association Standards of Practice for the APN

Standards of practice are directed toward setting minimum levels of acceptable performance. Standards of practice endeavor to provide clients with a means of measuring the quality of nursing care received. The American Nurses Association (ANA) defines a standard as an authoritative statement by which the quality of practice, service, or education can be judged (American Nurses Association, 2004).

The ANA developed general guidelines and conditions that can be used to determine whether a standard has been met. These conditions are frequently used by attorneys to examine the appropriateness of client care and to determine whether standards of nursing care were met in a specific situation. An example of one standard involves documentation of care and describes the collection of data about the health status of the client as a systematic and continuous process. The information is communicated to appropriate persons and is recorded and stored in a retrievable and accessible system (American Nurses Association, 2004). Documentation of chronic illness includes the assessment of the illness trajectory, with anticipated interventions along the path.

Since the development of standards of care in the 1970s, further work has been done with standards of care for APNs in various practice specialties. For more information on these specialties, contact the American Nurses Association.

Regulation of Practice

Regulation and validation of the practice of an APN is maintained primarily through the processes of credentialing and certification. The National Council of State Boards of Nursing defines *credentialing* as the validation of required education, licensure, and certification (Sheets, 1993). The purpose is to assure that the public is protected from the unsafe practices of a nonphysician health care professional. Credentialing also ensures compliance with federal and state laws related to nursing practice.

Certification for APN practice is obtained after completion of an advanced practice nursing program. It is a process by which nongovernmental associations certify that a nurse has met certain predetermined standards specific to advanced nursing specialties (Snyder et al., 1999).

Several professional organizations offer certification through written examinations to candidates who have submitted academic documentation verifying completion of a prescribed educational program. Examples of professional organizations that offer certification include the American Nurses Credentialing Center (ANCC), American Academy of Nurse Practitioners (AANP), and Association for Women's Health, Obstetrics and Neonatal Nursing (AWHONN). The Certification examinations are offered for a specific field of advanced study, such as, but not limited to, pediatrics, maternal/child, women's health, psychiatry/mental health, adult, family, or geriatric practice.

Some states require certification for advanced nursing practice, while other states subscribe to optional or voluntary certification. An example of a recent change is in North Carolina. Effective January 2001, all family NPs must be nationally certified to practice. Some states, such as Nevada, encourage but do not require certification for practice.

Models of Practice for Advanced Practice Nurses

All practice models have the same requirements for certification, and share similar professional legal/liability issues and educational preparation, but are different in the manner in which relationships with professionals are maintained. The three major models of practice are the independent practice model, the collaborative practice model, and the interdisciplinary care model.

Components of the independent model include ownership of the practice/office, full accountability for quality structure and activities, and financial/legal responsibility. This model is based on the delivery of nursing services provided by nurses in which nurses have full control (Lambert & Lambert, 1996).

The collaborative practice model is the nurse–physician joint practice. Joint responsibility for client care is based on each practitioner's education and ability. Complementary skills and common goals of practice are essential to the success of this model (Kyle, 1995).

In the interdisciplinary model, a team of specialists work together in a cooperative manner to provide comprehensive care of a client. The interdisciplinary model is an interactive one and is different from the multidisciplinary approach associated with individual specialists assessing the client. In this model, the APN works collaboratively with others in the care of the client.

Additional Roles for Experienced Advanced Practice Nurses

The complexities of chronic illness that may be presented to an APN for decision-making can be overwhelming to a novice practitioner. The development process for APN internship students and/or new APN graduates should include opportunities with preceptors and mentors. The experienced APN can be a role model while demonstrating the skills necessary when providing long-term supportive care to persons with chronic illness.

Serving as a Preceptor

An experienced APN can serve as a strong clinical role model, teacher, adviser, guide, and practitioner for students enrolled in APN programs. This is an active and purposeful role for both the APN and the student. The preceptor socializes the student into the occupational and social world of being an APN. The student learns a set of skills by observing, working with, and relating to a more experienced nurse practicing in an actual role (Douglass, 1996; Marquis & Huston, 1996).

Mentoring

Mentoring is crucial in the process of developing nonprofessionals into professionals, graduate students into specialists, and clinicians into academicians. Mentoring is an artful process of providing the "inside story" about the reality of the APN role.

The difference between a preceptor and a mentor is the personal interest in the long-range career development of the person in the subordinate role. A mentor provides a semiprotective environment in which the mentee or protégé can develop. A preceptor–preceptee relationship is time and role limited in that the preceptee will complete the current practicum and move to other preceptors and areas of practice (Gray & Anderson, 1991).

A Practice Scenario with a Clinical Nurse Specialist

The CNS is assigned to a client diagnosed with Type I diabetes mellitus who is admitted to the acute care setting for insulin regulation. Assessment includes a health history and an admission physical assessment to determine baseline health data. Assessment is the foundation of planning care for the client and integrating the health care agency's services to produce a successful outcome. Care will be coordinated between the physician and the staff with the CNS supervising the client's daily outcomes and discharge outcomes. Regular meetings occur between the CNS and the staff members, providing the day-to-day care, monitoring, instruction, and documenting of nursing interventions.

The CNS uses advanced skills and knowledge to coordinate the services of the health care agency and any projected homecare services that may be needed. Educational materials will be reviewed to determine educational level and understanding according to the unique needs of this client and/or family caregiver. The case manager and the CNS will evaluate any follow-up services provided. If adverse changes in the client's trajectory of recovery are noted, the CNS can arrange for additional interventions with the primary health care provider.

A Practice Scenario with a Nurse Practitioner

The NP examines an overweight client with a complaint of fatigue, loss of appetite, shortness of breath when walking to the kitchen, and a persistent, dull headache for the past few days. Following completion of a past and current health history, vital signs reveal that the client is afebrile, has a blood pressure of 160/100, a pulse rate of 94, and a respi-

ration rate of 24. The physical examination is completed, and vital signs are again taken after a 10-minute rest in a quiet, darkened room. The sitting blood pressure results are 158/98 in the left arm and 156/94 in the right arm. All other vital signs are within normal range. The NP reviews the findings from the history and physical examination. Laboratory and diagnostic studies are ordered from the outpatient department of the local hospital, with results to be called to the office for the NP to review as soon as possible.

Before the client leaves the office for the outpatient laboratory tests, instructions are given regarding food and fluid intake, activities management, and a strong recommendation that a call be made to the off-hours health care provider if any of the symptoms become worse or new symptoms develop. The client is scheduled to return within the next two days to have additional vital signs taken.

The NP reviews the information and orders with the physician as a diagnosis is being formulated. The NP will follow collaborative protocols in the management of this client.

Problems and Issues of Advanced Practice Nursing

Difficulty in Attracting Students and Faculty

Recruiting potential APN students and appropriately educated faculty is an ongoing issue. Newspapers and media news programs have continued to advertise the need for more nurses educated at an advanced practice level to meet the needs of the increasing elderly population and those needing long-term chronic disease management. However, APN programs have unfilled student openings in many parts of the United States. Reasons for this range from practice settings being in rural areas, where relocation of families may be unattractive, to difficulties in attracting active nurses into returning to graduate level studies. A new issue has evolved related to the acute care nursing shortage. Many hospitals are offering incentives to stay at the bedside and forgo advanced education. When an incentive to remain in an area that doesn't require additional time and energy as well as loss of income during schooling is available, deferring graduate studies can result.

Attracting faculty members with the education, experience, and desire to teach while maintaining a clinical practice has also been difficult. Universities are currently looking at creative ways to attract APN faculty. The commitments in an academic setting to teach and publish, in addition to maintaining a part-time clinical practice, may be overwhelming to an APN. Two organizations that are addressing this concern are the National Organization of Nurse Practitioner Faculties (NONPF) and the American Association of Colleges of Nursing (AACN).

Resistance from Physician Organizations

While the need is great for the mid-level primary care provider, resistance from some physician organizations remains. The concerns from these groups range from issues about APN practice preparation to a concern that only services with direct oversight by physicians should be permitted. Other objections have focused on the economic issues of reimbursement, contract issues for services, and liability issues (Archibald & Bainbridge, 1994).

Reluctance to permit APNs to have medical staff privileges and be allowed to admit clients varies across North America. Hospitals operate under a medical staff structure that requires the physicians to vote to accept new providers to the facility. When the climate is not favorable toward APNs, privileges are rarely granted.

Using Protocols or Guidelines in Practice

A majority of states have enacted a requirement that APNs work under a specific written set of protocols or guidelines that must be used in the treatment/therapeutics component of patient care.

Protocols and/or guidelines must reflect the current standard of care and be based on the available scientific knowledge that is practiced by the collaborating physician. Protocols establish the specific procedures to be followed in client-based assessment and in conducting research. These protocols provide a formula for obtaining subjective and objective data and conclude with making an assessment based on those data. This assessment leads to the development of a specific plan of care for the client's unique situation. When protocols are required, they must be followed accordingly, or the APN may be liable for negligence or malpractice (Hilgart & Karl, 1995). Practicing beyond the scope of the nurse practice act of a specific state can result in temporary or permanent loss of license to practice as an APN.

Although using protocols or guidelines has helped some APNs, it has hampered other APNs in their practices. A novice APN, newly graduated from a master's degree program, can benefit from following specific protocols to provide safe and effective patient care. However, experienced APNs often find protocols inflexible and unable to address unique client differences. Some practices use "guidelines" instead of protocols. With guidelines, there is more latitude for clinical decision making.

If specific protocols are not in place, the APN must contact the collaborating or consultative physician to discuss the case and receive verbal instructions on handling the client's care. If the physician cannot be reached, a delay in treatment may occur. In some cases, transporting the client to the closest health care facility with a physician in attendance is the only method of securing care for the client. This situation can lead to dissatisfaction from the perspective of both the client and the APN.

Expertise in clinical decision making evolves over time, and many APNs have significant knowledge with which to customize the care of each client instead of following exact "cookbook" plans of care. Using more flexible protocols or guidelines in practice may be the answer to the APN's concern about autonomy in practice.

Admitting Privileges in Acute Care Facilities

The privilege of admitting a client for care in an acute care facility requires maintaining records pertaining to education, skill attainment, and practice experience while meeting other requirements of the medical board of the facility. The term *clinical privileges* is often used in place of *admitting privileges.* Clinical privileges are frequently divided into two levels: First-level privileges are directed toward experience with specific procedures or skills; second-level privileges are related to a specific population of clients, diagnoses, and/or client care problem groups that are within the scope of practice for a specific practitioner (Meiner, 1998). Reluctance to permit APNs to have admitting or clinical privileges is a continuing issue throughout North America.

With clinical privileges for the APN come the legal implications of participating as medical staff in the medical staff organization. This organization has responsibilities to maintain a system for appointing staff, subjecting each member to periodic assessment and review to ensure that each practitioner remains clinically competent. Each member of the medical staff is an independent contractor, not an employee of the hospital or institution. Therefore, liability for legal claims remains with the practitioner and not as an agent of the facility. This status can be modified with a contract to the facility in which responsibility for practice is shared. The final responsibility is to abide by the medical staff organization rules and regulations (Orsund-Gassiot & Lindsey, 1991).

Reimbursement Issues in Advanced Practice Nursing

When the APN assumes responsibilities as an independent practitioner or collaborative practitioner in a physician practice, fee for service becomes a part of practice. Understanding the reimbursement procedures is essential for an APN's economic survival. APNs must know how to bill for reimbursement using the Current Procedural Terminology (CPT), and the International classification of Diseases (ICD-9) code (US Department of Health and Human Services [DHHS], 1996). The CPT is nomenclature for the reposting of physician services and procedures while the ICD-9 codes are diagnostic codes that classify morbidity and mortality (DHHS, 1996).

Medicare Title XVIII of the Social Security Act is a federal health insurance program for people age 65 years or older and for certain disabled people with chronic conditions. Medicare was designed to cover acute episodes of illness, not to provide coordinated care for chronic conditions. Many older adults have some form of "medigap" insurance, and this additional coverage takes care of preventive treatment and chronic illness management (Taylor & Schub, 1996).

The advent of diagnosis-related groups (DRGs) was implemented by Medicare to reduce the cost of health care services in the United States. With DRGs came capitation or limits on the payments that health care providers could charge for services rendered for each specific or combined patient diagnosis.

Reimbursement for services given in nursing homes, in rural settings, or in rural and underserved health clinics may be available to APNs. The reimbursement levels can depend on the type of APN practice, the setting of the practice, and the payment level. As a part of the Omnibus Budget Reconciliation Act (OBRA), NPs may be recognized as direct providers of services to nursing home residents. To receive payment, an NP must work for a physician, nursing home, or hospital and must have a collaborative relationship with a physician. The reimbursement goes to the NP's employer at less than that of the physician according to the Medicare fee schedule.

Medicare will make additional reimbursements to specific NPs and the CNS when their work is in collaboration with a physician. While claims may be submitted by the APN, they are reimbursed at a lower rate than the fee schedule for outpatient services and for inpatient services. Negotiations are continuing to equalize the pay structure for APNs according to physician reimbursement.

An additional form of reimbursement is available to APNs. Medicare defines "incident to" services as reimbursable activities performed in an ambulatory setting and meeting three guidelines:

1. Services must be within the APN's scope of practice.
2. The physician must be on site at the time that the service is being provided.
3. The service is related to the physician's plan of care for the client and is related to the primary condition for which the physician was first treating the client.

When managed care services are part of the client's reimbursement plan, the APN and the physician work together to provide the breadth of services needed. With the higher volumes of clients seen routinely, an effective and efficient distribution of services is provided. Health Maintenance Organizations (HMOs) hire an optimal balance of APNs and physicians to prudently spend the capitated money paid as premiums by the subscribers of the

organization (Green & Conway, 1995).

The newer insurance plans that assume Medicare funding with the additional health plan benefits provided by their company provide basic and extended health care services for subscribers. APNs are frequently assigned to manage these clients. Because these client groups are usually over age 65, chronic illnesses become the major diagnoses for management by the APN.

Prescriptive Authority

Each of the 50 states legislates rules and regulations that govern prescriptive authority of APNs. In 1971, Idaho became the first state to allow NPs to have limited prescriptive authority. During the subsequent years, state legislation has consistently expanded the prescriptive authority of APNs. However, each state has continued to individually determine the role and status of prescriptive authority with or without collaborative practice agreements between the physician and the APN (Carson, 1993; Safriet, 1992). Table 20-2 depicts the range of prescriptive authority of APNs.

Although the process concerning prescriptive authority varies among states, the majority of states

---

TABLE 20-2

Types of Prescriptive Authority of APNs

- Prescriptive authority
  - Controlled substances
    - independent of physician involvement
    - physician involvement required
      - delegation of writing prescriptions
      - collaborative practice limitations
      - specific protocols required
      - protocols on file with the Board of Nursing and/or Board of Pharmacy, with or without Board of Medicine file or approval
  - Non-controlled substances only
    - physician involvement required
    - collaborative agreement required
    - approved by Board of Nursing and/or Board Pharmacy, and/or Medical Board (Board of Healing Arts, or other official name)
- No statutory prescribing authority

require a three-tier granting authority. The state's Board of Nursing, Board of Medicine, and Board of Pharmacy (boards may be titled differently in various states) compose most joint committees working with granting prescriptive authority for APNs (Pearson, 1997). Some states automatically include prescriptive authority in the licensure of APNs. Other states require APNs to have a separate license to prescribe medication.

In some states, there are different rules and regulations regarding prescriptive authority for urban versus rural areas of a state, which affects the practice of the APN who may have prescriptive authority in a rural, undeveloped part of a state but is unable to provide the same level of care to clients in a clinic for the underserved in the middle of a city. In particular, this factor affects the practice of the gerontological nurse practitioner. With older adults consuming nearly 35 percent of all prescription medications (three times the rate of younger groups), prescriptive authority is central to that practitioner's practice.

Each year, the January issue of *The Nurse Practitioner* updates information from each state related to legislative issues affecting advanced nursing practice. This update includes issues of contracts, collaborative practice models, prescriptive authority allowances, and other matters directly pertaining to the law and advanced nursing practice.

Cultural Perspectives of Advanced Practice Nursing

The pluralistic society of North America represents multiple racial and ethnic groups. Each group has an identity that exists through practices based on the particular culture's belief system. When clients seek health care, they bring a set of values and beliefs about health and illness that may be dissimilar to the health care provider's beliefs (Spector, 1996). The APN working in culturally diverse settings needs to be cognizant of the various racial and ethnic groups that may present as clients. Preparation for the cultural diversity of patients through reading, discussion, and formal educational classes is essential in providing health care that will have positive outcomes for both the client and the provider.

Although nurturing care is identified as a female role in most societies, medical treatment may be viewed as a male role within the same ethnic group. Conversely, male or female APNs may be able to ascertain information from a client or family with more thoroughness than may a physician. This is often related to fear of the medical authority of "the doctor."

Whether the client seeks a specific type of health care provider or simply seeks help with a problem, the APN must be knowledgeable of diverse cultures. The "sick role" may vary widely from one racial/ethnic group to another. The needs of the client should be met without forcing the belief system of Western medicine on the client.

Interventions

Gaining Acceptance by Other Disciplines

Moving the role of the APN from a nearly invisible role to one that is recognized by the public and other disciplines continues to be a top priority for organizations that represent APNs. The benefits of having health care provided by APNs must be better publicized to receive needed recognition. Continuing to provide high-quality, professional, personal, and cost-effective care will assist in this effort. Media efforts must continue to tout the abilities and high-level care being provided by APNs.

During the past two decades, the physician assistant (PA) role has been more visible to the health care community and public than has the APN role. Although there is some overlap between these two roles, the nursing focus remains the strength of the APN.

Opening an Advanced Practice Nursing Practice

New businesses open and close at an alarming rate. The reasons for many failures in private business are poor planning and insufficient funds. Prior to beginning any business, a research study of the need for the service and the number of clients that might be available or interested in the service must be done. If the indications of this study are favorable, a full business plan needs to be developed. The business plan is the document that secures funding to open, operate, and grow the business over the first difficult years.

When the potential clientele of a practice is identified, the location of the office must be the next consideration. Individuals with chronic illnesses have limited energy and endurance to travel long distances to their health care provider. Therefore, a practice that is directed toward such individuals needs to be located within a short traveling distance of apartments or communities where significant numbers of elderly clients live. An office located near public transportation is essential. Placement of an office in an inner-city site proximate to senior housing complexes is one example of a selective location.

The message that will be directed to potential clients needs to be addressed. Focus groups of providers, administrators, and potential clients can assist in identifying issues and approaches that are desired for a specialty practice in a given location. An independent practice needs to consider the reasons that potential clients need the type of services that the practice will provide. The answers to that inquiry can serve as the foundation for a marketing approach (Lambert & Lambert, 1996). Reasons for marketing nursing and the APN role are included in Table 20-3.

Financially, health care practices are expensive to open and maintain. There needs to be significant reserve capital to meet expenses while billing procedures are initiated with third-party payers. Some insurance companies take months to reimburse for services. Medicare and Medicaid may take even longer to pay for services rendered.

Mentally, developing a new business is stressful. Securing a sound support system is essential to maintaining confidence during those first years in business. Finding a mentor that provides guidance when various decisions are in question can be the essential piece to making a new business work.

Policy Development

Policy is defined as a guiding principle designed to influence the decisions and actions of an organization. Further, it is a statement of decision-making criteria used to achieve efficiency in recurring situations by establishing routines for such decisions.

The APN must become politically active and involved in political decision making. When salient issues related to the advancement of APN practice are being discussed in a political arena, the need to become politically active is essential. However, being proactive by first identifying problems, followed by an action plan, is the preferred way to effect change, rather than waiting until an issue becomes a public debate.

TABLE 20-3

Reasons for Marketing Nursing and the Role of the Advanced Practice Nurse

1. In response to national concerns for quality in health care
2. In response to business concerns for rising health care costs
3. To increase the public's awareness of the APN role in health care
4. To provide information needed to obtain reimbursement for APNs
5. To identify new areas of practice for nurses, such as
   a. APN health care in assisted-living facility
   b. faculty-based practice for an APN in teaching
   c. APN consultant role in acute care settings

SOURCE: From Rubotzky, A. M. (1998). Marketing strategies. In A. S. Luggen, S. S. Travis, & S. Meiner (Eds.), *NGNA core curriculum for gerontological advanced practice nurses*, (pp. 251–253). Reprinted by permission of Sage Publications, Inc. Thousand Oaks, CA: Sage.

A Client with Congestive Heart Failure and the Nurse Practitioner

Mr. James is an 86-year-old patient of D. Markim, MD, and S. Miner, APN. He is hard of hearing but does not like to wear his hearing aid. Since he was widowed five years ago, he eats his meals in a neighborhood diner, where he socializes with other gentlemen his age.

Four months ago, he was admitted to the local hospital with congestive heart failure (CHF). He received emergent treatment and recovered after a five-day stay. His medication regime consists of a combination of diuretics, antihypertensives, and antiinflammatory medications. His co-morbidities include status post myocardial infarction, hypertension, non–insulin-dependent diabetes mellitus, arthritis, chronic constipation, macular degeneration, and a significant hearing loss.

The NP will manage Mr. James' health care through a number of interventions in a variety of settings. One goal of care will be to prevent placement in a long-term care facility. The overall goal of care is to prevent readmission to acute care due to exacerbation of symptoms related to his CHF.

In addition to the health history and physical examination, an evaluation of Mr. James' current health beliefs and practices, life-style, and willingness to modify those areas that are identified as nonsup-

portive of the treatment plan will be made. Examples of nonsupportive areas would be frequent intake of foods high in sodium and/or smoking. Assessment of the client's pharmacotherapeutics' practices would include both prescription and over-the-counter medicines.

The NP reviews all of the data to identify any precipitating causes that could exacerbate Mr. James' heart failure. Treatment for the precipitating causes would be initiated immediately. Correction of the underlying causes of heart failure would be addressed next, followed by control of the CHF state through reduction of cardiac workload, control of excess retention of salt and water, and enhancement of cardiac contractility.

The program of client management would include office visits on a monthly basis, supplemented with weekly telephone calls by the NP to Mr. James' home. These calls will review records of self-care that Mr. James will keep. For his condition, recording of daily weights is required. Typical questions will address fatigue, weakness, abdominal symptoms, cerebral symptoms, and respiratory symptoms. At the first indication of a problem, an office visit would be scheduled immediately.

APNs possess the skills to become active in political action and policy development. Throughout nursing education and practice, the art of communication is essential to successful client outcomes. With an understanding of the health care delivery systems, the ability to motivate others, strong organizational skills, and a commitment to health promotion and disease prevention, the APN is prepared to make an impact on health care policy (see Chapter 26, on politics and policy).

In addition, there is a continued need for nursing organizations' lobbying efforts to continue to support APN legislation. Through support of professional organizations such as the American Nurses Association, American College of Nurse Practitioners, American Association of Nurse Practitioners, and specialty organizations representing the CNS, CRNA, and CNM practitioners, legislators will receive information about the needs of the public and the benefits of APNs providing care.

A Client with Polypharmacy and the Clinical Nurse Specialist

On admission to the local hospital, Mrs. Rhodes' daughter states that her mother is losing weight and seems to be depressed. The admitting physician is concerned about an electrolyte imbalance that could be treated during an observation 23-hour stay.

Mrs. Rhodes relocated to a senior housing complex six months ago to be near her daughter, her only child. Mrs. Rhodes cannot recall the name of her previous provider. Her daughter had not been involved in her health care before this recent move, so she was not able to add any information regarding her mother's previous health care provider.

When Mrs. Rhodes does not pick up the pen and begin to write on the information sheet given to her by the receptionist, the daughter takes the material from her mother and completes the brief medical history questionnaire. Mrs. Rhodes continuously looks across the room at a television set while her daughter finishes the data sheet. She does not answer the verbal questions that are asked by her daughter.

The family interview with the CNS elicited little information from Mrs. Rhodes. The daughter volunteered information about herself. She is married and has three teen-age children living at home. She works day-hours Monday through Friday in a technically demanding office. Her husband does not like her absence from home during the evenings. While she tries to be with her mother as often as possible, that time only amounts to a couple of hours one evening a week and Sunday mornings. The daughter has noticed that her mother seems distant and noncommunicative lately and appears to have lost weight during the past few weeks. She believes that her mother is just depressed over moving away from her home of many years.

Outcomes

As more adults attain the age of 65, and even more the age of 85, APNs will routinely see older clients in all health care settings. It is likely that these older adults will have not one but many chronic illnesses that need ongoing management. The outcome for health management of persons with chronic illnesses is to reduce the number of hospitalizations and/or admissions to long-term care facilities through better disease management. Client education and health promotion activities can accomplish this goal through timely, well-planned interventions and follow-up illness prevention care.

The APN is an excellent health care professional to support the management of chronic care with a focus on health promotion. The ultimate goal of the APN in a practice involved with clients with chronic illnesses is to have positive health outcomes with increased quality of life for each client.

Study Questions

1. Differentiate the processes of certification from accreditation as applied to the education of APNs.

2. Discuss the benefits of the mentoring relationship in the development of a specific career path.

During the medication review, Mrs. Rhodes denies taking any medication. The daughter tells the CNS that her mother does take pills from several little bottles on her kitchen table on Sunday mornings while she is visiting. The mother says she takes aspirin sometimes but nothing else. The medication review is incomplete pending a brown bag/medication examination to be done as soon as the daughter can pick up the medicines from Mrs. Rhodes' apartment.

The result of examining the brown bag that was brought in later in the day revealed 24 bottles of prescription medications and six bottles of over-the-counter (OTC) medicines. Four different physicians prescribed the drugs over a two-year period. Several containers held the same medicine but with different brand names. Also, two of the OTC bottles contained two of the prescription drugs in lower dosages.

The CNS determined that Mrs. Rhodes was taking overdoses of several medicines, which could be the cause of her confusion and loss of appetite.

The CNS contacted the physician with the results of her evaluation of the drugs and set up a plan of recording signs and symptoms of complications that could occur as some of the dosages of medications were reduced or discontinued. The staff nurses were informed of the plan of care and instructed on documentation on a special form.

With her current condition, Mrs. Rhodes is admitted beyond the 23-hour admission. During her brief stay of three days, the CNS works with the case manager to initiate home health care visits with home-maker services. Transportation is arranged with the local Area on Aging office to assure return visits to the physician for follow-up.

3. What roles are exhibited by a preceptor in a clinical setting?
4. Identify the organization that mandates ethical responsibility in the support of client advocacy by RNs, including APNs?
5. Identify the items that need to be submitted to a medical staff board in order to be reappointed for admitting/practice privileges as an APN.
6. List the requirements for continuing education that are necessary to maintain standards of practice as an APN.
7. Name the various governing bodies that have the responsibility and authority to implement rules and regulations regarding prescriptive privileges for APN practice.
8. Reimbursement services for APNs are rarely equal to those for physicians. Discuss how this difference affects the APN's practice within a group of physicians.
9. Identify the benefits of APN practice in the care of chronic illnesses across the life span.

References

American Association of Colleges of Nursing. (1994). *Annual report: Unifying the curricula for advanced practice.* Washington, DC: Author.

American Nurses Association. (2003). *Nursing's social policy statement* (2nd ed.). Washington, D.C.: ANA.

American Nurses Association. (2004). *Nursing: Scope & standards of practice.* Washington, D.C.: ANA.

Archibald, P., & Bainbridge, D. (1994). Capacity and competence: Nurse credentialing and privileging. *Nursing Management, 25* (4), 49–56.

Carson, W. (1993). *Prescriptive authority information packet.* Washington, DC: American Nurses Association, Nurse Practice Council.

Craven, R. F. (1998). Core curriculum for NP/CNS education. In A. Luggen, S. Travis, & S. Meiner (Eds.), *NGNA core curriculum for gerontological advanced practice nurses.* Thousand Oaks, CA: Sage.

Douglass, L. M. (1996). *The effective nurse: Leader and manager* (5th ed.). St. Louis: Mosby.

Gray, W., & Anderson, T. (1991). *Mentoring style for college students.* Vancouver, BC: International Center for Mentoring.

Green, A. H., & Conway, C. (1995). Negotiating capitated rates for nurse managed clinics. *Nursing Economics, 13* (2), 104–106.

Hilgart, C. M., & Karl, M. H. (1995). Developing clinical protocols and guidelines for APN practice. In M. Snyder & M. Mirr (Eds.), *Advanced practice nursing: A guide to professional development,* (pp. 93–101). New York: Springer.

Kenney, J. W. (1999). *Philosophical and theoretical perspectives for advanced nursing practice* (2nd ed.). Sudbury, MA: Jones & Bartlett.

Kyle, M. (1995). Collaboration. In M. Snyder & M. Mirr (Eds.), *Advanced practice nursing: A guide to professional development.* New York: Springer.

Lambert, V. A., & Lambert, C. E. (1996). Advanced practice nurses: Starting an independent practice. *Nursing Forum, 31* (1), 11–21.

Luggen, A. S., Travis, S. S., & Meiner, S. (Eds.) (1998). *NGNA core curriculum for gerontological advanced practice nurses.* Thousand Oaks, CA: Sage.

Marquis, B. L., & Huston, C. J. (1996). *Leadership roles and management functions in nursing: Theory and application* (2nd ed.). Philadelphia: Lippincott.

McKenna, H. (1997). *Nursing theories and models.* New York: Rutledge.

Meiner, S. (1998). Clinical privileges. In A. Luggen, S. Travis, & S. Meiner (Eds.), *NGNA core curriculum for gerontological advanced practice nurses.* Thousand Oaks, CA: Sage.

Orsund-Gassiot, C., & Lindsey, S. (1991). *Handbook of medical staff management.* Gaithersburg, MD: Aspen.

Pearson, L. J. (1997). Annual update of how each state stands on legislative issues affecting advanced nursing practice. *Nurse Practitioner, 22* (1), 18–86.

Robinson, D. & Kish, C.P. (2001). *Core concepts in advanced practice nursing.* St. Louis: Mosby.

Rubotszy, A.M. (1998) Marketing strategies. In A. Luggen, S. Travis & S. Meiner (Eds.) *NGNA Core Curriculum for gerontological advanced practice nurses,* (pp. 251–253). Thousand Oaks, CA: Sage.

Safriet, B. J. (1992). Health care dollars and regulatory sense: The role of advanced practice nursing. *Yale Journal on Regulation, 9,* 417–487.

Sheets, V. R. (1993). Second licensure? ANA and NCSBN debate the issue. *The American Nurse, 25,* 8–9.

Snyder, M., Mirr, M., Lindeke, L., Fagerlund, K., et al. (1999). Advanced practice nursing: An overview. In M. Snyder & M. Mirr (Eds.), *Advanced practice nursing: A guide to professional development* (2nd ed.), (pp. 1–24). New York: Springer.

Spector, R. E. (1996). *Cultural diversity in health and illness* (4th ed.). Stamford, CT: Appleton & Lange.

Taylor, R. S., & Schub, C. (1996). Medicare risk plans: The health plan's view. In P. R. Kongstvedt (Ed.), *The managed health care handbook* (3rd ed.), (pp. 715–740). Gaithersburg, MD: Aspen.

United States Department of Health and Human Services (1996). *International classification of diseases* (9th ed.). Los Angeles, CA: Practice Management Information Corporation.

CHAPTER 21

Complementary, Alternative and Integrative Therapies

Linda A. Moore ▪ Kathryn Jones

Introduction

Alternative and complementary treatments are often sought by individuals independent of their allopathic providers. An alternative or complementary therapy may be a healthy intervention but considered "unapproved" by allopathic providers. However, times are changing, and many allopathic providers are integrating alternative and complementary therapies with western allopathic (evidence-based) treatments to improve client outcomes. Complementary and alternative medicine (CAM) practitioners wish to work cooperatively with traditional health care professionals to develop a holistic, client-centered approach to care within an integrated health care system (Barrett et al., 2004). Maximizing the body's healing ability by combining traditional approaches to care with alternative therapies can better treat the whole person through physical, mental and spiritual methods rather than just the pathological process (Barnes, Powell-Griner, McFann, & Nahin, 2004). A quote by Henry David Thoreau may best describe complementary and alternative medicine. "Nature is doing her best each moment to make us well. She exists for no other end. Do not resist. With the least inclination to be well, we should not be sick." (cited in Pizzorno & Murray, 1999, p. 3.).

While much of the past literature has referred to alternative therapies, this chapter will use the word "alternative" when specifically described as such in the literature; however, medical schools that teach concepts of complementary/alternative therapies have chosen to use the term *integrative medicine* when such therapies are used in combination with traditional western, allopathic medicine.

Alternative and complementary therapies are not new and have been utilized for thousands of years. In the past these treatments were sole therapies for disease before antibiotics, physical therapy, chiropractic, and other treatment modalities were available. Some 'old' therapies are now receiving a second look. As an example, bloodletting is gaining resurgence for polycythemia, but it has also been used in treating epilepsy, pneumonia and hydrocephalus (Byard, 2001). The bloodletting of ancient times was probably the precursor of the current concepts of therapeutic phlebotomy (i.e.hemochromatosis, in which excessive iron is removed from the blood) and plasmaphoresis (Rakel, 2000). Leeching is being studied and utilized for its hemolytic treatment and for improving venous supply for free-flap skin grafts (Thearle, 1998).

Complementary and alternative (CAM) therapies are increasing in popularity in the United States.

Whether this interest is related to the cost of traditional health care, difficulty getting an appointment in a timely manner for a non-acute problem, or the recommendation of a friend about the success of a particular remedy, the interest is there. Of importance to the health care professional is how these alternative therapies may interact with traditional, evidenced based Western medicine

Recent surveys estimate that from 50 to 70 percent of adults in the United States use one or more alternative therapies (Fontaine, 2005). Other researchers have found that total visits to alternative care providers exceed visits to conventional practitioners (Bodane & Brownson, 2002; Eisenberg et al., 2001; Kaler & Revella, 2002; Kessler, Davis, & Foster, 2001). It is estimated that over $30 billion is spent annually on various alternative therapies (Ambrose & Samuels, 2004), and with continued use of the internet and increased availability of information, this dollar amount will continue to rise.

This chapter will focus on some of the more popular complementary and alternative therapies that may be used as integrative therapies. "Walking in balance," the Native American culture philosophy of peaceful coexistence and harmony with all aspects of life (Fontaine, 2005), best describes how complementary and alternative therapies should blend with traditional Western medicine.

Why Individuals Seek Integrative/Complementary Treatments

Clients with chronic illness live with varied symptoms such as chronic pain, shortness of breath, fatigue, or abdominal discomfort. Traditional or allopathic medicine may offer short term relief to a certain degree, but tends to fall short of long term relief or cure. The three most common conditions for which adults use CAM are back pain or discomfort (16.8%), head or chest cold (9.5%) and neck pain (6.6%) (Barnes et al., 2004).

Many potential clients of healthcare believe that the goal of their health care professional is to

offer drug therapy at the expense of alternative therapies such as psychotherapy, social approaches, nutritional, herbal, and natural remedies, rehabilitation, general hygienic measures, or non-patentable drugs. The client perception is that pharmaceutical companies, physicians and health care professionals make a profit prescribing drugs (Whitaker, 1995). These inaccurate client perceptions may cause a sense of distrust in the health care professional, and cause the client to further reject treatments offered by allopathic providers. Once the client and family trust and confidence is lost, it is difficult if not impossible to re-establish that relationship. Belief and confidence in the practitioner is crucial for adherence and treatment success. Trust has to be maintained in the very industry that was thought to treat and preserve life, the medical field. Other countries (i.e., Australia, Germany) have already recognized collaboration between practitioners using CAM and 'regular' doctors in order to provide safe and effective management for clients (Cohen, 2004).

In the United States, CAM practitioners confront barriers when working with providers of traditional medicine. Barrett et al. (2004) interviewed 32 CAM practitioners to identify the positives and negatives of integrating conventional medicine and complementary medicine. While CAM practitioners wanted to collaborate with traditional medicine, there were barriers to accessing health care facilities, and negative attitudes and beliefs from 'regular' practitioners, all impediments to integrating CAM with Western medicine

The Centers for Disease Control (CDC) conducted a survey of the most commonly used complementary and alternative medicines (CAM). The survey utilized the data from the 2002 National Health Interview Survey (NHIS). Over 31,000 interviews were conducted with individuals over the age of 18 years of age who had used CAM within the past 12 months. The results indicated that over 60% of adults surveyed used some form of complementary or alternative therapy (Barnes et al., 2004) (see Table 21-1). Areas of high use included:

TABLE 21-1

Prayer	45.2%
Prayer specifically for one's own health	43.0%
Prayer by others for one's own health	24.4%
Prayer groups for one's own health	9.6%
Healing ritual for one's own health	2.0%
Nonvitamin, nonmineral, natural products	18.9%
Deep breathing exercises	11.6%
Meditation	7.6%
Chiropractic care	7.5%
Yoga	5.1%
Massage	5.0%
Diet-based therapies	3.5%
Progressive relaxation	3.0%
Megavitamin therapy	2.8%
Guided imagery	2.1%
Homeopathy	1.7%
Tai chi	1.3%
Acupuncture	1.1%
Energy healing/Reiki	0.5%

SOURCE: Barnes et al., 2004, p. 8

Percentages exceed 100% because a number of individuals used more than one therapy.

Problems and Issues Related to Complementary and Alternative Therapies

There are many issues surrounding treatments with complementary and alternative modalities. Seeking and finding a reputable and competent clinician in this arena can be daunting. Some treatments conflict with spiritual, social, familial values, traditional medical therapies and beliefs. For example, research with cannabis extracts (marijuana) has met with opposition due to the social aspects of encouraging the use of an illegal substance. However, research has found that cannabis extracts can improve neurogenic symptoms that have been unresponsive to traditional therapies (Wade, Robson, House, Makela, & Aram, 2003; Smith, 2004). Additionally, this socially unacceptable therapy has been found to decrease intraocular pressure and thereby aid in the treatment of glaucoma (Duke, 1997).

Some alternative therapies may be incongruent with allopathic treatment plans and be dangerous. Combining certain herbals/supplements with prescribed medications may have potential risks if this information is not shared with the client's health care professional (Barnes et al., 2004).

In addition to the concern about herbals and interactions with traditional therapies, it has also been found that some individuals experience increased anxiety while practicing relaxation techniques. Lazarus and Mayne (1990) found that relaxation techniques had some limitations and side effects that needed to be considered. Others have written about side effects and negative responses to techniques for stress management (Astin, Shapiro, Eisenberg, & Forys, 2003; Woolfolk & Lehrer, 1993).

Many available alternative therapies and modalities have no credible scientific basis, and therefore insurance companies may not recognize those treatments as reimbursable benefits. Clients presume that herbs for prevention and treatment purposes are safe because they consider these therapies as "natural"; however, that is certainly not always the case. A lack of published research with alternative therapies leaves practitioners and insurance companies in a gray area of treatment/non-treatment from these therapies (Zink & Chaffin, 1998). However, a lack of published research may not affect a client's usage of such therapies. In a study of clients with confirmed tissue biopsies for cancer, 8% to 10% of clients had sought alternative therapies immediately (Cassileth, 1999; Cassileth & Deng, 2004).

Although the United States is just now recognizing the value of integrating CAM with traditional therapies, European countries, such as Germany, have already found these therapies to be beneficial. Dr. Niki Knold, a German physician, explains that alternative therapies are used before traditional medications (personal conversations, September, 2003, December 2003, and June 2004; Blumenthal, 2000). If integrative therapies are to be considered beneficial, it is important that insurance companies see that value as well. One of the first insurance companies that has supported integrative/complementary therapies is Blue Cross and Blue Shield. They developed ALT MED BLUE which provides a 25% reduction in the cost of selected integrative therapies such as: massage, chiropractic care, stress management, biofeedback, yoga, acupuncture, guided imagery, and nutrition education (www.bcbsnc.com/blueextras/altmed). Other insurance companies may provide similar programs in response to public outcry for treatment alternatives that have scientific and clinical data supporting outcomes.

Previous arguments by insurance companies have suggested that allopathic providers do not accept complementary therapies. This thinking forces clients to substitute alternative care with, perhaps, expensive medications that their insurance will cover. This mindset prevents the client from having choices since they become responsible for the full cost of treatment. One example is the client with chronic back pain. Chiropractic care is scientifically reputable, has been replicated in numerous studies, and may provide better relief than pain medications and muscle relaxants (Carey, Garrett, Jackson & Hadler, 1999). As with any therapy or medication, insurance companies decide the coverage, if any. Reimbursement may be considered by insurance companies on a case-by-case basis depending on the diagnosis and recognized data that supports the therapy. This process can be time consuming and requires a tenacious client and health care professional to pursue insurance coverage for an alternative treatment.

Clients don't always consider the cost or interactions when selecting vitamins, herbals, or other therapies and that they may have to cover the entire expense for "non-proven" therapies. An example of this is the herb, hawthorn. This herb has been useful in treating hypertension. According to Dr. Julian Whitaker, a noted "wellness" MD in California, hawthorn (Crataegus monogyna) reduces angina attacks by dilating coronary vessels, and has been used in the treatment of heart failure (Whitaker, 1995, p.157). However, its cost and interaction with other anti-hypertensives has the potential to be very detrimental (Duke, 1997).

Use of complementary and integrative therapies is reaching a wider audience since the National Institutes of Health have recognized the need for further documented benefits or the lack of significant effects. Acceptance of complementary therapies by health care professionals benefits both the client and the provider and allows individuals to inform the provider about currently used therapies to ensure that there are no interactions with therapies.

Evidence-Based Practice

The missions of the National Center for Complementary and Alternative Medicine (NCCAM) at the National Institutes of Health (NIH) have been to: 1) explore complementary and alternative practices using rigorous scientific methodology; 2) to train researchers; and 3) to provide the public with authoritative information (P.L. 102-170, October 1991). By 2004 eighteen research centers were established to explore the safety and efficacy of various therapies (http://nccam.nih.gov). To expand the knowledge base of alternative and complementary therapies, NCCAM supports a broad-based portfolio of research with educational grants, contracts and research funding (The NIH Almanac-Organization, National Center for Complementary and Alternative Medicine, www.nih.gov, 2004), all to expand evidence based practice using alternative and complementary therapies.

In addition to the NCCAM, the NIH Office of Dietary Supplements supports and conducts research related to the role of dietary supplements on health. The Office of Dietary Supplements (ODS) originated from the Dietary Supplement Health and Education Act of 1994 (P.L. 103-417, DSHEA) and was developed to explore the role of dietary supplements in improving health care through scientific study (dietary-supplements.info.nih.gov). Further research is necessary due to the phenomenal increase in the number of self-help books found in American households, information on the internet and the proliferation of health food stores that provide information without research evidence (Office of Dietary Supplements, http://dietary-supplements. info.nih.gov).

While research continues to support a scientific basis for alternative therapies, clinical evidence has long been a method of informal documentation often times based on limited case studies. With the addition of the NCCAM at NIH, more evidence-based practice will be identified in using various therapies. In evaluating resources, one must be cognizant of research methodology to better analyze the information being presented. Often a marketing expert, not a researcher, is the one convincing the reader of the success of the therapy.

Qualitative research is being accomplished to determine individuals' perceptions and their responses (Astin et al., 2003) and the use of some complementary treatments has been validated from these experiences (Barnes et al., 2004). However, use of some complementary therapies has been based largely on clinical effects—in other words, an individual's perception of the therapy. If the modality seems to work for a number of persons, the person using the modality will continue.

Complementary and Alternative Interventions

Alternative and complementary therapies may augment allopathic care. In cancer, clients may benefit from dietary changes, exercise, and different herbs (Redd, Montgomery & DuHamel, 2001; Syrjala, Donaldson, Davis, Karppa, & Carr, 1995). Clients with cardiac disease may benefit from prayer that decreases the length of their hospital stay and affects their mortality and morbidity in a positive manner (Harris et al., 1999). It is beneficial to utilize all treatment modalities that can facilitate healing, stimulate immune function and reduce inflammation.

Studies (Astin, 1998; Quinn, 2000) have demonstrated specific reasons why consumers choose alternative therapies. Reasons include: seeking a degree of wellness not supported in traditional medicine; quality of life issues; involvement in the decisions about health and care; lack of effectiveness from conven-

tional medicines; avoiding toxicities of conventional medicine; and identifying a healing system that is a part of one's cultural background. Health care professionals need to have a level of understanding of the various types of therapies that clients may use.

Holistic Health Care

Holistic care considers all aspects of the mind, body and spirit. Currently, there are few educational institutions that are educating physicians in the use of complementary and alternative health care practices. However, centers of integrative health have expanded throughout the country to provide individuals with an alternative way of managing their health through using traditional western medicine and complementary and integrative care. In November 2004, there were 25 academic health centers that were part of the Consortium of Academic Health Centers for Integrative Medicine (Consortium of Academic Health Centers, www.pcintegrativemedicine.org/documents/ConsortiumSummary. pdf). The mission of the Consortium is to educate the public and conduct research regarding integrative medicine. Top medical schools in the Consortium include Harvard, Duke University, and Georgetown.

Nursing has continued to move toward a caring and healing model (Watson, 1997). Nursing is a combination of science and art. The science component has been more widely studied, and advances described in the literature. The art of nursing is less clearly defined. Nurses who practice care in a holistic manner consider the whole individual and include health and wellness within the context of the illness. It must be recognized that individuals make choices about their care and these choices affect their health/wellness continuum. It is imperative that the nursing professional be attuned to a client's perceptions, values, beliefs, attitudes, stages of change and the barriers to motivation to help move individuals to their maximum wellness potential (Gaydos, 2005).

Some alternative and complementary therapies describe the concept of body and mind interaction in terms of an aura or the energy field that surrounds the individual. Nursing has recognized the importance of the cultural aspects of care and the holistic concept of mind, body and spirit in the development of nursing art and science. Nursing theories have focused on this concept of holistic care and energy fields with the most well known being Martha Rogers and her nursing theory of unitary human beings and the use of therapeutic touch (Rogers, 1990). There is a certificate program in Healing Touch for Health Care Professionals offered by the American Holistic Nurses Association (AHNA), and this program has expanded the concept of therapeutic touch (Fontaine, 2005).

Cultural Integration

The inclusion of complementary and integrative health is an area that may be associated with one's culture and ethnic background. Included within culture is the concept of spirituality. Many alternative therapies have originated through traditions of spirituality (Krippner, 1995). Most spiritual traditions share the concept that energy is the link between the spirit and the physical being (Fontaine, 2005). Each culture has a different view of this energy and describes it in terms of the connection to providing wholeness in one's life.

Many American populations continue to utilize aspects of their ancestry for healing and comfort. These modalities can be spiritual, nutritional, behavioral, and familial. Familiarity can be very comforting when one is challenged with a life-threatening illness. Laying on of hands, spiritual prayers, and other rituals can provide significant change in outcomes for clients. There is profound comfort and rest when clients relinquish control to their "higher power". Ayurveda, practiced in India, is one example of how a traditional modality is practiced at the national level within the Federal health system of India (Barnes et al., 2004).

Many integrative therapies originated thousands of years ago and date back to spiritual customs of various groups. Yoga, originally from India, is one example and focuses on unification of the mind, body and inner spirit with the universe (Sivananda Yoga Vedanta Center, 1998).

Chakras (the Hindu concept of energy) describes seven energy centers that provide the electromagnetic activity and the circulation of vital energy (Shang, 2001). This concept is described by several South American cultures and many Eastern cultures. The seven chakras are vertically aligned through the center midline of the body and each represents a focal point relating to physical, emotional and spiritual aspects of one's life. The purpose of chakras is to maintain equilibrium of health, and individuals skilled in the techniques of working with chakras can feel if the energy source is not in balance (Shang, 2001; Slater, 1995) .

This energy concept has expanded to western culture with a program by Dr. Dean Ornish to reverse coronary artery blockage. Ornish (1999) uses the heart chakra and integrates diet, exercise, support groups and meditation into his program.

Several of the CAMs practiced today relate to specific cultures. Ayurveda is practiced at the national level in India, and Kampo is the herbal medicine system practiced in Japan. Additionally, the multiple therapies from China (i.e., acupuncture, acupressure, herbal medicine, tai chi, and qi qong) are a part of the national system of health care in their countries (Barnes, et al., 2004).

While the United States is in the infancy of evaluating complementary and alternative therapies, European countries have been consistently at the forefront regarding alternatives to care. The most reputable source is from Germany with the Commission E reports of alternatives (Blumenthal, 2000).

The United States provides a source titled *PDR on Herbals* (2000). This volume is similar to the traditional *Physicians Desk Reference* (PDR).

Selecting a Practitioner

There are inconsistencies in licensure and certification for many practitioners of integrative treatments. For example, a licensed, (graduate from a board-certified massage school) massage therapist can legitimately perform a massage, but it would be best if the therapist had a national certification. This certification recognizes a standard knowledge-base for all massage therapists. There are state-by-state regulations for licensure and practice. The various states' boards of medicine and the state laws provide detailed information on the registration, licenses required to practice various forms of alternative and complementary therapies (www.healthy.net/public/legal-lg/regulations/acustlaw.htm).

It is difficult for the average health care consumer to decide what provider is reputable and skilled. As previously discussed, word of mouth and recommendations by trusted healthcare professionals are excellent sources for referral. Certification boards and schools which teach a certain modality are other sources for reputable providers. Some insurance companies have limits on coverage as they do with physical/occupational therapy and will cover only a certain number of visits for therapies (i.e., acupuncture, massage). Clients may need to check with their individual insurance companies as to reimbursement.

Reputable and Competent Clinicians

As with allopathic medicine, there are "specialists" in integrative therapies. Many clients have been to a "specialist" in allopathic medicine, and the same experts exist within complementary medicine. Complementary practitioners may specialize in one or two therapeutic options. There are healthcare professionals who overlap in their skills, such as a medical doctor or nurse practitioner who is also certified in acupuncture or acupressure. Verification of credentialing and/or certification before utilizing complementary providers is essential. Build a network of reputable integrative providers and share it with your colleagues.

There are certain statements by alternative care providers that are danger signals that the provider should be avoided. Tiedje (1998) offers these guidelines:

■ If they say they have all the answers;
■ If they maintain that theirs is the only effective therapy;

■ If they promise overnight success;
■ If they refuse to include other practitioners as part of the healing team; and
■ If they seem more interested in money than in people's well-being.

Treatment Modalities

Healthcare professionals should assist clients in making decisions that will be therapeutic and beneficial for their particular symptoms or diagnosis. Considering the therapies in Table 21-2 requires recognizing the basic program of naturopathic healing as explained below by Murray & Pizzorno (1991).

1. The elimination of evil habits "over-eating, alcoholic beverages, drugs, tobacco, tea, coffee, cocoa, meat eating, sexual and social aberrations, improper hours of living . . ." (Murray & Pizzorno, 1991, p. 5).
2. Corrective Habits: "Correct breathing, correct exercise, right mental attitude. Moderation in the pursuit of health and wealth" (Murray & Pizzorno, 1991, p.5).
3. New Principles of Living: "Proper fasting, selection of food, hydrotherapy, light and air baths, mud baths, osteopathy, chiropractic and other forms of mechanotherapy . . ." (Murray & Pizzorno, 1991, p. 5).

For this chapter, alternative therapies have been grouped into several systems of care. This list is not all-inclusive, but provides an overview.

Manual Healing Therapies

There are a number of therapies involving physical touch that have continued for generations. ***Selected examples*** of these as noted in Table 21-2 are discussed in this section.

Chiropractic Medicine Chiropractic practice considers vertebral manipulation an important practice to prevent and improve chronic pain, decrease per-

TABLE 21-2

Complementary and Alternative Modalities and/or Integrative Modalities

Category of Modality	Specific Modalities
MANUAL HEALING THERAPIES	Chiropractic Osteopathy Massage (Myofascial, Rolfing, Shiatsu, Swedish) Therapeutic Touch Laying on of hands Acupressure Acupuncture Reflexology Craniosacral therapy
MIND/BODY THERAPIES	Yoga/ Tai Chi Meditation Hypnosis Light therapy Color and/or Music Therapy Relaxation
SPIRITUAL	Prayer Pet Therapy Shamanism Imagery Ayurveda
ENERGY THERAPIES	Biofeedback Reiki Magnets Crystals Aroma therapy Polarity

NUTRITION AND SUPPLEMENTS	Diets (Low sodium for cardiac/
	   Hypertensive, Calorie and carbohydrate controlled for diabetes
	     mellitus
	   Low fat diets for cholesterol management
	   Weight control includes numerous diets (Weight Watchers, South
	     Beach, Atkins, Zone)
	Herbals
	Vitamins, minerals and specific foods
	Homeopathy
	Chelation Therapy

MOVEMENT THERAPIES	Kinesiology Dance Aquatherapy Tai Chi

sistent drug use and avoid certain surgeries with regular treatments. Research indicates that a majority of clients seek chiropractic care for musculoskeletal conditions of the back and neck (Hurwitz, Coulter, Adams, Genovese & Shekelle, 1998). The majority of this care is reduction of mal-alignment of the spinal bones. Most clients continue with their primary care provider while seeing a chiropractor for specific treatments (Sherman et al., 2004). In a study by Sherman et al. (2004), chiropractic has been used mostly by individuals with back pain (54%). Most respondents in this study indicated they would "very likely" try chiropractic, acupuncture or massage for back pain if their physician thought it was a reasonable treatment modality or if they did not have to pay an out of pocket expense (Sherman et al., 2004).

Doctors of Osteopathy   Osteopathy originated in the US in the last of the nineteenth century (Goldberg et al., 1994). Osteopaths are trained in allopathic principles; however, osteopaths treat the whole person instead of one system or a specified ailment. Osteopaths believe the structure of the body is intimately related to its function. Many forms of movement modalities may be incorporated into the healing plan. Osteopaths can prescribe medications as an adjunct to their movement and manipulation therapies. Traditionally, the osteopath blends conventional medicine with manipulative treatments to provide a comprehensive treatment plan. (Goldberg et al., 1994). Typically they use manual medicine techniques to relieve pain, restore range of motion and enhance the body's capacity to heal. Doctors of Osteopathic Medicine (D.O.s), like their medical counterparts, must pass a national or state board examination in order to obtain a license to practice medicine. There are over 37,000 D.O.s in all 50 states and the District of Columbia (American Association of Colleges of Osteopathic Medicine, 2004).

Mind/Body Therapies

A number of these therapies had their beginnings thousands of years ago in Asian countries

(Barnes et al., 2004). Some of the more common therapies will be discussed, while others in Table 21-2 can be reviewed in other sources.

Yoga   Yoga centers on meditation, breathing and postures (Oken et al., 2004). There are several techniques of yoga practiced with the most common in the United States being Iyengar yoga. This form uses a stationary position and then alternates isometric contraction and relaxation of various muscle groups (Oken et al., 2004). Oken et al. experimental study (2004) of 69 clients with multiple sclerosis using yoga, exercise class and a control group found that fatigue was decreased compared with the exercise class and the control group (p < 0.001).

Studies have shown some success with yoga in treating carpal tunnel syndrome. Symptoms were significantly improved when compared with wrist splints or the placebo effect, and there was a significant reduction of pain and increase in grip strength (Garfinkel et al., 1998).

Meditation   In 2002 National Health Interview Survey (NHIS), meditation was listed with the third highest use therapy after prayer and deep breathing exercises (Barnes et al., 2004). Research has documented physiologic effects from the practice of meditation (Goldberg et al., 1994). These effects include decreased blood pressure, decreased heart and respiratory rates, decreased oxygen consumption, increased elimination of carbon dioxide, increase in the number of alpha brain waves, and decreased plasma cortisol (Goldberg et al., 1994; Jevning, Wallace, & Beidebach, 1992). Astin et al. (2003), in a meta analysis of mind-body research, reported that meditation therapy had provided positive response to pain and treatment-related symptoms of cancer. Others have found evidence of decreasing risk factors in cardiovascular disease through the use of meditation and specifically, transcendental meditation (Parati & Steptoe, 2004; Walton, Schneider, & Nidich, 2004).

Hypnosis   Hypnosis is an ancient treatment modality dating back to ancient Greece where priests would give advice to persons while they were sleeping (Nash, 2001). Hypnosis is defined as a technique in which a trancelike state allows the individual to be more responsive to suggestions by another. There is a change in perception, memory and voluntary control of action (Goldberg et al., 1994). Research has indicated that brain activity of the hypnotized person is that of a fully awake individual and that there are specific changes in the activation and deactivation of specific brain structures (Feldman, 2004). Individuals may seek assistance from a hypnotist to manage smoking cessation, weight loss, stress management, insomnia, blood pressure control, and for improving memory.

There is board certification for hypnotherapists, which is the preferred word for the neurobiological and sociocognitive perspectives of hypnosis (Feldman, 2004; Friend, 1999; Gruzelier, 2000). Reviews of research conducted with hypnosis (Green & Lynn, 2000) have provided mixed reviews for specific uses such as smoking cessation. Other uses of hypnosis and existential psychotherapy have been found to be beneficial in the treatment of clients with terminal illnesses and intractable pain. Chronic substance abusers have also benefited from hypnosis training. A study by Pekala and associates (2004) found that self-hypnosis training and continued practice of it decreased the relapse of drug usage and improved the participants' self-esteem.

Therapeutic Touch

Therapeutic touch (TT) originates from the concept that an energy field extends around the individual (Krieger, 1979). The focus of the therapeutic touch and energy fields is that a transfer of energy occurs from the person acting as healer to help the person alter the energy pattern to a better state (Krieger, 1979). This transfer of energy helps correct imbalances and aids healing. Research has been conducted with therapeutic touch (TT) to include effects on pain, relaxation, decreasing anxiety, and improving rest (Gagne & Toye, 1994; Heidt, 1990; Hughes, Meize-Growchoski, & Harris, 1996; & O'Mathúna, 2004). The use of TT has been examined as a method of pain relief, especially with post-operative pain and headaches (O'Mathúna, 2004; Kelly, Sullivan, Fawcett, & Samarel, 2004).

Light Therapy Seasonal affective disorder (SAD) is depression that occurs during the long winter days when there is decreased sun and light. Further study into the alterations of mood indicate that not only is there evidence of depression, there is also lethargy, inability to concentrate and difficulty sleeping which are usually symptoms attributed to depression (Eagles, 2004; Johnson, 2000). SAD affects approximately 4-6 persons per 100 people and usually females over the age of 20. Therapy can be from a light box source or from a high-intensity fluorescent lamp that does not emit ultraviolet rays (Keegan, 2001). The process of exposure to white light has been effective. Szabo et al. (2004) found that light therapy increased static visual contrast sensitivity in clients and improved SAD. Sher et al. (2001) reported that after two weeks of a daily one hour regimen of light therapy, atypical depressive symptoms improved. It is suggested that long-term response to light therapy may be predicted by the early responses (Sher et al., 2001).

Spiritual Therapies In 2000 the National Institutes of Health initiated a five-year study to determine whether prayer intervention improves the health of clients with cancer. Since African American (AA) women are more likely to use spiritual healing than white women, the project has focused on AA women in the early stages of breast cancer. Dr. Diane Becker of Johns Hopkins University and Dr. Harold Koenig of Duke University have been the co-investigators on this study entitled "Centering Prayer." With CDC's study indicating that prayer is the most commonly used complementary therapy, it is important to determine the clinical and spiritual benefits of this modality (Barnes et al., 2004).

McCaffrey and colleagues (2004) found that faith is a critical part of health care and that physicians must consider this in their plan of care. Intercessory prayer (praying for others) has been suggested as an effective adjunct to standard medical care in one study of clients in a coronary care unit (Harris et al., 1999). The Cochrane Library provides an analysis of the research conducted with intercessory prayer and notes that over 1400 subjects have been studied in the use of prayer. While the review did not find that physiological outcomes were significantly improved, it was noted that the effects were psychologically beneficial (Roberts, Ahmed, & Hall, 2004).

Guided imagery has been associated with spiritual models of therapy. Lewandowski (2004) studied guided imagery to treat pain, and found that it appeared to have a potential useful effect for chronic pain sufferers. Antall & Kresevic (2004) have used guided imagery to manage pain in elderly clients following orthopedic surgery with both clinically and statistically significant results. Van Kuiken (2004) conducted a meta-analysis to determine the significance of guided imagery. Ten studies indicated that guided imagery had a positive effect over the first 5–7 weeks.

Energy Therapies

Biofeedback Biofeedback is useful in assisting individuals to take conscious control of autonomic processes. The electronic equipment in biofeedback uses physiological parameters (i.e., muscle tension, brain wave patterns, skin resistance, heart rate, and blood pressure) to provide information about responses to visualization, muscle stimulation, imagery or relaxation techniques (Keegan, 2001). In addition to its use in stress reduction and the reduction of blood pressure and pulse, biofeedback has been used in the management of urinary incontinence. Initial studies used biofeedback to treat incontinence following prostatectomy (Jackson, Emerson, Johnson, Wilson & Morales, 1996). Additional research has expanded its use to stress incontinence in which vaginal probes are used to monitor muscle tension (Davila & Guerette, 2004).

Reiki Reiki originated approximately 5000 years ago in Tibet, but the concept and its use was renewed in the 1800s in Japan (Gallob, 2003). In the Japanese language, reiki means "universal life energy," and it is based on the concept of unseen energy flows that occur in all living things. Reiki has been used to heal the body, emotions, mind, and spirit. Reiki used light hand placement to channel healing energies (Keegan, 2001).

Nutrition and Supplements

Vitamins, Minerals and Specific Diet Foods.

Antioxidants. An on-going study at the National Center for Complementary and Alternative Medicine (NCCAM) is evaluating natural antioxidants in the treatment of multiple sclerosis (MS). The specific treatments include ginkgo biloba, alpha-lipoic acid, vitamin E, selenium and essential fatty acids. Client outcomes of this study will be measured by the effects on MS lesions as seen by gadolinium-enhanced magnetic resonance imaging (http://www.clinicaltrials.gov/show/NCT00010842, September 2004).

Basic information has been published by the National Multiple Sclerosis Society on the use of vitamins, minerals and herbs in the treatment of MS. The National Multiple Sclerosis Society has several brochures on supplements and these can be obtained through the organization. Additionally, an introduction to vitamins, minerals, and herbs in MS is available on the internet (http://www.nationalmsscoiety.org/Brochures-Vitamins.asp, September 2004).

Vitamins have been used for generations to help maintain the body in healthy balance. With the increased availability of fast foods, today's generation is more likely to consume a diet that does not meet all of the vitamin essentials. The NCCAM has multiple clinical trials underway to document the effects of certain vitamins and minerals. The entire list of studies can be found on the NIH webpage. In 2004, more than 32,000 participants were recruited to be subjects in a five-year study to examine selenium and Vitamin E. Outcomes will be measured on the prevention, quality of life, and correlation with the incidence of prostate cancer and other disease processes such as Alzheimer's disease, macular degeneration, and cardiovascular events. (http://clinicaltrials.gov/show/NCT00056392).

The use of antioxidants has received wide discussion and evaluation in recent years. A nationwide clinical trial, supported by the National Eye Institute of NIH, and reported in the *Archives of Ophthalmology* in 2001, indicated that individuals at high risk for age-related macular degeneration could decrease this risk by 25% with a high-dose combination of vitamin C, vitamin E., beta-carotene, and zinc. These same nutrients had no effect on the development or progression of cataracts according to the Age-Related Eye Disease Study (AREDS, 2001).

A study initiated in 2004 study is evaluating the results of Vitamin E in aging individuals with Downs' syndrome. It has been hypothesized that Vitamin E can improve quality of life in persons with Downs' syndrome (http://clinicaltrials.gov/show/NCT00056329, September 2004). Other research sponsored by NCCAM is examining the effect of high doses of Vitamin E on carotid artherosclerosis (http://www.clinicaltrials.gov/show/NCT00010699, September 2004).

The use of Vitamin B_2 (Riboflavin) has demonstrated significance but low efficacy as a preventative treatment for migraine headaches. Research has compared the efficacy of riboflavin with selective serotonin reuptake inhibitors (SSRIs), calcium channel antagonists, gabapentin and topiramate (Silberstein & Goadsby, 2002). Use of riboflavin has been suggested for prevention of headaches; however, it is noted that significant research is lacking using controlled studies. Mauskop (2001) indicated that while the quantitative research has not been done, there are case studies and a smaller number of clinical evidence that supports the use of 200 mg riboflavin twice a day to prevent headaches.

Other Supplements

Glucosamine and Chrondroitin Conflicting research results have led the NCCAM to support a study that evaluates the use of the dietary supplements, glucosamine, chrondroitin, and a combination of glucosamine and chrondroitin when compared with Celecoxib and a placebo. Results

focus on outcomes in individuals with osteoarthritis and evaluate the reduction of pain and improvement in movement. Data analysis has been completed, and the report is due for publication in the near future. However, one issue with the study is that it was only six months in length and cannot speak to long term benefits (http://nccam.nih.gov/news/19972000/121100/qa.htm, September 2004).

Diets, Food Sources and Herbals "We are what we eat" is a commonly accepted phrase regarding choosing diets and food sources. This chapter does not include all of the available diets because many books are written on specific diets; however, diets cannot be overlooked when exploring the concept of alternative and complementary therapies.

In addition to specific diets, there are various food sources that have been investigated to determine either positive or negative aspects on disease processes or interaction with treatment modalities. Cranberry juice is one example of a supplement that has been studied for its physiological effect on urinary tract infections (UTI). Originally, it was hypothesized that cranberry juice changed the pH of urine. Instead, it was found that cranberry juice actually decreased the adherence of bacteria to cells thus helping with the prevention of UTIs (Raz, Chazan, & Dan, 2004). Grapefruit juice is an example of a food source that may have a negative effect with certain medications (Lilley, 1998; Blumenthal, 2000).

Several remedies have been suggested by urologists for treatment of the symptoms of an enlarged prostate gland. The most popular therapy is saw palmetto berry (Serenoa repens). It does not reduce the size of the prostate gland, but it assists in managing symptoms (Blumenthal, 2000). Research has been mixed on the results of the use of saw palmetto, and it is speculated that the results may be due to the amount of herbal used, the lack of controls and the length of the studies (Braeckman, 1994; Strauch et al., 1994). Review in *Clinical Evidence Concise* (2003) reported that saw palmetto improves symptoms compared with a placebo, and there was no difference in symptom scores between saw palmetto and finasteride, a commonly prescribed medication for benign prostatic hypertrophy (BPH).

Much has been discussed regarding herbals in the management of chronic conditions, and health care professionals need a reliable source for this information. Examples of successful clinical outcomes with herbals that have not been documented in the research literature include feverfew for migraines, chitosan for weight loss, evening primrose oil for premenstrual syndrome and for schizophrenia, Ginkgo biloba for intermittent claudication, melatonin for jet lag and peppermint for irritable bowel syndrome (Goldberg et al., 1994). In the true spirit of alternative medicine, Thomas Edison is quoted by naturopathic providers as saying "The doctor of the future will give no medicine, but will interest his patients in the care of the human frame, in diet, and in the cause and prevention of disease" (Goldberg et al., 1994).

Movement Therapies

Kinesiology Kinesiology is the study of muscles and their movements. With this information, practitioners analyze muscle function, posture, gait, and other movement activities that may affect health (Keegan, 2001). Currently, the research related to applied kinesiology is in its infancy (Gin & Green, 1997). Numerous articles about kinesiology have been published, but results are not conclusive at this point because there has been limited replication of studies (Schmitt & Leisman, 1998; Monti et al., 1999). Applied kinesiology uses acupressure to "reflex points" at specific muscles (Keegan, 2001).

Tai Chi While Tai Chi is considered a mind/body therapy due to the concentration and the focusing required of an individual, it, in fact, can likewise belong to movement therapies. As with mind/body therapies, movement therapies deal with increasing mental awareness of the body to improve posture and enhance muscle groups (Keegan, 2001). Tai Chi is a therapy with extensive flowing moves with graceful movements for health and meditation as well as self-defense (Keegan, 2001). History of this Chinese therapy dates back to 3000 BC and has been noted in cave paintings. Tai Chi, meaning big energy, is exactly that, generating and feeling energy through movement. This form of exercise has been documented to be beneficial in helping elderly clients with balance and movement (Wolf et al., 1993; Wolfson et al., 1993). In addition to improvement in balance, results from a randomized trial found that Tai Chi had a positive effect on blood pressure in older adults (Young, Appel, Jee, & Miller, 1999). Lan and associates (1999) likewise found the positive benefits of Tai Chi on cardiorespiratory function of adults following coronary artery bypass surgery.

Qigong Qigong has it historical roots in China and has been used for over 7000 years (Kemp, 2004). The intent is to balance the flow of vital energy (chi) along the acupuncture meridians or energy pathways. The primary focus of Qigong is "to reduce stress, improve blood circulation, enhance immune function and treat a variety of health conditions" (Keegan 2001, p. 199). Qigong differs from Tai Chi in that it includes breathing and relaxation exercises, meditation and massage along with other natural methods (Keegan, 2001). To obtain maximum benefits, one should enroll in a program and continue on a consistent basis because it may take months to obtain desired benefits.

Outcomes

By developing increased awareness of alternative and complementary therapies, clinicians can work together to provide an integrative approach to health care. Without a clear understanding of both traditional, western medicine and various CAM therapies, an individual may select one or the other without recognizing the value (either positive or negative) of each. Some have delayed traditional cancer therapy in favor of alternatives and others have chosen not to use researched treatments (i.e., diet therapy, meditation, biofeedback, yoga) to improve quality of life during cancer treatment (Cassileth, 1999; Cassileth & Deng, 2004). It is anticipated with additional research studies sponsored by NIH, more alternative and complementary therapies will become a part of integrative health care. The desired outcome of combining therapies is to treat the "whole" person within a holistic care framework. It is each health care professional's responsibility to assess and understand alternative and complementary therapies that are used by their clients and to anticipate interactions with traditional medicine. One issue is that it is difficult to track outcomes, especially when alternative therapies are used with traditional, western therapies (Lewis, deVedia, Reuer, Schwan, & Tourin, 2003).

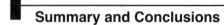

Summary and Conclusions

This chapter is not all inclusive of complementary, alternative and integrative therapies, but is meant to stimulate interest in further exploration of the kinds of therapies that clients use and the need for obtaining evidence that provides current and reliable information. An excellent start is accessing the National Institutes of Health for Complementary and Alternative Therapies (NCCAM) and the Office of Dietary Supplements.

Study Questions

1. How do complementary and alternative therapies differ from traditional western medicine?
2. Why do most people seek complementary therapies?
3. Compare costs of complementary therapies versus traditional medicine.
4. How does the nurse respond to clients describing the use of alternative therapies?
5. What are the benefits to incorporating complementary therapies with traditional medicine?
6. How can allopathic providers utilize alternative therapies in their practices?
7. What are 2 governmental sources for reviewing pertinent data and information on CAM therapies?
8. Describe two movement therapies.
9. Do insurance companies recognize CAM as legitimate alternatives or complements to allopathic treatment? Do they reimburse for these CAM treatments?

References

Age Related Eye Disease Study Group (2001). A randomized, placebo-controlled, clinical trial of high-dose supplementation with vitamins C and E and beta carotene for age related cataract and vision loss: AREDS report no. 9. *Archives of Ophthalmology, 119,* (10), 1439–1452.

Ambrose, E. T., & Samuels, S. (2004). Perception and use of herbals among students and their practitioners in a university setting. *Journal of the American Academy of Nurse Practitioners, 16* (4), 166–173.

American Association of Colleges of Osteopathic Medicine (2004). History. http://www.aacom.org/om.history. html. (Retrieved, 12/23/2004).

Antall, G. F. & Kresevic, D. (2004). The use of guided imagery to manage pain in an elderly orthopaedic poluation. *Orthopaedic Nursing, 23* (5), 335–340.

Astin, J. A. (1998). Why patients use alternative medicine: Results of a national study. *The Journal of the American Medical Association, 279,* 1548–1553.

Astin, J. A., Shapiro, S. L., Eisenberg, D. M., & Forys, K. L. (2003). Mind-body medicine: State of the science, implications for practice. *Journal of the American Board of Family Practice, 16,* 131–147.

Barnes, P. M., Powell-Griner, E, McFann, K., & Nahin, R. L. (2004). *Complementary and alternative medicine use among adults: United States, 2002.* U.S. Department of Health and Human Services: Centers for Disease Control and Prevention, National Center for Health Statistics, Number 343, May 27, 2004.

Barrett, B., Marchand, L., Scheder, J., Appelbaum, D., et al. (2004). What complementary and alternative medicine practitioners say about health and health care. *Annuals of Family Medicine, 2* (3), 253–259.

Blue Cross/Blue Shield of North Carolina. (www.bcbsnc.com/blueextras/altmed), retrieved 1/03/05.

Blumenthal, M. (Ed.). (2000). *Complete German commission E monographs.* Austin, TX: American Botanical Council.

Bodane, C., & Brownson, K. (2002). The growing acceptance of complementary and alternative medicine. *The Health Care Manager, 20* (3),11–22.

Braeckman, J. (1994). The extract of Serenoa repens in the treatment of benign prostatic hyperplasia: A multicenter open study. *Current Therapeutic Research, 55,* 776–785.

Byard, R.W. (2001). Bloodletting and leeching: Instruments of healing or torture? *The Medical Journal of Australia, 175,* 665 (www.mja.com.au/public/issues, retrieved, 12/21/2004).

Carey, T. S., Garrett, J. M., Jackson, A. C., & Hadler, N. (1999). Recurrence and care seeking after acute back pain: Results of a long term follow up study. *Medical Care,* 37(2), 157–164.

Cassileth, B.R. (1999). Evaluating complementary and alternative therapies for cancer patients. *CA: A Cancer Journal for Clinicians, 49* (6), 362–375.

Cassileth, B.R., & Deng, G. (2004). Complementary and alternative therapies for cancer. *Oncologist, 9* (1), 80–89.

Clinical Evidence Concise (2003). London: BMJ Publishing Group.

Cohen, M.M. (2004). CAM practitioners and "regular" doctors: Is integration possible? *Medical Journal of Australia, 180* (12), 645–646.

Consortium of Academic Health Centers for Integrative Medicine. www.pcintegrativemedicine.org/documents/ConsortiumSummary.pdf, retrieved 1/4/2005.

Davila G.W., & Guerette, N. (2004). Current treatment options for female urinary incontinence—A review. *International Journal of Fertility in Women's Medicine, 49* (3), 102–12.

Deng, G., Cassileth, B. R., & Yeung, K. S. (2004). Complementary therapies for cancer-related symptoms. *The Journal of Supportive Oncology, 2* (5), 419–426.

Duke, J. A. (1997). *The Green Pharmacy.* Emmaus, PA: Rodale Press.

Eagles, J. M. (2004). The seasonal health questionnaire is more effective at detecting seasonal affective disorder than the seasonal pattern adjustment questionnaire. *Evidence-Based Mental Health, 7* (3), 71.

Eisenberg, D. M., Kessler, R. C., Van Rompay, M. I., Kaptchuk, T. J., et al. (2001). Perceptions about complementary therapies relative to conventional therapies among adults who use both. *Annals of Internal Medicine, 135* (5), 344–351.

Feldman, J.B. (2004). The neurobioloby of pain, affect and hypnosis. *American Journal of Clinical Hypnosis, 46* (3), 187–200.

Fontaine, K. L. (2005). *Complementary & Alternative Therapies for Nursing Practice* (2nd ed.). Upper Saddle River, NJ: Pearson, Prentice Hall.

Friend, B. (1999). So you want to be a . . . hypnotherapist. *Nursing Times, 95* (7), 32–33.

Gagne, D., & Toye, R. (1994). The effects of therapeutic touch and relaxation therapy in reducing anxiety. *Archives of Psychiatric Nursing, 8* (3), 184–189.

Gallob, R. (2003). Reiki: a supportive therapy in nursing practice and self-care for nurses. *Journal of New York State Nurses Association, 34* (1), 9–13.

Garfinkel, M. S., Singhal, A., Katz, W. A., Allan, D. A., Reshetar, R., & Schumacher, H.R. (1998). Yoga-based intervention for carpal tunnel syndrome: a randomized trial. *Journal of the American Medical Association, 280* (18), 1601–1603.

Gaydos, H. L. B (2005). The art of holistic nursing and the human health experience. In B. Dossey, L. Keegan, & C. Guzzetta (Eds.), *Holistic Nursing: A Handbook for Practice.* Sudbury, MA: Jones & Bartlett.

Gin, R. H., & Green, B. N. (1997). George Goodheart, Jr., D. C. and a history of applied kinesiology. *Journal of Manipulative Physiological Therapeutics, 20* (5), 331–337.

Goldberg, B. et al. (1994). *Alternative Medicine: The Definitive Guide.* Fife, Washington: Future Medicine Publishing, Inc.

Green, J. P., & Lynn, S. J. (2000). Hypnosis and suggestion-based approaches to smoking cessation: An examination of the evidence. *International Journal of Clinical and Experimental Hypnosis, 48* (2), 195–224.

Gruzelier, J.H. (2000). Redefining hypnosis: Theory, methods and integration. *Contemporary Hypnosis, 17* (2), 51–70.

Harris W. S., Gowda, M., Kolb, J. W., Strychacz, C. P., et al. (1999). A randomized controlled trial of the effects of remote, intercessory prayer on outcomes of patients admitted to the coronary unit. *Archives of Internal Medicine, 159,* 2273–2278.

Heidt, P. R. (1990). Openness: A qualitative analysis of nurses' and patients' experiences of therapeutic touch. *Image: The Journal of Nursing Scholarship, 22* (3), 180–186.

Hughes, P., Meize-Growchowski, R., & Harris, C. (1996). Therapeutic touch with adolescent psychiatric patients. *Journal of Holistic Nursing,14* (1), 6–23.

Hurwitz, E. L., Coulter, I. D., Adams, A. H., Genovese, B. J., et al. (1998). Use of chiropractic services from 1985 through 1991 in the United States and Canada. *American Journal of Public Health, 88* (5), 771–776.

Jackson, J., Emerson, L., Johnson, B., Wilson, J., & Morales, A. (1996). Biofeedback: A noninvasive treatment for incontinence after radical prostatectomy. *Urologic Nursing, 16* (2), 50–54.

Jevning, R., Wallace, R. K., & Beidebach, M. (1992). The physiology of meditation: A review. *Neuroscience Behavior Review, 16* (3), 415–424.

Johnson, R. M. (2000). Diagnosing and managing seasonal affective disorder. *Nurse Practitioner, 25* (8), 56, 59–62, 68–70.

Kaler, M. M., & Revella, P. C. (2002). Staying on the ethical high ground with complementary and alternative medicine. *Nurse Practitioner, 27* (7), 38–42.

Keegan, L. (2001). *Healing with Complementary & Alternative Therapies.* Albany, NY: Thomson Learning.

Kelly, A. E., Sullivan, P., Fawcett, J., & Samarel, N. (2004). Therapeutic touch, quiet time and dialogue: Perceptions of women with breast cancer. *Oncology Nursing Forum, 31* (3), 625–631.

Kemp, C. A. (2004). Qigong as a therapeutic intervention with older adults. *Journal of Holistic Nursing, 22* (4), 351–373.

Kessler, R. C., Davis, R. B., & Foster, D. A. (2001). Long-term trends in the use of complementary and alternative medicine in the United States. *Annals of Internal Medicine, 135,* 262–268.

Krieger, D. (1979). Therapeutic touch and contemporary applications. In H. A. Otto & J. W. Knight (Eds.), *Dimensions in Holistic Healing: New Frontiers in the Treatment of the Whole Person,* (pp. 297–303). Chicago: Nelson-Hall.

Krippner, S. (1995). A cross-cultural comparison of four healing models. *Alternative Therapies in Health and Medicine, 1* (1), 21–29.

Lan, C., Chen, S. Y., Lai, J. S., & Wong, M. K. (1999). The effect of Tai Chi on cardiorespiratory function in patients with coronary artery bypass surgery. *Medicine and Science in Sports and Exercise, 31* (5), 634–638.

Lazarus, A. A. & Mayne, T. J. (1990). Relaxation: Some limitations, side effects, and proposed solutions. *Psychotherapy, 27,* 261–266.

Lewandowski, W. A. (2004). Patterning of pain and power with guided imagery. *Nursing Science Quarterly, 17* (3), 233–241.

Lewis, C. R., deVedia, A., Reuer, B., Schwan, R., & Tourin, C. (2003). Integrating complementary and alternative medicine (CAM) into standard hospice and palliative care. *American Journal of Hospice and Palliative Care, 20* (3), 221–228, 240.

Lilley, L. L. (1998). Grapefruit and medication. *American Journal of Nursing, 98* (12), 10.

Mauskop, A. (2001). Alternative therapies in headache: Is there a role. *Medical Clinics of North American, 8* (4), 1077–1084.

McCaffrey, A. M., Eisenberg, D. M., Legedza, A. T., Davis, R. B., et al. (2004). Prayer for health concerns: results of a national survey on prevalence and patterns of use. *Archives of Internal Medicine, 164* (8), 858–862.

Monti, D. A., Sinnott, J., Marchese, M., Kunkel, E. J., et al. (1999). Muscle test comparisons of congruent and incongruent self-referential statements. *Perceptual and Motor Skills, 88* (3), 1019–1028.

Murray, M., & Pizzorno, J. (1991). *Encyclopedia of Natural Medicine.* Rocklin, CA: Prima Publishing.

Nash, M. (2001). The truth and the hype of hypnosis. *Scientific American, 285,* 46–49, 52–55.

Oken, B. S., Kishiyama, S., Zajdel, D., Bourdette, D., et al. (2004). Randomized controlled trial of yoga and exercise in multiple sclerosis. *Neurology, 62,* 2058–2064.

O'Mathúna, D. P. (2004). Therapeutic touch for pain. *Alternative Therapies in Women's Health, 6* (3), 17–24.

Ornish, D. (1999). *Love and Survival: The Scientific Basis for the Healing Power of Intimacy.* New York: Harper Collins.

Parati, G., & Steptoe. A. (2004). Stress reduction and blood pressure control in hypertension: A role for transcendental meditation? *Journal of Hypertension, 22* (11), 2057–2060.

Pekala, R. J., Maurer, R., Kumar, V. K., Elliott, N. C., et al. (2004). Self-hypnosis relapse prevention training with chronic drug/alcohol users: Effects on self-esteem, affect, and relapse. *American Journal of Clinical Hypnosis, 46* (4), 281–297.

Physician's Desk Reference on Herbals, (2nd ed). (2000). Montvale, N.J.: Medical Economics Company.

Pizzorno, J., & Murray, M. (1999). *Textbook of Natural Medicine, Volume I and II.* New York: Churchill Livingstone.

Quinn, J. F. (2000). The self as a healer: Reflections from a nurse's journey. *AACN Clinical Issues, 11* (1), 17–26.

Rakel, R. (2000). *Saunders Manual of Medical Practice.* Philadelphia: Saunders.

Raz, R., Chazan, B., & Dan, M. (2004). Cranberry juice and urinary tract infection. *Clinical Infectious Disease, 38* (10), 1413–1419.

Redd, W. H., Montgomery, G. H., & DuHamel, K. N. (2001). Behavioral intervention for cancer treatment side effects. *Journal of the National Cancer Institute, 93,* 810–823.

Research, Research Centers Programs, funded Research Centers http://nccam.nih.gov. (Retrieved 12/23/04).

Roberts, L., Ahmed, I., & Hall, S. (2004). Intercessory prayer for the alleviation of ill health. *The Cochrane Library, 2004,* (4).

Rogers, M. E. (1990). Nursing science of unitary, irreducible, human beings: Update 1990. In E. A. M. Barrett, (Ed.), *Visions of Rogers' Science-Based Nursing.* New York: National League of Nursing.

Sand-Jecklin K., Hoggatt B., & Badzek L. (2004). Know the benefits and risks of using common herbal therapies. *Holistic Nursing Practice, 18* (4), 192–8.

Schmitt, W. H., Jr., & Leisman, G. (1998). Correlation of applied kinesiology muscle testing findings with serum immunoglobulin levels for food allergies. *International Journal of Neuroscience, 96* (3/4), 237–244.

_____ Selecting a Complementary and Alternative Medicine (CAM) Practitioner. nccam.nih.gov/health/practitioner/index.htm. (Retrieved 12/23/2004).

Shang, C. (2001). Emerging paradigms in mind-body medicine. *Journal of Alternative and Complementary Medicine, 7* (1), 83–91.

Sher, L., Matthews, J. R., Turner, E. H., Postolache, T. T., et al. (2001), Early response to light therapy partially predicts long-term antidepressant effects in patients with seasonal affective disorder. *Journal of Psychiatry and Neuroscience, 26* (4), 336–338.

Sherman, K. J., Cherkin, D. C., Connelly M. T., Erro, J., et al. (2004). Complementary and alternative medical therapies for chronic low back pain: What treatments are patients will to try? *BMC Complementary Alternative Medicine, 4*:9 http: www.biomedcentral.com/1472-68882/4/9, (retrieved 12/22/04)

Silberstein, S. D., & Goadsby, P. J. (2002). Migraine: Preventive treatment. *Cephalalgia, 22* (7), 491–512.

Sivananda Yoga Vedanta Center (1998). What is yoga? In I. Whitelaw & I. Lyford (Eds.) *Yoga: Mind & Body.* New York: D.K. Publishing

Slater, V. E. (1995). Toward an understanding of energetic health, Part 1: Energetic structures. *Journal of Holistic Nursing, 13* (3), 209–224.

Smith, P.F. (2004). Medicinal cannabis extracts for the treatment of multiple sclerosis. *Current Opinion of Investigational Drugs, 5* (7), 727–739.

Strauch, G., Perles, P. Vergult, G., Gabriel, M., et al. (1994). Comparison of finasteride (Proscar) and Serenoa repens (Permixon) in the inhibition of 5a-reductase in healthy male volunteers. *European Urology, 26,* 247–252.

Syrjala, K. L., Donaldson, G. W., Davis, M. S., Karppa, M. E., et al. (1995). Relaxation and imagery and cognitive-behavioral training reduce pain during cancer treatment: A controlled clinical trial. *Pain, 63,* 189–198.

Szabo, Z., Antal, A., Kalman, J., Keri, S., et al. (2004). Light therapy increases visual contrast sensitivity in seasonal affective disorder. *Psychiatry Research, 126* (1), 15–21.

Thearle, M. J. (1998). Leeches in medicine. *Australia, New Zealand Journal of Surgery, 68,* 292–295.

The NIH Almanac-Organization, National Center for Complementary and Alternative Medicine. www.nih.gov/about/almanac/organization/NCCAM.htm; (retrieved December 23, 2004).

The Office of Dietary Supplements. http://dietary-supplements.info.nih.gov/About/about_ods.aspx; (retrieved 12/23/2004).

Tiedje, L. B. (1998). Alternative health care: An overview. *Journal of Obstetric, Gynecologic and Neonatal Nursing, 27* (5), 557–562.

Van Kuiken, D. (2004). A meta-analysis of the effect of guided imagery practice on outcomes. *Journal of Holistic Nursing, 22* (2), 164–179.

Wade, D. T., Robson, P., House, H., Makela, P., et al. (2003). A preliminary controlled study to determine whether whole-plant cannabis extracts can improve intractable neurogenic symptoms. *Clinical Rehabilitation, 17,* 21–29.

Walton, K. G., Schneider, R. H., & Nidich, S. (2004). Review of controlled research on the transcendental meditation program and cardiovascular disease. Risk factors, morbidity and mortality. *Cardiology in Review, 12* (5), 262–266.

Watson, J. (1997). The theory of human caring: Retrospective and prospective. *Nursing Science Quarterly, 10* (1), 49–52.

Whitaker, J. (1995). *Dr. Whitaker's Guide to Natural Healing.* Rocklin, CA: Prima Publishing.

Wolf, S. L., Kutner, N. G., Green, R. C., & McNeely, E. (1993). The Atlanta FICSIT study: Two exercise interventions to reduce fragility in elders. *Journal of the American Geriatrics Society, 41* (3), 329–332.

Wolfson, L., Whipple, R., Judge, J., Amerman, P., et al. (1993). Training balance and strength in the elderly to improve function. *Journal of the American Geriatrics Society, 41* (3), 341–343.

Woolfolk, R. L. & Lehrer, D. M. (Eds.) (1993). *Principles and Practice of Stress Management* (pp. 139–168). New York: Guilford Press.

Young, D.R., Appel, L.J., Jee, S., & Miller, E.R. (1999). The effects of aerobic exercise and Tai Chi on blood pressure in older people: Results of a randomized trial. *Journal of the American Geriatrics Society, 47* (3), 277–284.

Zinc, T., & Chaffin, J. (1998). Herbal "health" products: What family physicians need to know. *American Family Physician, 58* (5), 1133–1140.

Internet Sources

http://www.clinicaltrials.gov/show/NCT00010842, September 2004. Natural Antioxidants in the Treatment of Multiple Sclerosis.

http://clinicaltrials.gov/show/NCT00056329, September 2004. Vitamin E in Aging Persons with Down Syndrom.

http://nccam.nih.gov/news/19972000/121100/qa.htm, September 2004. Questions and Answers: NIH Glucosamine/Chrondroitin Arthritis Intervention Trial (GAIT).

http://www.nationalmssociety.org/Brochures-Vitamins.asp, September 2004. National Multiple Sclerosis Society, Vitamins, Minerals, and Herbs in MS: An Introduction by A. Bowling and T. Stewart.

http://ods.od.nih.gov/factstheets/cc/vita.html, September 2004. Vitamin A and Carotenoids.

http://ods.od.nih.gov/factstheets/cc/vitb6.html, September 2004. Vitamin B_6.

http://ods.od.nih.gov/factstheets/cc/vitb12.html, September 2004. Vitamin B_{12}.

http://www.clinicaltrials.gov/show/NCT00010699, September 2004. Effect of High Dose Vitamin E on Carotid Atherosclerosis.

http://www.bravewell.org , The Consortium of Academic Health Centers for Integrative Medicine.

http://www.consumerlab.com. An independent laboratory that provides current information on therapies. There is a subscription cost.

http://www.healthy.net/public/legal-lg/regulations/acustlaw.htm provides information related to laws of each state.

PART IV

Impact of the System

CHAPTER 22

Home Health Care

Margaret M. Patton ▪ Gwendolyn F. Foss

Community based nurses are in an optimal position to identify and promote adaptation to chronic disease processes, resulting in fewer limitations.

Lundy & Janes (2001)

Introduction

Home health nursing is a dynamic specialty requiring outstanding knowledge and skill in assessing, intervening, and evaluating nursing actions (Hitchcock, Schubert & Thomas, 2003, p. 478). Home health care has achieved great popularity because of its holistic approach in helping clients manage their health care needs in the home setting. Home health nursing care is very much in keeping with nursing's focus of health by helping individuals to reach their optimum level of wellness and independence. Though most often associated with the Medicare-eligible elderly client, home care is provided to a much more diverse population that includes high-risk infants and persons of all age groups who have chronic illnesses or disabilities.

With the advent of Medicare, regulations were established that determine who is eligible to receive reimbursable home care services. Generally all third party payors adhere to Medicare regulations as the eligibility and payment standard for home care

agencies. In the event that the services received by a client are being privately paid, agencies are permitted, within specific state stipulations, to establish what the criteria for care will be within their own organizations. Agencies adhering to the Medicare Guidelines to receive Medicare and Medicaid payment are classified as "Certified." "Non-certified" home health agencies render home health care privately without consideration of the Medicare Guidelines, and thus receive no payment from Medicare. However, as a quality measure, private payment agencies often follow the standards of adequate care as established by Medicare.

Between 1980 and 1996, the home health care industry demonstrated a 400 percent increase in Medicare-sponsored home care alone. During that time period, the number of agencies certified to bill Medicare rose by 200 percent (Montauk, 1998). This was a direct result of many reimbursement changes affecting hospitals in the early 1980s. In a direct effort to control the cost of care in acute care hospitals, Congress passed a law in 1983, the Social Security Amendments of 1983 as they were called, to initiate the prospective payment system for inpatient services and to end the payment for a service after it is rendered to the client (Stanhope & Lancaster, 2002). Thus, the federal government authorized the shift from a cost-based system to a prospective payment system called diagnosis-related groups (DRGs). DRGs are a patient classification system defining 468 illness categories and the related and necessary health care services that are Medicare reimbursable. With reimbursement for hospital care now predetermined by client diagnosis, hospitals responded to the significant revenue reductions by decreasing the average length of stay for clients. The direct consequence was shorter hospital stays. With shorter hospital stays, home health and nursing home costs increased dramatically. According to the Health Care Financing Administration (HCFA), which was then the federal government's Medicare management agency, Medicare A expenditures increased from less than 50 billion dollars in 1980 to well over 200 billion dollars by 1997 (Stanhope & Lancaster, 2002).

Between 1993 and 2000, the number of home health agency employees increased by 26%, according to the National Association of Home Care (NACH) (2001). That was the apex of home health costs because what followed, with the passage of the Balanced Budget Act of 1997, forced home care costs to begin to decrease. Over the next 3 years with the Interim Payment System, followed by the introduction of the Prospective Payment System, the management of care required that the home care nurse administer the care by balancing both clinical and economic demands. Home care nurses have reduced their home visits by the number of visits in a given time period and the frequency of those visits and in

their overall management of each case, have reduced the visits of other disciplines, as well (Maurer & Smith, 2005).

The elderly population was affected most by the reimbursement changes. This population has the greatest incidence of disability and chronic illness and uses more health care services than the younger populations (Lundy & Janes, 2003). When DRGs started decreasing the amount of time and money that could be spent on clients with chronic illness in the hospital setting, home health care agencies increasingly provided care for clients who still needed nursing care. Hospitals developed a dependence on both certified home health agencies and skilled nursing facilities to provide needed acute, skilled posthospital care to clients who were being discharged from the hospitals "sicker and quicker" (Stanhope & Lancaster, 2002).

A home health agency may choose to participate in the Medicare program and can receive payment from Medicare for those clients who meet the eligibility criteria (Table 22-1). Agencies choosing not to participate in the Medicare program follow their respective state-established regulations that govern the provision of home care services.

Historical Perspectives

During the Renaissance (1500-1700 A.D.) society began to modify its belief that disease was punishment for sin and began to take care of its citizens

---

TABLE 22-1

Prerequisites for Medicare Entitlement for Home Health Care

- Client is under the care of a physician
- Client requires skilled nursing, physical therapy, occupational therapy, or speech therapy on an intermittent basis
- Client qualifies for Medicare
- Care is medically reasonable and necessary
- Client is homebound
- Client's needs can be met on an intermittent or part-time basis
- Client resides in a home or facility that does not perform skilled care
- A plan of care is rendered under the guidance of a physician

SOURCE: From Montauk (1998).

by promoting their health and welfare. Of particular interest was the growing concern for taking care of the ill and the infirm in their homes (Hitchcock et al, 2003). St. Vincent de Paul and the Sisters of Charity in France and the Irish Sisters of Charity are early examples of this change. Few people could afford hospital care; support from societal agencies reinforced the care that the family gave to an ill member (Lundy & Janes, 2001).

Perhaps the best-known and best-documented historical account of visiting nursing services is attributed to William Rathbone, a wealthy British businessman and philanthropist who founded the first district nursing association in England. Working with Florence Nightingale, he advocated for district nursing throughout England (Stanhope & Lancaster, 2002). Influenced by the impressive nursing care provided to his ill wife, Rathbone is credited with developing a concern for the sick-poor in Liverpool, England. In the mid 1880s, he established the first visiting nursing service for those who could not pay for such services. The effective approach of combining therapeutic nursing care and education for healthful living practices resulted in the establishment of a permanent district nursing service in that city. With the further help of Florence Nightingale, Rathbone founded a visiting nurses training school to ensure that nurses had the necessary knowledge and skills to work successfully in a community setting (Hitchcock et al., 2003).

The visiting nurse model established in England was soon adapted by the United States as a means of addressing some of the more serious public health problems of the nineteenth century. Large American cities, in particular, faced many new challenges associated with the increasing numbers of immigrants entering the country. Poverty-stricken communities with congested living conditions quickly gave rise to epidemics of infectious diseases such as tuberculosis, small pox, scarlet fever, typhoid, and typhus (Schoen & Koenig, 1997). During the second half of the nineteenth century, with increased urbanization resulting from the Industrial Revolution, jobs for women steadily and rapidly increased. As it became more acceptable for women to work outside the home, the first nursing schools based on the Nightingale Model opened in the United States in 1870. Community health nursing began in order to address the worsening urban health care needs, especially since the availability of acute hospital services was limited, and, in addition, many people preferred to be treated at home (Stanhope & Lancaster, 2002).

Concerned about the substandard living conditions of the poor in the late 1800s and the potential impact of illness and disease on the greater society, philanthropists in the cities of Philadelphia, Boston, and New York provided financial support for visiting nurses to provide care, cleanliness, and character to the homes of the sick-poor. The first visiting nurse associations to provide care in the needy person's home were established in the United States in Buffalo (1885); Philadelphia (1886); and Boston (1886). Charitable activities, supported by the wealthy people, funded both settlement houses and the early visiting nursing associations. One of the early settlement houses in the U.S. began through the efforts of Lillian Wald and Mary Brewster (Stanhope & Lancaster, 2002).

The expanded concept of public health nursing was revolutionized by the socially conscious leadership of Lillian Wald and Mary Brewster (Hitchcock et al., 2003). Lillian Wald is credited with developing the title, public health nurse, and with that title the focus of nursing care was broadened to encompass not only the health of individuals but the health, social, and economic needs of the community as a whole. Wald and Brewster are best known for having co-founded, in 1893, the first organized public health nursing agency, New York City's Henry Street Settlement. The visiting nurse services of the settlement house have been described as a unique combination of social work, nursing, and social activism (Schoen & Koenig, 1997). The women concentrated on public education to bring about improvement in areas of maternal and child health, communicable disease control, nutrition, and mental health. Wald and Brewster greatly influenced the social advocacy role of modern day public health nurses (Hitchcock et al., 2003).

The roles of the visiting nurse and public health nurse became more distinct by the late 1920s. Visiting nurses, employed by the private sector and financed by charity and public contributions, clearly were the "hands-on" providers of bedside nursing care in the home setting. Public health nurses, employed primarily by government health departments, focused their attention on promoting health and preventing disease in the broader community. Though their areas of concentration differed, both groups of nurses functioned independently in the delivery of nursing care outside of an institutional setting and shared the common goal of promoting, maintaining, and restoring health in the community (Hitchcock et al., 2003) (Table 22-2).

Successes achieved by the collective efforts of visiting nurses, public health nurses, and public health services created a shift in the focus of health care in the first half of the twentieth century. With mass immigration no longer occurring (resulting in fewer hazards of communicable diseases threatening the community) and the simultaneous increase in technological advances, new medications, and employer-paid health insurance, the focus of health care moved increasingly away from public health concerns and more toward acute care services. Hospitals were increasingly becoming the primary providers of health care. During the 1930s and 1940s, fewer clients received care from visiting nurses (Reichley, 1999). However, hospitals quickly realized that although

---

TABLE 22-2

Similarities and Differences between Public Health Nursing and Home Health Nursing

Similarities

Setting	Nursing care is provided to clients in their residences or in a community environment.
Independent nature of practice	Nurses practice independently outside of institutions.
Control and environment	Client is active participant in care decisions. Control is shifted to the client. Environment empowers the client.
Family-centered care	The family is considered as a unit of care. Family members contribute significantly to client care.
Broad goals	Public health and home health services strive to promote, maintain, and restore health in the community.

	PHN	HHN
Differences		
Focus of intervention	Population	Individual/family
Caseload acquisition	Case finding in community at large	Referral by physician
Interventions	Continuous	Episodic
Orientation	Wellness	Illness
	Primary prevention	Secondary prevention
		Rehabilitation
		Tertiary prevention
Entry into services	Risk potential	Medical diagnosis
	Social diagnosis	

PHN: Public Health Nursing; HHN: Home Health Nursing.

Source: From *Community Health Nursing*, 2nd edition by Hitchcock © 2003. Reprinted with permission of Delmar Learning, a division of Thomson Learning: www.thomasrights.com.

they were the providers of acute care, they were also becoming the providers of care for individuals with long-term chronic disorders. As a result, hospitals began searching for ways to control the increasing costs incurred by chronic illness care.

Establishment of New York City's Montefiore Hospital Home Care Program in 1947 provided one alternative to care of clients needing health care interventions but not in an acute care setting. The Montefiore Program, entitled a "Hospital Without Walls," created a model of hospital-linked, home-delivered care utilizing the professional services of physicians, nurses, and social workers (Gunderson, 1999). This hospital-based home care model served as the catalyst for the resurgence of home health care as we know it today (Reichley, 1999). By comparison, the cost of home care during that time averaged $3 a day, while the cost of hospital care averaged $10 to $12 per day (Reichley, 1999). The focus for home care from Montefiore was not only the client's illness, with its subsequent chronic state, but also their holistic needs. Social workers addressed the client's social needs, and were interested in the client's family, their overall well-being, and their role in providing for the client's health care (Lundy & Janes, 2001).

For more than half a century, the home care services provided by visiting nurses were funded solely by philanthropists, public charities, and contributions raised by VNAs. In 1966, the federal government began providing for home care services as a benefit of the new legislation known as Medicare. Medicare allowed for the expansion of home care services to many people, particularly the elderly who did not have access to such care. In 1973, the Medicare home care benefit was expanded to include disabled Americans regardless of age.

Accompanying the Medicare funding stream were strict regulations for client eligibility, home care practice, and reimbursement mechanisms. Although the home care benefit was designed to extend care to more people, access was difficult because only certain types of agencies could provide care, and restrictions limited who was eligible for care, which services clients could receive, and length of service. An additional burden on home care agencies was a complex billing system that often resulted in extensive payment delays.

Home care advocates became increasingly concerned that the narrowness of home care legislation limited services as a means of avoiding the excessive costs of providing the full range of services that many clients needed (Reichley, 1999). Over time and through legal efforts, advocacy, and awareness campaigns, supporters of the home care industry met success in loosening the restrictions. In the late 1980s, access to care was easier, eligibility requirements were less restrictive, and billing processes were more efficient. With Medicare dollars more available to support home care services, the increase in home care agencies certified to bill the Medicare program more than doubled between the mid-1980s and the mid-1990s (Reichley, 1999). However, the next influential event was the passage of the Balanced Budget Act of 1997. In an effort to balance the federal budget, Congress targeted home health care as a place to reduce expenditure by reducing the amount of care delivered and thus, the cost. Data had been collected for over a year via the OASIS system, a data collection instrument designed to link outcomes of home care to the management of the delivery of the care (Lundy & Janes, 2003).

The passage of the Balanced Budget Act of 1997 (BBA) imposed stricter limits on Medicare reimbursement for home care services. The increased money and the easier regulations of the 1980s and 1990s for the provision of home care were gone. The BBA narrowed the definition of "home-bound" resulting in people no longer being eligible for home care if they were able to leave home for *any* reason other than medical services (Maurer & Smith, 2005). The number of persons eligible for Medicare home care funding declined by 50% between 1997 and 2000 (USDHHS, 2002).

Model of Home Health Care

Home health care originally used an acute care/rehabilitative model, and as such, traditionally did not attend to the needs of chronically ill individuals. Consequently, chronic illness management in home care has led to frequent, high-cost hospitalizations and emergency room visits. Analysis of health care spending reveals that 78% of all health care dollars are associated with chronic illnesses (Anderson & Horvath, 2004).

Similarly, the predominant medical model of care is to treat individuals with specific diagnoses rather than managing multiple diagnoses and coordinating all of a client's needs (Anderson & Horvath, 2004). Although causes of death from chronic diseases have now increased to 70% of all deaths (National Center for Chronic Disease Prevention and Health Promotion, 2004), there has been significant increase in healthy aging and in the number of healthy years a person may expect to live (Rice & Fineman, 2004). These trends suggest the need for shifting from an acute care medical model to a preventive and chronic-care model for home health (Anderson & Horvath, 2004). Such a model must include informal caregivers as consumers of care, for they are the ones who provide the bulk of care to individuals with chronic illnesses who live at home. Ignoring the needs of families and caregivers increases their stresses and burdens.

Over the past thirty years, advocates for the elderly and disabled have successfully advocated for consumer-directed services in home and community settings. Consumers of home care desire and have achieved increasing degrees of decision-making power (Benjamin, 2001). Medicare enforces consumer-directed services in home health care by stating that the locus of decision for care is with the patient. A social-psychological model of empowerment supports this trend. When using an empowerment model, individuals/caregivers with chronic illnesses are encouraged to achieve maximum mastery over their own lives (Leino-Kilpi & Kuokkanen, 2000). When the focus is on supporting individuals to achieve mastery over their own lives, ethnically diverse individuals and families are encouraged to achieve mastery in ways that are consistent with their cultural values and family processes rather than conforming to agency mores.

Applying Nursing Theory to Home Health Care

Advocacy for disadvantaged populations arises from the roots of home health care nursing. Nurses

use their power to facilitate actions of the client that will increase the degree of mastery they have over their lives (Leino-Kilpi & Kuokkanen, 2000). Goals of home health nursing include providing the knowledge, materials, and training for caregivers and family to foster maximum independence and self mastery. Three nursing theories illustrate how nurses can empower families in home health care.

Imogene King's Open Systems Model focuses on goal attainment through the interaction and relationship of the nurse and the client. King's theory includes client's rights to participate in the goal-setting process. The nurse and the client make decisions about goals, obtain a mutual agreement on how to achieve the goals, and then implement or make the transactions toward goal attainment. The final stage of the process is evaluation of whether goals were or were not attained or met (King, 1996). This process is illustrated when the nurse evaluates the client's needs and functional ability and establishes a plan of care with interventions and goals (titled Form 485) with the client. Progress toward the goals and the client's wishes are measured periodically. Plans are revised as indicated.

Madeline Leininger's Culture Care Diversity and Universality recognizes that the cultural perspective of the client must be understood in order to produce a therapeutic outcome (Leininger, 1996). To provide culturally appropriate care, the nurse learns an individual's worldview or perspective, and assesses the family's environment, their values, their spiritual, political, socio-economic, language, educational, and cultural systems (Leininger, 1996). The process of learning about the family requires that the nurse take a participant approach, listening and observing the culture while in a client's home. The client's perspective and participation are important in the development of a culturally appropriate home health plan of care. Consistent with a model of empowerment, the nurse and the client, or family group, make mutual decisions about appropriate home health goals and interventions.

Orem's Self-Care Deficit Theory includes three categories that define the client's level of self-care ability and self-care deficits, or dependence for care. These categories are wholly compensatory, partly compensatory, and supportive-educative (Taylor et al., 2002). The wholly compensatory client is totally dependent for care, and in the home setting may be dependent on family and informal caregivers. The client and caregiver in the supportive-educative category needs assistance in locating community resources and education about care of the chronic illness. The plan of care for a partly compensatory client is based on the client's self-care limitations and is designed to help the client compensate for identified limitations and thus achieve the highest degree of mastery possible (Orem, 1997). When done in participation with the client, assessment of the self-care deficits and development of a plan of care can be used to identify goals of care and intermediate steps to achieve the greatest degree of self-mastery possible.

The Language of Home Health Care

Several definitions are important in determining eligibility of clients and subsequent reimbursement by the home health care agency. These terms are defined by federal Medicare regulations and include *homebound*, *primary services*, *continuing services*, and *dependent services*.

Federal Medicare regulations include the qualifications of clients for coverage of home health services. The client must be confined to the home or to an institution that is not a hospital or SNF. *Home confined* does not mean the client must be bedridden. *Homebound*, or *home confined*, is defined as an inability to leave the home normally and that leaving would be taxing and require considerable effort and assistance. When the client does leave the home, the absences are infrequent and of relatively short duration or to receive medical care. The client must be under the care of a physician and in need of skilled services on an intermittent visit, not continuous, basis. Intermittent services are provided on visits to the home, with a physician's certifying order for the number of visits from each service to be made during a week or month and for the total duration or number of weeks for the home health services. These skilled services are the *primary services* and include nursing, physical therapy (PT), speech therapy, and occupational therapy (OT), which must be initiated in conjunction with the client's receipt of another *primary service* and may continue even though other service is no longer necessary until the goals for that discipline have been met (Medicare Conditions of Participation, 1996).

Occupational Therapy in home health care is considered a *continuing service*, meaning that the involvement of OT in the client's care depends on an initial *primary service*. However, once the primary service of nursing, physical therapy, or speech therapy has been initiated, the occupational therapist can continue working with the client after the other services are no longer needed, a *continuing service*.

In addition to primary skilled services, home health aide and social work services are covered as *dependent services* under Medicare regulations. The client must require a skilled service to receive home health aide or social work services, and once the skilled service is no longer required, the home health aide and social work services are not covered. These *dependent* services can also be continued if OT (a *continuing service*) is to be provided to the client.

The Home Health Care Team

The multiple practitioners on the home health care team have the knowledge and skills to identify client needs and address those needs through management of complex plans of care (Marelli, 1998). Specific characteristics of the successful home health care practitioner include a strong grasp of the rules and regulations that govern home health care, the ability to pay incredible attention to detail, well-developed interpersonal skills, strong clinical skills, a working knowledge of the changing economics of health care, and the ability to effectively prioritize and time-manage challenging tasks and responsibilities.

Home health care practitioners and standards of practice are governed by state and federal legislation. Individual state regulations must be met for basic licensing of all home health agencies. If participation in the Medicare reimbursement program is desired, there are also federal regulations that govern Medicare certification and coverage of services (Conditions of Participation and HHA-11, respectively) that must be met. These federal mandates, along with individual state licensing or certification requirements, help ensure that home health care practitioners are well qualified to provide their specialized services.

The home health care team consists of physicians, nurses, physical therapists, occupational therapists, speech therapists, medical social workers, and home health aides. Each member of the team possesses a special set of skills that collectively supports a comprehensive approach to assist the client in meeting his or her care needs.

Physician

The physician is the leader of the home care team and assumes primary responsibility for the client's care. In this capacity, he or she is responsible for managing the client's medical and/or psychiatric problems, establishing and approving a plan of care for the client, evaluating the quality of care being provided, and maintaining close communication with the other members of the team. When the client needs additional supportive resources (such as durable medical equipment, other medical supplies, or services from health care specialists), the physician authorizes such resources. It is essential that the physician assume an active role in the client's care by being available and responsive to the client and the health care team (Unwin & Jerant, 1999).

Registered Nurse

The registered nurse is the primary caregiver member of the home care team. To be reimbursed by insurance companies, the nurse must provide at least one of the following activities during a home visit: assessment of the client's condition, teaching the client about his or her specific care needs, and providing hands-on technical care. Technical care can include the expertise needed to assist clients and caregivers with specialized care needs. These needs could include home intravenous therapy, pain management devices, ventilation management, total parenteral nutrition, or specialized wound care management.

Physical Therapist

The overall goal of PT is to promote rehabilitation and prevent disabilities. To achieve this goal, the physical therapist generally focuses on client needs involved with mobility and gross motor activities. Musculoskeletal and neurological disorders are common types of conditions requiring PT intervention. Specific treatment modalities include therapeutic exercises, range of motion, balance and transfer techniques, bed mobility, strength and gait training, ultrasound, whirlpool therapy, and all electrical modalities. Physical Therapy is considered a primary service, and the therapist can initiate home health care services and complete the initial assessment. Following the evaluation visit, and with consultation from the physician, a plan of care is developed that is tailored to the client's needs.

Speech Therapist

Another home health care service recognized as a primary service is speech therapy. Speech therapists, also referred to as speech–language pathologists, provide specialty care to clients with speech, language, or swallowing disorders. The speech therapy assessment identifies the nature and severity of a client's need for a speech therapy component of the plan of care. Treatment modalities may include multisensory language stimulation; auditory, tactile, and visual cues; speech melody and rhythm practice; compensatory movements; and techniques. As mentioned, the speech therapist may also be involved with the diagnosis and treatment of swallowing disorders.

Occupational Therapist

Occupational therapy involves working with a client's functional abilities. The OT assessment is designed to identify and intervene with difficulties in performing activities of daily living (ADLs), fine motor activities, personal care activities, or instrumental activities of daily living (IADLs) such as grocery shopping, household maintenance, and money management. Impairments in these areas are often the product of acute injury or normal aging or may be associated with developmental disabilities. The occupational therapist focuses on reeducation of routine ADL tasks, perceptual-motor activities, vision training, fine motor coordination activities, safety training, or work simplification and energy conservation techniques. The occupational therapist also recommends the use of assistive devices or adaptive equipment. The physical therapist and occupational therapist need to coordinate the client's plan of care to avoid duplication of service, because oftentimes there is some overlap in services.

Social Worker

Social work services are often requested in a variety of situations when resources are unavailable to meet a client's basic needs, a high-risk potential for abuse or neglect exists, the safety of a client's care or home environment is questionable, caregiver stress has become overwhelming, an alternative living arrangement needs to be explored, and so forth. The social work assessment and plan of care concentrate on the client's social, emotional, and financial needs so the client can maintain or achieve independence at home. Social workers assist clients and caregivers with these issues through education and counseling, referrals to appropriate community resources, crisis intervention, and stress relief modalities, including identifying resources for financial, housing, or placement assistance.

As with all other services, physician authorization is necessary prior to using social services. Coordination with other members of the team is essential because social work interventions cannot continue once other providers are no longer involved in the client's care.

Home Health Aide

The paraprofessional role of the home health aide is highly regarded by the home health care team because aides provide the actual hands-on, personal care and ADL assistance to clients. Tasks that the home health aide is allowed to perform include personal care (hygiene care, feeding transfer and mobility assistance, and exercise maintenance under the supervision of a skilled therapist) and household services (light housekeeping, personal laundry, and grocery shopping). Home health aide services are included as part of the home care benefit when the client is physically or mentally unable to perform self-care activities and when there is no available caregiver willing or able to provide the necessary care. Home health aide services must be initiated by nursing or other primary therapy staff, all of whom can provide mandated semimonthly supervision visits.

Problems and Issues of Home Health Care

The home health care industry currently faces a number of challenges. While hospitals depend heavily on home care to provide effective, cost-controlled services, the home health care industry must deliver quality services under new regulations with decreased available resources and reimbursements.

Limited Reimbursement

Because Medicare is the major payor of home health care, any changes in Medicare reimbursement greatly affect the home health care industry. The reader is cautioned to remember that much of what applies to Medicare beneficiaries also applies to other clients who receive home health care, especially when receiving service from a certified agency.

The need to control Medicare spending began in the mid-1980s as a result of escalating acute care costs. The introduction of DRGs in hospitals imposed a reimbursement cap on client care that resulted in significantly reduced hospitalization periods for acutely ill clients. During this same time period, the federal government was being legally challenged by home health care industry advocates to loosen tight restrictions on the home health care benefit for Medicare recipients. The home health care industry won its case, allowing expansion of home care services (Reichley, 1999). However, despite the "loosening" of tight restrictions of eligibility in the receipt of Medicare benefits, the law governing Medicare did not change.

This turning point in the Medicare program allowed a significant number of funds to better provide for clients' home care needs. As might be expected, available funding created a tremendous growth spurt for service providers who wanted to enter the home care arena, given that Medicare was now fully reimbursing home care agencies for their operational costs. Home care, previously provided by VNAs or public health agencies, was now being offered by hospital-based and free-standing, for-profit agencies. By the mid-1990s, an estimated 10,000 home health care agencies had received certification to participate in the Medicare benefit and bill for services (Reichley, 1999).

Over a 5-year period, as the number of Medicare-certified home health agencies grew, there was an astronomical rise in Medicare outlays. Continuing growth rates of 23 to 30 percent per year led to predictions of Medicare home health expenditures reaching 100 billion dollars by the year 2000 (Remington, 2000). To restrain these spiraling costs, governmental controls were set in motion that resulted in a dramatic altering of home care services and led to profound revenue reductions (Grindel-Waggoner, 1999). Consequently, there was a dramatic drop of 45 percent in payments from 1997 through 1999. Per individual, expenditures decreased from $4,969 in fiscal year 1997 to $4,052 in fiscal year 1998 to $3,110 in fiscal year 1999 (Zhu, 2004). Unable to continue operations with such profound revenue reductions, approximately 2,500 home health agencies closed nationwide by 1999 (Malugeni, 1999).

The Operation Restore Trust Project

During the peak of the Medicare expenditure period, the outpouring of Medicare funds into the home health care system invited governmental speculation that agency noncompliance with Medicare regulations was an issue. In response to the compli-

ance issue, a comprehensive health care federal/state antifraud waste and abuse initiative began in 1995. The project became known as Operation Restore Trust (ORT).

For the next two years (1995–1997), five states (California, Florida, Illinois, New York, and Texas) were investigated and audited for Medicare fraud and abuse. Expansive investigative authority was given to ORT staff, many of which were agents of the Federal Bureau of Investigation. The investigation involved Medicare clients, their caregivers, physicians, and home health agency employees, along with clients' medical and billing records.

Overall results of ORT investigations revealed fraudulent and abusive patterns of practice that spanned all the targeted states. The most common practices were (1) illegal billing to the Medicare program, (2) billing of services to clients who did not meet eligibility criteria, and (3) illegally referring clients for home care services in exchange for funds or other products of value ("kickbacks"). Based on these findings, the ORT project was expanded nationwide and stringent compliance guidelines were initiated for home health agencies. Agencies found to be involved with serious fraud and abuse activities were prosecuted aggressively. Once again, countless home health care agencies, reeling under the increased burden of intensive self-audit or feeling the effects of the government imposed audit of the ORT project, closed their doors forever.

The Balanced Budget Act

Not only responding to ORT findings, but also needing to restrain the growth and cost of the home health care benefit, the federal government enacted cost-containing legislation in 1997 as part of the Balanced Budget Act (BBA) (Health Care Financing Administration, 1997). The BBA included several components that affected home health care services. For example, venipuncture services were discontinued for clients who had no other skilled need other than the actual blood draw. Clients, especially those residing in rural areas, were forced to seek alternate ways to access venipuncture services, such as mobile laboratories, more frequent trips to physicians' offices, or visits to laboratory facilities, or consider stopping medical therapy.

Changes in Reimbursements The most significant effect of the Balanced Budget Act (BBA) of 1997 was the legislation that moved home health care from a cost-based reimbursement system to a prospective payment system (PPS). One of the goals of this legislation was to control Medicare spending by transitioning agencies from their current reimbursement system, *cost-based, fee-for-service* (FFS), to a more stringent one, the *Prospective Payment System* (PPS). This change was complex and included an intermediate step, the *Interim Payment System* (IPS).

The first phase of cost control, the IPS, was designed to bridge the gap between the FFS system and the PPS. It placed stringent limits on the dollar amount agencies would receive over a 12-month period for each Medicare client. Once the PPS was in place, it eliminated both the FFS system and the IPS. Many home health agencies did not successfully survive this transitional phase; they closed their doors to certified home health care. Closing their doors to certified care did not negate the continuation of their private or non-certified business. Agencies continued to make home care available to patients and families but did not bill Medicare because they no longer qualified for Medicare reimbursement. When a client's care could no longer be billed to Medicare, rather than just leaving the patient without any home care, the client could independently pay the agency. This arrangement provided an alternative to third-party reimbursed care. Since the inception of IPS, followed by PPS, many long-term care patients have paid their own bills for care. As Medicare defines its payment criteria, it was never intended to pay for care other than short-term, acute, intermittent, and skilled.

Potential for Client Abandonment With the advent of the IPS, providing home care services for clients who needed large numbers of visits created a costly situation. To achieve needed cost control,

home health agencies turned their attention to informing clients and their informal caregivers about the urgency of either assuming primary financial responsibility for care or finding other providers. Clients had difficulty understanding these changes because their eligibility for services had not changed, and they had little understanding that the actual change related strictly to the reimbursement mechanism. To adapt to these drastic changes in care was overwhelming and confusing. If a home health agency determined that a client could no longer be served because of costs, the agency was responsible for providing advanced notice to the physician and client and was required to assist with finding other sources of care. To do otherwise, the agency found itself at risk for charges of client abandonment. The definition of abandonment is the cessation of services by an agency to a client who continues to require care and for whom no provision has been made, nor has the patient received proper and timely notice of impending discharge from service.

Many clients rapidly exceeded their per-beneficiary limits for the year, and home health agencies realized that any overpayment on their Medicare-capped annual reimbursement allowance meant a repayment to the federal government. It was estimated that 75 percent of home health agencies exceeded their Medicare reimbursement limits the first year of the IPS (NAHC Report, 1998).

Because of the severe limits placed on reimbursement, some home health agencies were selective about who was accepted for services. The ideal candidate for home care services was the client with less intense care needs and whose cost of care was unlikely to exceed the IPS cap. In choosing such clients, the agency was at the same time carefully preventing any future risk of potential client abandonment. As a result, the client with the greatest needs often was unable to receive care. With severely restricted Medicare reimbursement, government legislation indirectly encouraged agencies to steer away from clients with high-cost care needs and essentially constructed a system of penalizing agencies that chose to care for such clients (Majorowicz, 1999).

Prospective Payment System: Moving toward Capitation In the capitated payment system, a specific dollar amount per client is given to a health care provider for delivery of services. The health care provider, in turn, becomes the coordinator of the individual's care and assumes responsibility for managing cost, risk, resources, and outcomes of care (Remington, 2000). The transition of the home care industry to the PPS billing clearly represents movement toward a managed care, capitated environment.

The government's goal is to develop a reimbursement system that pays home care agencies equitably under the PPS. Under this system, home health agencies are paid on a 60-day episode of care, not by individual home visits, as previously done. The initial payment is 60 percent of the total cost,

with 40 percent paid later. Both payments for all subsequent episodes are divided equally.

Actual reimbursement amounts are determined by clinical assessment of the client's needs using the mandated assessment tool, *Outcome Assessment System and Information Set* (OASIS). The 79-question OASIS assessment tool was designed to establish a national standard for collecting home care outcome data that can be used to evaluate home care services on an industry-wide basis and collect demographic, clinical, and functional client care data to use in calculating PPS payments to home health agencies.

The actual charges that can be submitted by an agency are determined by the OASIS clinical scoring system, which assigns points to select items in the OASIS data set plus assigns additional points if therapy services are needed. The OASIS scoring system

---

PPS Case Study in Home Health

Mr. S., a 75-year-old widowed gentleman, is being discharged to his daughter's (Mrs. H.) home following a 5-day hospitalization for a cerebral vascular accident (CVA). Prior to the hospitalization, Mr. S. lived independently in his home. Mrs. H., a married mother of two children, desires to care for Mr. S. in her home rather than pursue nursing home placement. With this choice, Mrs. H. is taking an unpaid leave of absence from her factory job. This income loss will be an unplanned financial impact on the family. Mrs. H. has no previous experience caring for a chronically ill person.

The home health agency received a referral from the hospital to provide home health care services for Mr. S. The referral is for nursing care, therapy services, social work, and personal care for the rehabilitation of Mr. S. to optimal functional ability post-CVA. Mr. S.'s left hemisphere CVA with right hemiparesis has affected his ex-

pressive speech; cognitive ability, with loss of memory; and functional ability. He is now nonambulatory and requires assistance for bed mobility and transfers. He requires maximum assistance with grooming, bathing, and eating. The 24-hour-a-day responsibility will be a demanding and difficult responsibility for Mrs. H. Long-term planning of Mr. S.'s care will need to be addressed, because Mrs. H.'s leave of absence from work is temporary.

Ms. Thomas, RN, BSN, makes the initial home visit. Ms. Thomas conducts a comprehensive assessment and collects the OASIS data, since it is required on admission to service, as well as other designated events in the regime of home care. The OASIS measures Mr. S.'s functional status and ability and the level of assistance required with grooming, bathing, toileting, transfers, ambulation, and eating. Mr. S.'s speaking and cognitive ability needs for is intended to calculate Medicare payments based on the severity and acuity of the client's condition, and in this way, the provision is for higher payment for sicker clients. There are no limitations on the number of 60-day episodes of care that a client can receive. Full implementation of the PPS, utilizing the OASIS data set, occurred on October 1, 2000 (Health Care Financing Administration, 2000). The influence of the implementation of the PPS in home health has been more stringent regulations about which services will be reimbursed, and for how long, in some instances. This may well limit access to care for certain vulnerable groups, such as the frail elderly, chronically ill individuals whose care is largely home-based, and people who are HIV positive. According to Stanhope and Lancaster in their book addressing community oriented practice, the goal is to ensure that care is appropriate, rather than limiting access. Nurses and other health care providers must work even more closely with families to determine the kinds of services needed to foster self-care and the optimal timing of these services (2002). The major barrier that home health practitioners confront daily is that some of the neediest patients, chronically ill and elderly, may experience limitations in their access to care.

Increased Documentation Although the PPS sounds like a solution to the spiraling costs of home care, it has drawbacks. One of these is the increase in the amount of required paperwork. The OASIS assessment tool is used with all home care clients except for antepartum and postpartum clients, clients less than 18 years of age, and clients not receiving

home medical equipment are assessed for OASIS documentation. During the initial assessment visit, a plan of care (Form 485) is developed with Mrs. H.'s and Mr. S.'s input for nursing and home health aide visits for personal care and bathing. Interventions are discussed and goals are developed for the number of visits per week for each of the visiting disciplines for the next 60 days. Nursing interventions will include instruction on the aspects of the chronic illness and care, such as skin care, nutrition and hydration, elimination, and signs and symptoms of complications. After the home visit, Ms. Thomas discusses the plan of care with Mr. S.'s physician.

Evaluation visits are scheduled: PT for therapeutic exercises to the right lower extremity, ambulation, and mobility training; OT for exercises to the right upper extremity and ADL training; and ST for speech and communication therapy. Each practitioner will develop a plan of care with interventions and goals with Mrs. H. and Mr. S. The social worker will make a home visit to help Mrs. H. and Mr. S. make long-range plans and identify community resources that can assist with Mr. S.'s care and the stressful impact to Mrs. H. related to the demands of Mr. S.'s care and the changes in Mrs. H.'s household.

The OASIS data for clinical, functional, and therapy services scores are used to determine the home health resource grouper (HHRG) used to calculate the amount of the Medicare PPS payment for the 60-day episode. For effective and efficient use of limited resources in the PPS model, coordination of care is extremely important so that there is no duplication or overlap of care and services. Each team member must be aware of the collective goals for the client's care to ensure the best outcome possible for the client.

professional health care services. Home care agencies have expressed great concern about the additional time, paperwork, and cost superimposed by OASIS (Schroeder, 2000). Data collection must be done upon admission to the home health agency and following any significant change in the client's condition or plan of care (Health Care Financing Administration, 1998). Once collected, the data must be entered and locked in an approved OASIS computer software system within seven days. The OASIS data are electronically submitted to the government at least monthly.

The routine home care admission packet contains at least 15 documents, and obtaining the information to complete the document can be extremely demanding and exhausting for clients, who are often quite ill. In addition, this increased paperwork burden is placed on clinical staff who must implement and document a new set of assessment questions multiple times during the course of the client's care. Other agency staff assumes the burden of reviewing the clinician's work and making sure errors or omissions are promptly addressed for data entry and ultimate submission to governmental offices.

To accommodate the cost and time considerations associated with OASIS compliance regulations, home health agencies have had to adjust their operational systems and budgets. Agencies without computer systems have had to secure such systems. Data entry staff has been hired. All staff and clients have had to be educated about the purpose and use of the OASIS data set.

Skewed Outcome Data   One significant problem that has become apparent during implementation of the OASIS is the consistency and reliability of the collected data (Citarella, 2000). Initial attention was placed on gathering and submitting data on time rather than on the reliability of data. Citarella (2000) asserts that the biggest challenge under PPS is the lack of standardization. Without standardization, wide variations can occur in how clinicians interpret OASIS questions and how answers are selected. The lack of standardized measures to assure that a client's condition is assessed and recorded in a consistent

and accurate manner can affect client care reimbursements and create inconsistent and skewed data outcome reports (Citarella, 2000).

Compliance Pitfalls   In the past, reimbursement systems involving the Medicare program did not allow home health agencies to make a profit. With the introduction of the PPS, this has changed. Well-designed and efficiently delivered home care services could result in retained revenues if the client's care does not require full use of allocated funding (Randall, 2000). The potential for making a profit can become an incentive for some agencies to disregard governmental compliance guidelines. Infractions might include (1) "upcoding," inflating a client's acuity level for the purpose of receiving more reimbursement than is warranted; (2) underserving clients, providing care that falls below standards; (3) inappropriate admissions, admitting clients for service who do not meet or only marginally meet criteria; (4) denial of admission for care, for fear that a client's care needs will exceed the allowable reimbursement; and (5) inappropriate referral practices, offering something of value, such as payments or free services, in exchange for client referrals (Randall, 2000). Agencies choosing to participate in such practices risk government prosecution for violation of abuse or fraud laws.

Insufficient Staffing of Home Health Agencies
Across all health care settings, there is an insufficient number of nursing personnel. Common factors contributing to the decline in the nursing work force include an aging work force; greater opportunities for individuals in other professions; fewer nurses working, secondary to higher family incomes generated by a healthy economy; and declining enrollment in nursing programs.

In home health agencies, staffing has decreased because of the nursing shortage in general and because of staff choosing to leave their positions in the wake of the changes that have occurred in the home care arena. In some states, recruitment difficulties are compounded by the requirement that nurses have prior professional experience for a specified period of time before being hired as home health care nurses. Many home health agencies prefer previous work experience in medical-surgical nursing because the demands of today's home care market have created a significant need for highly skilled clinicians who are proficient with technology (Malugani, 1999). Salaries have increased in the acute care settings to attract more nurses, while salaries in the community health arena have not commensurately increased in given geographic areas. The shortage of nurses has reached a crisis level in many home health agencies.

An insufficient nursing staff prevents home health agencies from accepting clients needing service. If home health agency services cannot be secured for a client, the client may be required to remain in the hospital longer or seek care from a clinic, a physician's office, or an emergency room; consider nursing home placement; or return home without essential in-home health care support.

Conflict with Hospice Nursing When end-of-life care is needed, clients and their caregivers may be referred to a hospice program, another service provided in the client's home. The philosophy of hospice care is to provide comfort measures, pain and symptom control, and emotional and spiritual support to enhance quality of life during the terminal phase of illness. Services provided are similar to those of home health care but are utilized only during the terminal phase of illness, a period of time that can extend for several months and is usually intended to be within a six-month timeframe. Unlike home health services, hospice care can also be provided in inpatient facilities. This holistic approach to care is further extended to family members and caregivers who can receive supportive bereavement care following the client's death (Hitchcock et al., 2003).

The hospice team also consists of physicians, nurses, therapists, social workers, and home health aides. This team can provide many of the services that a home health agency provides. Hospice programs also include bereavement counselors, volunteers, and other specialized care providers. Hospice programs, like home health programs, are heavily regulated and subject to strict criteria to qualify for Medicare or other reimbursement.

For the hospice team to function, home health care referrals are made when staff identify an end-of-life client need that cannot be adequately addressed by the home care agency. Unfortunately, there is a tendency for home care agencies to make such referrals 48 to 72 hours prior to a client's anticipated death. Such late referrals often occur because a client will not accept hospice care until then. However, at other times, it occurs because the home care agency determines that this is when hospice services can best be utilized (Schim et al., 2000). Home health agencies have the prerogative to retain patients rather than referring them to hospice because they provide income. Anecdotal reports confirm that this does happen. Such very short service periods deprive the client and family of receiving the benefits of comprehensive hospice care.

It is often difficult to determine when a chronically ill patient should be referred to hospice. The intent of hospice is not to provide long-term, chronic care; referral of the patient too early is a disservice to the patient, the family, and the agency. Medicare addresses this in its criterion of the physician's certification that requires the physician to state that the patient is expected to die within six months. However, it is often a difficult decision for the physician, as well as a difficult acceptance for the patient and family to progress from the chronic illness state to one of terminal illness and expected death. In addition to all the personal reasons to be at home during the terminal phase of an illness, the cost differential to Medicare is an incentive. According to the Center to Advance Palliative Care, the average cost of hospice care at home is $107.00 per day, compared to $476.00 per day in the hospital, and $624.00 per day for continuous home care (von Gunten, Ferris, Portenoy, & Glajchen, 2001).

Use of Family Caregivers As a consequence of limited home care resources, there is a growing reliance on family members or other informal caregivers for provision of long-term care. Guided by formal caregivers (health team members), clients and their caregivers may find themselves in a position of experiencing improved health behaviors and health status or stabilization of chronic conditions. Simultaneously, this care is cost effective because informal caregivers are mostly unpaid.

With such responsibility and the desire to avoid hospitalization or long-term care, informal caregivers must not overlook that there is considerable risk or cost to their social, emotional, physical, and financial well-being (Montauk, 1998). Family caregivers often provide 24-hour care, which may turn part of the household into a patient care facility (Marelli, 1998). The resultant stress creates a disequilibrium in family functioning because of such factors as role changes, strained relationships, loss of space, dwindling funds, and shifting of family priorities to caregiving activities (see Chapter 11, on family caregivers). The basic demanding nature of any caregiving role may be compounded by the additional responsibilities of employment, child rearing, and other household tasks (Hitchcock et al., 2003). The untoward consequences of the caregiver burden may result in vulnerability to injuries, exhaustion, social isolation, and despair.

▎ Interventions

Home health agencies are known for their resilience. With a commitment to the population they serve and a determination to stay in business, these agencies have developed strategies to turn challenge into opportunity. A few of these strategies are noted here. Regardless of who is responsible for payment of home care, one theme is common to all settings: the expectation that a caregiver (or caregivers) is (are) available to provide the majority of the client's care.

Diversifying Home Care Services

Until stringent limitations were placed on Medicare reimbursement, home health agencies worked hard to maintain a high percentage of Medicare clients. In the past, the greater the number of visits that could be provided, the stronger the agency's revenue base, due to the favorable reimbursement paid by Medicare. Now, with new regulations and cost-containment measures firmly in place, the Medicare market is no longer attractive. Expansion into other areas of service delivery, such as managed care, pharmacy services, adult day care, or private duty nursing, allows a more varied pool of revenue sources. Venturing into these broader markets requires that home health agencies educate themselves on the varying regulations as well as operational and fiscal systems that are particular to each new venue, because the classic Medicare rules and regulations most likely will not apply. For example, many home health agencies have established contracts with managed care organizations (HMOs) as part of their diversification strategy. Home care nurses, who traditionally assumed primary care management responsibilities for their clients, have had to adapt to sharing this care management role with nurses in the HMO organization, who are also charged with similar care management responsibilities (Brown & Neal, 1999).

Changing the Model of Care Delivery

Survival strategies from a fiscal and clinical perspective have resulted in many home health agencies consolidating into larger, more efficient organizations covering expansive geographical areas (Nugent, 1999). Changes such as these are accompanied by new models of care delivery, because the agency's traditional service delivery methods no longer fit. Several examples of new models include managed care teams, self-directed work teams, or productivity engineered work teams. These models were developed proactively by home health agencies in anticipation of sharply declining home care revenue (Brown & Neal, 1999; Stafford, Seemons & Jones, 1997; Oriol, 1997). The commonality among these care delivery models is that all value a highly structured team approach to coordinate client care, with a shared outcome being the delivery of high-quality care at the lowest possible cost.

Counterbalancing the Staffing Shortage

Physician home visits have largely been replaced by the advent of home health care agencies. In fact, most recent data indicate that less than 1 percent of clients receive home visits from physicians (Unwin & Jerant, 1999). In support of more physician home visits, it is stressed that both client preferences and major changes in the health care system have created an increased need for physician involvement because of the increasing medical complexity of client needs, fewer hospital admissions, and shortened hospital stays (Unwin & Jerant, 1999). It is recommended that physicians consider an expanded use of the telephone and advanced communication technologies, such as two-way video conferencing (telemedicine), to complement or replace the need for in-person home visits.

A significant addition to the home health care team is the advanced practice nurse (APN). In view of the current shortage of home care nurses, the time required in the home to address clients' complex medical needs, and the pressures of meeting industry productivity standards of at least five or six clients a day, the skills of the APN can provide significant support to clients and agency staff (Pierson & Minarik, 1999) (see Chapter 20, on the advanced practice nurse in chronic illness).

The APN is able to conduct extensive assessments of a client, and, under a physician protocol, the APN may order appropriate diagnostic tests and initiate early treatment (Kane, Ouslander & Abrass, 1999). The APN can provide follow-up care and resources on a longer term basis than can home care nurses. APNs are in a position to provide greatly needed, in-depth services to frail elders and persons with chronic disorders.

One barrier to incorporating more APNs into the home care arena is the lack of payment sources that cover the cost of their services. Most insurance companies do not include the services of APNs as a covered home health benefit. As home health agencies continue to search for ways to offset the costs of services by an APN, some agencies have already im-plemented creative approaches, such as securing community-based grants and contracting out their APNs as health consultants to other providers (Pierson & Minirak, 1999).

Changes in Nursing Education

With health care moving away from acute care and toward home- and community-based services, the shortage of highly skilled home care nurses has attracted attention from several directions. In the nursing education arena, for example, preparation for community practice in the community has traditionally been concentrated in baccalaureate nursing programs, while associate degree programs focused their curricula heavily on the preparation of nurses to work in more acute care settings. Recognizing the declining need for acute care nurses and the rising demand for nurses who possess the knowledge and skills to work successfully in a community setting, associate degree nursing programs are beginning to revise their curricula to prepare future nurses accordingly (Jamieson, 1998). As these programs expand their curricula, they face the challenge of integrating concepts such as health promotion; disease prevention; community-based client education; holistic, psychosocial, and environmental assessments into their programs without lengthening the associate degree program (Jamieson, 1998).

Avoiding Legal and Compliance Pitfalls

With limited human resources, home care agencies must exercise caution and discretion in admitting clients to their service. They do so by giving serious consideration to factors such as complexity of the client's medical needs, safety issues, the social support system, and the agency's ability to provide the necessary resources for the length of time the client may need them. Through such actions, agencies reduce the risk of inviting circumstances that might lead to client abandonment. In addition, home health agencies are cautioned to reject any desire or temptation to influence increased profits through questionable practices such as upcoding, which might generate concerns about fraud and abuse.

Computerization

Reimbursable home health services include skilled nursing, PT, OT, speech therapy, home health aides, medical social work, and the newly acquired responsibility of managing supplies specific to the client's condition. With home health's clinical side now driving financial reimbursement, it becomes imperative that all home health agencies construct a model of care that successfully blends their clinical and business operations.

The billing expertise of a home health agency's staff will depend on Medicare's reimbursement structure. With billing processes fully dependent on clinical documentation, timeliness of paper flow has great influence on the agency's cash flow. All staff must develop an appreciation for the fact that delayed paperwork is likely to translate into a cash-flow problem.

Innovative home health agencies have included in their planning process the need for transitioning staff from manual to computerized data collection and transmission systems. Client documentation that previously required days to complete is now instantly transmitted. Having the ability to transmit and receive data on a daily basis not only simplifies the billing process, but also allows efficient tracking of the client's care and staff visits. Consequently, claims can be sent in on time, preventing lags in the billing system and delayed payments (Lewis, 2000).

An electronic record system allows maximum efficiency in accessing OASIS data for both clinical and billing purposes. It continues to be a challenge for the home health industry to ensure consistency and reliability of OASIS data for equitable reimbursement and accurately recording clinical outcomes. It is recommended that reliability studies of the OASIS be done to establish standardization of OASIS outcomes (Citarella, 2000).

Legislation

Since passage of the BBA in 1997, a priority of the home care industry has been to prevent further reductions in service and to restore the Medicare home health benefit. In 2000, Congress approved the Beneficiary Improvement and Protection Act (BIPA) as an amendment to the Social Security Act. One of the changes in BIPA is a clarification of the *homebound* definition for home health. Under BIPA, absences from home to receive health care treatment, to receive therapeutic adult day care, or any absence that is of an infrequent or short duration, such as religious service attendance, do not disqualify a person from being considered homebound (Department of Health and Human Services, 2001). This act will restore $21 billion, over a 5-year period, to hospitals, home health agencies, nursing homes, and other providers whose budgets were reduced as a result of the 1997 BBA (California Association for Health Services at Home, 2000b). The act includes the delay of a 2001 proposed budget cut to 2002 and clarification allowing the use of telemedicine in home care settings.

Medicare Modernization Act of 2003

In 2003, Congress modified the 1965 Medicare Act in an effort to offer better health care benefits and more choices in health care coverage. Medicare Part D now includes prescription drug and preventive benefits. People with low incomes are the targeted beneficiaries of these new entitlements. This is not intended or expected to have any specific effect on home health care, but it may well affect patients with chronic illnesses who struggle to pay for necessary medications. Medicare-approved drug discount cards are available from 2004 until the actual Medicare drug benefits begin in 2006 (Centers for Medicare and Medicaid Services, 2004). Medicare Part D is expected to provide drug discounts of between 10 and 15% off the purchase price (Markey, 2004).

The Medicare Advantage plan, replacing Medicare + Choice, the managed care plan option, another addition of the new Medicare Law, is one of the choices for seniors to choose, along with other choices of Medicare enhanced fee-for-service (EFFS), or a prescription drug plan (PDP) (Maurer & Smith, 2005). The intent of this plan is to manage Medicare costs by increasing the use of established provider networks. Medicare beneficiaries enrolled in managed care are expected to double within six years (Markey, 2004). The enactment of Medicare as a managed care provider will have far reaching implications to home care provisions for clients with chronic illness. This Act will further affect health care services to senior citizens by providing new enrollees into Medicare with an initial physical examination and other primary prevention services. These new services should help improve health promotion and disease prevention areas in Medicare (Maurer & Smith, 2005).

Supporting Family Caregivers

The prediction of an increasing demand for informal caregiving is not capturing the attention of national and state legislators. The need to control the escalating costs of long-term care provides a major incentive for developing programs that offer family caregiver support and respite care. Receiving care in one's own home environment affords familiarity, comfort, and a sense of well-being. Many family caregivers find that providing home health care gives them a sense of empowerment as they remain directly involved in the care of their loved ones. Additionally, the trust and rapport that develop in the health care partnership between informal and formal caregivers boost the family caregiver's confidence in effectively attending to client needs. An equal partnership is promoted between the client and his or her caregiver and the health care teams so that common goals are established. The ultimate goal, of course, is that, with appropriate resources and health education, the informal caregivers will develop the skills necessary to successfully manage the client's care independently in the home setting.

As with the development of any type of public policy, the effectiveness of program planning depends heavily on the target population's perception of its needs and how those needs can best be met. The Federal Health Protection and Assistance for Older Americans Act of 1999 incorporates several proposals for caregiver support, including a tax credit for long-term care. Financing for the caregiver was finally allocated in 2000 as an amendment to the Older Americans Act (Department of Health and Human Services 2001). Funds are available to provide caregiver support measures that extend beyond the monetary tax credit to help fortify, sustain, and maintain caregivers. Services include providing respite resources, access to networks of caregiver support services, and tax incentives for employers who develop programs that support caregiving employees. The funding for this amendment is administered through state agencies. All services are directly to support home and community-based services to families caring for frail older members (Maurer & Smith, 2005).

Outcomes

The desired outcomes for the role that home health care plays in the management of the long-term client with chronic illness client seem initially to be quite apparent. The positive effects of the health care delivered in the home to the client, as well as the positive effects of the caregiver support mechanisms in order to keep the patient at home and not necessitating institutionalization, are beyond any doubt. However, the urgency of establishing outcome criteria that are stable and dependable in order to measure outcome attainment is essential to knowing if the positive effects are really happening to the advantage of the client and caregiver or simply because there is no alternative to the provision of care.

Maurer and Smith have established nine Possible Outcome Measures for evaluating the outcome attainment judged by changes in the population, the health care system within the community, or the environment. The identified outcome measures include 1) knowledge; 2) behaviors, skills; 3) attitudes; 4) emotional well-being; 5) health status (epidemiology); 6) presence of health care system services and components; 7) satisfaction or acceptance regarding the program interventions; 8) presence of policy allowing, mandating, funding; and 9) altered relationship with physical environment (p. 403).

Evaluating the outcomes of care rendered by any of the disciplines participating in home health care for the first five measures is inclusive in the care itself. The professionals and paraprofessionals who work within the home care teams function within and by delivering care using these first five principles, thus making their use as measurement variables relatively easy and functional. The last four outcome measures, however, have been a continuous struggle for home health care throughout the twentieth and now the twenty-first century. These four measures are unpredictably influenced by the ups and downs of financial support, government regulations, management control in home health itself, and in the institutional care that passes clients on to in-home care.

With the establishment of capitation payment and agencies learning how best to serve the client within this system, along with increased Medicare support to both the individual client and to the caregiver, the desired outcomes of home health care should become more realistic. These outcomes should be more attainable, too. Outcome evaluation analysis will hopefully be demonstrating the home health care process resulting in appropriate, adequate, and effective patient care because it is the best way to serve this patient and not because there was no alternative.

▌ Summary and Conclusions

The home health industry is challenged to skillfully manage the risk, cost, resources, and outcomes of client care. To prepare for the delivery of efficient, high-quality, cost-effective services under the PPS, home health agencies are developing strategic plans that will prepare them for survival in a tightly controlled economic environment. All agency staff needs a thorough education to be familiar with the new rules and regulations for agency operations and

how each staff member's skills and talents will be used to achieve agency goals. All clinicians need educational sessions on accurate, thorough client assessments and the importance of rapid and accurate submission of these data, considering the attachment of reimbursement to assessment.

In addition, home health agencies are now responsible for utilization management and will need to develop "tool kits" designed to promote efficiency. In the past, these agencies based their operations on the concept that more care meant more reimbursement, but the new payment system limits the amount of money that will be paid per client while expecting that the quality of care be maintained. Resources such as protocols, care maps, and clinical pathways will become more useful, along with the incentive to explore advanced technologies such as point-of-service computers and telemedicine devices. From a comprehensive perspective, the PPS can be measured by an agency's skill in implementing a strategy that integrates the domains of quality care and client satisfaction with fewer client visits, high staff production and morale, and timely completion and submission of documentation within a tight budget.

It is essential that physicians, clients, and their caregivers become integral components of **this** process, and they must be educated to the importance of their contributions in home health care, particularly as Medicare-reimbursed home health care moves into the managed care arena. As supervisors of client care, physicians need to provide more guidance and medical direction necessary for effectively addressing client care needs. This requires more open, positive communication patterns between the physician and the home health agency.

Positive client outcomes require that home care agencies become more aware of the roles that clients, family, and caregivers have prior to the client being admitted for service. Families and caregivers need to know the significance of their roles in the plan of care and must be informed early on as to the agency's expectations of their involvement with the client's care. In turn, the client's family must understand what can and cannot be expected from agency services.

A chronology of the home health industry since 1965 gives testimony to its remarkable resilience in times of adversity. Through restrictive eligibility requirements, allegations of fraud and abuse, and recent reimbursement limitations, home health agencies continue to rebound to fulfill the goal of supporting client and caregiver self-determination in managing client care needs at home. There is no doubt that these agencies will continue to be in great demand, and skillful adaptation to today's economic environment will determine their success.

Note

The Authors would like to thank Deborah Card and Wanda Huffstetler for their work on this chapter in the 5th edition.

Study Questions

1. Describe how Medicare regulations affect the delivery and reimbursement of home health care services.
2. Discuss the definition of *homebound* and how that definition might affect an individual's ability to go to church regularly and provision of their health care.
3. Differentiate between primary, continuing, and dependent services.
4. Describe the historical under-pinnings of home health care.
5. Discuss the pros and cons of having new graduates of nursing programs employed by a home health care agency.
6. Discuss the reality of providing quality, effective home health care services within the current health care system.
7. Explain how a home health care agency balances the need for services versus the realities of reimbursement.
8. Discuss the differences between the reimbursements for Medicare supported home care and hospice care and patient care considerations.

References

Anderson, G., & Horvath, J. (2004). The growing burden of chronic disease in America. *Public Health Reports, 119* (3), 263–270.

Benjamin, A. (2001). Consumer-directed services at home: A new model for persons with disabilities. *Health Affairs, 20,* (6), 80.

Brown, N., & Neal, L. (1999). Development of a managed care team in a traditional home healthcare agency. *Journal of Nursing Administration, 27,* 43–48.

California Association for Health Services at Home. (2000a). DHS comes through for home health, *16* (12).

Centers for Medicare and Medicaid Services. (2004). The Facts about Upcoming New Benefits in Medicare. US Department of Health and Human Services Available at http://www.medicare.gov/Publications/Pubs/pdf/11054.pdf

Citarella, B. (2000). Preparing for PPS: Developing a comprehensive education program. *The Remington Report: Business and clinical solutions for home care and post-acute markets,* July/August, 16–18.

Department of Health and Human Services. *Federal Register, 63* (2) (1998).

Department of Health and Human Services. *Federal Register, 65* (2000).

Department of Health and Human Services. (2001). Administration on Aging: Older Americans Act amendments of 2000. Available on-line at: http://www.aoa.dhhs.gov.

Grindel-Waggoner, M. (1999). Home care: A history of caring, a future of challenges. *MedSurg Nursing, 8,* 118–122.

Gundersen, L. (1999). There's no place like home: The home health care alternative. *Annals of Internal Medicine, 131,* 639–640.

Health Care Financing Administration. (1997). Department of Health and Human Services. *Federal Register, 62* (6).

Hitchcock, J., Schubert, P., & Thomas, S. (Eds.). (2003). *Community health nursing: Caring in action.* (2nd ed). Albany, NY: Delmar.

Jamieson, M. (1998). Expanding the associate degree curriculum without adding time. *Nursing and Health Care Perspectives, 19* (4), 161–163.

Kane, R., Ouslander, J., & Abrass, I. (1999). *Essentials of clinical geriatrics* (2nd ed.). New York: McGraw-Hill.

King, I. M. (1996). The theory of goal attainment in research and practice. *Nursing Science Quarterly, 9,* 61–66.

Leininger, M. M. (1996). Culture care theory, research, and practice. *Nursing Science Quarterly, 9,* 71–78.

Leino-Kilpi, H., & Kuokkanen, L. (2000). Power and empowerment in nursing: three theoretical approaches. *Journal of Advanced Nursing, 31,* 235–241.

Lewis, A. (2000). Prospective pay the easy way. *The Remington Report, 8,* 5–7.

Lundy, K., & Janes, S. (2001). *Community health nursing: Caring for the public's health.* Sudbury, MA: Jones & Bartlett.

Lundy, K., & Janes, S. (2003). *Essentials of community-based nursing.* Sudbury, MA: Jones & Bartlett.

Majorowicz, K. (1999). Coordinating the medicare home health benefit. *CME Resource,* 17–42.

Malugani, M. (1999). No place like home: Always adaptable, home care faces the future. *Nurseweek, 12* (24), 1, 18.

Manger, D., & Fredette, S. (2000). New graduates can succeed in home care. *Journal of Nursing Scholarship, 32,* 6.

Marelli, T. (1998). *Handbook of home health standards and documentation guidelines for reimbursement.* St. Louis: Mosby.

Markey, C. (2004). Understanding the Impact of the New Medicare Law on Home Health Patients. *Home Healthcare Nurse, 22,* 378–379.

Maurer, F., & Smith, C. (2005). *Community/public health nursing practice.* St. Louis: Elsevier Saunders.

Montauk, S. (1998). Home health care. *American Family Physician, 58,* 1609–1614.

National Center for Chronic Disease Prevention and Health Promotion. (2004). Indicators for Chronic Disease Surveillance. *MMWR, 53, (RR11),* 1–6. Available at http://www.cdc.gov/mmwr/preview/mmwrhtml/rr5311a1.htm

Nugent, D. (1999). Providing solutions for the growing trend toward home health care. *Health Management Technology, 20,* 28.

Orem, D. E. (1997). Views of human beings specific to nursing. *Nursing Science Quarterly, 10,* 26–31.

Oriol, M. (1997). Specialty team development: One agency's formula. *Home Healthcare Nurse, 15,* 505–508.

Pierson, C., & Minarik, P. (1999). APNs in home care. *American Journal of Nursing, 99,* 22–23.

Randall, D. (2000). Compliance issues for home health agencies under the new medicare PPS system. *The Remington report: Business and clinical solutions for home care and post-acute markets, November/December,* 16–18.

Reichley, M. (1999). Advances in home care: Then, now and into the future. *Success in Home Care, 3* (6), 10–18.

Remington, L. (2000). PPS is making people run out of excuses for a change. *The Remington report: Business and clinical solutions for home care and post-acute markets, July/August,* 13–15.

Rice, D. P., & Fineman, N. (2004). Economic implications of increased longevity in the United States. *Annual Review of Public Health, 25,* 457–473.

Schim, S., Jackson, F., Seely, S., Grunow, K., et al. (2000). Knowledge and attitude of home care nurses toward hospice referral. *Journal of Nursing Administration, 30,* 273–277.

Schoen, M., & Koenig, R. (1997). Home health care nursing: Past and present. *Medsurg Nursing, 6* (4), 230–234.

Schroeder, B. (2000). Medicare OASIS for home health. *Nurseweek, 13* (4), 12–13.

Stafford, D., Seemons, D., & Jones, J. (1997). Case management through productivity engineering. Part 1: Development of the intensity of home care acuity scale. *Home Health Care Manager Practice, 9* (4), 1–5.

Stanhope, M., & Lancaster, J. (1998). *Community health nursing: Process and practice for promoting health.* St. Louis: Mosby.

Stanhope, M. & Lancaster, J. (2002). *Foundations of community health nursing: Community-oriented practice.* St. Louis: Mosby.

Taylor, S. G., Compton, A., Eben, J. D., Emerson, S., et al. (2002). Dorothea E. Orem: Self-care deficit theory of nursing. In A. M. Tomey, & M. R. Alligood (Eds.), *Nursing theorists and their work,* (pp. 175–194). St. Louis: Mosby.

US Congress (2000b). *Congress considers BBA relief. 16* (10), 1, 4.

Unwin, B., & Jerant, A. (1999). The home visit. *American Family Physician, 60,* 1481–1490.

von Gunten, C., Ferris, F., Portenoy, R., & Glajchen, M. (2001). Medicare Hospice Benefit Reimbursement Rates (Eds.), *CAPC Manual: How to Establish A Palliative Care Program.* New York: Center to Advance Palliative Care.

Zhu, C. (2004). Effects of the Balanced Budget Act on Medicare Home Health Utilization. *Journal of American Geriatrics Society, 52,* 989–994.

CHAPTER 23

Palliative Care

Barbara M. Raudonis

Death is inevitable. Severe suffering is not.

Kathleen Foley

Introduction

The aging American population will eventually experience one or more chronic illnesses with which they will live for years before death (Morrison & Meier, 2004). Four chronic diseases, heart disease, cancer, cerebrovascular disease, and chronic respiratory disease, are the leading causes of death for older adults (Centers for Disease Control, National Center for Health Statistics, 2002). These chronic diseases share protracted illness trajectories that include phases of decline resulting in progressively advanced disease and disability. Individuals with illness trajectories such as those associated with chronic disease can benefit from palliative care.

Historical Perspectives

Palliative care has its roots in the hospice movement; thus a discussion of hospice is pertinent to discussing palliative care. Hospice is both a philosophy of care and an organized form of health care delivery. The Latin origin of the word *hospes* relates to hospitality. During the Middle Ages, pilgrims to the Holy Lands stopped at way stations for food, water, and respite. These way stations (hospices) were also centers of refuge for poor, sick, and dying people.

Dame Cicely Saunders is considered the founder of the modern hospice movement. Educated as a nurse, social worker, and physician, she founded St. Christopher's Hospice in Sydenham, England, in 1967. St. Christopher's Hospice was the first research and teaching hospice, and it is known for innovations in pain and symptom management, providing a holistic approach to care, home care, family support throughout the illness and bereavement follow-up (Lattanzi-Licht, Mahoney, & Miller, 1998). The services provided by St. Christopher's Hospice evolved over time to meet the needs of patients and families, and now include in-patient care, home care, and a day center. In the United Kingdom (UK) hospice and palliative day care is the fastest growing, but least researched, component of palliative care services (Hearn & Myers, 2001).

Hospice and palliative day care is a complex service with the goal of improving the quality of life of terminally ill individuals through a variety of programs in an individualized, flexible, and non-medical environment (Hearn & Myers, 2001). In the UK, no eligibility criteria related to prognosis exist to access services. Therefore, clients may be admitted early in their illness trajectory. Early entry enables them to participate in activities such as arts and crafts projects and outings. The traditional services offered include a review of symptom control and medications, respite for relatives and friends, companionship of people with similar problems, counseling and support and help with personal hygiene (Haywood House, 1996; St. Christopher's Hospice, 1996). St. Christopher's Hospice continues to serve as a prototype for hospice and palliative care throughout the world. However, Dame Saunders cautions not to clone St. Christopher's, but to refine the principles of hospice and palliative care within the cultural context of the needs of the individuals served.

Two years after the opening of St. Christopher's Hospice, Elisabeth Kubler-Ross's book *On Death and Dying* (1969) was published. One of the outcomes of her seminal work was the identification of the stages of dying. More importantly, her work initiated a national dialog regarding the needs of the dying.

Florence S. Wald, a nurse and pioneer in the hospice movement in the United States, strengthened her vision for improving the quality of life for terminally ill persons during a visit to St. Christopher's Hospice. After conducting a needs assessment for hospice care in Connecticut, Wald opened the first hospice program in the United State in 1974. The Connecticut Hospice was established as a home-care program (without in patient beds) and became a model of care for the entire United States. As services evolved, inpatient beds were added, and the Connecticut Hospice became the first independent hospice inpatient facility in the country (Lattanzi-Licht et al., 1998). Wald's work for the next 30 years led the way in translating the English hospice philosophy and models of care into the American hospice movement. She is considered the "mother of hospice and palliative nursing care in the United States" by the Hospice and Palliative Nurses Association and Foundation. She became the first

recipient of the Hospice and Palliative Nurses Association 'Leading the Way Award' in January, 2004 (Hospice and Palliative Nurses Association, 2005).

The National Hospice and Palliative Care Organization (NHPCO) (2005) estimated in 2003 there were 3,300 operational hospice programs throughout the United States with an estimated 950,000 patients being served by these programs. These figures illustrate the enormous growth and progress in hospice care since 1974. However, in 2003 for all Americans who died, approximately 50% died in a hospital. These numbers suggest that hospice care is still a "best kept secret."

During the 1990s, two reports further influenced the hospice and palliative care movement in the United States. Those reports, the SUPPORT study (*Study to Understand Prognosis and Preferences for Outcomes and Risks of Treatments*) (1995) and the Institute of Medicine (IOM) report, *Approaching Death: Improving Care at the End of Life* (1997) were pivotal in bringing the status of end of life care to the forefront of health care.

SUPPORT Study

The SUPPORT study (SUPPORT Principal Investigators, 1995) was funded by the Robert Wood Johnson Foundation for $29 million to study the process of dying in five American teaching hospitals. The study involved approximately 9,000 participants with congestive heart failure (CHF), chronic obstructive pulmonary disease (COPD), colon cancer, lung cancer, and liver failure. Findings revealed that greater than 50% of clients had serious pain during the last three days of life. In addition, there was poor communication between doctors and clients about their goals of care, accompanied by substantial emotional suffering of clients, families, and healthcare professionals. Thirty-one percent of the families lost most of their life savings in providing care for their loved ones. The findings from this study sparked a groundswell of initiatives in research, education, and practice with the goal of changing the culture of death and dying in the United States.

IOM Report

The second landmark study was the Institute of Medicine's Committee on Care at the End of Life report, *Approaching Death: Improving Care at the End of Life* (Field & Cassel, 1997). The committee found four broad deficiencies in the care of individuals with life-threatening and incurable illnesses. These deficiencies included:

- Too many people suffer needlessly at the end of life both from errors of omission—when caregivers fail to provide palliative and support care known to be effective—and from errors of commission—when caregivers do what is known to be ineffective and even harmful;
- Legal, organizational, and economic obstacles conspire to obstruct reliably excellent care at the end of life;
- The education and training of physicians and other health care professionals fail to provide them with the knowledge, skills, and attitudes required to care well for the client who is dying; and
- Current knowledge and understanding are inadequate to guide and support the consistent practice of evidence-based medicine at the end of life (pp. 264-265).

Healthcare professionals, clients, families, health plan administrators, agency administrators, and policy makers must work together to influence and change attitudes, policies, and actions to surmount the deficiencies in palliative care (Field & Cassel, 1997). The report concluded with optimism that a "vigorous societal commitment . . . would motivate and sustain individual and collective efforts to create a humane care system that people can trust to serve them well as they die" (Field & Cassel, 1997, p. 13).

Clinical Practice Guidelines for Palliative Care

The SUPPORT study and the IOM work led to recognizing the need to integrate palliative care into health care of individuals with chronic, debilitating and life-limiting illnesses. This need resulted in the National Consensus Project for Quality Palliative Care (NCPQPC) and the establishment of Clinical Practice Guidelines (National Consensus Project for Quality Palliative Care, 2004).

The Clinical Practice Guidelines promote consistent high standards of palliative care. In addition, individual providers regardless of setting can use the guidelines to provide palliative approaches in their daily clinical practice across the health care continuum (NCPQPC, 2004). The National Institutes of Health (NIH) recognized the need to evaluate the current science regarding end-of-life care and convened the first State-of-the-Science Conference on Improving End-of-Life Care in December 2004.

Clinical Specialty of Palliative Care

Palliative care is a broad term used to describe the care provided by an interdisciplinary team consisting of physicians, nurses, social workers, chaplains, and other health care professionals to clients with long term illnesses.

Palliative Medicine

Palliative medicine is an accepted medical specialty in the United Kingdom, Australia, Hong Kong, Taiwan, and Romania. In 1987 the United Kingdom adopted the following definition of palliative medicine:

> . . . is the study and management of patients with active, progressive, far-advanced disease, for whom the prognosis is limited and the focus of care is the quality of life (Derek, Hanks, Cherny, & Calman, 2004).

In the United States, the American Board of Hospice and Palliative Medicine (ABHPM) incorporated and initiated its first certification examination in 1996 (ABHPM, 2005). The American

Academy of Hospice and Palliative Medicine's (AAHPM) mission is dedicated to excellence in and advancement of palliative medicine (AAHPM, 2005). Members include physicians and other medical professionals. The AAHPM has since updated their definition of palliative medicine as follows:

The specialty of Palliative Medicine is the study and treatment of patients living with life-threatening or severe advanced illness expected to progress toward dying and where care is particularly focused on alleviating suffering and promoting quality of life. Major components are pain and symptom management, information sharing, advance care planning, and coordination of care, including psychosocial and spiritual support for patients and their families. The special needs of the pediatric and geriatric populations and patients' cultural contexts are considered when formulating a comprehensive treatment plan.

The palliative medicine physician serves as a consultant to other physicians but is often the principal treating physician and may provide care at various levels. Activities include but are not limited to, directing treatment, prescribing medication, prescribing palliative services, performing pain relieving procedures, counseling patients and families, participating on a multidisciplinary team, coordinating care with other health care providers, and providing consultative services to public and private agencies pursuant to optimal healthcare delivery to the patient (AAHPM, 2005).

Palliative Care Nursing

Palliative care nursing parallels the continuing development of the art and science of palliative care. The scope of palliative care nursing involves the "provision of evidence-based physical, emotional, psychosocial, and spiritual care to individuals and families experiencing life-limiting progressive illness" (Hospice and Palliative Nurses Association & American Nurses Association, 2002, p. 5). This care is provided across settings and throughout the illness trajectory, the client's death and the family's bereavement. There are two levels of hospice and palliative care nursing practice: generalist and advanced. Advance practice nurses, registered nurses, licensed practical/vocational nurses, and nursing assistants can all become certified through the certification examinations offered by the National Board for Certification of Hospice and Palliative Nurses (NBCHPN).

Differentiating Hospice Care and Palliative Care

It is critical to differentiate between hospice care and palliative care in the context of clinical practice. The terms hospice and palliative care are frequently used interchangeably. Palliative care is a broader concept and includes the entire continuum of care. Hospice care is palliative care, but not all palliative care is hospice care.

Hospice is a specific type of palliative care, and in the United States it is generally considered a philosophy or program of care rather than a building of bricks and mortar. Hospice programs provide state-of-the-art palliative care and supportive services to dying persons and their families. This comprehensive care is available 24 hours a day, every day of the year in community-based settings, homes and facility-based care settings. A medically directed interdisciplinary team (clients, family members, professionals and volunteers) provide physical, psychosocial, and spiritual care during the final phase of an illness, the process of imminently dying, and the period of bereavement (Standards and Accreditation Committee, 1999). In hospice care the dying person and the family are the unit of care. Client and family values direct the care. However, the current Medicare hospice benefit eligibility criteria for hospice services include a terminal diagnosis and a six month prognosis. In addition, it requires that clients discontinue curative or life-prolonging treatments to access comprehensive hospice care (Lynn, 2001).

The three outcomes of hospice care include: 1) self-determined life closure; 2) safe and comfortable dying, and 3) effective grieving (Standards and Accreditation Committee, 1997). Humane, holistic, comprehensive plans of care involving an interdisciplinary health care team are critical to maintain quality of life for the person and family making the transition to end of life. In the United States, hospice is the gold standard for end of life care (Billings, 1998).

One of the first definitions of palliative care accepted throughout the world was developed by the World Health Organization (1990). Subsequent definitions have been developed or refined by the National Hospice and Palliative Care Organization (NHPCO), the American Academy of Hospice and Palliative Medicine (AAHPM) and the Center to Advance Palliative Care (CAPC) (See Table 23-1).

Although it appears that hospice and palliative care have much in common, there are two major distinctions. First, palliative care *permits* the continued use of life-prolonging therapies. For the client with cancer, it might include radiation therapy or chemotherapy. Secondly, palliative care is integrated throughout the course of a chronic, progressive, and incurable disease, from diagnosis through death, rather than during the final six months of life. The chronic illness experience of clients and their families demonstrates the need for comprehensive palliative care early in the disease trajectory (Portenoy, 1998).

In response to the need for broadening the scope of palliative care, the Last Acts Palliative Care Task Force reformulated palliative care to include all persons with serious or life-threatening illness. The Last Acts Palliative Care Task Force developed five palliative care precepts or principles of care (see Table 23-2). Integration of these precepts into clinical practice enables clinicians to provide a continuum of care otherwise unavailable to clients with advancing illness and their families (Cumming & Okun, 2004).

Palliative Care and Chronic Illness

Chronic illness is never completely cured, and it involves the "total human environment for sup-

portive care and self-care, maintenance of function and prevention of further disability" (Curtin & Lubkin, 1995, pp. 6–7). Symptoms may increase or decrease during phases of stability, exacerbation, remission, and eventually death (Corbin, 2001).

Palliative care seeks to treat, reduce, or prevent symptoms of diseases, relieve suffering and improve the client and family's quality of life without effecting a cure. It is not restricted to dying hospice clients (Field & Cassel, 1997). The principles of palliative care extend to broader populations that can benefit from holistic, comprehensive plans of care involving interdisciplinary health care teams from the time of diagnosis and throughout the disease processes and illness trajectory.

According to von Guten, (2001) Palliative Care is interdisciplinary care that focuses on relieving suffering and improving quality of life. This simple definition illustrates the fit between chronic illness and palliative care, making it clear that persons with chronic illness can benefit from palliative care.

Problems and Barriers Related to Palliative Care

Barriers to clients receiving palliative care exist for many reasons. The major underlying resistance to palliative care stems from a medical philosophy that emphasizes cure and prolongation of life over quality of life and relief of suffering (Morrison & Meier, 2004). Insurance reimbursement also forces consumer choice between cure and comfort care. Medicare only reimburses for curative treatment, leaving the Medicare hospice benefit to cover comfort care (Fisher, Wennberg, Stukel, Gottlieb, Lucas, & Pinder, 2003).

The SUPPORT study (1995) findings identified several problems related to palliative care. Client suffering included dying in pain with severe symptoms. Poor communication between clients, families and their physicians led to undesired resuscitation efforts and extensive use of hospital resources.

Communication is a core skill of palliative care. However, many clinicians are uncomfortable sharing bad news and poor prognoses. Recent studies

---

TABLE 23-1 ——

Definitions of Palliative Care

World Health Organization (WHO)

The active total care of clients whose disease is not responsive to curative treatment. Control of pain, of other symptoms, and of psychological, social, and spiritual problems is paramount. The goal of palliative care is achievement of the best quality of life for clients and families. It affirms life and regards dying as a normal process. Palliative care neither hastens nor postpones death. It emphasizes relief from spiritual aspects of client care and offers a support system to help the family cope during the client's illness and in their own bereavement.

National Hospice and Palliative Care Organization (NHPCO)

The treatment that enhances comfort and improves the quality of an individual's life during the last phase of life. No specific therapy is excluded from consideration. The test of palliative care lies in the agreement between the individual, physician(s), primary caregiver, and the hospice team that the expected outcome is relief from distressing symptoms, the easing of pain, and/or enhancing the quality of life. The decision to intervene with active palliative care is based on an ability to meet the stated goals rather than affect the underlying disease. An individual's needs must continue to be assessed and all treatment options explored and evaluated in the context of the individual's values and symptoms. The individual's choices and decisions regarding care are paramount and must be followed

American Academy of Hospice and Palliative Medicine

Palliative Care is comprehensive, specialized care provided by an interdisciplinary team to patients and families living with a life-threatening or severe advanced illness expected to progress toward dying and where care is particularly focused on alleviating suffering and promoting quality of life. Major concerns are pain and symptom management, information sharing and advance care planning, psychosocial and spiritual support, and coordination of care.

Center to Advance Palliative Care

Palliative care aims to relieve suffering and improve quality of life for patients with advanced illness, and their families. Palliative care is provided by an interdisciplinary team and offered in conjunction with all other appropriate forms of medical treatment.

Palliative care programs structure a variety of hospital resources—medical and nursing specialists, social workers, clergy—to effectively deliver the highest quality of care to patients with advanced illness. Vigorous pain and symptom control is integrated into all stages of treatment.

The palliative care approach decreases length of hospital and ICU stays and eases patient transitions between care settings, resulting in increased patient and family satisfaction and compliance with hospital care quality standards. Successful palliative care programs have used an array of delivery systems, from consultative services to inpatient units.

SOURCES: WHO (World Health Organization). (1990). *Cancer pain relief and palliative care.* WHO Technical Report Series 804 (p.11). Geneva: WHO.
National Hospice and Palliative Care Organization (NHPCO). Retrieved on January 10, 2005 from http://www.nhpco.org
American Academy of Hospice and Palliative Medicine (AAHPM). Retrieved on January 10, 2005 from http://www. nhpco.org
Center to Advance Palliative Care (CAPC). Retrieved on January 10, 2005 from http://capc.org

suggest that "patient-centered" interviews are associated with improved levels of satisfaction on the part of patients and their families (Dowsett, Saul, Butow, et al., 2000; Steinhauser, Christakis, Clipp, McNeilly, McIntyre, & Tulsky, 2000).

The Institute of Medicine (IOM) (Field & Cassel, 1997) work, *Approaching Death: Improving Care at the End of Life*, revealed a critical need for improvement in the education and training of health care professionals in palliative care and end of

TABLE 23-2

Precepts of Palliative Care

1. Respecting patient goals, preferences, and choices
2. Providing comprehensive caring
3. Utilizing the strengths of interdisciplinary resources
4. Acknowledging and addressing caregiver concerns
5. Building systems and mechanisms of support

From: Lomax, K.J., & Scanlon, C. (1997). *Precepts of palliative care* (Last Acts Task Force on Palliative Care). Princeton, NJ: The Robert Wood Johnson Foundation/Last Acts

life care. Health care professionals have traditionally received inadequate education and training in effectively managing pain and other symptoms. They also lack the skills and confidence to address the psychological, social and spiritual aspects of care (Sullivan, Lakoma, & Block, 2003).

Nursing curricula and textbooks have been found to be deficient in palliative and end of life content and clinical learning opportunities. If nurses are not taught that their professional role includes providing quality palliative care and end of life care, then they cannot practice it (Ferrell, Virani, & Grant, 1999). In response to these identified issues, resources for teaching palliative care nursing to students and practicing nurses have been and continue to be developed and disseminated. Essential nursing competencies in end-of-life care were proposed and disseminated by the American Association of Colleges of Nursing (AACN) in the document entitled "Peaceful Death" (1998). Matzo and Sherman (2001) used the AACN competencies as the framework for their nursing textbook entitled: *Palliative Care Nursing: Quality Care to the End of Life.* Ferrell and Coyle (2001) wrote a comprehensive volume entitled the *Textbook of Palliative Nursing.* Recognizing the special needs of older adults, Matzo and Sherman also authored a textbook entitled *Gerontologic Palliative Care Nursing* (2004).

Prognostication in chronic, debilitating and life-threatening illness presents a major challenge for health care professionals and is a barrier to adequate palliative care (Christakis & Lamont, 2000). Our current health care system forces clients and families

to choose between curative treatment and comfort care. However, there is growing recognition that palliative care is needed from the time of diagnosis through the process of dying (Foley, 2001). Reiterating von Guten's (1999) definition of palliative care: interdisciplinary care focused on the relief of suffering and improving quality of life, removes any burden of prognostication and the requirement of a terminal diagnosis.

The public's lack of understanding related to the options available to dying clients and their families results in delayed access to hospice and palliative care services (Field & Cassel, 1997). Surveys consistently indicate that clients prefer to die at home. However, in 2003, for all Americans who died, approximately 25% died at home, 25% died in a long term care facility, and approximately 50% of deaths occurred in a hospital (National Hospice and Palliative Care Organization, 2005). Consumers' and communities' lack of understanding of what comprehensive palliative care programs offer, and poor communication about client and family preferences and denial of death, all impede timely referrals to palliative care services [End of Life Nursing Education Consortium (ELNEC) Curriculum, Module 1, 2000].

Family Caregiving Burden

In palliative care, the client and family are the unit of care. Family caregivers provide supportive care throughout the chronic illness trajectory, in all care settings, and for all types of needs (McMillan, 2004). The caregiver's burden is increasingly significant as more complex health care moves into the home setting. Evidence is growing that extended time as a caregiver can negatively impact the physical, social, and emotional well-being of caregivers (Pinquart & Sorenson, 2003). Some caregivers experience sustained stress related to highly stressful times of caregiving, and this negatively impacts their bereavement process (Schultz, Mendelsohn, Haley, et al., 2003; Schultz, Newsom, Fleissner, DeCamp, & Nieboer, 1997).

Successful intervention studies have been carried out to decrease caregiver burden with caregivers of clients with Alzheimer's disease, but little has been done with caregivers of hospice and palliative care clients. The NIH Consensus Statement on Improving End of Life Care (2004) concluded that more randomized clinical trials examining decreasing caregiver burden are needed. Studies are needed to determine which caregivers are at greatest risk for distress and specific interventions most likely to relieve the distress.

Interventions

The IOM report developed seven recommendations (see Table 23-3) to address the four identified areas of deficiency in palliative and end of life care. Change is occurring, due in part to the increased involvement of health care consumers in the 21st century about the issues related to quality of care, quality of life, advance care planning and the burdens of caregiving (Berry, 2004).

Approximately 100 articles have been published based on the findings of the SUPPORT study. Implications of the data for future reform suggest that individual, client-level decision-making may not be the most effective strategy for improving end-of-life care. The SUPPORT investigators recommend system-level innovations and quality improvement in routine care as potentially effective strategies for change (Lynn et al., 2000).

Interventions for palliative care must relate to the domains of its science and practice. Researchers (Emanuel & Emanuel, 1998; Steinhauser et al., 2000; and Teno, 2001) and professional organizations such as the National Hospice and Palliative Care Organi-

---

TABLE 23-3

Recommendations from the IOM Committee on Care at the End of Life

1. People with advanced, potentially fatal illnesses and those close to them should be able to expect and receive reliable, skillful, and supportive care.
2. Physicians, nurses, social workers, and other health professionals must commit themselves to improving care for dying patients and to using existing knowledge effectively to prevent and relieve pain and other symptoms.
3. Because many deficiencies in care reflect system problems, policymakers, consumer groups, and purchases of health care should work with health care providers and researchers to:
   a. strengthen methods for measuring the quality of life and other outcomes of care for dying patients and those close to them;
   b. develop better tools and strategies for improving the quality of care and holding health care organizations accountable for care at the end of life;
   c. revise mechanisms for financing care so that they encourage rather than impede good end-of-life care and sustain rather than frustrate coordinated systems of excellent care; and
   d. reform drug prescription laws, burdensome regulations, and state medical board policies and practices that impede effective use of opioids to relieve pain and suffering.
4. Educators and other health professionals should initiate changes in undergraduate, graduate, and continuing education to ensure that practitioners have the relevant attitudes, knowledge, and skills to care well for dying patients.
5. Palliative care should become, if not a medical specialty, at least a defined area of expertise, education, and research.
6. The nation's research establishment should define and implement priorities for strengthening the knowledge base for end-of-life care.
7. A continuing public discussion is essential to develop a better understanding of the modern experience of dying, the options available to dying patients and families, and the obligations of communities to those approaching death (pp. 270–271).

SOURCE: Field M.J. & Cassel, C.K. (Eds.). (1997) *Approaching Death: Improving Care at the End of Life.* Reprinted with permission from the National Academy of Sciences. Courtesy of the National Academies Press, Washington D.C.

zation (2002) and the American Geriatrics Society (Lynn, 1997) have published standards of care, as well as philosophical or conceptual frameworks describing proposed domains of end-of-life care (Ferrell, 2004).

A major advancement of the science and practice of palliative care occurred with the release of the Clinical Practice Guidelines by the National Consensus Project for Quality Palliative Care (NCP) (2004). Groups that participated in the NCP were the American Academy of Hospice and Palliative Medicine, the Center to Advance Palliative Care, the Hospice and Palliative Nurses Association, the Last Acts Partnership, and the National Hospice and Palliative Care Organization. The purpose of the NCP was to establish Clinical Practice Guidelines that promoted consistent, high quality care, and guided the development and structure of new and existing palliative care services. The two-year consensus process involved reviewing 2,000 articles from the literature, 31 consensus documents and standards, and peer review by 200 experts in the field (Ferrell, 2004). The purposes of the Clinical Practice Guidelines for Quality Palliative Care are to:

- Facilitate the development and continuing improvement of clinical palliative care programs providing care to patients and families with life-threatening or debilitating illness.
- Establish uniformly accepted definitions of the essential elements in palliative care that promote quality, consistency, and reliability of these services.
- Establish national goals for access to quality palliative care.
- Foster performance measurement and quality improvement initiatives in palliative care services (Ferrell, 2004, p.30).

Recognizing a need for clarity in the definitions of key concepts or domains of end-of-life care and a framework for advancing research and practice, the NCP developed the following domains.

- Domain 1: Structure and processes of care
- Domain 2: Physical aspects of care

- Domain 3: Psychological and psychiatric aspects of care
- Domain 4: Social aspects of care
- Domain 5: Spiritual, religious, and existential aspects of care
- Domain 6: Cultural aspects of care
- Domain 7: Care of the imminently dying patient
- Domain 8: Ethical and legal aspects of care

Determining Goals of Care

The domains identified by the NCP (above) guide decision-making regarding research, practice, and policy. Each domain is an area for an intervention for improving end of life care and meeting the needs of palliative care clients and their families. Palliative care interventions logically flow from goals of care. Therefore, the first step in palliative care is to establish the goals of care (Morrison & Meier, 2004). In the context of chronic, debilitating, and life-threatening illness, realistic and attainable goals of care that relieve pain and other symptoms, improve quality of life, limit the burden of care, enhance personal relationships, and provide a sense of control are crucial to dying persons and their families (Steinhauser et al., 2000; Singer, Martin, & Kelner, 1999).

Health care professionals must work with clients and their families to establish appropriate goals of care. Using open-ended and probing questions may be helpful when interviewing the client (Morrison & Meier, 2004). Examples of possible questions include: "What makes life worth living for you?" "Given the severity of your illness, what are the most important things for you to achieve?" "What are your most important hopes?" "What are your biggest fears?" and "What would you consider to be a fate worse than death?" (Quill, 2000).

Goals of care are dynamic and change across the trajectory of the disease (EPEC Project, 2004; Quill, 2000). Meier, Back, and Morrison (2001) describe some of the warning signs of ineffective or contradictory goals as frequent or lengthy hospitalizations, physician feelings of frustration, anger, or powerlessness, and feelings of caregiver burden.

Assessment and Treatment of Symptoms

A core principle of palliative care is comprehensive care that includes the relief of pain and other symptoms (Steinhauser et al., 2000). Effective symptom management begins with a thorough assessment. Research findings support the practice of routine and standardized symptom assessment with validated instruments (Morrison & Meier, 2004). Benefits attributed to routine assessments include identification of overlooked or unreported symptoms (Bookbinder, Coyle, Kiss, et al., 1996; Manfredi, Morrison, Morris, Goldhirsch, Carter, & Meier, 2000). Dissemination and increased use of the same validated instruments will facilitate the comparison of findings across practice settings and research studies. The Center to Advance Palliative Care (www.capc.org) and Brown University's Center for Gerontology and Health Care Research provide access to clinically useful instruments through their respective Web sites. Brown's Web site features a tool kit of instruments to measure end-of-life care. (www.chcr.brown.edu/pcpc/toolkit.htm).

The nursing assessment of clients receiving palliative care is the same as a standard nursing assessment. However, the palliative care assessment focuses on enhancing the client's quality of life. Ferrell's (1995) quality of life framework is useful in organizing the assessment according to four domains: physical, psychological, social, and spiritual well-being. Based on the changing needs of clients and families across the trajectory of the chronic illness, quality of life should be assessed four times: 1) at the time of diagnosis; 2) treatment, post-treatment; 3) long term survival or terminal phase; and 4) active dying. A comprehensive assessment serves as the foundation for goal-setting, developing a plan of care, implementing interventions, and evaluating the outcomes and effectiveness of care (Glass, Cluxton, & Rancour, 2001).

The prevalence of symptom burden for clients at the end of life is high. Assessment and management of symptoms have been studied most thoroughly in clients with cancer according to the NIH State of the Science Consensus Statement on Improving End-of-

Life Care (2004). Clients with other life-limiting illnesses, such as congestive heart failure, have their own challenges. Regardless of the diagnosis, there are symptoms common to advanced disease. These common symptoms include: anorexia and cachexia, anxiety, constipation, depression, delirium, dyspnea, nausea, and pain (Morrison & Meier, 2004). It is beyond the scope of this chapter to describe in detail the assessment and management recommendations for these symptoms; however, there are numerous resources in the literature with specific protocols and interventions Examples include the AGS Panel on Persistent Pain in Older Persons (2002); Block (2002); Casarett & Inouye (2001); Luce & Luce (2001); and Strasser & Bruera (2002).

Palliative care is needed across the lifespan, and assessments and interventions should be tailored to the specific population served. Often the literature categorizes adults as a homogenous group needing palliative care. Experts in gerontology, however, are calling for recognition of the unique palliative care needs of older adults (Cassel, 2003). Amella (2003) described the common goal of helping clients experience the best quality of life as the touchstone for collaboration between geriatric and palliative care nurse specialists. Symptoms of illness and dying may appear differently, for longer periods of time, and in greater numbers in older adults (Amella, 2003). Pain, confusion, dyspnea, fatigue, satiety and anorexia, gastrointestinal distress, infection, fever and fears and depression are symptoms that can present differently in older adults.

At the other end of the lifespan, initiatives are underway that address palliative care in children. In 2003, the IOM released its latest report, *When Children Die: Improving Palliative and End-of-Life Care for Children and Their Families.* The report identified challenges which can be used to focus efforts and resources to improve palliative care for children and their families (see Table 23-4).

Advance Directives

Following the establishment of the goals of care, the next logical intervention is the completion of ad-

Four Basic Challenges to Improve Pediatric Palliative Care

1. Children should have care that is focused on their special needs and the needs of their families.
2. Health plans should make it easier for children and families to get palliative care.
3. Health care professionals should be trained to give palliative care to children.
4. Researchers should find out more about what care works best for children.

SOURCE: Field M.J. & Behrman, R.E. (Eds.). (2003). When children die: Improving palliative and end-of-life care for children and their families. Reprinted with permission from the National Academy of Sciences. Courtesy of the National Academies Press, Washington, D.C..

vance directives. Goals of care reflect the values, beliefs, and culture of the person with a serious, life threatening illness. Numerous studies (Miles, Koepp, & Weber, 1996) report that most people do not have advance directives and the documents that do exist are ineffective in improving communication between clients and their physicians (Morrison & Meier, 2004). Other authors report that advance directives are ineffective in the decision-making related to cardiopulmonary resuscitation (Teno et al., 1997). Morrison and Meier (2004) suggest that as the number of advance directives increases, more consumers and health care professionals will become familiar with the documents, thus improving their effectiveness. The current literature suggests that the focus of advance care planning should shift to determining an acceptable quality of life and goals of care (Fried, Bradley, Towle, & Allore, 2002; Meier, & Morrison, 2002). This type of discussion is the critical element, not the mere completion of the forms.

It is also important to be knowledgeable of your state's required documents and process for the completion of advance directives. The process and forms vary from state to state. The names of the documents may also vary. The two basic forms are: 1) Power of Attorney for Health Care: A document that appoints an agent or proxy who becomes the decision maker when the individual can no longer do so: and 2) Directive to Physician (Living Will): A document that gives direction to a physician regarding the type of care/procedures that are wanted or not wanted (artificial nutrition, hydration, or mechanical ventilation etc.) if the individual cannot speak for him/her self.

Psychosocial, Spiritual and Bereavement Needs

Psychosocial, spiritual and bereavement care are key components of palliative care. Professional and accrediting bodies such as JCAHO now require documentation of spiritual assessments of clients.

Members of interdisciplinary palliative care teams assess and intervene to meet the spiritual and psychosocial needs of clients and their families. Bereavement support is part of the follow-up care after an individual dies. Research demonstrates that family members with spiritual and psychological distress are more likely to experience extended or a complicated grief and bereavement process (McClain, Rosenfield, & Breitbart, 2003).

Acknowledgement of spiritual distress, alone, can be an intervention. However, a common language and mutual comfort must be present for a meaningful exchange to occur (Chochinov, 2004). Helping clients die with dignity is a basic tenet of palliative care. Empirical work with dying clients found that the paradigm of dignity which includes matters of spirituality, meaning, purpose, and other psycho-social issues related to dying was acceptable language and a topic for discussion (Chochinov, Hack, Hassard, Kristjanson, McClement, & Harlos, 2004). This work is adding to the growing empirical evidence that palliative care is more than symptom management and must include the spiritual, psychosocial and existential concerns.

Chochinov's research team developed a Dignity Model (2004) which serves as the basis for the psychotherapeutic intervention, Dignity Therapy. The phase I data from this work is undergoing analysis at the present time. Those results will be the basis for a randomized clinical trial which will "attempt to further establish the efficacy of this approach to addressing suffering, distress, or paucity of meaning and purpose in patients nearing death" (Chochinov et al., 2004, p.140).

Culture and Palliative Care

Culture is a defining component of the human experience. Each individual's culture provides the sense of security, belonging, and guidelines regarding how to live and die (End of Life Education Consortium (ELNEC)) (2000). Cultural diversity refers to differences between people based on shared teachings, beliefs, customs, language and so forth, that influence both an individual's and family's response to illness, treatment, death, and bereavement (Showalter, 1998). Despite the enormous differences among individuals, an understanding of common cultural characteristics is helpful in providing culturally sensitive and effective care (Kemp, 1999). It is beyond the scope of this chapter to describe all the cultural perspectives of individual populations regarding dying, death, and bereavement. However, it is important to be aware of the principles of providing culturally sensitive, quality palliative care for clients and their families. Table 23-5 outlines ten principles of culturally sensitive care originally developed by the Council on Social Work Education (CSWE) Faculty Development Institute, 2001 (cited in Sherman, 2004).

Sullivan (2001) identified Latino views regarding end-of-life care. Data were obtained using focus groups in Latino communities. The Latino participants believed: they could not communicate effectively with health care providers due to language barriers; they did not understand the concept of informed consent even with the use of interpreters. Latinos believed it is the responsibility of the family to care for their relatives and should not send them away to nursing homes. Consequently, these participants did not want to die in nursing homes. Most of the participants were unaware of hospice services or had inaccurate information. Religious beliefs, primarily reliance on God and fatalism, were critical components of their decision-making regarding end-of-life care. Racial discrimination and cultural insensitivity were perceived by many of the participants.

TABLE 23-5

Principles of Culturally Sensitive Care

Health care providers should:
1. Be knowledgeable about cultural values and attitudes.
2. Attend to diverse communication styles.
3. Ask the patient for his/her preferences for decision-making early in the care process.
4. Recognize cultural differences and varying comfort levels with regard to personal space, eye contact, touch, time orientation, learning styles, and conversation styles.
5. Use a cultural guide from the palliative care patient's ethnic or religious background.
6. Get to know the community, its people, and its resources available for social support.
7. Create a culturally friendly physical environment (ex. decorate facilities with artwork or pictures valued by the cultural groups to whom care is most commonly provided).
8. Determine the acceptability of patients' being physically examined by a practitioner of a different gender.
9. Advocate for availability of services, accessibility in terms of cost and location, and acceptability of services that are compatible with cultural values and practices of the person served.
10. Conduct a self-assessment of the health care provider's own beliefs about illness and death.

Adapted from: Council on Social Work Education (CSWE) Faculty Development Institute, 2001 as cited in Sherman, D. W. (2004). Cultural and spiritual backgrounds of older adults. In M. L. Matzo & D. W. Sherman (Eds.) *Gerontologic palliative care nursing.* (p.11). St. Louis: Mosby.

Several beliefs in the Hispanic culture influence the experience of palliative care for individuals. Many Hispanic families will assume the responsibility of caring for their dying member at home based on their belief in strong family support to include extended family members. The dying member is protected from the prognosis. A major challenge to thorough pain assessment in palliative care is the reluctance of Hispanics to acknowledge, report, or describe pain, as stoicism is highly regarded. However, moaning is acceptable but can not serve as a valid indicator of the severity of pain (Kemp, 1999). Although death is an adversity, funerals are an integral part of family life, lasting several days. The Day of the Dead is celebrated in November on the same day as All Souls Day is celebrated in the Catholic religion. Day of the Dead is a day of celebration with special foods and decorating of the graves.

Education for Healthcare Professionals

AACN and City of Hope National Medical Center received major funding from the Robert Wood Johnson Foundation for the development and dissemination of the End-of-Life Nursing Education Consortium (ELNEC) Curriculum. Curricula for bac-

calaureate, graduate, continuing education/in-service, pediatric, oncology, and geriatric nurses and nurse educators have been developed. Train-the-Trainer methodology has been used to disseminate the knowledge. A quarterly newsletter "ELNEC Connections" is sent to all ELNEC trainers. The newsletter provides updates, on-going resources and project ideas from the ELNEC staff as well as trainers throughout the country. Collegial sharing is in the spirit of improving and disseminating the science and art of palliative care nursing. One of the outcomes of the project was the award-winning series on palliative care that was published in the *American Journal of Nursing* for two and a half years and included 17 articles.

Physicians have a parallel program: The EPEC Project: Education on Palliative and End of Life

---

Case Study

Casey is a 70-year-old man who resides in an apartment with his 63-year-old wife. They have been married 45 years. Casey has a 10-year history of Parkinson's disease. He has osteoarthritis in his back, coronary artery disease, hypertension, and dry macular degeneration in his left eye. His medications have kept him stable and able to enjoy his daily life. He is able to perform all of his own activities of daily living. The Parkinson's disease continues to progress slowly requiring him to use a cane.

Spontaneously one day, he developed severe, acute pain in his right shoulder. His wife took him to an orthopedic surgeon to have the shoulder evaluated. The diagnosis was a torn rotator cuff. The surgeon explained that if they were going to perform surgery they needed to do it soon. Then Casey's wife explained the co-morbidities: Parkinson's and coronary artery disease. It was then explained that rehabilitation after the surgical repair would be quite intense

and painful. Casey's wife was very concerned that he would not have the stamina for the rehab, that he might develop pneumonia after surgery and would experience intense pain.

The decision was made to confer with Casey's neurologist and cardiologist. Casey was still able to perform his own ADL's but eating was more awkward since he was right handed. Pain was controlled with extra strength Tylenol. The final decision was to forgo the surgical repair. The risk-benefit ratio was not worth it. The cardiologist and the neurologist agreed.

Three months later Casey had full range of motion in his right shoulder without any pain. The tear had spontaneously healed. Everyone was very pleased!

Questions:

1. Would you describe this situation as palliative care? If so, why? If not, why not?
2. What would have been your recommended plan of care for Casey?

Care. However, the mission is to educate ALL health care professionals on the essential clinical competencies in palliative care. Conferences using the Train-the-Trainer methodology is also used. In addition, the entire curriculum is now available on-line (see www.epec.net).

Another very useful resource for health care professionals is the End of Life/Palliative Education Resource Center found at www.eperc.mcw.edu. Its purpose is advancing end of life care through an on-line community of educational scholars. Case studies, presentations, and articles are a few of the resources available.

Research

The continued evolution of palliative care to meet the needs of an aging population rests in part with outcomes research. The question becomes whether the research, education, and clinical interventions funded to improve end of life care were effective. Measuring the effectiveness of palliative care to evaluate the effectiveness of care is a challenge that requires both prospective and retrospective studies (Steinhauser, 2004). Four challenges exist related to outcome measurement in palliative care:

1) End of life is a complex multidimensional experience in which understanding of the interrelatedness of domains is unclear.
2) The period "end of life" is ill-defined.
3) Both patient and family are the unit of care, yet little is known about the correlation of the trajectories of their experience.
4) Patients, the primary focus of care, are often unable to communicate in the last days or weeks, rendering their subjective experience unevaluable (Steinhauser, 2004 p. 33).

Outcome research in palliative care is in the early stages of development. There is consensus about the broad domains related to end of life: physical or psychosocial symptoms, social relationships, spiritual, or philosophical beliefs, hopes, expectation and meaning, satisfaction, economic considerations, and

caregiver and family experiences. Quality of life is also considered an outcome, but quality of life needs a clearer definition and consistent measurement in order to strengthen the relationship.

Outcomes

The Center to Advance Palliative Care (CAPC) has identified outcomes of palliative care (www.capc.org). They include: 1) Relief of pain and other distressing symptoms; 2) Clear communication and decision-making regarding goals of care and development of treatment plans; 3) Completion of life-prolonging or curative treatments; 4) Increased patient and family satisfaction; and 5) Ease of referral to appropriate care settings to achieve the goals of care, resulting in reduced hospital and ICU length of stay and cost.

Summary and Conclusions

Although palliative care has been established as a legitimate area of practice, much work remains to be done. In concluding this chapter, a conceptual framework recently published by Nolan and Mock (2004) entitled: *Integrity of the Person: A Conceptual Framework for End-of-Life Care* is described. The framework is organized around the core concept of the integrity of the human person and the relationship of the health care professional to the patient, and it builds on the earlier work of Pellegrino (1990). The framework involves relationships among the following components: External Factors–the integrity of the health professional, organizational culture and health care resources; Internal Factors–spiritual domain, psychological domain, physical domain, functional domain, and community culture and family. Completing the framework are patient care goals and the outcomes of care. Although end of life appears to be a prominent part of the framework, Nolan and Mock (2004) use the IOM's definition of end of life that extends the illness trajectory to include "the period of time during which an individual copes with declining health from an ultimately terminal illness—from a serious though perhaps chronic illness or from the frailties associated with advanced age even if death is not clearly imminent." (Lunney, Foley, Smith, & Gelband, 2003, p. 22).

The multidimensional nature of the framework provides a structure for future research related to the factors that influence the integrity of the person, client care goals and outcomes of care. In essence, this framework summarizes the major concepts about palliative care. In addition, the framework provides a foundation to passionately go forward in clinical practice, teaching, and research to build the science and the care to relieve suffering and improve quality of life.

Study Questions

1. Discuss the differences in the definitions of palliative care listed in Table 23-1.
2. Describe how the goals of care might differ for an 85-year-old man diagnosed with congestive heart failure at the time of diagnosis and in an advanced stage of the illness.
3. Discuss the meaning of the statement: hospice care is palliative care, but not all palliative care is hospice care.
4. Differentiate between hospice and palliative care.
5. List the domains of end-of-life care developed by the National Consensus Project.
6. Identify barriers to palliative care for an individual with a serious, life-limiting illness.
7. Identify the components of Ferrell's framework/model for quality of life.
8. What is your vision of palliative care?
9. Discuss how stoicism may impact palliative care for a Latino grandmother.
10. List three on-line resources to use to continue your education in palliative care.
11. Go on-line and find support information appropriate for the family caregiver of a palliative care patient.
12. Describe how you could you use *Integrity of the Person: A Conceptual Framework for End-of-Life Care* as an organizing framework for your future clinical practice.

References

AGS Panel on Persistent Pain in Older Persons. (2002). The management of persistent pain in older persons. *Journal of the American Geriatrics Society, 50*: Supplement:S205–S224.

Amella, E. J. (2003). Geriatrics and palliative care: Collaboration for quality of life until death. *Journal of Hospice and Palliative Nursing, 5*(1), 40–48.

American Academy of Hospice and Palliative Medicine (AAHPM) *About AAHPM.* Retrieved on January 8, 2005 from http://www.aahpm.org/positions/definition.html

American Board of Hospice and Palliative Medicine (ABHPM). *Certification.* Retrieved January 8, 2005 from http://www.abhpm.org

Berry, P. H. (2004). Promoting quality of life during the dying process. In M. L. Matzo & D. W. Sherman (Eds.). *Gerontologic palliative care nursing.* (pp.1–2). St. Louis: Mosby.

Billings, J. A. (1998). What is palliative care? *Journal of Palliative Medicine, 1*(1), 73–81.

Bookbinder, M., Coyle, N., Kiss, M., et al. (1996). Implementing national standards for cancer pain management: Program model and evaluation. *Journal of Pain and Symptom Management, 12*, 334–347.

Block, S. D. (2000). Assessing and managing depression in the terminally ill patient. *Annals of Internal Medicine, 132*, 209–218.

Casarett, D. J., & Inouye. S. K. (2001). Diagnosis and management of delirium near the end of life. *Annals of Internal Medicine, 135*, 32–40.

Cassel, C. K. (2003). Foreword. In R. S. Morrison, & D. E. Meier (Eds.). *Geriatric palliative medicine* (pp vii–ix): Oxford, UK: Oxford University Press.

Center for Disease Control, National Center for Health Statistics (September 16, 2002). *National Vital Sta-*

tistics Report, 50 (15). Retrieved August 10, 2004 from www.cdc.gov/nchs/fastats/deaths.htm

Center to Advance Palliative Care (CAPC). Retrieved on January 10, 2005 from http://capc.org

Chochinov, H. M. (2004). Interventions to enhance the spiritual aspects of dying. *National Institutes of Health state-of-the science conference on improving end-of-life care program & abstracts.* Bethesda, MD: U.S. Department of Health and Human Services, National Institutes of Health.

Chochinov, H. M., Hack, T., Hassard, T., Kristjanson, L. J., et al. (2004). Dignity and psychotherapeutic considerations in end-of-life care. *Journal of Palliative Care, 20* (3), 134–142.

Christakis, N., & Lamont, E. B. (2000). Extend and determinants of error in doctors' prognoses in terminally ill patients: Prospective cohort study. *British Medical Journal, 320,* 469–473.

Corbin, J. (2001). Introduction and overview: Chronic illness and nursing. In R. Hyman & J. Corbin (Eds.), *Chronic illness: Research and theory for nursing practice* (pp. 1–15). New York: Springer.

Council on Social Work Education (CSWE) Faculty Development Institute. (2001) as cited in Sherman, D. W. (2004). Cultural and spiritual backgrounds of older adults. In M. L. Matzo & D. W. Sherman (Eds.) *Gerontologic palliative care nursing.* (p. 11). St. Louis: Mosby.

Cumming, K. T., & Okun, S. N. (2004). Community-based palliative care for older adults. In M. L. Matzo, & D. W. Sherman (Eds.), *Gerontologic palliative care nursing* (pp. 52–65). St. Louis: Mosby.

Curtin, M., & Lubkin, I. (1995). What is chronicity? In I. Lubkin (Ed.), *Chronic illness: Impact and interventions* (3rd ed.) (pp. 3–25). Sudbury, MA: Jones & Bartlett.

Derek, D., Hanks, G., Cherny, N., & Calman, K. (2004). Introduction. In D. Doyle, G. Hanks, N. Cherny, & K. Calman (Eds.), *Oxford textbook of palliative medicine* (3rd ed.) (pp.1–4). Oxford, UK: Oxford University Press.

Dowsett, S. M., Saul, J. L., Buttow, P. N., et al. (2000). Communication styles in the cancer consultation: Preferences for a patient-centered approach. *Psychooncology, 9,* 147–156.

Emanuel, E. J., & Emanuel, L. L. (1998). The promise of a good death. *Lancet, 351*(Supplement 2), S1121–S1129.

End of Life Nursing Education Consortium (ELNEC) (2000). *Module 1: Nursing at the end of life.* American Association of Colleges of Nursing and City of Hope National Medical Center.

End of Life Nursing Education Consortium (ELNEC). (2000). *Module 5: Cultural considerations in EOL care.* American Association of Colleges of Nursing and City of Hope National Medical Center.

EPEC Project: Education on Palliative and End-of-Life care. (Accessed May 25, 2004, at http://www.epec.net).

Ferrell, B. R. (1995). The impact of pain on quality of life: A decade of research. *Nursing Clinics of North America, 30,* 609–624.

Ferrell, B. R. (2004). Overview of the domains of variables relevant to end-of-life care. *National Institutes of Health state-of-the science conference on improving end-of-life care program & abstracts.* Bethesda, MD: U.S. Department of Health and Human Services, National Institutes of Health.

Ferrell, B. R., & Coyle, N. (2001). *Textbook of palliative nursing.* Oxford, UK: Oxford University Press.

Ferrell, B., Virani, R., & Grant, M. (1999). Analysis of end-of-life content in nursing textbooks. *Oncology Nursing Forum, 26* (5), 869–876.

Field, M. J., & Behrman, R. E. (Eds.). (2003). *When children die: Improving palliative and end-of-life care for children and their families.* Washington, DC: National Academy Press.

Field, M. J., & Cassel, C. K. (Eds.). (1997). *Approaching death: Improving care at the end of life.* Committee on Care at the End of Life, Division of Health Care Services, Institute of Medicine. Washington, DC: National Academy Press.

Fisher, E. S., Wennberg, D. E., Stukel, T. A., Gottlieb, D. J., et al. (2003). The implications of regional variations in Medicare spending: Health outcomes and satisfaction with care. *Annals of Internal Medicine, 138,* 288–298.

Foley, K. (2001). Preface. In K. M. Foley & H. Gelband (Eds.), *Improving palliative care for cancer* (pp. xi–xii). Washington, DC: National Academy Press.

Fried, T. R., Bradley, E. H., Towle, V. R., & Allore, H. (2002). Understanding the treatment preferences of seriously ill patients. *New England Journal of Medicine, 346,* 1061–1066.

Glass, E., Cluxton, D., & Rancour, P. (2001). Principles of patient and family assessment. In B. R. Ferrell & N. Coyle (Eds.) *Textbook of palliative nursing.* Oxford, UK: Oxford University Press.

Haywood House. (1996). *Day care at Haywood House, City Hospital* (pamphlet). Nottingham, England: Author.

Hearn, J., & Myers, K. (2001). *Palliative day care in practice.* Oxford, UK: Oxford University Press.

Hospice and Palliative Nurses Association & American Nurses Association, (2002). *Scope and standards of hospice and palliative nursing practice.* Washington, D.C. Author.

Hospice and Palliative Nurses Association (2005). Florence Wald. (Retrieved January 5, 2005 from http://www. hpna.org/FlorenceWald_home.asp).

Kemp, C. (1999). *Terminal illness: A guide to nursing care* (2nd ed). Philadelphia: Lippincott.

Kubler-Ross, E. (1969). *On death and dying.* New York: Macmillan.

Lomax, K.J., & Scanlon, C. (1997). *Precepts of palliative care* (Last Acts Task Force on Palliative Care). Princeton, NJ: The Robert Wood Johnson Foundation/ Last Acts

Luce, J. M., & Luce, J. A. (2001). Perspective on care at the close of life: Management of dyspnea in patients with far-advanced lung disease: "Once I lose it, it's kind of hard to catch it . . ." *Journal of the American Medical Association, 285,* 1331–1337.

Lunney, J. R., Foley, K. M., Smith, T. J., & Gelband, H. (2003). *Describing death in America: What we need to know.* Washington DC: National Academy Press.

Lynn, J. (2001). Serving patients who may die soon and their families: The role of hospice and other services. *Journal of the American Medical Association, 285,* 925–932.

Lynn, J., Arkes, H. R., Stevens, M., Cohn, F., et al. (2000). Rethinking fundamental assumptions: SUPPORT's implications for future reform. *Journal of the American Geriatrics Society, 48* (5), S214–S221.

Manfredi, P. L., Morrison, R. S., Morris, J., Goldhirsch, S. L., et al. (2000). Palliative care consultations: How do they impact the care of hospitalized patients? *Journal of Pain and Symptom Management, 20,* 166–173.

Matzo, M. L., & Sherman, D. W. (2004). *Gerontologic palliative care nursing.* St. Louis: Mosby.

Matzo, M. L., & Sherman, D. W. (2001). *Palliative care nursing: Quality care at the end of life.* New York: Springer.

McClain, C. S., Rosenfield, B., & Breitbart, W. (2003). Effect of spiritual well-being on end-of-life despair in terminally ill cancer patients. *Lancet, 361,* 1603–1607.

McMillan, S. C. (2004). Interventions to facilitate family caregiving. *National Institutes of Health state-of-the-science conference on improving end-of-life care program & abstracts.* Bethesda, MD: U.S. Department of Health and Human Services, National Institutes of Health.

Meier, D. E., & Morrison, R. S. (2002). Autonomy reconsidered. *New England Journal of Medicine, 346,* 1087–1089.

Meier, D. E., Back, A. L., & Morrison, R. S. (2001). The inner life of physicians and care of the seriously ill. *Journal of the American Medical Association, 286,* 3007–3014.

Miles, S.H., Koepp, R., & Weber, E.P. (1996). Advance end-of-life treatment planning: A research review. *Archives of Internal Medicine, 156,* 1062–1068.

Morrison, R. S., & Meier, D.E. (2004). Palliative care. *New England Journal of Medicine, 350,* 2582–2590.

National Consensus Project for Quality Palliative Care. (2004). *Clinical practice guidelines for quality palliative care.* Brooklyn, NY: National Consensus Project for Quality Palliative Care. Available at: www.nationalconsensusproject.org

National Hospice and Palliative Care Organization (2005). *Hospice facts and figures.* (Accessed January 5, 2005, at http://www.nhpco.org).

National Hospice and Palliative Care Organization. (2002). *Standards of Practice for Hospice Programs.* Arlington, VA: National Hospice and Palliative Care Organization.

National Institutes of Health (December, 2004). *National Institutes of Health State-of-the Conference Statement: Improving End-of-Life Care.* (Draft Statement released December 8, 2004). Washington, DC: National Institutes of Health.

Nolan, M. T., & Mock, V. (2004). A conceptual framework for end-of-life care: A reconsideration of factors influencing the integrity of the human person. *Journal of Professional Nursing, 20* (6), 351–360.

Pellegrino, E. (1990). The relationship of autonomy and integrity in medical ethics. *Bulletin of PAHO, 24,* 361–371.

Pinquart, M., & Sorenson, D. (2003). Differences between caregivers and noncaregivers in psychological health and physical health: A meta-analysis. *Psychology and Aging, 18,* 250–257.

Portenoy, R. K. (1998). Defining palliative care. *Newsletter.* Department of Pain Medicine and Palliative Care, *1*(2). Beth Israel Medical Center, New York.

Quill, T. E. (2000). Perspectives on care at the end of life: Initiating end-of-life discussions with seriously ill patients: Addressing the "elephant in the room." *Journal of the American Medical Association, 284,* 2502–2507.

Schulz, R., Mendelsohn, A.B., Haley, W.E., Mahoney, D. et al. (2003). End of life care and the effects of bereavement among family caregivers of persons with dementia. *New England Journal of Medicine, 349,* 1936–1942.

Schulz, R., Newsom, J. T., Fleissner, K., DeCamp, A. R., et al. (1997). The effects of bereavement after family caregiving. *Aging and Mental Health. 1*, 269–282.

Sherman, D. W. (2004). Cultural and spiritual backgrounds of older adults. In Matzo, M. L, & D. W. Sherman (Eds.). *Gerontologic palliative care nursing* (p. 11). St. Louis: Mosby.

Showalter, S. (1998). Looking through different eyes: Beyond cultural diversity. In K. Doka & J. Davidson (Eds.), *Living with grief when illness is prolonged* (pp. 71–82). Washington, DC: Hospice Foundation of America.

Singer, P. A., Martin, D. K., & Kelner, M. Quality end-of-life care: Patients' perspectives. *Journal of the American Medical Association, 281*, 163–168.

St. Christopher's Hospice. (1996). *St. Christopher's Hospice Day Center* (Handout). Sydenham, England: Author.

Standards and Accreditation Committee. (1999). *Hospice standards of practice*. Arlington, VA: Hospice and Palliative Care Organization.

Steinhauser, K. E. (2004). Measuring outcomes prospectively. *National Institutes of Health state-of-the science conference on improving end-of-life care program & abstracts*. Bethesda, MD: U.S. Department of Health and Human Services, National Institutes of Health.

Steinhauser, K. E., Christakis, N. A., Clipp, E. C., McNeilly, L., et al. (2000). Factors considered important at the end of life by patients, family, physicians, and other care providers. *Journal of the American Medical Association, 284*, 2476–2482.

Strasser, F., & Bruera, E. D. (2002). Update on anorexia and cachexia. *Hematology and Oncology Clinics of North America, 16*, 589–617.

Sullivan, A.M., Lakoma, M.D., & Block, S.D. (2003). The status of medical education in end-of-life care: A national report. *Journal of General Internal Medicine, 18*, 685–695.

SUPPORT Principal Investigators. (1995). A controlled trial to improve care for seriously ill, hospitalized patients: The Study to Understand Prognoses and Preferences for Outcomes and Risks of Treatments (SUPPORT). *Journal of the American Medical Association, 274*, 1591–1598.

Teno, J. (2001). Quality of care and quality indicators for lives ended by cancer. In K.M. Foley & H. Gelband (Eds.), *Improving palliative care for cancer*. Washington, DC: National Academy Press.

Teno, J., Lynn, J., Wenger, N. et al. (1997). Advance directives for seriously ill hospitalize patients: Effectiveness with the patient self determination act and the SUPPORT intervention. *Journal of the American Geriatrics Society, 45*, 500–507.

von Guten, C., & Romer, A.L. (2001). Designing and sustaining a palliative care and home hospice program: An interview with Charles von Guten. *Innovations in end-of-life care*, 1999; *1*(5), www.edc.org/lastacts [hard copy of article]

World Health Organization. (1990*). Cancer pain relief and palliative care* (Technical Report Series 804) (p.11). Geneva, Switzerland: World Health Organization.

Internet Resources

http://www.epec.net
http://www.aacn.nche.edu/elnec
www.hpna.org
www.nhpco.org
www.nationalconsensusproject.org
www.ons.org

www.ampainsoc.org
http://www.guideline.org
http://prc.coh.org
http://www.palliative.org (Edmonton Assessment Tools)
Toolkit of Instruments to Measure End of Life Care (TIME)
      http://www.chcr.brown.edu/pcoc/toolkit.htm

CHAPTER 24

Long-Term Care

Susan J. Barnes

Introduction

Improvements in health practices, pharmaceutical advances, technological advances in medical care, and nursing innovations have significantly increased life expectancy. Florida, Iowa, Pennsylvania, and West Virginia report that 15 percent or more of their population is 65 or older (Federal Interagency Forum on Aging, 2004). This trend will continue, with those over 65 making up an increasingly significant part of the population (Administration on Aging, 2004). Increasing longevity in the population brings with it the increased chance for individuals to develop chronic illness and frailty. This issue is significant enough that the 2005 White House Conference on Aging is slated to address aging trends as baby boomers prepare for retirement. The topics of this conference are promoting dignity, healthy independence, and economic security of older persons (White House Conference on Aging, 2004).

For many individuals, the aging process is accompanied by one or more chronic illnesses. Some measure of self-care deficit is likely to develop with chronic illness, and this self-care deficit is a precursor to accessing long-term care (LTC) services. Once the individual with chronic illness can no longer in-dependently manage self-care, daily activities, and home maintenance, LTC services can provide assistance and ensure some quality of life for the client.

LTC is a broad concept that covers a wide spectrum of services. It is useful to think of LTC as a continuum, on which services can range from intermittent community-based care delivered to the individual who has a minor degree of self-care deficit to the most restrictive residential facilities for those with profound medical conditions (Figure 24-1). LTC includes a range of services that address the health care, personal care, psychiatric and social needs of individuals who lack some capacity for self-care. Often LTC services are used to augment those services provided by family members. Ideally, the formal LTC services can enable individuals and their families to maintain independence as long as possible.

LTC may be needed for a variety of reasons. The physiological and functional changes that occur with aging may lead to gradual decline, and for some clients, that may mean accessing LTC services. The client with a gradual decline may benefit from community-based services such as receiving Meals on Wheels. If gradual decline continues, further access of community-based LTC services may be incremental. However, for many frail elders or others with chronic illness, progression may not occur

FIGURE 24-1

Long-Term Care Continuum in Terms of Intensity

Least Intense ↑↓ **Most Intense**	Community Based Services	Meals on Wheels
		Homemaker Services
		Parish Nurse Programs
		Home Health
		Rehabilitation Outpatient
		Community Mental Health Services
		Senior Citizen Centers
	Acute Care Services	Community-Based Senior Renewal Programs
		Respite
		Day Care for Elders
		Hospice
		Acute Care Rehabilitation or Skilled Nursing Facility
		Assisted Living, Group Homes, Adult Foster Homes
		Long-Term Rehabilitation Center
	Residential Services	Nursing Home
		Inpatient Psychiatric Unit

NOTE: Many services provide similar or overlapping services.

smoothly or predictably because of exacerbations of existing disease or an acute illness. Often the nurse's role is to determine what functional difficulties exist and then assist the individual and their family to access appropriate community services. The provision of ongoing care in LTC settings is complicated by many factors. The complex medical conditions of many LTC recipients, plus the multifaceted access and funding issues of formal care provision, present an intimidating maze for both health care practitioners and clients in LTC. Being aware of the challenges assists the care professional to construct a meaningful health care milieu for clients requiring such services.

Historical Perspectives

Caring for a client with complex health needs over a long period of time continues to be a challenge for the health care system. Throughout history, consideration given to the quality of care for the elderly is seen as a reflection of societal values (Koop & Schaeffer, 1976). In societies with more fluid resources, vulnerable populations such as the frail elderly or chronically ill are better cared for because of the availability of assistance with health care (Kalisch & Kalisch, 2004). History has demonstrated that in societies under the strain caused by famine, war, or social upheaval, the vulnerable may not be able to survive because of malnutrition, lack of health care, and the lack of ability of the family unit to provide support (Kalisch & Kalisch, 2004).

Review of LTC in the United States reveals several significant events in the past century that have led to our current system of providing care. Prior to the twentieth century, elders in the United States were usually cared for within extended family units (DeSpelder & Strickland, 2002). Those without family to care for them might have gone to a facility supported by a religious organization or by charitable citizens, such as a poor house or almshouse. Changes in medical care altered hospital stays and allowed LTC to evolve, with group rest homes and private charitable homes providing care for chronically ill, dependent persons. Because life expectancies continued to increase, the demand for LTC accompanied that increase (Lekan-Rutledge, 1997). Political response came in the form of the enactment of the Social Security Act in 1932, which provided services for the elderly and chronically ill. In 1951, the first White House Conference on Aging was held. The first conference (now held every 10 years) focused on issues that affected the quality of life of the aged person.

Title XVIII of the Social Security Act, which passed in 1965 and was a part of the "Great Society" of President Lyndon B. Johnson, provided medical insurance for the elderly (Medicare) and further involved the federal government in health care (Centers for Medicare and Medicaid Services, 2004). Medi-

care opened the door for the government to dictate regulations and set the standard for care in formal caregiving settings. Evolution of the system included a recent restructuring of Health Care Financing Authority into the Centers for Medicare and Medicaid Services with the emphasis on improving the overall process of coordinating care of complex illness in the context of managed care (Whitehouse on Aging, 2004). At the same time, in 1965, public policy was altered by the enactment of the Older Americans Act, which established aging networks throughout the states and funded community-based health services.

Part of the Social Security Amendments of 1965 was Title XIX, Medicaid, to provide medical and health-related services for individuals and families with low incomes. Medicaid, a cooperative work between each state and the federal government, is the largest source of funds for services to the poor. Each state establishes its own eligibility standards, sets the rate of payment for services, and administers its own program (Centers for Medicare and Medicaid Services, 2004). Further changes in LTC were accomplished by Title XX of the Social Security Act Amendments, which made in-home services for medically indigent more widely available. In 1972, legislation was established that paid for intermediate care. The Omnibus Reconciliation Act, passed in 1987, included the Nursing Home Reform Act, which established high quality of care as a goal, along with the preservation of residents' rights in LTC facilities. Changes included that comprehensive assessments of all nursing home residents were to be done to determine functional, cognitive, and affective levels of the residents and to be used in planning care. In addition, more specific requirements for nursing, medical, and psychosocial services were designed to attain and maintain the highest possible mental and physical functional statues by focusing on outcomes (such as incontinence, immobility, pressure sores). Resident rights were also clearly defined (Harrington, Carrillo & Crawford, 2004).

As our culture has evolved over the past 50 years, the family structure has been modified by the increasing number of women who work outside the home and are unavailable to care for aging parents (Lekan-Rutledge, 1997). Current cultural values have made it less common for extended families to live together. The Hispanic and Asian cultures often include extended families, with several generations living in the same household or nearby, which makes it possible for family members to look after the interests of vulnerable elder members and limits the need for formal LTC services (Leininger, 2002). However, current U.S. values emphasize single-family dwellings, dual-income families, and transient life-styles, which have led to families no longer residing in the same area but geographically separated by great distance. This culturally driven environment has created a high demand for services from an already inefficient LTC care system.

The Continuum of Care

Community-Based Long-Term Care

The range and type of organizations providing assistive and nursing services to individuals living in the community are broad. Access to this system is often confusing to health care professionals, as well as to the client and family. The current trend is toward using a case management approach to more effectively coordinate services and to ensure that individuals receive services in a timely manner. Case management may also include the goal of allowing an individual with chronic illness to remain in the community as long as possible. Services may include nutrition centers or meal provision, homemaker provision, visiting nurse services, or home health services. Related services for the frail elder or individual with chronic illness include legal services, aid to the aged, adult protective services, area council of government services, ombudsman programs, senior citizen centers, and elder advocacy groups. For elders, home health care services funded by Medicare require that the individual be able to increase their functional capacity or have rehabilitation potential. Otherwise, the elder must pay privately for such services. Other private pay services are developing in

many areas across the country to provide respite for family caregivers in the area of providing respite, homemaker services, shopping services, etc.

Residential Long-Term Care Settings

LTC facilities are formal, organized agencies in business to provide care for individuals who cannot care for themselves but who do not require hospitalization. LTC facilities fulfill two important roles in the residents' lives: The facility is both a home and a health care agency. The challenge of constructing an appropriate care setting for the individual with chronic illness with minimal funding and a for-profit motive is not an easy task. There are three common types of residential LTC facilities: group homes, assisted-living centers, and nursing homes.

For the vast majority of individuals with chronic illness, the decision to move to a residential LTC facility is a difficult decision based on declining health, inability to provide self-care, and the exacerbation of chronic illnesses and frailty by accident or aging. In many instances, family members are involved in the decision and influence the final move to the LTC facility. Individuals living in LTC facilities—residents—are, by definition, a vulnerable population group and may require an advocate in some form. Many factors unique to the individual client require consideration in order to provide appropriate nursing care. Complex medical conditions, psychosocial needs and rapid changes in personal living arrangements can overshadow the personhood of the individual. Because of the loss of power in the fragile elderly client, rights can be inadvertently violated not only by caregivers and institutional governance, but also by an individual's own family.

Group Homes Group homes exist throughout the United States and are regulated by the state agency responsible for supervision of health care, usually a division of the state health department. These homes can be family or corporately owned businesses and are often located in an environment that is homelike, such as a multi-bedroom dwelling or premanufactured home. Other names for group homes include: *personal care homes, foster homes, domiciliary care homes, board and care homes*, and *congregate care homes.*

The concept of personal care or domiciliary care homes, in general, is not unlike the old-time rooming houses of the nineteenth and early twentieth centuries. Individuals may live in such environments supported by private pay (from their own resources or extended family resources) or, in some states, paid by the state welfare or LTC system. The home manager is responsible for overseeing nutritional intake, medication management, general safety of the residents, and cleaning and laundry services. The nonspecialized group home environment may be very desirable for clients with less complicated medical conditions.

Assisted-Living Centers   One of the fastest growing health care industries today is the assisted-living center. Assisted-living centers are for individuals who can pay privately for services. Medicare or Medicaid does not pay for assisted-living arrangements. This phenomenon of self-pay is made possible by many post-retirement individuals who have accrued significant retirement income. Assisted-living homes resemble handicapped-accessible apartment complexes, with the additional services of meal preparation, bathing assistance, medication management, and group activities to encourage socialization. Residents of these facilities may or may not be able drive an automobile. Of note is the fact that corporately owned centers may have only one registered nurse (RN) consultant for several hundred residents across several facilities. On the premises is one licensed practical nurse (LPN) for eight hours a day, five days a week. This person is responsible for all health concerns and medication management and may be assisted by minimally trained medication aides. This organizational structure is possible by the fact the facility is based on a social model of care rather than a health care institutional model.

Being a resident in an assisted-living facility may be very comfortable for the older client. Residents retain a great deal of autonomy, personal space is protected, and arrangement of apartment space can be achieved with personal items and preferences. This setting is ideal for those with minimal needs for assistance and the ability to pay for such assistance.

Skilled Nursing Facilities or Nursing Homes   *Nursing home* is a term used to refer to a facility that has either skilled nursing services (SNFs) and/or intermediate care. Nursing homes are LTC facilities for chronically ill, medically frail, and disabled persons. The level of care can be described as residential, long-term, non-emergent, custodial care. A number of facilities may include an intermediate care or rehabilitation unit for individuals who need assistance in increasing self-care abilities.

The majority of such agencies are "for profit." Exceptions are agencies generally associated with churches or other nonprofit organizations such as the Veterans Affairs Administration. All agencies that receive income from the Center for Medicare and Medicaid Services (CMS) are required to meet minimum state and federal standards. Standards address nutritional and fluid intake; provision of social interaction and activities; support services, such as physical therapy, rehabilitation therapy, housekeeping, and laundry services; and so forth. There is a continuing concern by those employed in LTC settings that facility structure and staffing are often based on minimal standards that contain costs instead of what is desirable or needed for the client. However, as the Baby Boom generation ages, it is expected that its interest in this issue will influence the creation of higher standards, and quality of care may improve in LTC facilities.

Approximately five percent of the elderly population resides in nursing homes in the United States, and 28 percent pay for their own care (CMS, 2004). Care in nursing homes may be funded by the individual (self-pay), insurance, Medicare, or Medicaid. To be eligible for Medicaid payment for residential care, the client must have limited assets with which to pay for the services required. Often, an LTC resident will enter a nursing home, paying for services until their estate is spent down, and then Medicaid pays for care until the client's death (AARP, 2002).

The care provided for individuals in a SNF is generally custodial care. Rehabilitative services are provided for those who have the capacity to regain function. Because the institutionalized individual may require a great deal of help with the physical aspects of care, such as bathing, dressing, eating, and space maintenance, the cognitive needs (emotional, psychological, and spiritual) may be considered less important. Activity programs are sometimes geared only toward one segment of the facility population. Care in LTC settings should include not only appropriate physical care, but also appropriate cognitive stimulation.

Long-Term Care Recipients— A Vulnerable Population

Vulnerable individuals are those who are at increased risk for loss of autonomy, loss of self-will, injustice, loss of privacy, and increased risk for abuse. A vulnerable adult is defined as a individual who is either being mistreated or is in danger of mistreatment and who due to age and/or disability is unable to protect him/herself (Teaster, 2002). A vulnerable individual can be described as one who has been judged by someone to be a nonperson. In a culture that values youth, energy, strength, and work ability, many devalue an elder or one with a chronic illness because of the loss of valued, but superficial, qualities. The care provider in LTC is charged with maintaining an environment that supports the unique personhood of the client.

Many individuals requiring LTC have already lost some autonomy and self-will because of illnesses that affect the individual's ability to make decisions or carry out intentional behavior. Vulnerability is of special concern in these individuals. Decisions must be made for them regarding many aspects of life, such as eating, bathing, medication administration, socialization, and exercising religious practices.

■ Problems and Issues in Long-Term Care

There are a number of issues in LTC, and they range from overall system issues to individual treat-

ment issues for clients in the system. The issues mentioned in this chapter are not an exhaustive list, but can be considered an introduction to current problems.

Provision of Care

Along the continuum of LTC, provision of care problems include organization of services and access to care, gaps in public policy, funding, staffing, and standards. Specific issues vary within individual states or communities. It is imperative that the professional nurse involved in LTC is cognizant of the local and state issues that affect delivery and quality of LTC services. Being a political activist in order to further the issues of the recipients of LTC is important.

Organization of Services

In community-based LTC, the array of services in a given community may not be organized according to any hierarchy. Each specialized service, such as home care, elder daycare, hospice, or nutrition programs, was most likely begun in response to a specific need or business opportunity in the community. It is often necessary for a program of LTC to be pieced together from a number of different organizations to meet one client's needs. This is especially true for those who are community-dwelling residents.

Partial help with this problem comes from the United Way, a nonprofit service-based agency. The United Way publishes a resource book in larger cities that describes community programs and services. This resource book assists clients, family, and care providers in identifying appropriate services, phone numbers, and eligibility requirements. Many times, individuals with chronic illness and their families are not aware that when they are involved with one system (such as a nursing home), they have access to other services (such as hospice). This publication can be obtained by calling the local United Way Office.

Individuals with chronic illnesses often view access to the LTC system as complicated and overwhelming. Those with chronic illnesses and their families may have a limited amount of energy to invest in problem solving and identifying the best options. Oftentimes, access to the LTC system is controlled by gatekeepers who have minimal training and experience with complex medical conditions. Rules may be seen as arbitrary and appear to exclude the very individuals intended to benefit from programs.

With the utilization of more case management for individuals with chronic illness, whether through the local or federal Veterans Affairs Administration, state health and human services divisions, or private insurance companies, some progress is being made in assisting community-dwelling individuals to more effectively access LTC services. However, for most clients and families, access to the LTC system remains confusing and complex.

Gaps in Public Policy

Related to organization of LTC services are the gaps in policy. Despite the creation of significant public policy, as discussed in the historical overview, no overall umbrella of comprehensive care exists. There are many individuals who fall outside of policy parameters and cannot benefit from services. Pharmaceutical costs, extended home health care, and rehabilitative services are problematic for many in LTC. As a result, clients either self-pay, if possible, or go without services or medications. Because of recent legislative changes, in 2006 many will be eligible for a discount on medication cost with a prescription benefit card. However, it is unclear how much financial assistance will be provided.

Funding

Gaps in service and public policy are both related to funding issues. One hundred two billion dollars were spent by state and federal agencies to pay for nursing home care in 2002 (Harrington, Carillo, & Crawford, 2004). In addition, approximately 28 percent of residents in nursing homes and other residential care facilities pay privately for their care (CMS, 2004). Private insurance and nonprofit

organizations also provide services for those in need of LTC. However, beyond the nursing home setting, piecing together a comprehensive LTC program for a frail elder with comorbidities who wishes to remain in the community is challenging. Certification for eligibility for certain benefits, such as extended home care, is strict. Recertification is often difficult and for a limited amount of time only.

Resources, whether private or public, are limited. Community-dwelling elders may be eligible for Medicare to pay for certain services, such as home health care, but only as long as some rehabilitation progress can be documented. Once progress stops, and the condition is considered chronic, the individual must pay privately for rehabilitative and home services. For individuals who have lived through the Great Depression, World War II, and other historical events that have required genuine frugality, spending nearly $100 to pay for less than an hour of a home visit from an agency RN is not an option. Many elders from working class backgrounds do without needed care rather than pay privately.

In some states, PACE (Program of All Inclusive Care for the Elderly) is available to assist those who wish to remain at home as long as possible (National PACE Association, 2004). The number of states with participating organizations has increased from 13 to 17 in the last five years. Those currently enrolled include: California, Hawaii, Illinois, Kansas, Maryland, Massachusetts, Michigan, New Mexico, New York, Ohio, Oregon, Pennsylvania, Tennessee, Texas, Virginia, Washington, and Wisconsin. Continuing evaluation of this program in terms of cost benefit to the funding agencies may make it available on a wider scale. However, for the time being, the program is limited in scope. Other programs are being developed to try to enhance autonomy and quality of life for seniors living at home such as the Oklahoma Advantage Program.

It is important to consider the entitlement to care that elders and those with chronic illness possess because of Social Security programs. These programs were designed to provide some comfort and security to the older individual. One view is that society has an obligation to provide for those in need, particularly the elderly, because of the labor and service that they have provided (Tobin & Salisbury, 1999). Another view is that society is obligated to provide care for frail and chronically ill elders because of the sanctity of all human life, and not simply because of work undertaken during the adult life. Philosophical origins play an important part not only in the establishment and continuation of programs, but also in setting standards for ongoing programs.

Staffing

Health care agencies that receive Medicare and Medicaid funding are licensed by each state or are accredited by a recognized accrediting agency. Each agency must meet requirements in staffing. Two main issues in staffing are the training of the staff member and the staff-to-client ratio.

Standards for required staff training are often minimal. For example, medication aides working in an assisted-living center may be required to attend a six-week training course, yet the medication regimes for the assisted-living center clientele may be extremely complex. For proper medication management, much more time is required to educate a person on the pharmacological effects of medications, side effects, and complications. Although assisted-living centers are required to have an RN available, that one RN may act as a consultant for multiple centers under the same ownership umbrella. The actual individual who "supervises" the medication aides may be an LPN who works a forty-hour week.

Qualifications for a home manager in an assisted-living center are minimal and may be as little as attending a state-sponsored seminar lasting two weeks or less, with yearly continuing education. The majority of staff working in such facilities may be minimally trained personnel, and client safety is a legitimate concern.

Staffing challenges in providing home health care are also significant. State requirements vary for home health aides, but no training program is more than eight to 12 weeks in length. Often, aides are trained and then expected to work independently, with little supervision.

Staffing in nursing homes is a continuing issue. There is conclusive evidence that a positive relationship exists between nursing staffing and quality of nursing home care. The decreasing levels of RN staffing is of growing concern, and yet reimbursements and prospective payments have been reduced in some cases, making it impossible to increase the number of RNs in residential facilities.

Nursing homes have a minimum client-to-staff ratio that is rarely exceeded in for-profit agencies. This ratio may be marginally adequate for routine care, but when a resident becomes ill and requires additional nursing care, the staffing patterns may not be adequate to manage the situation (Kayser-Jones, 1999). If more than one resident is ill, such as during a respiratory infection outbreak, staff capabilities are stretched to the limit, and once again, client safety could be in jeopardy. To complicate this situation, there is a projected shortage of health care professionals. Half of the registered nurse workforce is at least 45 years old. The U.S. Bureau of Labor Statistics estimates that employers will need to find replacements for 331,000 RN's by 2008. Currently, less than 1% of RNs are certified in geriatrics (Gerontological Society of America, 2004).

Standards

Residential and community-based LTC facilities that accept government payments are regulated by federal and state mandates. Agencies and institutions in LTC that receive outside funding are required to meet certain standards and undergo regular inspection (Harrington et al., 2003).

Requirements change frequently. Part of the responsibility of the chief nursing administrator of an LTC facility is to be aware of and implement changes that are necessary due to new state and federal requirements. In home health agencies, the number and type of visits that can be reimbursed by insurance or Medicare are limited. If evidence in regard to why the visits were made and what health-related goal was achieved is unclear, the payer may bill the agency back for those services, which can be financially devastating to an organization.

Nursing homes undergo an initial survey to become certified and then undergo inspection at least every 15 months (CMS, 2004). State surveyors evaluate both process and outcomes of nursing home care in several areas (Table 24-1). If deficiencies are found, follow-up surveys may be conducted. Agencies must demonstrate that the staff meets educational requirements, that residents are being given adequate care, and that documentation is appropriate. Standards may allow gross issues to be ignored, while minute details are examined. Requirements vary for various types of agencies and are quite complicated.

Standards address issues such as nursing hours per client, nursing assessments, care plans, accidents, number of pressure sores, use of physical restraints, nutrition, and housekeeping services. Additionally, facilities are to provide care for residents in a manner that maintains dignity and respect by providing grooming, appropriate dress, and promotion of independence in dining; allowing private space and property; and interacting respectfully.

TABLE 24-1

Nursing Home Quality Indicators

Domain	Quality Indicator	Resident Risk Category
Accidents	Incidence of new fractures	
	Prevalence of falls	
Behavior/emotional patterns	Prevalence of behavior symptoms affecting others	High risk
	Prevalence of symptoms of depression	Low risk
	Prevalence of symptoms of depression without antidepressant therapy	
Clinical management	Use of 9 or more medications	
Cognitive patterns	Incidence of cognitive impairment	
Elimination/ incontinence	Prevalence of bladder or bowel incontinence	High risk
	Prevalence of occasional or frequent bladder or bowel incontinence without a toileting plan	Low risk
	Prevalence of indwelling catheter	
	Prevalence of fecal impaction	
Infection control	Prevalence of urinary tract infections	
Nutrition/eating	Prevalence of weight loss	
	Prevalence of tube feeding	
	Prevalence of dehydration	
Physical functioning	Prevalence of bedfast residents	
	Incidence of decline in late-loss ADLs	
	Incidence of decline in range of motion	
Psychotropic drug use	Prevalence of antipsychotic use, in absence of psychotic or related conditions	High risk Low risk
	Prevalence of antianxiety/hypnotic use	
	Prevalence of hypnotic use more than two times in last week	
Quality of life	Presence of daily physical restraints	
	Presence of little or no activity	
Skin care	Prevalence of stage 1–4 ulcers	High risk Low risk

Source: From Nursing Home Quality Indicators Development Group, Center for Health Systems Research and Analysis (Marnard, 2002).

Harrington et al. (2004) points out that quality of care provided in nursing homes has long been a matter of great concern to consumers, professionals, and policy makers. If the regulation and inspection process is ignored, LTC residents may suffer. Examples of system failures can be found at both the local and state levels. Deficiency reports are readily available online through the Center for Medicare and Medicaid Services. The RN is at times required to act as an advocate for the residents and to ensure compliance with minimal standards.

Ethical Issues in Long-Term Care

Some issues associated with LTC are ethically based. Because of the high degree of professional independence afforded to employees of the LTC system and the vulnerability of many of the clients, decision making can be problematic. Dealing with individuals who are chronically ill or who are frail requires a solid understanding of the ethics involved in health care. Principles upon which decisions should be made include autonomy, nonmaleficence, beneficence, and justice (Beauchamp, 2001) (see Chapter 18, Ethics in Chronic Illness). The manner in which these principles are executed in the professional nurse–client relationship can make a visible difference in the quality of life of the LTC resident.

Client Autonomy versus Dependence

One principle of critical importance in LTC is autonomy. Autonomy is sometimes misapplied or ignored (Kane, Freeman, Chaplan, Asashar & Uru-Wong, 1990). It is possible for an individual to gradually lose increments of their autonomy because of limitations imposed by sensory deprivation, immobility, weakness, and cognitive impairment (Mezey, Mitty & Ramsey, 1997). Almost without thinking, a caregiver begins to take over a client's decision-making. The client moves toward developing a self-care deficiency that is actually a result of interaction with the caregiver. This loss of autonomy and development of excess disability is a problem for LTC clients. Excess disability is the dependence of a client on a caregiver to perform a task the client has the ability to perform

(Dawson, Wells & Kline, 1993). Depression, learned helplessness, perception of locus of control, and the sick role contribute to the development of excess disability (Salisbury, 1999). An example of excess disability is dressing assistance provided to nursing home residents. Aides often do the dressing activities for residents in order to save time, instead of allowing the residents to perform the activity at their own pace (Beck et al., 1997). This action moves the resident toward unnecessary and unwanted dependence.

Custodial Care versus Life Enhancement

Using basic ethical principles, an issue arises whether providing minimal physical care for those with chronic illness is acceptable versus providing more comprehensive care extending beyond custodial physical care. This is particularly challenging in a residential LTC environment. As a result of regulation, funding, and staffing patterns for Medicare/Medicaid residential facilities, the goal inadvertently becomes custodial care.

Physical issues of the resident are important, but those issues should not be the only focus. Mental health needs should also be considered in the chronically ill and elderly populations. With limited attention to these needs, the client is at risk of suffering boredom, anxiety, and, consequently, depression. Suicide rates of elder men are the highest in the nation (Shalala, 2000). Appropriate referral is a responsibility of the nurse who detects symptoms of emotional difficulties. Signs of depression include feeling nervous, empty, guilty, tired, restless, irritable, and unloved, and that life is not worth living. Physical symptoms associated with mental health problems include eating more or less than normal, sleep disturbances, headaches, stomachaches, and an increase in chronic pain (Varcarolis, 2002). If these symptoms are present in an LTC client, services are available to provide assistance.

End-of-Life Decision Making

For many with chronic illness, end-of-life decision making is complex. When an individual in frail health, possibly nearing the end of life, suffers an acute crisis, the individual, the family, and the caregiver may be faced with deciding whether to treat and to what extent to treat. There isn't a decision-making algorithm that is suitable for every person, and each individual's unique circumstances and situation must be considered. Decisions related to treating infections in a terminal individual or similar situations must be made with all involved individuals. Religious, social, and cultural values are of the utmost importance and must be given due consideration by all health care team members. The signing of an advanced directive records personal wishes regarding end-of-life decision-making. However, many compounding factors may affect the effectiveness of the advanced directive.

Assessing the situation using the concept of futile care can augment decision-making. There are a number of ways to define futile care, but principles that may be included are: treatment does not achieve the patient goals; treatment that is unsuccessful most of the time; treatment outside accepted standards (Ferrell & Coyle, 2001).

Abuse and Neglect of Vulnerable Adults

The number of abuse occurrences involving the elderly and other vulnerable adults is estimated to be 750,000 to 1.2 million cases annually in the United States (Fulmer, 1999). In 2000, 472,813 cases of abuse were reported, with 4,857 of those cases being substantiated (Teaster, 2002). Abuse can be categorized as domestic or institutional. Within these categories, physical, sexual, emotional/psychological abuse may occur as well as neglect, self neglect, abandonment, and financial exploitation. Because of longer life expectancies for those with chronic illness, it is very likely that incidents of abuse will increase (Teaster, 2002). The individual with chronic illness, if cognitively competent, may be hesitant to discuss the mistreatment because of the fear of loss of the relationship or other reprisal by the perpetrator. If the individual is not capable of expressing information regarding the abuse, identification may be by forensic evidence. Fulmer (1999) discusses three main types of abuse: physical abuse, neglect, and exploitation.

Physical abuse is the actual assault of an individual, and evidence exists with the presence of unexplained bruises, fractures, cuts, or burns in various

stages of healing. The victim of such treatment is in danger and requires immediate advocacy.

Neglect is defined as the lack of provision for basic necessities, such as food, water, and medical care. Neglect may be evidenced by poor hygiene, malnutrition or dehydration, pressure ulcers, and reports of being left in an unsafe condition or being left without resources to obtain necessary medications. Neglect can take place because of willful intention or because home management has become overwhelming to the client's aging spouse or family. Neglect can include self neglect which is defined as when individuals lose the will or the ability to properly care for themselves. Abandonment is the extreme form of neglect.

The third type of elder abuse, *exploitation,* is defined as the use of an elder's resources without knowledge or consent for the gain of another. Signs of elder exploitation include the disappearance of monetary resources or the "taking over" of personal belongings without permission or consent (Fulmer, 1999).

Each state has a Department of Adult Protective Services (APS) whose purpose is to protect the rights and health of older people and people with disabilities who are in danger of being mistreated or neglected, unable to protect themselves and have no one to assist them. APS is responsible for receiving the report of abuse, investigating the report, assessing the individual's risk, developing and implementing case plans, service monitoring, and evaluation. Some agencies may provide more in depth services including housing, medical care, social support, economic and legal services (National Association of Adult Protective Services Administrators, 2005).

Health care professionals and paraprofessionals such as RNs, physicians, nurse aides, and homemaker aides are mandated by law to report suspected adult or elder abuse.

Adjustment to Long-Term Care

Adjustment to LTC for the community-based elder involves learning the expectations of the agency and making provisions for compliance with those expectations. If delivery of Meals on Wheels requires that someone answer the door between 11:30 and

12:00 noon, Monday through Friday, the individual must be prepared to do so or risk losing the service. If a requirement for home health services is that the client is homebound, this may be difficult for a client who has become accustomed to playing bridge on Wednesday afternoon or going to church on Sunday.

Retired individuals may make an autonomous decision to move to an assisted-living facility. The comfort of such an environment subsequently makes it difficult for the individual to perceive the need for further transition when continued deterioration in health status requires more intensive nursing care. Individuals tend to delay for as long as possible leaving an assisted-living center to go to an SNF. This delay often leaves them vulnerable to complications arising from lack of appropriate care.

Admission to a nursing home for any individual can be very distressing. From the individual's perspective, the move to a nursing home may symbolize the reality of the loss of health, autonomy, economic power, productivity, and independence (see the case study concerning Mary Gray). Adjustment to such facilities may evoke a mix of emotions. The stress of going into a facility in which one is surrounded by strangers can be difficult. In addition, the individual must adjust to schedules determined by others, instead of following routines established throughout a lifetime. In many nursing homes, eating and bathing schedules are relatively fixed. Although not ideal, the resident is often the one who must change expectations to make allowance for the workload of the nursing home staff.

Interventions

Theoretical Framework for Practice

Nurses working in LTC settings have unlimited opportunities to implement theory in interactions with clients. Nurses draw from physiological theory, pharmacological theory, and theories of communication, caring, bereavement, ethics, and transcultural nursing. Using a theoretical framework to plan and implement nursing care in an

LTC setting helps the nurse to avoid doing things simply 'because they have always been done that way'. The main purpose for use of a theoretical framework is to guide one's practice. Mid-range theories are those defined as specific to particular caregiving situations and which have measurable outcomes. Theoretical frameworks give direction in the choice of interventions so that nursing care is most appropriate for the client. Several frameworks are appropriate for LTC. One example is "The Needs-Driven Dementia-Compromised Behavior Model." It can assist the care professional in understanding how to better interact with dementia clients (Algase et al., 1996). This model states that problematic behaviors in dementia clients are a result of needs that, when identified, can be addressed by the care provider, thereby avoiding a crisis. Such frameworks are helpful in assisting the care provider in solving problems encountered in the clinical area when dealing with LTC clients (Peterson & Bredow, 2004).

Admission and Assessment in the Long-Term Care Setting

Accessing community-based LTC services may seem a natural and necessary transition for an elder needing help with either rehabilitation or assistance with other aspects of care. For others, accessing services may create significant emotional turmoil. Once a frail elder can no longer stay in the community environment, the individual and family may decide that a move to another environment that provides needed services is necessary. For those who can afford assisted living, this option may be less emotionally traumatic. Individuals feel they have retained a great deal of autonomy while paying for the services that they can no longer perform, such as food preparation, laundry, housekeeping, and medication management.

The decision to move to a nursing home is usually made after much consideration by the client and family. The transition may be made more smoothly when the client retains as much participation in the process as possible. The client should be allowed to have input into choosing the facility and in planning the move. Retention of personal items gives the elder a better sense of self in the new facility. The predictability of the move, the reason for the move, and the degree of control the elder client retains in the decision-making process all affect the outcome (Reinardy, 1995).

During the admission process to a LTC facility, the care provider will complete a battery of paperwork that documents the client's condition and reason for admission. An accurate assessment of the client is the critical beginning for the client's experience in the LTC system. In residential nursing homes, this assessment is important because of the potential to enhance health, as opposed to the creation of excess disability (Dawson, Wells & Kline, 1993). It is imperative that the admission process not be limited to completing paperwork but include gaining insight into the client to provide individualized care.

The information that the nurse gathers during the admission process is the basis for appropriate care planning activities. There are several tools available that assist in admission assessment of the physical, functional, psychological, and social status of the LTC client (Sehy & Williams, 1999).

Based on the Nursing Home Reform Legislation in 1987, the Minimum Data Set (MDS) for Resident Assessment and Care Screening was developed for use by nursing homes. It provides extensive data about individual clients, but it also makes possible the establishment of a nationwide database regarding nursing home residents. Information requested by the MDS covers the areas of the resident's functional, medical, cognitive, and affective status at the time of admission and periodically thereafter (Sehy & Williams, 1999). This type of information also helps in tracking the improvement or decline of a resident over time. In the initial or follow-up assessment, the assessment protocol summarizes vulnerable aspects of the client's life that may require special care planning, interventions, and reporting of progress or problems in the resident's chart. The reliability of the information obtained varies with the knowledge the administrator has about the client. Other assessment tools are available and can provide more specific or multidimen-

sional information. Tools can help the nurse determine functioning in cognitive, communication, behavioral, social support domains. Other instruments measure vision, personality, depression, affect, comorbidity, and quality of life (Teresi & Evans, 1997). Examples of individual tools that are readily available in the literature include the Katz Index of Activities of Daily Living (Katz et al., 1970), Older American Resources and Services (OARS) (Duke University, 1978), the Beck Depression Rating Scale (Beck et al., 1979), and the Arthritis Impact Measurement Scale (AIMS) (Meenan, 1985).

Preservation of Autonomy as a Nursing Intervention

Health care professionals dealing with clients in LTC have special responsibilities in protecting and preserving their clients' autonomy (American Nurses Association, 2004; Mysak, 1997). The concept of autonomy is rooted in the idea of self-rule. There is a great deal of discussion related to client rights, autonomy, and personal rights. To more fully understand the concept of autonomy, the caregiver is encouraged to think about autonomy from the client's perspective when making caregiving decisions.

The role of the nurse in providing LTC along the continuum of care is to preserve the autonomy of the client. At the same time, the client must be protected from harm. Balancing these issues is not always easy. It is imperative that the care provider not assume that because an individual has lost some physical autonomy, such as requiring personal assistance with daily hygiene, that the individual has given up his or her autonomy. Promotion of autonomy is accomplished by allowing the individual to make as many decisions as possible. In decisions that can impact health or health care, the nurse must provide the appropriate information to enable the client to make an informed decision. Obviously, when competence is in question, the designated family member or legal guardian must be informed and allowed to make decisions.

It is important to understand that an individual's decision-making capacity does change during chronic illness and frailty (Mezey, Mitty & Ramsey, 1997). The law in some states define the line of authority for decision making when competence is in question. For example, in research dealing with clients with dementia, the client's representatives must be informed and give written consent for the individual's participation, but the patients, too, must be given information regarding participation and assent obtained. When a person has lost some degree of autonomy, the nurse must act in a judicious way that protects the individual from harm or exploitation.

It is also possible for someone who has legally lost autonomy (been declared incompetent) to continue to make some decisions. An example of this might be when a person with advanced dementia decides to walk the halls. This autonomous decision-making is appropriate as long as other principles, such as the client's safety and the safety of others, is considered. It is the nurse's responsibility to recognize an individual's capacity for autonomy and preserve that capacity as much as possible (Mezey, Mitty & Ramsey, 1997; Roberto et al., 1997). Sometimes, the nurse must compromise what he or she perceives to be the best treatment in order to incorporate client preferences. An example would be a client's bathing twice a week as opposed to more frequent bathing. In that case, the nurse might alter other interactions, such as frequency of spot baths or application of lotion to ensure skin integrity, while respecting the autonomy of the client.

Enablement of the client is one way of improving care for the cognitively impaired individual

Mary Gray

Mary Gray is an 83-year-old widow who has lived alone for 19 years. For 51 years, she lived in the same neighborhood and in the same house. During the majority of those years, she was an active senior and had many lifelong friends with whom she spent time. In the past five years, Mary developed an anemia related to malnourishment. Mary's chronic conditions included urinary incontinence, degenerative joint disease in the hips and knees, vision changes, and moderate hearing loss. These conditions slowly progressed, decreasing her ability to take care of herself. Mary had wisely recognized her decline in ability to drive and consequently had resorted to walking to the grocery store once a week and carrying home one bag of groceries. Walking to the grocery store had been a pattern of life in earlier years when her family had only one car. However, this restriction in this time of her life was a contributory factor in the development of malnourishment.

Approximately 18 months ago, Mary developed shortness of breath, fatigue, and weight loss. Assisted by an elderly neighbor, she managed a trip to the clinic where laboratory work and physical examination confirmed that she was malnourished. Mary qualified for homemaker services for 90 days. During this time, her condition improved, based on the assistance she received in buying groceries and preparing nutritious meals. Toward the end of the first 90 days, Mary was diagnosed with a urinary tract infection, allowing a recertification of home health care, based on medication teaching and monitoring, for a few more weeks. Homemaker services continued also for an additional six weeks. At the end of this time, Mary's health status had significantly improved. However, when the homemaker service stopped, she was no longer able to purchase groceries. Her condition began to decline, based, in part, on her poor nutri-

(Dawson, Wells & Kline, 1993). This perspective focuses on how the disease affects the client's abilities to carry out day-to-day activities. The purpose of this nursing care is to determine the client's remaining abilities and to enhance those abilities. Three areas of human behavior considered by this approach are self-care, social interaction, and interpretive abilities. This approach specifically targets the prevention of excess disability in the client. In the area of self-care, when the client is having difficulty achieving purposeful behaviors, certain nursing interventions have been identified that can assist the caregiver in enhancing the client's abilities. These include object cueing, touch, direct physical assistance, and verbal prompting (Dawson, Wells & Kline, 1993). When a client with dementia loses many of the skills required for daily activity, there is the possibility of retention of some significant skill or pleasure, such as a music-related activity or game playing. The nurse should help preserve those abilities as much as possible by providing opportunities for their expression (Beatty, 1999; Greiner et al., 1997).

Abuse in the home or in a residential facility is an extreme threat to the autonomy of the client. If the nurse providing care is the first one to observe signs and symptoms of mistreatment, reporting these observations to Adult Protective Services (or other public agency, as designated in the particular state) is required by law (Fulmer, 1999). In the home, the home health care nurse may be the one in a position to discover abuse and act as the primary advocate to prevent further abuse. The nurse may work

---

tional intake. During a probable hypoglycemic state, Mary fell and broke her hip, requiring surgery and admission to a residential LTC facility for rehabilitation. Mary demonstrated difficulty adjusting to the nursing home and was placed on antidepressive medications that altered her affect. Friends avoided coming to visit, not only because of their own advanced age and driving difficulties, but also because "Mary just didn't seem like Mary." With the increased social isolation from her friends, Mary began to show signs of increased forgetfulness and disengagement. She received an additional diagnosis of senile dementia because of a cursory examination by a family physician and because the physician was under the mistaken premise that the diagnosis might help the reimbursement rate of the nursing home. Mary seldom engaged in conversation with staff and purposefully avoided interactions with other residents.

A gerontological clinical nurse specialist (GCNS) was asked to consult on the nursing home wing where Mary lives. The GCNS not only conducted a thorough assessment of Mary, but also spent time observing her behavior and talking to her. The information and observations gathered by the GCNS led her to believe that Mary's short-term memory loss and flat affect might be from a combination of overmedication and depression. Mary's medication was adjusted, and she began to see a professional counselor twice a week at the nursing home. Mary improved, and her memory loss became less pronounced. She began to discover old acquaintances and also to make new friends in the nursing home. The quality of her life improved significantly through socialization and activities in her new environment. After nine months, Mary no longer needed counseling, and her adjustment to the nursing home was greatly enhanced.

with various agencies to ensure that appropriate intervention is made. Because elder mistreatment is often subtle, the nurse must be persistent in reporting signs until action is taken. If abuse or neglect of the community-based client is profound, a move to residential care may need to occur.

Advocacy: The Role of the Ombudsman

The LTC ombudsman is an advocate charged with the protection of the rights of all LTC clients. Although important for all clients, this individual is particularly helpful in advocating on behalf of those in residential facilities. The LTC ombudsman is an individual hired by a state LTC service agency under the auspices of the state or local health department or the statewide aging services. The purpose of the ombudsman is to advocate for residents' rights and quality care, educate consumers and providers, resolve residents' complaints and provide information to the public. Volunteers who report to the ombudsman supervisor may do many of the actual investigations. The complaints may come from the LTC resident, concerned family, or caregivers. Findings must be reported to the client and/or family, and, most importantly, the ombudsman is responsible for achieving an equitable settlement between the resident and the LTC facility. The role of the ombudsman is founded in ethical principles and is implemented on behalf of the vulnerable client. Updates on the organizational activities contacts can be found at the Ombudsman website at http://www.ltcombudsman.org.

Adjustment

Admission to a nursing home may be one of the most traumatic life transitions. The nurse needs to assist in making the adjustment of the client to the facility as smooth as possible. The client experiencing psychological and emotional difficulty during the admission and transition into any LTC facility needs support from the attending nursing staff. The use of therapeutic communication techniques by the staff in addition to spending adequate time with a transitioning resident can make a difference in the level of anxiety and stress experienced. If indicated, the nurse should initiate a referral for the resident to be seen by mental health services. These services are generally an underused resource for elders.

One of the most enduring aspects of human behavior is the requirement for socialization. In making the transition to the nursing home, the resident needs the opportunity to socialize and choose friends. In small communities, residents often know each other prior to admission, which is an advantage. In most environments, however, the new resident of the facility will need to make new friends. The nurse can help by introducing residents and encouraging participation in group activities, in which opportunities for socializing are possible. This socialization process can positively influence the adjustment to a residential facility.

Nursing Care

Nursing care is the primary service provided by residential LTC facilities. The further one progresses along the LTC continuum, the more intense are the nursing care needs. Figure 24-2 lists the most common conditions of nursing home residents in the United States and the percentage of residents who have those conditions. There are many issues that impact the quality of life in individuals with chronic illness, and these issues should not be ignored during the provision of routine daily care. The nurse should never lose touch with the personhood of the client, and needs to provide personal, caring, sensitive interactions.

Activities of Daily Living

Whether considering quality of life or Maslow's hierarchy of needs, issues of daily living begin with meeting physiological needs. Adequate food and fluid intake is basic to survival for the individual with chronic illness. Although this view may seem simplistic, adequate nutrition is often a key issue in

FIGURE 24-2

Percentage of the Most Frequently Occurring Health Conditions for Nursing Home Residents under Age 65 and Age 65 and over: United States, January 1, 1996

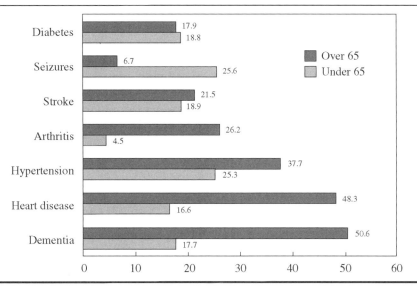

NOTE: The most frequently occurring conditions for nursing home residents under age 65 are seizures, hypertension, stroke, diabetes, and dementia. The most frequently occurring conditions for residents age 65 and over are dementia, heart disease, hypertension, arthritis, and stroke.

SOURCE: Center for Cost and Financing Studies, Agency for Health Care Policy and Research: Medical Expenditure Panel Survey Nursing Home Component, 1996.

entering the LTC continuum. Meals on Wheels and homemaker services provide adequate nutrition in the community. Whether in the community or in a nursing home, it is important to realize that the presence of food does not guarantee that the individual will have adequate intake. The client should be properly evaluated for difficulties that have an impact on the ability to eat, including dental problems, swallowing disorders, digestive disorders (including related factors such as hiatal hernia or gastric reflux), and mobility.

If the client is in a residential facility and food and water are placed in the client's room but out of reach, although this act fulfills regulatory requirements, it does the client little good. Additionally, water

and other fluids are sometimes placed in containers that are too large or too heavy to be lifted by the client.

Pain Management

The science of pain management has advanced significantly over the past two decades (Celia, 2000). It is important for the nurse in LTC to adequately assess pain and to provide adequate treatment of that pain (Ferrell & Coyle, 2001). Of particular importance is assessing clients' suffering from the pain associated with arthritis, osteoporosis, or neuralgia. A great deal of information is available on appropriate pain management strategies, and the nurse dealing with such clients should access this body of literature. When implementing pain management strategies in the LTC setting, follow-up is critical. Pain relief varies for many reasons, and pain may not be relieved by a method that was previously successful for the client. When pain is chronic and affects the ability of the client to function, current treatment strategies include routine regular administration of medication to manage the pain. Breakthrough pain, or pain experienced intermittently when a client is on routine pain medication, is then treated with "as needed" medication. Addiction is not generally considered to be a major problem for elders suffering from chronic pain, but tolerance can be problematic (see Chapter 4, on chronic pain).

For individuals unable to verbally express pain, its presence is noted in other ways. Evidence of pain may include facial expression (grimacing), body position, bracing, guarding, and rubbing of the painful body part. Alternative methods of dealing with pain should be considered. Massage, heat, cold, and support mechanisms such as knee or back braces may be helpful. The quality of life of the LTC client can be greatly affected by pain. With current advances in pharmacology and treatment, most pain can be managed effectively.

Disease Prevention/Health Promotion

Few preventive health measures are funded by Medicare. However, current development in Medicare policy indicates that preventive measures may be given an increasingly higher priority in the future. An important preventive health measure provided along the LTC continuum is the provision of flu and pneumonia vaccines to clients. A vaccination program in residential facilities is essential; in such settings, infections such as influenza can spread rapidly and cause significant deaths among the frail elderly. These types of infections may affect a number of residents at one time and place a difficult burden on staff to deal with a number of acutely ill clients. Admission of clients to acute care settings in such circumstances is not unreasonable to ensure that all clients receive adequate nursing care during an outbreak of illness.

Preventive screenings are generally not performed in residential facilities, and reimbursement is not usually available. Part of the discussion and logic regarding this situation centers on the practical application of the screening results. In a frail elder with multiple medical conditions or with dementia, the decision to treat a condition such as cancer may not be a reasonable option. A person who has chronic illness may not be able to withstand the trauma of surgery or have the required recuperative powers. Kidney and liver function may not be at a level adequate to tolerate chemotherapy. It may be decided that palliative care is more appropriate. It is essential to know what advanced directives are in place with residents in LTC facilities to assist in dealing with acute crises and chronic health problems.

Cognitive Impairment

Individuals in LTC may suffer cognitive impairment from a variety of pathological processes. Individuals with closed head injuries, central nervous system involvement from infections, stroke, or dementia from a number of pathological processes such as Alzheimer's disease, Pick's Disease, Lewy Body Disease, etc. often, need LTC. With each decade of extended life, there is an increase in the number of individuals suffering changes in cognitive function. The first and foremost consideration in dealing with cognitively impaired individuals is the determination of whether the cognitive impairment is due to delirium or dementia. Appropriate evaluation of the condition can prevent an unnecessary death. Delirium is an acute condition brought on by one or more conditions that have altered brain functioning. The chief symptoms include sudden disturbance in consciousness and/or cognition. The underlying condition can be a single or combination of conditions, which include but are not limited to fever, infection, allergic reaction, malnutrition, vitamin deficiency, drug toxicity (over the counter or prescription), drug interactions, food supplement toxicity, hyper- or hypoglycemia, and hypoxia. The underlying condition can be life threatening and must be corrected or the incident may result in death. If the nurse providing care in the LTC setting determines that a client is suffering from delirium, it may be necessary to arrange transportation to an acute care facility where appropriate emergent care can be provided.

Because of the physiological changes that occur with aging, the signs of delirium in a frail elder may develop over a period of days as a subclinical condition worsens to a crisis point. Also, in a patient who has a complicated medication regime, mental confusion can occur subltly. The astute nurse will make the appropriate observations to detect delirium even when the symptoms are subtle. In a client population with fluctuating cognition, such as at many residential facilities, detection of delirium becomes more challenging.

Dementia differs from delirium in that the condition is chronic and the underlying pathological process is progressive and irreversible. It is estimated that five percent of individuals over age 65, and 20 percent of those over age 80, suffer from dementia (Raskind & Bower, 1996). In addition, it is estimated that between 40 percent and 80 percent of those living in nursing homes have a cognitive impairment (Raskind & Bower, 1996).

Dementia is defined as the development of multiple cognitive deficits manifested by memory impairment and other problems, such as aphasia (inability to speak), apraxia (loss of ability to use familiar objects or carry out purposeful movements not due to loss of sensory ability), and agnosia (loss of ability to determine the significance of sensory input, such as recognition of a familiar face or voice) (American Psychiatric Association, 1994; Abrams, Beers & Berkow, 1995). Primary dementias have no cure, and although a large investment is being made in drugs that could affect the progression of disease, little success has been achieved.

It is estimated that as much as 70 percent of dementia care is delivered in the home by a family caregiver. In the community LTC setting, the role of the nurse is to support the family caregiver with problem solving or identifying resources such as respite care, adult day care, or the local chapter of the Alzheimer's Association. The nurse may play a key role in the decision-making that takes place when caregiving for a demented loved one is negatively affecting the health of the spousal caregiver (Maas, Reed, Park, Specht, Schutte, Kelley, Swanson, Tripp-Reimer, & Buckwalter, 2004). When caregiving becomes overwhelming at home, the decision to place the individual with dementia in a residential facility is appropriate.

Initial careful evaluation of individuals with chronic cognitive changes is necessary so that, later, changes can be detected and appropriate care given (Teresi & Evans, 1997). Many nurses working in the LTC setting rely on intuitive detection of cognitive changes, but this method can be improved by the inclusion of an objective measure of cognition such as the Mini Mental Status Exam (MMSE) (Folstein, Folstein & McHugh, 1975), the Dementia Rating Scale (Alexopoulos & Mattis, 1991), the Blessed Dementia Scale (Blessed, Tomlinson & Roth, 1968), or the Cognition Assessment (Matteson, Linton & Barnes, 1996; Barnes, 2002).

Nursing interventions that deal with dementia generally address one or more of three symptom domains: cognitive, functional, and/or behavioral. All clients with dementia demonstrate functional difficulties, while only some demonstrate behavioral problems. Dealing with individuals suffering from permanent cognitive impairment takes patience and understanding. It is important that the caregiver not lose sight of the client perspective. It is more important to validate the client's personhood rather than to insist that he or she achieve "reality orientation." The client may find comfort in some behavior, such as carrying a doll, and this behavior, although not grounded in immediate reality, is grounded in the reality of a universal human behavior regarding caring for others, specifically infants. The case study regarding Mr. Hurley demonstrates this principle, but applications are as varied as the number of clients.

The activity director is responsible for providing activities for residents, and this includes activities for those with cognitive impairment. The nurse needs to work closely with the activity director to meet the needs of the clients and to find appropriate and enjoyable activities for those with dementia.

Approximately ten percent of nursing homes and even some assisted-living centers have special care units for dementia clients (Rhoades & Krauss, 1999). The environment in such settings allows for safe wandering. Ideally, the staff has received training specific to caring for clients with dementia. The units are generally set up with consideration given to lighting, color, noise levels, congregate areas, and room set-ups. Such considerations are used to make the environment more pleasant for the residents. Although some of the considerations may have scientific evidence to support their use, much is based on trial and error.

Risk-Reduction and Safety Issues

One of the most important functions of the nurse in an LTC setting is to reduce risk and ensure client safety. In a community setting, part of the home assessment includes a thorough examination of the environment to detect possible hazards and correct them. The most obvious hazards include throw rugs, electrical cords strung across traffic areas, worn or broken steps, loose tiles in the shower, and similar environmental conditions.

In residential settings, the nurse has similar responsibilities to ensure client safety. One important safety issue is the use of restraints. Originally, restraints were thought to prevent injury to clients and were applied to ensure patient safety through limiting movement. Research has demonstrated, however, that restraints do the opposite and are likely to cause injury (Lekan-Rutledge, 1997). Currently, restraints cannot be applied without a physician order, and the trend is a restraint-free environment. The most current reports regarding restraint use are available online (CMS, 2004).

Palliative Care

There is a point in the life of each client at which the focus of care is no longer considered curative or custodial. Palliative care is a philosophical approach of viewing a client, as well as a treatment modality for those at the end of life. When chronic illnesses become overwhelming, the care should, in the interest of the client, become palliative, with the intent of providing comfort care. In the terminal phase of life, appropriate care includes pain relief, comfort, and emotional and spiritual support for the client and family (Tarzian, 2000). Hospice services are a type of palliative care. The general requirement for Medicare reimbursement for hospice service is that the individual has 6 months or less to live. Determination of the terminal phase of an illness is difficult, particularly in noncancer clients. It is possible to have hospice come into nursing homes to augment and oversee comfort care. In palliation, physiological needs are met and aggressive measures are taken for pain relief. A holistic view of the client should be maintained, and the personhood of the client is of primary consideration in this type of nursing care. The client and family can be referred for grief counseling related to the experience of incurable illness (Ferrell & Coyle, 2001).

Death is a natural part of life, and the nurse should be prepared to facilitate the client's passing and provide support to the family survivors (DeSpelder & Strickland, 1996). Once hospice services are begun for community-dwelling elders, other LTC services may not be allowed by reimbursement policy.

Interest in and information on palliative care are increasing. During the next decade, it is expected that knowledge on palliative and end-of-life care will increase and this treatment methodology will advance (see Chapter 23, on palliative care).

Research in Long-Term Care

The science of caring for those who have chronic illness is changing rapidly. A number of nurse researchers have focused research programs dealing with chronic illness and issues related to the nursing home experience (Cornelia Beck, Jeanne Kaiser-Jones, Terri Fulmer, etc). Research in LTC care settings is essential if the complex problems of clients

Mr. Hurley

Mr. Hurley is a 78-year-old man who resides in an Alzheimer's special care unit. He spends most of the time wandering the halls in what appears, to the casual observer, to be a bizarre posture. He walks slowly, leading with the right foot, and is bent over, staring at the ground. Mr. Hurley has one hand extended and makes a rolling motion between his thumb and index finger after each step. He then takes his left foot and slides it across the floor in front of him. A new nursing assistant, Jane, is hired to work on this unit. Jane has had no previous experience in caring for dementia clients. Mr. Hurley's behavior is disturbing to the new aide, who, with all good intentions, tries to "orient Mr. Hurley to person/place/time" and to get him to stop pacing the halls and participate in a group activity. Mr. Hurley's reaction is, at first, avoidance of the aide. As she becomes more persistent, Mr. Hurley comes closer to a crisis. The day LPN notices the interactions taking place between Jane and Mr. Hurley. She explains to Jane that Mr. Hurley worked for over 40 years as a truck farmer and his behavior is most likely a remnant of actions performed while planting seeds in the field. Mr. Hurley does not want or need to be redirected, and it is best for his reality to be validated by allowing him to continue the motions as long as he is content. Jane learns the difference between reality orientation and validation through her experience with Mr. Hurley.

---

are to be addressed appropriately (Baldwin & Nail, 2000). Research often begins with clinical observations of problems or recurring events that require solutions. Nurses in a clinical role should not ignore the opportunity to define a problem and propose a solution. A novice researcher may partner with a more experienced researcher to develop an idea into a researchable question. Regional research organizations such as the Southern Nursing Research Society, the Midwest Nursing Research Society, and Sigma Theta Tau, are available to provide assistance. In addition, funding for such inquiry is increasing (Grady, 2000)

Outcomes

Desired outcomes for LTC clients are as multi-faceted as the clients. Simple medical models are rarely sufficient to state desired outcomes for those with complicated chronic medical conditions (Mold, 1995). It is not sufficient to consider the quality of life based on absence of sickness, but to consider the overall well-being of the client. Outcomes will vary along the LTC continuum. For community-based clients, the overall outcome may be to remain in their homes as long as possible. Interventions to support that outcome may include client and family teaching on medication management, safety issues, or wound care. Rehabilitation may be a desired outcome for a community-based client following hospitalization.

For the resident in an LTC facility, outcomes are different and may include a reduction in the exacerbations of a chronic illness such as congestive heart failure. A client in the rehabilitative area of the facility may have as an outcome to live independently again. Outcomes for others may be to function at the highest potential with the limitations imposed by the chronic illness. A decrease in pain and/ or nausea might be an appropriate outcome for an individual in palliative care. Living each day with optimal quality of life is an outcome for most clients in LTC.

▌ Summary and Conclusions

Providing appropriate, timely and specialized care for individuals in long term care can be complex and multifaceted. The nurse responsible should perform not only as a skilled care provider but as a source of information and referral to ensure that all available resources are used for the client. In depth knowledge of the pathophysiology and treatment of the chronic disease conditions form the basis for practice. However, just as significant a role for the nurse includes advocacy for the client. Because of the nature of the long term care client, role expectations of the nurse will frequently include that of patient liaison. Preservation of client autonomy and the presence of client vulnerability drive the need for ongoing awareness of ethical issues on the part of the nurse.

In order to maintain the highest professional standards of care, the nurse should update his or her own knowledge base on a regular basis by accessing continuing education offerings, reading journal and text publications, and accessing resources online. Excellent online resources include sites such as Centers for Medicaid and Medicare Services, the National Long Term Care Ombudsman Resource Center, National Association for Adult Protective Services, Association of Retired Persons, and the pages for the state long term care authority in which the nurse practices.

Study Questions

1. What is the broad definition of *long-term care*?
2. What are the major problems facing both caregivers and clients in today's long-term care continuum?
3. Discuss the ethical principle of autonomy when constructing an appropriate plan of care for a long-term care recipient.
4. Does the consideration of autonomy vary depending on whether a client dwells in the community or in a residential facility?

5. What constraints do nursing home administrators face when providing residential care for Medicare and Medicaid recipients?
6. What are some of the precipitating factors for an individual to access the long-term care system?
7. What are the three types of elder abuse, and what signs would a caregiver notice to indicate that an individual is a victim?

References

AARP. (2002). Understanding Long-term Health Care. Available on-line at http://www.aarp.org/financial-insurance/a2002-08-13-Insurance.LongTermCare.html

Abrams, W. B., Beers, M. H., & Berkow, R. (Eds.). (1995). *The Merck manual of geriatrics* (2nd ed.). Whitehouse Station, NJ: Merck.

Administration on Aging. (2004). Aging News. http://www.aoa.gov/press/news.

Alexopoulos, G. S., & Mattis, S. (1991). Diagnosing cognitive dysfunction in the elderly: Primary screening tests. *Geriatrics, 46* (12), 33–38, 43–44.

Algase, D., Beck, C., Kolanowski, A., Whall, A., et al. (1996). Need-driven dementia-compromised behavior: An alternative view of disruptive behavior. *American Journal of Alzheimer's' Disease, 11* (6), 10–19.

American Nurse's Association. (2004). *Code of ethics with interpretive statements.*Washington, DC: ANA Publications.

American Psychiatric Association (1994). *Diagnostic and statistical manual of mental disorders* (4th ed.). Washington, DC: American Psychiatric Association.

Baldwin, K. M., & Nail, L. M. (2000). Opportunities and challenges in clinical nursing research. *Journal of Nursing Scholarship, 32* (2), 163–166.

Barnes, S. J. (2002) "Cognition Assessment in Elders with Dementia: Testing with Developmental Tasks." Presentation at Southern Nursing Research Society Annual Meeting, February 8, 2002, San Antonio, Texas.

Beatty, W. (1999). Preserved cognitive skills in dementia: Implications for geriatric medicine. *Journal: Oklahoma State Medical Association, Reprint, 92* (1).

Beauchamp, T. L. (2001). *Principles of biomedical ethics* (5th ed.). New York: Oxford University Press.

Beck, A. T., Rush, A. J., Shaw, B. F., & Emery, G. (1979). *Cognitive therapy of depression.* New York: Guilford.

Beck, C., Heacock, P., Mercer, S. O., Walls, R. C., et al. (1997). Improving dressing behavior in cognitively impaired nursing home residents. *Nursing Research, 46* (3), 126–132.

Blessed, B., Tomlinson, B., & Roth, M. (1968). The association between quantitative measures of dementia and of degenerative changes in the cerebral gray matter of elderly subjects. *British Journal of Psychiatry, 114,* 797–811.

Celia, B. (2000). Age and gender differences in pain management following coronary artery bypass surgery. *Journal of Gerontological Nursing, 26* (5), 7–13.

Center for Medicare and Medicaid Services (CMS). (2000). Medicare 2000: 35 years of improving Americans' health and security: Profiles of Medicare beneficiaries. Washington, DC: U.S. Government Printing Office.

_____. (2004) State operations manual. http://www.cms.hhs.gov.

_____. (2004). *Restraint reduction newsletter.* Available online at http:www.hcfa.gov.

Dawson, P., Wells, D., & Kline, K. (1993). *Enhancing the abilities of persons with Alzheimer's and related dementias: A nursing perspective.* New York: Springer.

DeSpelder, L. A., & Strickland, A. L. (2002). *The last dance: Encountering death and dying* (6th ed.) Boston: McGraw Hill.

Duke University Center for the Study of Aging and Human Development (1978). *Multidimensional functional assessment: The OARS methodology.* Durham, NC: Duke University.

Federal Interagency Forum on Aging (2004). *Older Americans 2004: Key indicators of well-being.* Federal Interagency Forum on Aging-Related Statistics. Available on-line at http://www.agingstats.gov.

Ferrel, B. & Coyle, N. (2004). *Textbook of palliative nursing.* Oxford: Oxford University Press.

Folstein, M. R., Folstein, S. E., & McHugh, P. R. (1975). Mini-mental state: A practical method for grading the cognitive state of patients for the clinician. *Journal of Psychiatric Research, 12,* 189–198.

Fulmer, T. T. (1999). Elder mistreatment. In J. T. Stone, J. F. Wyman, & S. A. Salisbury (Eds.). *Clinical gerontological nursing: A guide to advanced practice* (2nd ed.), (pp. 665–674). Philadelphia: Saunders.

Gerontological Association of America and Merck Institute of Aging & Health. (2004). The state of aging and health in America. Published report.

Grady, P. (2000). Prologue from the Director, National Institute of Nursing Research. http://ninr.nih.gov/ninr/research/diversity/mission.html

Greiner, F., English, S., Dean, K., Olson, K. A., et al. (1997). Expression of game-related and generic knowledge by dementia patients who retain skill at playing dominoes. *Neurology, 49,* 518–523.

Harrington, C., Carrillo, H., & Crawford. (2004). Nursing facilities, staffing, residents, and facility deficiencies, 1996 through 2003. Service Employees International Union. Available online at www.cmms.hhs.gove/medicaid/service/nursinfac04.

Kalisch, P. A., & Kalisch, B. J. (2004). *American nursing: A history* (4th ed.). Philadelphia: Lippincott Williams & Wilkins.

Kane, R., Freeman, I., Chaplan, A., Asashar, M., et al. (1990). Everyday autonomy in nursing homes. *Generations, 14* (Suppl), 69–71.

Kane, R. L., & Kane, R. A. (1982). *Values and long-term care.* Lexington, MA: Lexington Books.

Katz, S., Downs, T. D., Cash, H. R., & Grotz, R. C. (1970). Progress in development of the index of ADL. *Gerontologist, 10,* 20–30.

Kayser-Jones, J. (1999). Inadequate staffing at mealtime: Implications for nursing and health policy. *Journal of Gerontological Nursing, 9,* 14–21.

Koop, C. E., & Schaeffer, F. (1976). *Whatever happened to the human race?* Old Tappan, NJ: Fleming H. Revell.

Leininger, M. (2002). Culture care theory: A major contribution to advance transcultural nursing and practices. *Journal of Transcultural Nursing, 13* (3), 189–192.

Lekan-Rutledge, D. (1997). Gerontological nursing in long-term care facilities. In M. Matteson, E. McConnell, & A. Linton (Eds.), *Gerontological nursing: Concepts and practice* (2nd ed.), (pp. 930–960). Philadelphia: Saunders.

Maas, M.L., Reed, D., Park, M., Specht, J.P., et al. (2004). Outcomes of family involvement in care interventions for caregivers of individuals with dementia. *Nursing Research, 53* (2), 76–86.

Marnard, B. (2002). Nursing home quality indicators. Washington, DC: AARP.

Matteson, M. A., Linton, A. D., & Barnes, S. J. (1996). The cognitive developmental approach to dementia. *Image, 28* (3), 233–240.

Meenan, R. F. (1985). New approaches to outcome assessment: The AIMS questionnaire for arthritis. *Advances in Internal Medicine, 31,* 167–185.

Mezey, M., Mitty, I., & Ramsey, G. (1997). Assessment of decision making capacity: Nursing's role. *Journal of Gerontological Nursing, 23* (3), 28–34.

Mold, J. W. (1995). An alternative conceptualization of health and health care: Its implications for geriatrics and gerontology. *Educational Gerontology, 21,* 85–101.

Mysak, S. (1997). Strategies for promoting ethical decision making. *Journal of Gerontological Nursing, 23* (1), 25–31.

National Association of Adult Protective Services Administrators (2005). http://www.elderabusecenter.org/default.cfm?p=naapsa.cfm.

National PACE Association. (2004). Report on Model State Practices for PACE. Available online at http://www.natlpaceassn.org/content/states/.

Peterson, S. J., & Bredow, T. S. (2004). *Middle range theories: Application to nursing research.* Philadelphia: Lippincott, Williams and Wilkins.

Raskind, M., & Bower, P. (1996). Alzheimer's disease: A diagnosis and management update. *Federal Practitioner, 7,* 24–35.

Reinardy, J. R. (1995). Relocation to a new environment: Decisional control and the move to a nursing home. *Health & Social Work, 20* (1), 31–38.

Rhoades, J. A., & Krauss, N. A. (1999). *Nursing home trends 1987 and 1996.* Rockville, MD: Medical Expenditure Panel survey, Agency for Health Care Policy and Research Publication No. 99-0032.

Roberto, D. A., Wacler, R. R., Jewell, M. A., & Rickard, M. (1997). Resident rights: Knowledge of and implementation by nursing staff in long term care facilities. *Journal of Gerontological Nursing, 23* (12), 32–37.

Salisbury, S. A. (1999). Iatrogenesis. In J. T. Stone, J. F. Wyman, & S. A. Salisbury (Eds.), *Clinical gerontological nursing: A guide to advanced practice* (2nd ed.), (pp. 369–383). Philadelphia: Saunders.

Sehy, Y. B., & Williams, M. P. (1999). Functional Assessment. In W. C. Chenitz, J. Takano Smith, & S. A. Salisbury (Eds.), *Clinical gerontological nursing: A guide to advanced practice* (2nd ed.), (pp. 175–199). Philadelphia: Saunders.

Shalala, D. (2000). Message from Donna E. Shalala, Secretary of Health and Human Services. Available on-line http://www.surgeongeneral.gov/Library/MentalHealth/home.html.

Tarzian, A. J. (2000). Caring for dying patients who have air hunger. *Journal of Nursing Scholarship, 32* (2), 137–143.

Teaster, P. B. (2002). A response to the abuse of vulnerable adults: The 2000 survey of state adult protective services. Washington, DC: The National Center on Elder Abuse.

Teresi, J. A., & Evans, D. A. (1997). Cognitive assessment measures for chronic care populations. In J. A. Teresi, M. P. Lawton, D. Holmes, & M. Ory (Eds.), *Measurement in elderly chronic care populations,* (pp. 1–23). New York: Springer.

Tobin, P., & Salisbury, S. (1999). Legal planning issues. In J. T. Stone, J. F. Wyman, & S. A. Salisbury (Eds.), *Clinical gerontological nursing: A guide to advanced practice* (2nd ed.), (pp. 31–44). Philadelphia: Saunders.

Varcarolis, E. M. (2002). *Foundation of psychiatric mental health nursing: A clinical approach.* Philadelphia: Saunders.

White House Conference on Aging. (2004). Online at: www.whitehouse.gov.

CHAPTER 25

Rehabilitation

Robin E. Remsburg ▪ Barbara Carson

Introduction

Rehabilitation refers to services and programs designed to assist individuals who have experienced a trauma or illness that results in impairment that creates a loss of function (physical, psychological, social, or vocational). Rehabilitation also refers to a philosophical approach of care in promoting recovery from acute illnesses and chronic diseases (Pryor, 2002).

The primary goal of rehabilitation, whether from a program/service perspective or a philosophical perspective, is to achieve the highest level of independence possible for the client. Rehabilitation should be considered as part of the overall plan of care for most acute illness episodes and throughout the duration of most chronic illnesses.

Optimal functioning is highly individual; therefore, the rehabilitation process begins with identification of the individual's values and goals. The individual's strengths, e.g., what he/she can do, are assessed and interventions that build upon these strengths are initiated to assist the individual in reaching their highest level of function. For some, that may include returning to previous employment and functioning in the same job as prior to illness. For others, the highest level of independence may be feeding oneself unassisted, being able to use a "sip and puff" wheelchair, or being able to stay in one's home with some assistance. For each rehabilitation client, the goals will be different; but for all, the overarching goal is to return to the highest level of functioning possible in a setting of the client's choice.

A major outcome of the rehabilitation process is resocialization. Resocialization is the process by which individuals are reintegrated into society after a condition or situation alters their previous roles. Within a rehabilitation setting, resocialization is a continuing goal. Rehabilitation professionals work with the disabled client or individual with chronic illness and their family to achieve reintegration into society. This reintegration may be physical, social, emotional, or vocational, but the resocialization process deals with all aspects of an individual's life.

The goals of rehabilitation are accomplished through a variety of interventions designed to restore initial function and abilities, teach alternative techniques, or provide assistive/adaptive and prosthetic/orthotic devices that overcome impairments or augment function, and to make environmental modifications that reduce barriers to independent functioning. Examples include:

- An individual with osteoarthritis with a total knee replacement, through a regimen of progressive resistance exercise and pain management including ice packs and the use of nonsteroidal anti-inflammatory drugs, may regain most of his/her joint function and return to their previous level of function.

■ An adult with type II diabetes with a below the knee amputation may, with the use of a prosthetic device, crutches, or a wheelchair, be able to resume most previous activities.

■ An older adult with a right-hemisphere cerebrovascular accident (CVA) may learn alternative dressing, bathing, and ambulation techniques; may use assistive devices such as a reaching device, a button fastener, a plate guard, and a wheelchair, and have modifications made to the environment, e.g. grab bars in the bathroom, a raised toilet seat, a wheelchair ramp, all to accomplish their activities of daily living independently.

Because rehabilitation is a comprehensive process involving all aspects of an individual's life, an interdisciplinary team concept of care is essential. No one discipline can provide all the expertise necessary in the rehabilitation of a client. An interdisciplinary team of professionals working together to develop and provide ongoing evaluation of a plan of care is necessary to achieve optimal outcomes. Participation of the client and family in the rehabilitation process is crucial to its success. It is expected that the client and family will attend team meetings, assist in goal setting, and be active participants in care.

There are a number of chronic conditions that may benefit from rehabilitation services. A partial list includes neuromuscular diseases such as multiple sclerosis (MS) and Parkinson's disease; cancer; cardiac and pulmonary conditions; musculoskeletal conditions such as rheumatoid arthritis or osteoarthritis; trauma including spinal cord or traumatic brain injuries; burns; cerebrovascular accidents (CVAs); and orthopedic conditions such as disk disease, joint replacements, or fractures. Although the above mentioned conditions are dissimilar in many ways, they are similar in their ability to affect function, cause disability, and decrease independence.

Definitions

Rehabilitation

There are a number of terms specific to rehabilitation that need to be defined before relating them to chronic illness. Many authors have defined rehabilitation (see Table 25-1), and there is considerable overlap among these definitions. Most definitions emphasize the dynamic interaction among the individual and his/her personal characteristics, the disease or health condition, the environment, and the resulting impairment.

Vocational Rehabilitation

Vocational rehabilitation refers to specific programs that are designed to assist the disabled individual return to gainful employment and develop financial independence (Lysaght, 2004; Kielkofner, Braveman, Finlayson, Paul-Ward, Goldbaum, & Goldstein, 2004; O'Neill, Zuger, Fields, Fraser, & Pruce, 2004; Targett, Wehman, & Young, 2004).

Rehabilitation Nursing

The Association of Rehabilitation Nurses (ARN) (2000) defines rehabilitation nursing as a specialized practice requiring specialized skills and knowledge for assessing, planning, implementing, and evaluating care of the rehabilitation client. The roles of the rehabilitation nurse include: caregiver, teacher, case manager, counselor, and advocate.

The standards and scope of practice for rehabilitation nurses and advanced rehabilitation nurses are included in *Standards and Scope of Rehabilitation Nursing Practice* (2000) and *Scope and Standards of Advanced Clinical Practice in Rehabilitation Nursing* (1996).

Restorative Care

The purpose of restorative care is to actively assist individuals in long-term care settings to maintain their highest level of function and to assist residents in retaining the gains made during formal therapy

TABLE 25-1

Definitions of Rehabilitation

Source	Definition
Rusk (1965)	Ultimate restoration of a disabled person to his or her maximum capacity: physical, emotional, and vocational
Krussen, Kottke & Ellwood (1971)	The process of decreasing dependence of the handicapped or disabled person by developing, to the greatest extent possible, the abilities needed for adequate functioning in the individual situation
Dittmar (1989)	The process by which an individual's movement toward health is facilitated
Hickey (1992)	A dynamic process by which a person achieves optimal physical, emotional, psychological, social, and vocational potential and maintains dignity and self-respect in a life that is as independent and self-fulfilling as possible
National Council on Rehabilitation (1994)	Restoration of the handicapped to the fullest physical, mental, social, vocational, and economic usefulness of which they are capable
Institute of Medicine, Brandt & Pope (1997)	The process by which physical, sensory, or mental capacities are restored or developed. This is achieved not only through functional change in the person, such as strengthening injured limbs, but also through changes in the physical and social environments, such as making buildings accessible to wheelchairs. Rehabilitation strives to reverse what has been called the disabling process, and may therefore be called the enabling process.
Commission on Accreditation of Rehabilitation Facilities CARF (2000)	The process of providing those comprehensive services deemed appropriate to the needs of persons with disabilities in a coordinated manner in a program or service designed to achieve objectives of improved health, welfare, and realization of the person's maximum physical, social, psychological, and vocational potential for useful and productive activity

(Resnick & Remsburg, 2004; Nadash & Feldman, 2003; Resnick & Fleishall, 2002). Restorative care does not include procedures or techniques carried out by or under the direction of a qualified therapist, but instead nursing interventions that promote the resident's ability to adapt and adjust to living as independently and safely as possible in the long-term care setting (CMS, 2002). Restorative care maximizes an individual's abilities, focuses on what the individual can do, and "seeks to create independence, improve self-image and self-esteem, reduce the level of care required, and eliminate or minimize the degrading features of long-term care such as restraints, incontinence, and supervised feeding" (Atchinson, 1992, p. 9).

Restorative care includes the following activities: walking and mobility exercises, dressing, grooming, eating, swallowing, transferring, amputation/prosthesis care, communication skills, and teaching/practicing self-care skills such as diabetic manage-

ment, ostomy care, or self-administration of medication (Remsburg, 2004). While the definition of restorative care has considerable overlap with the definition of rehabilitation, restorative care is targeted at individuals who are not candidates for formal rehabilitation therapy, lack potential for substantive improvement or who have reached their optimal level of function.

Classification Systems

Rehabilitation models can assist us in understanding how disabling conditions develop, progress, and can be reversed or effectively managed. Numerous classification systems are used by professionals to describe and document the rehabilitation process (WHO, 1980; Pope & Tarlov, 1991; Brandt & Pope, 1997; WHO, 2002). Frequently used systems include the Functional Limitations System (FLS), the Institute of Medicine's Enabling–Disabling Model, and the WHO International Classification of Functioning, Disability, and Health (ICF). Although the Institute of Medicine (IOM) recommends the use of the Enabling–Disabling Process Model, and the WHO recommends the use of the IFC to facilitate communication regarding diagnosis, care and treatment, other rehabilitation professionals may use other models. Therefore, it is essential that rehabilitation professionals identify and articulate which classification system is being used in their practice. The use of standard terminology, common definitions, and assessment strategies will also promote theory-based research and guide the development and application of effective treatments and prevention strategies.

The Enabling-Disabling Process   The Enabling-Disabling Process is a framework for professional rehabilitation practice that addresses the individuality and uniqueness of each rehabilitation client. The framework was developed from the landmark work of the Institute of Medicine (IOM) in 1997. This work, *Enabling America*, urged the adoption of a new conceptual framework that better addressed the enablement-disablement process (Brandt & Pope, 1997; Pellmar, Brandt & Baird, 2002). The IOM defines rehabilitation as:

> . . . the process by which physical, sensory or mental capacities are restored or developed. This is achieved not only through functional change in the person, such as strengthening injured limbs, but also through changes in the physical and social environments, such as making buildings accessible to wheelchairs. Rehabilitation strives to reverse what has been called the disabling process, and may therefore be called the enabling process
>
> Brandt & Pope, 1997, p. 12–13

Unlike other models that present disability as a deficit of the individual, the Enabling-Disabling Model recognizes the contextual aspects of disability and the dynamic interaction between the individual and his/her environment (Lutz & Bowers, 2003). The five basic concepts of the Enabling-Disabling Process include pathology, impairment, functional limitation, disability and society limitation (Pope & Tarlov, 1991; Brandt & Pope, 1997). A complete description of these concepts is found in Table 25-2.

The Enabling-Disabling Process is a model for rehabilitation that conveys the idea that not all pathologies result in disability and any two people with the same impairment may have different levels of disability, e.g., one client may have severe disability and another client may not have a disability. Inherent personal characteristics in interaction with the client's environment along with the degree of insult inflicted by the disease, trauma, or congenital condition can result in vastly different outcomes for clients with the same medical diagnosis. Developing effective rehabilitation strategies involves understanding the contextual aspects of disability.

The contextual aspects of disability refers to the biological, environmental and lifestyle/behavioral factors that can influence each stage of the disabling process. Biological factors include comorbidities, physical condition, and genetic makeup. Environmental factors include societal prejudices, availability of services, and reimbursement mechanisms. Lifestyle and behavioral factors include use of cigarettes and alcohol, and diet and exercise.

International Classification of Functioning, Disability and Health (ICF)   In 2001, the World Health Organization (WHO) approved the International Classification of Functioning, Disability and Health (ICF). This new classification was a major revision of the 1980 WHO International Classification of Impairments, Disabilities, and Handicaps (ICIDH), which was widely used for many years to describe the disability process (WHO, 2002). Functioning and disability are viewed as a dynamic interaction between the individual's health conditions and contextual factors. Contextual factors are personal and environmental. Function/disability can be expressed in two

TABLE 25-2

Concepts of the Enabling– Disabling Process

Pathophysiology	Impairment	Functional Limitation	Disability	Societal Limitation
Interruption of or interference with normal physiological and developmental processes or structures	Loss and/ or abnormality of cognition, and emotional, physiological, or anatomical structure or function, including all losses or abnormalities, not just those attributable to the initial pathophysiology *Level of Impact*	Restriction or lack of ability to perform an action in the manner or within a range consistent with the purpose of an organ or organ system	Inability or limitation in performing tasks, activities, and roles to levels expected within physical and social contexts	Restriction, attributable to social policy or barriers (structural or attitudinal), that limits fulfillment of roles or denies access to services and opportunities that are associated with full participation in society
Cells and Tissues	*Organs and Organ Systems*	*Function of the Organ and Organ System*	*Individual*	*Society*
Structural or Functional	Structural or Functional	Action or Activity Performance or Organ or Organ System	Task Performance by Person in Physical, Social Contexts	Societal Attributes Relevant to Individuals with Disabilities
Patient Example: Lacunar infarct of the cerebellum (right hemisphere) related to microvascular changes associated with chronic hypertension	Neuromotor function of the brain plegia,	Left hemiparesis or difficulty with spatial–perceptual tasks, difficulty sequencing, memory deficits	Deficits in ambulation, self-care, shopping, work	Lack of adaptations in the work environment that would enable person to continue employment

SOURCE: From NCMRR (1993); Whyte, J. (1998). Enabling America: A report from the Institute of Medicine on rehabilitation science and engineering. *Archives of Physical Medicine and Rehabilitation, 79*(11), 1477–1480. Reprinted with permission from Elsevier.

ways. It can indicate a problem, e.g., impairment, activity limitation, or participation restriction, or it can indicate the lack of a problem, unimpaired functioning. Within the concept of functioning/disability are two components, body functions and structures and activities and participation. Body functions refer to physiological functions of body systems (including psychological functions), e.g., mental, sensory, and voice functions, cardiovascular, hematologic, immune and respiratory systems. Body structures refer to anatomical parts of the body such as organs, limbs and their components, e.g., eye, ear, cardiovascular system, respiratory system, musculoskeletal system. Activities refer to problems in body function or structure such as a significant deviation or loss, e.g., anxiety, paralysis, loss of sensation of extremities. Participation refers to involvement in a life situation, e.g., socialization, religious activities, employment. Environmental factors are aspects of the physical, social, and attitudinal environment in which individuals live and conduct their lives, e.g., climate, terrain, social attitudes, institutions, and laws. An overview of the ICF can be found in Table 25-3.

Excess Disability

Excess disability refers to an inability to perform an activity that is above and beyond the usual disability associated with the impairment. Both formal and informal caregivers can inadvertently contribute to excess disability. Care patterns, such as providing too much assistance or an inappropriate type of assistance can increase clients' dependency. Excess disability is a major problem in the long-term care setting (Blair, 1995; Osborn & Marshall, 1993; Rogers et al., 1999; and Tappen, 1994). Factors influencing excess disability include: a desire of the caregiver to be helpful; lack of knowledge and skill of the caregiver; and lack of time and staff can result in increased dependency among impaired clients, e.g., it saves time for staff to do something for a client than take the time for the client to do it independently. Over time, disuse can result in increased impairment and disability and increased caregiver demands; therefore, identification of appropriate types and amount of assistance is critical in assisting impaired individuals to reach and maintain their optimal level of function (Rogers, Amador & Bryan, 2000).

TABLE 25-3

Concepts of the International Classification of Functioning, Disability and Health (ICF)

Major Concepts			
Health Condition	*Impairment*	*Activity Limitation*	*Participation Restriction*
Diseases, disorders, and injuries, e.g., leprosy, diabetes, spinal cord injury.	Problems in body function or structure such as a significant deviation or loss, e.g., anxiety, paralysis, loss of sensation of extremities.	Problems in body function or structure such as a significant deviation or loss, e.g., anxiety, paralysis, loss of sensation of extremities.	Problems an individual may experience in involvement in life situations, e.g., unable to attend social events, unable to use public transportation to get to church, unable to perform job functions.
Example			
Spinal cord injury	Paralysis	Incapable of using public transportation	Unable to attend religious activities

SOURCE: From WHO (2002). Towards a common language for functioning, disability and health ICF. Available on line at: http://www3.who.int/icf/icftemplate.cfm?myurl=beginners.html&mytitle=Beginner%27s%20Guide

Historical Perspective

The history of rehabilitation (see Table 25-4) reflects society's apathy and insensitivity toward the young, old, poor, mentally impaired, and physically disabled, all of whom are at a disadvantage when compared with the general population. Primitive people, using the philosophy that only the fit should survive, abandoned the disabled and old. Even after such practices stopped, it was many centuries before people in disadvantaged positions received more than alms.

The 1800s generated interest in rehabilitation. Physical restoration was used in the training and care of crippled children, and the discipline of occupational therapy was born. The first medical social service department was established at Bellevue Hospital in New York City, and Lillian Wald began the first visiting nursing service (Dittmar, 1989).

War influenced the growth of rehabilitation. The return of injured soldiers provided the impetus for the establishment in 1918 of a national rehabilitation program for veterans of World War I. This first program, however, concentrated only on the physical aspects of disability. The disabled veterans of World War II received a more comprehensive program that included both physical and psychosocial rehabilitation. During this time, Dr. Howard Rusk demonstrated to the Army that rehabilitation, rather than convalescence, was essential for recovery (Kottke, Stillwell & Lehmann, 1990).

Rusk's pioneering work provided the impetus for the establishment of the American Academy of Physical Medicine and Rehabilitation in 1938 and the development of rehabilitation medicine as a board-certified specialty in 1947 (DeLisa, Currie & Martin, 1998). In 1974, the Association of Rehabilitation Nurses was created, followed closely by the establishment of rehabilitation as a specialty of nursing by the American Nurses' Association (Edwards, 2000).

Societal forces continue to expand rehabilitation practice. Industrial and vehicular accidents and trauma from leisure and sporting activities have increased the number of clients with disabilities. Additionally, advances in medicine and science have lengthened the life span of those with traumatic injuries and chronic diseases and provided more potential candidates for rehabilitation.

TABLE 25-4

Historical Events and Legislative Initiatives Affecting Rehabilitation

Date	Event/Initiative	Purpose
1910	"Studies of Invalid Occupation"	Published by nurse Susan Tracy; beginning of occupational therapy
1917	American Red Cross Institute for Crippled and Disabled Men personnel	Created to provide vocational training for wounded military
1918	Smith-Sears Legislation (PL 65-178)	Authorized Federal Board for Vocational Education to administer a national vocational rehabilitation service to disabled veterans of World War I
1920	Smith-Fess Legislation (PL 66-236)	Provided vocational rehabilitation services to people disabled in industry and otherwise
1930	Veteran's Administration (VA)	Created by Executive Order 5398 to care for those with service-related disabilities, signed by President Herbert Hoover. At this time there were 54 hospitals, 4.7 million living veterans.
1935	Social Security Act (PL 74-271)	Provided permanent authorization for the civilian vocational rehabilitation program
1938	American Academy of Physical Medicine	Organization formed; physical medicine and rehabilitation emerges as a specialty

continues

TABLE 25-4

Continued

Date	Event/Initiative	Purpose
1941	First comprehensive book on physical medicine and rehabilitation	Written by Frank Krusen, MD
1942	Sister Kenny Institute	Institute and Sister Kenny's research led to the development of the profession of physical therapy and provided support for physiatry as a specialty.
1943	Welsh-Clark Legislation (PL 78-16)	Provided vocational rehabilitation for disabled veterans of World War II
1943	United Nations Rehabilitation Administration	Organization established with representatives from 44 countries to plan care for disabled WWII veterans
1946	Department of Medicine and Surgery	A department within the VA established to provide medical care for veterans; succeeded in 1989 by the Veterans Health Services and Research Administration, renamed the Veterans Health Administration in 1991
1947	Bellevue Medical Rehabilitation Services	First U.S. rehabilitation program, established by Howard Rusk, MD
1947	American Board of Physical Medicine and Rehabilitation specialty	Board formed, and rehabilitation becomes a board-certified
1954	Hill-Burton Act (PL 83-565)	Provided greater financial support, research and demonstration grants, state agency expansion and grants to expand rehabilitation facilities
1958	Rehabilitation Medicine	H. Rusk and colleagues publish a rehabilitation text.
1965	Vocational Rehabilitation Act (PL 89-333)	Expanded and improved vocational rehabilitation services
1973	Rehabilitation Act (PL 93-112)	Expanded services to the more severely handicapped by giving them priority; affirmative action in employment and nondiscrimination in facilities
1974	Association of Rehabilitation Nurses	Organization formed; rehabilitation nursing emerges as a specialty
1975	Education for All Handicapped Act (PL 94-142)	Provided for a free appropriate education for handicapped children in the least restrictive setting possible
1975	National Housing Act Amendments (PL 94-173)	Provided for the removal of barriers in federally supported housing; established Office of Independent Living for disabled people in Department of Housing and Urban Development
1975	*Rehabilitation Nursing*	First issue published
1981	Rehabilitation Nursing: Concepts and Practice—A Core Curriculum	First core curriculum of rehabilitation nursing published
1982	Tax Equity and Fiscal Responsibility Act (TEFRA)	Originally designed to be a bridge from the old fee-for-service system to the DRG system; free-standing rehabilitation hospitals reimbursed based on reasonable costs (with limits)
1984	Diagnosis-Related Groupings (DRGs)	Established to decrease Medicare payments through the establishment of a prospective payment system for acute care

TABLE 25-4

Continued

Date	Event/Initiative	Purpose
1989	Omnibus Budget Reconciliation Act (OBRA)	Contained legislation on nursing home reform; required standards for nursing assistant education and certification; required Health Care Financing Administration (HCFA) to develop a standardized assessment instrument and move to from a fee-for-service system to a prospective payment system
1989	Department of Veteran's Affairs	VA becomes the 14th department in the President's Cabinet.
1990	Americans with Disabilities Act	Americans with Disabilities Act (PL 101-336); established a clear discrimination on the basis of disability
1997	Balanced Budget Act (BBA)	Enacted to restructure Medicare Part A reimbursement methods; mandated a prospective payment reimbursement system for rehabilitation hospitals and units
1999	Balanced Budget Act Amendment	Provided adjustments to PPS for skilled nursing facilities
2001	PPS for Inpatient Rehabilitation Facilities	PPS mandated by the 1997 BBA phase-in begins
2001	New Freedom Initiative	President George W. Bush launches a nationwide effort to remove barriers to community living for people of all ages with disabilities and long-term illnesses; goals of the initiative include increasing access to assistive technologies, expanding educational opportunities, and promoting full access to community life.
2003	PPS for Inpatient Rehabilitation Facilities	Phase-in complete; Case-mix groups (CMGs) are used as the basis for reimbursement.
2004	CMS modifies criteria used to classify inpatient rehabilitation facilities (IRF)	Phase-in begins for "75% rule." By 2007, 75% of population treated in the facility must match one or more specified medical conditions.

SOURCE: Adapted from the following sources: Larsen, P. (1998). Rehabilitation. In I. Lubkin & P. Larsen (Eds.), *Chronic illness: Impact and interventions* (4th ed.), p. 534; Easton, K. (1999). *Gerontological rehabilitation nursing*, pp. 32, 41. Philadelphia: WB Saunders; Kelly, P. (1999). Reimbursement mechanisms. In A. S. Luggen, & S. Meiner (Eds.), *NGNA core curriculum for gerontological nursing*, pp. 185–186. St. Louis: Mosby; Blake, D., & Scott, D. (1996). Employment of persons with disabilities. *Physical Medicine and Rehabilitation*, p. 182. Philadelphia: WB Saunders; Department of Veterans Affairs. (2000). Facts about the Department of Veterans Affairs. Available on-line at http://www.va.gov/press rel/FSVA2000.htm

Public Policy and Rehabilitation

Reimbursed rehabilitation services provided to the client with chronic illness vary greatly under Medicare, Medicaid, and private insurance. It is essential that health care professionals be knowledgeable of financing restrictions on rehabilitation.

Medicare   Medicare is a federal health insurance program that provides health care for individuals over the age of 65 and for disabled persons (CMS, 2005a). Medicare consists of two primary medical care benefits: hospital insurance (Part A) and supplemental medical insurance (Parts B and C). Medicare Part A covers inpatient hospital care, skilled nursing facility care, home health agency care, and hospice care. Medicare Part A covers the first 20 days in a skilled nursing facility (within 30 days of a hospitalization that lasted for at least three days) and then with co-payments for an additional 80 days. Medicare Part A covers home care for individuals certified by a physician as needing intermittent skilled nursing care, physical, occupational, or speech/language therapy, and considered home bound, i.e., normally unable to leave the house unassisted. Medicare Parts B and C, supplemental health insurance coverage, are optional and require payment of a monthly premium. Part B requires an annual deductible and covers 80% of the costs of physician services, and numerous non-physician services including physical and occupational therapy, durable medical equipment, and prosthetics and orthotic items. The Medicare Prescription Drug, Improvement, and Modernization Act of 2003 (MMA) replaced Part C, Medicare-Plus-Choice with Medicare Advantage, a managed care plan providing many preventative and well adult services and prescription drug benefits (Doherty, 2004; Emmer & Allendorf, 2004; Stuart, 2004). The enactment of the Medicare Modernization Act of 2003 provides Medicare beneficiaries enrolled in traditional Medicare part B an optional prescription drug benefit and have some primary prevention and adult well care services as well.

In the past, rehabilitation facilities have been reimbursed under the 1982 Tax Equity and Fiscal Responsibility Act (TEFRA), a cost-based system (Ross, 1992); however, the 1997 Balanced Budget Act mandated that inpatient rehabilitation units and hospitals receive reimbursement under a Prospective Payment System (PPS) beginning in 2003 (Federal Register, 2003; CMS, 2004c). Under PPS, Medicare pays a predetermined, fixed amount per discharge. Reimbursement is based on the client's impairment level, functional status, co-morbid conditions, and age (Grimaldi, 2002). The Functional Independence Measure (FIM) is used to determine the appropriate classification of a Medicare client into case-mix groups (CMGs) for payment under the prospective payment system (Stineman, 2002).

Additionally, in 2004, CMS modified the criteria used to classify a facility as an inpatient rehabilitation facility (IRF). The new criteria is being phased in over a four-year period beginning July

2004. To qualify as an IRF, a specified percentage of the total population treated in the facility (50% in 2004, 60% in 2005, 65% in 2006, and 75% in 2007) must match one or more medical conditions for which Medicare provides reimbursement (Federal Register, 2004; CMS, 2004b; CMS, 2005b). Medical conditions covered under the IRF rule include stroke, spinal cord injury, congenital deformity, amputation, major multiple trauma, femur fracture, neurological disorders (e.g., multiple sclerosis, motor neuron diseases, polyneuropathy, muscular dystrophy, and Parkinson's disease), burns, certain arthritis conditions and arthropathies, systemic vasculidities with joint inflammation, and knee or hip replacement.

Medicare pays for rehabilitation care provided in skilled nursing facilities as well as rehabilitation units and hospitals. Reimbursement is also provided under a PPS system. Per-diem payments for each client are case-mix adjusted using a resident classification system, resource utilization groups (RUGs) derived from assessment data collected via the Minimum Data Set (MDS). There are five RUG categories for patients receiving rehabilitation services that are based on the amount and type of rehabilitation required. RUG categories range from ultra high, treatment for a minimum of 720 minutes weekly including two disciplines—one at least five days per week and one three days per week—to low, treatment of 45 minutes weekly over at least three days.

Medicaid Medicaid is a federal-state matching entitlement program that pays for medical assistance for vulnerable and needy individuals and their families with low income and resources. Medicaid eligibility, services, and payments are complex and vary from state to state (Santerre, 2002). Broad national guidelines are set by the Federal statutes, regulations, and policies (CMS, 2005a). Each State: (1) establishes its own eligibility standards; (2) determines the type, amount, duration, and scope of services; (3) sets the rate of payment for services; and (4) administers its own program (CMS, 2004a; CMS, 2005a).

State Medicaid programs must offer the following: inpatient and outpatient hospital services, prenatal care. vaccines for children, physician services, nursing facility services for persons aged 21 or older, family planning services and supplies, rural health clinic services, home health care for persons eligible for skilled-nursing services, laboratory and x-ray services, pediatric and family nurse practitioner services, nurse-midwife services, federally qualified health-center (FQHC) services, and ambulatory services of an FQHC that would be available in other settings, early and periodic screening, diagnostic, and treatment (EPSDT) services for children under age 21. States may also receive Federal matching funds to provide certain optional services. Following are the most common of the thirty-four currently approved optional Medicaid services: diagnostic services, clinic services, intermediate care facilities for the mentally retarded (ICFs/MR), prescribed drugs and prosthetic devices, optometrist services and eyeglasses, nursing facility services for children under age 21, transportation services, rehabilitation and physical therapy services, and home and community-based care to certain persons with chronic impairments.

Workers' Compensation   Workers' compensation in the United States was created by the Federal Employees Compensation Act of 1914. By 1949, Workers' Compensation was available in all 50 states (Kiselica, Sibson, & Green-McKenzie, 2004). Workers' Compensation is a federally mandated and state run health and disability insurance program developed to provide benefits to disabled workers for injury or illness sustained on the job. The three types of benefits employees are eligible to receive include: (1) survivor benefits for employee spouse in the case of death; (2) hospitalization, medical, and rehabilitation expenses; and (3) compensation for wage-loss (Kiselica, Sibson, & Green-McKenzie, 2004).

In the 1960s and 1970s, concerns over inadequate coverage for workers and their families during periods of disability spurred expansion of workers' compensation programs, extending coverage to more workers and increasing the amount of benefits. By the 1980s and 1990s, the expansion of benefits and the escalating costs of health care services drove up the costs of programs for employers and insurers. Current programs use fee schedules, limited physician choice, restricted eligibility, lower benefits, and managed care to contain and reduce plan costs (D'Andrea & Meyer, 2004).

Private Insurance   Reimbursement for rehabilitation care, services, equipment, and devices by private insurance plans varies depending on the type of plan, i.e., fee-for-service, managed care (Health Insurance Association of America, 2002-2003). Most plans offer benefits for rehabilitation. Private insurers are applying more pressure to health care facilities to contain costs. As a result, companies have implemented strict utilization review and catastrophic case management programs (Kovacek & Kovacek, 1998). Often case managers are nurses who can justify services or choose to decline services for a client. Regular communication is needed with the case manager about client needs, client progress, and anticipated length of stay. Private insurance plans also vary in their coverage of inpatient rehabilitation; plans frequently reimburse facilities at a flat rate per day.

Social Security Disability Income   Social Security Disability Income (SSDI), established in 1956 under the auspices of the Social Security Disability Act of 1954, is a federally administered disability insurance program for individuals who are not able to work because of a disability (Social Security Online, 2005). Disabled individuals who have actively worked for at least five out of the preceding ten years, have remained unemployed for the previous six months, and have an income of less than $300 per month can qualify for supplemental income. This program is based on the individual's contributions to the Old Age, Survivors, and Disability Insurance (OASDI) or financial need. Recipients may receive a monthly stipend, Medicare Supplemental Insurance, and vocational rehabilitation coverage.

Supplemental Security Income (SSI) provides disability benefits for individuals who do not meet the work history criteria. This program is based on financial need and benefits include a monthly stipend, Medicaid Insurance Supplement, and vocational rehabilitation coverage (Social Security Online, 2005).

Disability Benefits for Veterans The Department of Veterans Affairs (VA) administers a federally-sponsored disability program for veterans who were disabled during their military service or for veterans with a non-service-connected injury who have a permanent and total disability (60% or more). Benefits of this program include a monthly stipend, medical care at VA facilities, prosthetic/orthotic devices, durable medical equipment, and home and motor vehicle modifications if appropriate (Department of Veterans Affairs, 2004).

Vocational Rehabilitation Vocational rehabilitation is one component of the rehabilitation process. Legislation pertaining to vocational rehabilitation was first introduced in 1918 when Congress enacted the Smith-Sears Act, which authorized national vocational rehabilitation services to disabled veterans of World War I. The Smith-Fess Act of 1920, mandated vocational rehabilitation and training for all individuals with disabilities, not just war-related disabilities (Buchanan, 1996). That act defined rehabilitation as "the rendering of a disabled person fit to engage in a remunerative occupation" (Athelstan, 1982, p. 163). The Rehabilitation Act of 1973 authorized funds for and supports state vocational rehabilitation programs that are designed to provide individuals with a disability, defined as a physical or mental impairment that results in a substantial impediment to employment or an individual whose employment outcome could be positively affected from vocational rehabilitation services (U.S. Department of Education, 2005).

Vocational rehabilitation includes an array of services that prepare and assist disabled individuals to engage in gainful employment consistent with their strengths, resources, priorities, concerns, abilities, capabilities, and informed choice. Services provided include counseling, medical and psychological services, job training and other individualized services that assist disabled individuals to obtain and retain employment (Lysaght, 2004; Kielkofner, Braveman, Finlayson, Paul-Ward, Goldbaum, & Goldstein, 2004; O'Neill, Zuger, Fields, Fraser, & Pruce, 2004; Targett, Wehman, & Young, 2004).

State vocational rehabilitation agencies are the main source of vocational services for individuals with chronic diseases or disabilities. The agencies are financed primarily by the federal government under the Rehabilitation Services Administration with a smaller percentage of funds coming from each state. The Department of Veterans Affairs also offers veterans with a service connected disability services to prepare for and find suitable employment (Department of Veterans Affairs, 2005).

Work provides a sense of contribution to society and personal accomplishment, and for many individuals, work is a major part of their identity. However, for the increasing number of chronically ill elderly in our society, vocational rehabilitation may not be appropriate. Though these individuals are excellent candidates for rehabilitation, employment is not a goal.

Americans with Disabilities Act The Americans with Disabilities Act of 1990 provides disabled individuals physical and vocational access to the private sector of business, industry, and education. Prior legislative efforts, the Rehabilitation Act of 1973 and its amendments, were concerned only with access to businesses, organizations, and institutions that received federal financial assistance; the private sector did not have to provide accessibility to the disabled. The ADA makes compliance to equal access mandatory for the private sector as well (U.S. Equal Opportunity Employment Commission, 2002).

The ADA defines three categories of disability that are protected: (1) a physical or mental impairment that substantially limits one or more of the major life activities of an individual; (2) a record of such an impairment; (3) being regarded as having such an impairment (PL 101-336). The ADA consists of four major titles that address access to employment, public services, public accommodations and services offered by private entities, and telecommunication relay services (see Table 25-5). The ADA

TABLE 25-5

The Americans with Disabilities Act

Title 1: Employment	Employers cannot discriminate against a qualified disabled job applicant or employee in any manner related to employment and benefits.
	Employers must make their existing facilities accessible and usable by individuals with disabilities.
	Accommodations in all aspects of job attainment and performance are required in order to place individuals on an equal plane with the nondisabled.
Title 2: Public Services	Qualified disabled individuals must have access to all services and programs provided by state or local governments. Public rail transportation must be made accessible to disabled individuals and supplemented with paratransit.
Title 3: Public Accommodations Services Operated by Private Entities	Virtually every entity open to the public must now be made accessible to the disabled. A study is to be conducted concerning accessibility of the over-the-road transportation.
Title 4: Telecommunications Relay	Telephone companies are required to furnish telecommunication devices to enable hearing- and speech-impaired individuals to communicate by wire or radio.

SOURCE: Reprinted from Watson, P. (1990). The Americans with Disabilities Act: More rights for people with disabilities. *Rehabilitation Nursing, 15*, 326. Published by the Association of Rehabilitation Nurses, 4700 W. Lake Avenue, Glenview, IL 60025-1485. Copyright © 1990 by the Association of Rehabilitation Nurses. Used with permission.

constitutes civil rights protection for the disabled individual with access to the private sector guaranteed by law.

Rehabilitation Issues and Challenges

Providing rehabilitation services can present many challenges for providers. Primary among these are the rising costs of care, caregiver burden, inequities among disabled Americans, inequities among the disabled, the negative image of disability, the changing composition of the disabled population, ethical issues, providing culturally competent care, inadequate documentation of rehabilitation outcomes, and formal and informal caregiver issues.

Rising Care Costs

Rising health care costs have made cost containment of health care a major social and political problem in the United States today. The cost of health care insurance alone has skyrocketed, and as a result, 16 percent of the U.S. population or 45 million Americans have no health insurance. Millions more have inadequate coverage (U.S. Census Bureau, 2004). The number of Americans with health care insurance through their employment is decreasing, while the number of Americans covered by government health insurance programs is increasing. The insured individual with chronic illness is facing reduced funding for fewer services as health care costs rise. Escalating costs make access to health care for the uninsured nearly impossible.

The provision of care to chronically ill or disabled persons is a major societal issue. Although the number of elderly with disabilities declined between 1980 and 1990 (Manton & Gu, 2001), almost 50 million Americans have some type of long-term condition or disability (U.S. Census Bureau, 2004). This represents over 19 percent of the 257 million people who are aged five and older in the civilian noninstitutionalized population—or nearly one person in five community dwellers. More than 18 million of those aged 16 and older have a condition that makes it difficult to go outside the home to shop or visit a doctor (nine percent of the 212 million people this age); more than 21 million of those aged 16 to 64 have a condition that affects their ability to work at a job or business (12 percent of the 179 million people this age). How our health care system will be able to support ongoing, cost-conscious services to someone who may be chronically ill for decades is a major challenge.

One basic question is 'what is the economic cost of dependency'? It is estimated that the U.S. government spends $200 billion a year on public assistance for persons with disabilities (Council of State Administrators of Vocational Rehabilitation, 2004–2005). As the population ages and medical advancements and technologies continue to increase longevity for the individual with chronic illness, the U.S. will continue to face an enormous economic burden of providing health care and livelihood for the disabled (Fried, Bradley, Williams, & Tinetti, 2001). The challenge for the future will be to find ways to decrease health care costs and improve disabled individuals' abilities to obtain work and earn a living wage.

Caregiver Burden

Family members constitute approximately 72 percent of both paid and unpaid caregivers of elderly persons with activity limitations due to chronic diseases (Shirey & Summer, 2000). Adult children assume responsibility for largest proportion of caregiving activities, 42 percent, followed by spouses who are responsible for 25 percent of caregiving activities. The impact of disability on the chronically ill individual and family is difficult to assess. Because each illness produces different deficits and each individual and family has a unique social system, the impact that results is unpredictable (Power, 1989). However, results from recent studies indicate that being a caregiver for someone with a chronic disabling disease or condition is an independent health

hazard for the caregiver. Caregiver burden, the effects of stressors on family members caring for physically or mentally ill persons, has been associated with emotional distress, anxiety, depression, poorer quality of life, poor immune function, and increased risk of death (Anderson, Linto, & Stewart-Wynne, 1995; Canam & Acorn, 1999; Brouwer, van Exel, van de Berg, Dinant, Koopmanschap, & van den Bos, 2004; das Chagas Medeiros, Ferraz & Quaresma, 2000; Grunfeld et al., 2004; Hughes et al., 1999; Kolanowski, Fick, Waller, & Shea, 2004; Lieberman & Fisher, 1995; Mills, Yu, Ziegler, Patterson, & Grant, 1999; Schulz & Beach, 1999; Shaw et al., 1999; Weitzenkamp et al., 1997; Wu et al., 1999).

Maintaining the health and well-being of caregivers is as important as maintaining the health and well-being of the rehabilitation client. Rehabilitation professionals need to include an assessment of caregiver burden in their plan of care for the client. Early identification and management of signs of caregiver stress may prevent some of the health problems associated with caregiving and help the family remain independent (see Chapter 11, Family Caregivers).

Inequities among Disabled Americans

A recent survey by the National Organization on Disability (NOD) reveals significant differences in the levels of participation among people with disabilities and other Americans in employment, income, education, socializing, religious and political involvement, and access to healthcare and transportation (National Organization of Disability, 2004). According to the survey, only 35% of disabled Americans work full or part-time compared with 78% of non-disabled Americans. Three times as many disabled Americans live in households with a total income less than $15,000. Twenty-two percent of disabled Americans report encountering job discrimination. Rehabilitation professionals need to actively participate at the community, state, and national levels in developing and implementing new initiatives and policies to address these gaps.

Mrs. Cole: Adjustment to a Life Altering Condition

Mrs. Cole was a healthy, energetic, independent woman living in her own home enjoying the fruits of her years of hard work. Although the loss of her family and many friends was difficult, it wasn't until she began losing her independence that she realized that she had few resources to enable her to continue to reside independently in the community. Mrs. Cole had been diagnosed with multiple sclerosis several years earlier, but initially the condition had little impact on her life. With no support system, she soon recognized that her debilitating and progressive condition was robbing her of her independence and drastic steps would need to be taken. She lost the use of her lower extremities, suffered visual field disruption, experienced occasional incontinence, had gradual muscle wasting and was in constant jeopardy for her safety.

Mrs. Cole decided to admit herself to a nursing facility where she could optimize and maintain what function she retained and possibly regain additional skills that would enable her to function more independently. Mrs. Cole had a basic course of occupational and physical therapy to reach mutually established goals, and then was followed up with daily restorative nursing care to maintain therapeutic gains. While Mrs. Cole had no family, facility staff and residents soon began to fill this void in her life. Mrs. Cole became the president of resident council and a spokesperson for resident rights. While Mrs. Cole's physical condition continues to deteriorate, her mind remains active. Mrs. Cole feels she is in control of her life despite her debilitating condition.

In the United States, disparities in health care quality and access exist among numerous minority groups, the poor, children, mentally ill, rural dwellers, the elderly, and the disabled (U.S. Department of Health and Human Services, 2003). Some studies indicate that the disabled face significant disparities in health care access and quality (Beatty, Hagglund, Neri, Dhont, Clark, & Hilton, 2003; Havercamp, Scandlin, & Roth, 2004; U.S. Department of Health and Human Services, 2003). Within the disabled population, some groups are subject to even greater disadvantage and disability (Fujiura & Yamaki, 1997; Kingston & Smith, 1997; Ostchega et al., 2000; Reichard, Sacco, & Turnbull, 2004; U.S. Department of Health and Human Services, 2003). Data from the third National Health and Nutrition Examination Survey (NHANES III) indicates that minorities including non-Hispanic Black and Mexican-American men and women generally report significantly more disability than non-minority

men and women, and the magnitude of disability is greater for minority women than for minority men (Ostchega et al., 2000). Non-elderly disabled Medicare beneficiaries are more likely to have lower income and difficulties accessing health care (U.S. Department of Health and Human Services, 2003). Among disabled elderly, minorities and individuals from poorer households are twice as likely to report problems with quality of health care. Twice as many Hispanic disabled elderly report having problems getting to the doctor compared to non-Hispanic whites. These studies indicate that further research is needed to understand why these disparities in health care exist and to find ways to address them.

Image of Disability

Much progress has been made in dispelling the myths and negative connotations associated with

Daniel: Technological Advances

Daniel was 21 years old when he had surgery for a benign gangiocytoma in the tectal region of the brain. Initially he was ventilator dependent, received nourishment through a gastrostomy tube, and had a Glasgow Coma Score of 10. Over a two-year period of physical, occupational, and speech therapy, Daniel made remarkable progress and achieved independence in locomotion through the use of a motorized wheelchair; however, he remained dependent on caregivers for most of his activities of daily living. With assistance in setting up his meals and the use of adaptive feeding devices, he was able to feed himself.

After several years of almost total dependence, Daniel had a series of surgeries to release contractures of his hands and ankles. Within four months of his ankle surgery, Daniel was able to take his first steps toward independence. Ten months later, Daniel was able to walk 100

feet with the use of a walker and minimal assistance from caregivers. In the early stages of his rehabilitation, he was able to feed himself; but now he is able to cook snacks for fellow residents in the Care Center with minimal assistance from the nursing supervisor. He has voiced a desire to become a chef. With the assistance of caregivers, Daniel has become the unofficial evening activity coordinator, planning holiday parties and other social activities for residents.

New surgical techniques and technological advances offer hope for further improvements in Daniel's functional abilities. Unfortunately, resources within the community for young people with this type of disability are limited, and this bright, energetic young man is forced to reside in a chronic medical facility but with continued improvement it is possible that some day he may be able to live and work in the community.

---

disability. The prevailing models of function and rehabilitation, the Enabling-Disabling Process and the International Classification of Functioning, Disability, and Health (ICF) try to eliminate the negative concept of handicap and include the concept of health in both the presence and absence of a disabling condition (WHO, 2002; Brandt & Pope, 1997). The changes in these rehabilitation models reflect the current belief that disability is a function of the interaction of the individual and the environment and not just a result of impairment of a body function. The models promote the idea that it is possible for an individual with a severe impairment to have no disability at all. These models encourage a positive image for individuals with impairments. Persons with impairments can lead full, productive, and satisfying lives. Disability frequently occurs when resources in the individual's environment fail

to accommodate the individual's needs. Health care providers, scientists, rehabilitation professionals, and community leaders need to promote this more positive image and work to enhance environment and community resources to meet the needs of impaired individuals.

The negative image of disability and the disabled is eroding as more individuals with impairments become involved in mainstream activities such as the arts, media, sports, and politics. Olympic runner Marla Runyon, the late actor/director Christopher Reeve, Pulitzer prize-winner journalist Charles Krauthammer, and Senator Max Cleland are just a few examples of individuals with disabilities who serve as excellent role models for disabled persons. Runyon, an Olympic runner who participated in the 2000 games in Sydney, Australia, is legally blind. Christopher Reeve, the actor who starred as Superman in the movies, was a ventilator-dependent quadriplegic, who continued with a full schedule of acting and directing movies throughout his life as a disabled person. Cleland, a three-limb amputee, served as a United States senator and director of the Department of Veterans Affairs. Krauthammer, quadraplegic from a spinal cord injury, attended medical school and residency training and then left medicine to become a journalist writing a weekly column for the Washington Post and participating as a panelist on *Inside Washington*, a political television talk show. These individuals, along with thousands of other Americans who are teachers, doctors, accountants, craftsmen, computer operators, mothers and fathers, represent a vast continuum of functional diversity of disabled people, who are independent, work every day, and make significant contributions to society.

Invisible disability, a condition that evidences no noticeable outward physical changes, is an issue associated with many chronic illnesses. In general, one thinks of a chronic illness or injury producing a visible disability. A visible disability is the emphysemic client with noticeable shortness of breath, walking with portable oxygen or an individual using a wheelchair or walker because of a neuromuscular disease. However, the impact on the individual and family of having an invisible disability may be just as devastating. Examples of invisible disabilities include cardiovascular disease, diabetes mellitus, multiple sclerosis in remission, or intractable pain. Although it may seem preferable to have no noticeable signs of disability, the invisible disability may provide the individual, family, and society with unrealistic expectations of the client. This ultimately may affect the psychosocial adjustment of the individual to the chronic illness. The uncertainty of his or her future health may be an additional burden.

Changing Composition of the Disabled Population

The composition of the disabled population is changing in three distinct ways: increases in the number of elderly with chronic diseases (Gregg et al., 2000; Spillman, 2003; SoRelle, 1999; Waidmann & Liu, 2000); children living with disabilities (Allen, 2004; Fujiura & Yamaki, 2000; Hogan, McLellan & Bauman, 2000; van Dyck, Kogan, McPherson, Weissman, & Newacheck, 2004; Wood, Marlow, Costeloe, Gibson & Wilkinson, 2000); and persons with disabling mental health conditions (Druss et al., 2000; Jans, Stoddard, & Kraus, 2004).

Although disability among older U.S. adults, as measured by limitations in instrumental activities of daily living, has declined since the early 1980s (Freedman, Martin, & Schoeni, 2002), Americans are living longer and extending the amount of time one can live with a chronic illness. Also, due to advances in medical treatment and technology, people with disabilities, e.g., cerebral palsy, spina bifida, postpoliomyelitis, are living longer (Klingbeil, Baer, & Wilson, 2004). Approximately 80% of all persons aged >65 years have at least one chronic condition, and 50% have at least two (National Center for Chronic Disease Prevention and Health Promotion, 1999). By the year 2050, nearly 20% of the U.S. population will be 65 years or older (Centers for Disease Control and Prevention, 2003). As U.S. adults live longer, the prevalence of Alzheimer's disease, which doubles every five years after age 65, also is expected to increase (National Center for Chronic Disease Prevention and Health Promotion, 1999). Approximately 10% of adults aged >65 years and 47% of adults aged >85 years suffer from this degenerative and debilitating disease (National Center for Chronic Disease Prevention and Health Promotion, 1999).

It is estimated that approximately 12.8 percent of the 35 million children under the age of 18 are disabled, with 1.9 percent having the disability classified as severe (McNeil, 1997; van Dyck, Kogan, McPherson, Weissman, & Newacheck, 2004). Children with disabilities have much higher health care use and expenditures than children without disabilities (Newacheck, Inkelas, & Kim, 2004). Parents of children with disabilities are less likely to work or will work fewer hours (Loprest & Davidoff, 2004). Among disabled children, the prevalence of unmet needs for assistive devices and services ranges from 6% for vision care to 25% for communication aids. Major areas of concern for disabled children include altered learning abilities, speech or language impairments, mental retardation, serious emotional disturbances, and orthopedic impairments.

Approximately 20 percent of individuals in the U.S. experience mental disorders in a given year, and it is estimated that mental disorders contribute to limitations in daily activities and functioning in three to seven percent of the population (Grant et al., 2004; Jans et al., 2004). Almost 31 million Americans have at least one personality disorder (e.g., obsessive-compulsive, paranoid personality, antisocial personality, schizoid personality, avoidant personality, histrionic personality, dependent personality). It is estimated that 12 to 17 million adults experience mood disorders annually (National Depressive and Manic-Depression Association, 1998; National Institute of Mental Health, 1998). Work participation rates for people under the age of 45 with mental disabilities are far below the rates of all same aged persons with other types of disabilities (Trupin, Sebesta, Yelin, & LaPlante, 1997).

Adequately meeting the acute and long-term health and social services needs of this diverse disabled population poses many challenges for health care professionals. Primary and secondary prevention strategies are needed to reduce the amount of time elderly persons must live with disability. Recent research indicates that disability can be postponed through healthier lifestyles (Hubert, Bloch, Oehlert, & Fries, 2002). New strategies are needed to prevent disabling conditions among children and minimize the disability in children with learning disabilities, speech or language impairments, mental retardation, serious emotional disturbances, and orthopedic impairments. Preventing and reducing disability among persons with mental illness will require continuing public education to help dispel the myths and negative stigma associated with this population, and will require earlier diagnosis and treatment.

Ethical Issues

In caring for rehabilitation clients, nurses are frequently confronted with ethical dilemmas. These dilemmas are created when a choice must be made between difficult alternatives or when conflicts exist among values and beliefs. The following ethical issues are faced by many rehabilitation professionals:

For children (Edwards & Reed, 2000; Kirschner, Stocking, Wagner, Foye, & Siegler, 2001)

- Withholding or withdrawing treatment
- Organ donation
- Research
- Genetic Screening
- Prenatal diagnosis

For adults (ARN, 1995; Edwards & Reed, 2000)

- Withholding or withdrawing treatment
- Difficulties determining decision-making capacity
- Pressures resulting from health care reimbursement changes
- Conflicts/disagreement among patient and family members regarding treatment options
- Use of alternative and complementary medicine and therapies
- Maintaining patients' rights, including adolescents and cognitively impaired
- Use of restraints
- Do-not-resuscitate orders
- Execution of advance directives
- Clients with self-destructive behaviors or suicidal gestures
- Health care reform and changes in how health care is performed and delivered
- Confidentiality
- Substance abuse
- Abuse
- Intimacy in the nurse/patient relationship

Health care professionals are increasingly turning to ethics committees to assist in decision-making (Hogstel, Curry, Walker, & Burns, 2004; Johnson, 2004; Hughes, 2004; Nelson, 2004). Members of ethics committees may include a physician, nurse, social worker, chaplain or clergy, administrator, an ethicist, an attorney, and someone from the community. These committees review the medical facts and records; consider the beliefs, interests and values of all people involved; propose alternative courses of action; and assist in determining the goal that is in the best interest of the client, including what he/she would want. As medical treatments and technology advance, new ethical concerns will continue to emerge; therefore, rehabilitation professionals need to develop resources and skills to assist them in facing challenges created by ethical dilemmas.

Cultural Competency

Rehabilitation professionals are providing care to a growing diversity of clients. Projections from the U.S. Census Bureau (1999) indicate that by 2050 the population will increase to 394 million, up from 263 million in 1995, and minorities will account for almost 90 percent of this growth. All racial and ethnic minority groups will increase faster than non-Hispanic whites, and Asians and Hispanics are the fastest growing groups. A major challenge for the future will be providing culturally sensitive rehabilitation care (Niemeier, Burnett, & Whitaker, 2003).

Culturally competent health care is defined as sensitivity to the differences between groups, to the differences in behavior, and to the attitudes and meanings attached to emotional events such as depression, pain and disability (Seibert, Stridh-Igo, & Zimmerman, 2002). Cultural sensitivity is defined as sensitivity to group beliefs, values, interpersonal styles, languages, and behavior. Important considerations in providing culturally competent care include: (1) identifying the client's preferred method of communication and obtaining translators if needed; (2) identifying and learning about the client's culture, e.g., belief systems; (3) respecting client beliefs and values that are different from caregivers; (4) identifying client or family misconceptions or unrealistic views about caregivers, treatments, or the recovery process (Balcazar, 2001; Seibert et al., 2002).

Culture and ethnicity influence how clients and their families perceive disability. Being sensitive to issues related to culture, race, gender, sexual orientation, social class, and economic class can influence clients' acceptance of rehabilitation services. Cir-cumstances, race, culture, language, experience, and belief may also affect clients' access to information and services, goals for rehabilitation and independent living, and the information sources and services that are deemed credible and useful (Campinha-Bacote, 2001; NCDDR, 1999).

Perceptions of disability vary among cultural groups. Although great diversity exists within various cultural groups, for example among various Hispanic subgroups, e.g., Cuban, Puerto Rican, Mexican populations, some commonalities have been identified (NCDDR, 1999). To illustrate cultural differences, examples for African American, Hispanic, Asian Pacific, and Native American cultures are described, although rehabilitation professionals are cautioned against assuming that these values and beliefs exist among these groups in their own practice. It is imperative that professionals learn about the ethnic and cultural groups they serve from the groups themselves

For African Americans, spirituality is important in ascribing cause and treating developmental and other disabilities. African Americans tend to rely heavily on community supports, and in particular their church. African Americans may also have a broader view of normalcy and wider range of expectations for developmental milestones of developmentally disabled children (NCDDR, 1999).

Hispanics rely heavily on families as a major support system and consider many disabling conditions as a reflection of individual differences, with families working to accommodate the differences. However, severe disability is a stigma for the traditional Hispanic family.

Great diversity exists among Asian cultures, e.g., Chinese, Japanese, Taiwanese, Korean, Philippine, though some commonalities are found. Asian Americans' beliefs in metaphysical forces influence their beliefs about causes of disability and treatment of disability. They may have feelings of guilt and shame in having a disability or having a family member with a disability. Asian Americans often seek traditional eastern medicine including herbal medicines in addition to western medicine and rehabilitation care.

Native American cultures believe in the interrelatedness of the body and spirit, often have culturally distinct communication styles, and rely on their extended community and kinship networks. Most traditional Native American languages do not have words for the disabled, but rather names that are descriptive of the disability are used. Native Americans with strong ties to tribal culture may seek folk healers.

Providing culturally competent care is complicated by the enormous diversity of the disabled and chronically ill population and the lack of diversity among rehabilitation providers [National Center for Dissemination of Disability Research (NCDDR, 1999)]. Additionally, the growing numbers of new immigrants, the acculturation of immigrants, and the blending of cultures will further challenge rehabilitation professions (NCDDR, 1999). Resources exist for rehabilitation professionals to assist them in understanding how ethnicity and culture influence the rehabilitation process [Center for International Rehabilitation Research Information Exchange (CIRRIE), 2002; National Clearing House of Rehabilitation Training Materials, 2003]. CIRRIE (2002) developed a series of monographs designed to provide useful information on cultural issues to rehabilitation professionals. These monographs provide information on 11 countries of origin of foreign-born population in the United States. Monographs are available for China, Cuba, Dominican Republic, El Salvador, India, Jamaica, Korea, Mexico, Philippines, Vietnam, and Haiti at hhtp://cirrie.buffalo.edu/mseries.html. More than 130 training programs for rehabilitation providers covering issues related to various racial groups and types of disabilities are available from The National Clearing House of Rehabilitation Training Materials (2003), which can be accessed at http://www.nchrtm.okstate.edu.

Inadequate Documentation of Rehabilitation Outcomes

Although rehabilitation professionals see how rehabilitation care makes a difference for their clients and observe increased function, independence, and quality of life in clients they serve, scientific data relating to treatment effectiveness and positive client outcomes are lacking (DeLisa et al., 1998; Doyle, 2002; Hahn & Cella, 2002). Many studies focus on discrete aspects of functioning, e.g., sensation return, changes in strength (Doyle, 2002; Gittler, McKinley, Stiens, Groah, & Kirshblum, 2002) rather than on total function. After receiving rehabilitation services does the client have better function; is quality of life improved; is the client more independent; are activities of daily living improved? Although research has demonstrated how interventions can modify a variety of factors that can affect functioning, more study is needed to determine whether incremental, discrete and short-term changes can affect overall function, morbidity and mortality (Pellmar et al., 2002).

Documentation of outcomes is critical as reimbursement for rehabilitation services provided under a prospective payment system (PPS). Rehabilitation providers will need to provide evidence of the quality of their care as well as the effectiveness of their services (Johnston, Eastwood, Wilkerson, Anderson, & Alves, 2005). Additionally, rehabilitation professionals will need to explore ways to reduce care costs while maintaining care quality and improving outcomes. Services and programs that fail to demonstrate the benefits of their services will not survive. Finally, consumer wishes need to be considered. What clients and families expect is paramount to the success of the rehabilitation process (Estores, 2003).

Formal and Informal Caregiver Issues

The growing numbers of individuals with chronic illnesses is increasing the demand for physicians and nurses trained in chronic illness and rehabilitation. The United States lacks qualified physiatrists (physicians with special training in rehabilitation) and nurses (DeLisa et al., 1998; Verville & DeLisa, 2001; Currie, Atchison, & Fiedler, 2002; Dean-Baar, 2003). Only one-half of the accredited medical schools in the country have physical medicine and rehabilitation departments within their schools (DeLisa et al., 1998). Even those departments have been allowed very little time to teach rehabilitation concepts. Few nursing schools have course work dedicated to rehabilitation care. Many rehabilitation nurses receive specialized training by becoming certified rehabilitation nurses (Association of Rehabilitation Nurses, 2005). Lack of exposure to rehabilitation care in medical and nursing schools, though, makes it difficult to interest physicians and nurses in careers in rehabilitation (Neal, 2001; Thompson, Emrich, & Moore, 2003).

The growing number of older adults with chronic illness is creating a demand for health professionals who are adequately trained in geriatrics. More than 35 million people in the United States are age 65 and older; older adults use 23 percent of ambulatory care visits, 48 percent of hospital days, and represent 83 percent of nursing facility residents (Kovner, Mezey, & Harrington, 2002; Mezey & Fulmer, 2002). Over half of nursing schools in this country have no full-time faculty certified in geriatric nursing; only three of the nation's 145 medical schools have geriatric departments, and fewer than ten percent require a geriatrics course. Health care professionals who are not trained in care of the elderly, often see the older client as having a lessened rehabilitation potential. With the increasing number of older persons with chronic illness, this bias must be eliminated. Rehabilitation potential is not age-dependent. Small gains or maintaining current levels of function in an older client may make a major difference, enabling a disabled older adult to live in his or her own home instead of a long-term care facility.

Another major caregiver issue that needs to be addressed is the growing number of disabled and chronically ill who have unmet needs for personal assistance (Kennedy, 2001; LaPlant, Kaye, Kang, & Harrington, 2004). It is estimated that 3.2 million adults with disabilities have at least one assistance deficit, usually involving IADLs like housework (Kennedy, 2001). Almost one million adults report one or more assistance deficits with basic ADLs. Compared to adults with met ADL needs, individuals with ADL assistance deficits are more likely to live

alone, to be in poor health, to be a member of a racial or ethnic minority, and to need help with multiple activities. Compared with the individual with unmet needs who lives with others, people with unmet needs who live alone are worse off; however, both groups are more likely than those whose needs are met to experience adverse consequences such as discomfort, weight loss, dehydration, falls, and burns (LaPlante, et al, 2004). Future studies are needed to explore the causes and costs of unmet need, and to identify ways to assist persons with unmet needs to obtain these services.

Interventions

The Rehabilitation Process

Rehabilitation is a philosophy as much as it is a set of techniques (Secrest, 2000). Basic to this philosophy is the concept of the dignity and worth of each person, whether disabled or able-bodied. Each individual is of value and brings different talents to life. Another concept of the rehabilitation philosophy is that increased independence of clients will increase quality of life. That is, self-care is an integral part of each individual, and with increasing self-care and independence, quality of life is enhanced.

Rehabilitative care should be initiated before the individual reaches the rehabilitation unit. Immediately upon admission to the acute care facility, planning for rehabilitative care should begin. As soon as the client's medical condition permits, therapy should be initiated.

Team Approach

When trying to meet the physical, social, emotional, economic, and vocational needs of clients, it is ludicrous to imagine that one or two disciplines could accomplish all necessary tasks. Comprehensive rehabilitation of the client with chronic illness relies on the expertise of a number of disciplines. A team approach is seen as a compromise between specialization of disciplines and the need for a comprehensive approach to care (Rothberg, 1981). It is an established practice of rehabilitation to use a "team" approach in caring for clients.

Rehabilitation teams may be either *multidisciplinary, interdisciplinary, or transdisciplinary*. Multidisciplinary teams consist of individuals from different disciplines who may or may not coordinate their efforts in the care of a client (Secrest, 2000). A team of this nature is merely a sum of each discipline and does not build on each other's strengths.

A newer team model is the transdisciplinary model, where each client has a primary therapist from the team, who can be a nurse, physical therapist, or occupational therapist. The primary therapist provides therapy based on advice and counsel from the team consisting of members from all disciplines (Secrest, 2000). This model provides for continuity of care, but may evoke concerns about licensure and accountability and might be best suited to clients who are stable and require long-term care services.

A common and often preferred rehabilitation team model is the interdisciplinary team (see Table 25-6). The interdisciplinary team approach is based on each discipline communicating on a regular basis and establishing common goals for clients (Secrest, 2000). The interdisciplinary team is synergistic, pro-

---

TABLE 25-6

Members of the Rehabilitation Team

Physiatrist
Certified rehabilitation registered nurse (CRRN)
Certified nursing assistant
Physical therapist
Physical therapist assistant
Occupational therapist
Certified occupational therapy assistant
Speech therapist/speech–language pathologist
Audiologist
Dietitian/nutritionist
Social worker
Psychologist
Therapeutic recreation specialist
Pastoral counselor
Prosthetist/orthotist
Case manager

---

ducing more than each discipline can accomplish individually (DeLisa et al., 1998). Common to such teams is consolidation and validation of knowledge; communication with the client, family, and health care providers; and collaboration of care.

The composition of the interdisciplinary rehabilitation team is influenced by several factors: the specific needs of the clients served, the philosophy of rehabilitation in that particular facility, financial resources, the availability of personnel, and state and federally mandated policies and requirements (Dittmar, 1989). The client and family are integral members of the rehabilitation team as well. They must be included in the development of a plan of care, and they are expected to be active participants of the team. Table 25-6 lists other potential team members in addition to the client and family members.

Evaluation of the Client

Primary to considering rehabilitation as an option for the client is determining his or her rehabilitation potential. This is an issue for both younger and older clients. Is there a potential to be semi-independent in mobility, or is there a potential to live at home with assistance? What support is needed and available in the community for the client to stay at home?

A key in determining rehabilitation potential is the client's motivation to be independent. Internal motivation of the client is essential to completing a program and attaining goals. External motivation may be enough initially, but will not carry the client through the program. Motivation is a factor with all rehabilitation clients (Kemp, 1986).

Rehabilitation Potential   Health care payors are willing to spend money on clients with the most rehabilitation potential. Unfortunately, there is not a clear-cut answer as to who that individual is. The one standard question in accepting a person into a rehabilitation program is, 'will the client be able to both physically and psychologically participate in the total rehabilitation program each day'? For inpatient rehabilitation facilities, this may consist of three hours of some type of therapy daily.

Each specific disease or condition has its clients who have "better" potential than others. For example, stroke rehabilitation clients have poorer outcomes and prognoses if they have had a previous stroke, are older, have bowel and bladder dysfunction, and visual-spatial deficits (Brandstater, 2005). Also integral to dealing with the stroke client are the ability to follow instructions, either verbal or gestural, and the extent of memory deficits. Kraft and Cui (2005) found that poor rehabilitation outcomes were associated with clients with MS who have severe tremors, poor coordination, or cognition and perception deficits. Although these criteria are often used by the rehabilitation team to make decisions regarding the client's rehabilitation potential, practitioners are finding that some clients with such deficits are able to participate in programs and experience improvements in functional status that can lower care-giving needs. For example, advancements in diagnostic techniques allow identification of dementia at much earlier stages than ever before. Because some individuals who are in earlier stages of dementia are able to participate in therapy, in 2001 the Centers for Medicare and Medicaid Services issued new guidelines on reimbursement for rehabilitation for persons with dementia (CMS, 2001).

The issue that makes determining rehabilitation potential so difficult is that one is dealing with unique human beings. Clients with supposedly poor potential can and do make progress, while those with excellent potential may do poorly. Rehabilitation potential should not be guided solely on the basis of presence or absence of a predetermined set of criteria; a thorough assessment of each client and his/her circumstances should inform decisions regarding initiating rehabilitation.

Strengths of the Client, Family, and Environment

An important early step in the evaluation process is the identification of the client's and family's strengths. What can the client do for him/herself? What resources does the family already possess? What are the client's personal goals and values?

Client and family rehabilitation goals are highly individualized and based on activities and functional abilities that are important to the client and family.

Functional Assessment   Evaluation of the client is an ongoing component in the rehabilitation process. Because the goal of rehabilitation is to increase functional performance and assist the client to an optimal level, it is essential to measure *functional outcomes* of the client. Rehabilitation uses the term functional assessment to describe such client evaluation. Granger (1998) defines functional assessment as "a method used to describe abilities and limitations individuals experience so that performance of the necessary activities can be measured" (p. ix). Completing a comprehensive functional assessment involves the use of a number of different assessment tools. The lack of an all-inclusive functional assessment tool often makes completing a comprehensive assessment challenging and time consuming.

Functional assessment tools include: (1) the development of a client problem list, (2) goal setting based on identified strengths and weaknesses of the client (3) evaluation of the client's progress and outcomes, (4) measurement of treatment interventions, (5) cost-benefit effectiveness of care, (6) assistance in the rehabilitation program's evaluation and audit, and (7) research.

In general, functional assessment tools are categorized by the domain of functioning or the complexity of functioning they assess (Ferrucci et al., 1995). *Complex functional* measures are multidimensional and evaluate basic physiological abilities such as hand/grip strength or a complex task such as dialing a telephone. *Domain-specific* measures are limited to a single domain, such as hand function, mental status, or mobility status. Methods used to assess function include traditional self-report questionnaire-based and performance-based tests, which allow for actual observation of function. Self-report measures reveal information about the individual's perception of their functional abilities and resulting disability. Performance-based methods demonstrate how an individual performs a task in a standardized manner and may include the amount of time it takes to complete the task as well as the number of repetitions of the task the individual is able to complete. Successful completion of the task, i.e., performance, is based/judged on pre-established objective criteria.

Functional assessment in rehabilitation often focuses on the client's ability to complete basic activities of daily living (ADL) such as eating, bathing, walking, and dressing. The *Barthel index* is an example of a self-report measure. Respondents are asked to rate their ability to perform various ADL activities, e.g. drinking from a cup or dressing the upper body, as "can do by myself, can do with help of someone else, or cannot do at all." This measure provides the clinician with information about how specific ADL tasks are accomplish by the individual, e.g., independently, with help, not at all (see Table 25-7). However the *Barthel index* does not reveal the difficulty or the amount of time that it takes or any assistive devices or strategies that are used to accomplish the tasks.

TABLE 25-7

The Barthel Index

	"Can Do by Myself"	"Can Do with Help of Someone Else"	"Cannot Do at All'"
SELF-CARE SUBSCORE			
1. Drinking from a cup	4	0	0
2. Eating 6	0	0	
3. Dressing upper body	5	3	0
4. Dressing lower body	7	4	0
5. Putting on brace or artificial limb	0	2	0 (N/A)
6. Grooming	5	0	0
7. Washing or bathing	6	0	0
8. Controlling urination	10	5 (accidents)	0 (incontinent)
9. Controlling bowel movements 10 5 0		(accidents)	(incontinent)
MOBILITY SUBSCORE			
10. Getting in and out of chair	15	7	0
11. Getting on and off toilet	6	3	0
12. Getting in and out of tub or shower	1	0	0
13. Walking 50 yards on the level	15	10	0
14. Walking up/down one flight of stairs	10	5	0
15. If not walking: Propelling or pushing wheelchair	5	0	0 (N/A)

Barthel total: Best score is 100; worst score is 0.

NOTE: Tasks 1–9, the self-care subscore (including control of bladder and bowel sphincters), have a total possible score of 53. Tasks 10–15, the mobility subscore, have a total possible score of 47. The two groups of tasks combined make up the total Barthel index, with a total possible score of 100.

SOURCE: From Granger, C., & Gresham, G. (1984). *Functional assessment in rehabilitation medicine*, p. 74. Baltimore: Williams & Wilkins. Used with permission.

In contrast, the *Functional Independence Measure (FIM)* is a widely accepted and used performance-based measure of ADLs (see Figure 25-1). The *FIM* is a seven-level ordinal scale with 18 performance items that are used to assess self-care, sphincter control, transfers, locomotion, communication, and

FIGURE 25-1

FIM™ Instrument

LEVELS		
	7 Complete Independence (Timely, Safely) 6 Modified Independence (Device)	**NO HELPER**
	Modified Dependence 5 Supervision (Subject = 100%+) 4 Minimal Assist (Subject = 75%+) 3 Moderate Assist (Subject = 50%+) **Complete Dependence** 2 Maximal Assist (Subject = 25%+) 1 Total Assist (Subject = less than 25%)	**HELPER**

	ADMISSION	DISCHARGE	FOLLOW-UP
Self-Care			
A. Eating			
B. Grooming			
C. Bathing			
D. Dressing - Upper Body			
E. Dressing - Lower Body			
F. Toileting			
Sphincter Control			
G. Bladder Management			
H. Bowel Management			
Transfers			
I. Bed, Chair, Wheelchair			
J. Toilet			
K. Tub, shower			
Locomotion	W Walk / C Wheelchair / B Both	W Walk / C Wheelchair / B Both	W Walk / C Wheelchair / B Both
L. Walk/Wheelchair			
M. Stairs			
Motor Subtotal Score			
Communication			
N. Comprehension	A Auditory / V Visual / B Both	A Auditory / V Visual / B Both	A Auditory / V Visual / B Both
O. Expression	V Vocal / N Nonvocal / B Both	V Vocal / N Nonvocal / B Both	V Vocal / N Nonvocal / B Both
Social Cognition			
P. Social Interaction			
Q. Problem Solving			
R. Memory			
Cognitive Subtotal Score			
TOTAL FIM Score			

NOTE: Leave no blanks. Enter 1 if patient not testable due to risk.

social cognition (Uniform Data Systems for Medical Rehabilitation, 1997). The *FIM* provides data on whether or not the client requires assistance in completing basic ADLs and instrumental activities of daily living (IADLs), e.g., complete independence, modified independence, modified dependence, and complete dependence, as well as the degree of assistance required, e.g., supervision, minimal moderate, maximal, or total assistance. The rehabilitation professional who completes the FIM evaluation observes how the client actually completes the various ADL and IADL tasks.

When assessing function in the elderly client, however, caution must be used. The above-mentioned tools, as well as many other functional assessment tools, were normed to a general population or to an injury-based rehabilitation population and may not provide an accurate representation of all persons with chronic illnesses. This is particularly true for the client over the age of 75 and for clients who are institutionalized.

Rehabilitation Nursing

As the field of rehabilitation grows, so does the expertise and specialization of the rehabilitation nurse. Many rehabilitation facilities and units have developed a variety of new rehabilitation specialty roles for nurses over the last several years. Some of these roles have been established to address the external pressures imposed by both private and public reimbursement systems to maintain or reduce health care costs. In 1984, the Association of Rehabilitation Nurses created a certification for registered nurses working with rehabilitation clients, certified rehabilitation registered nurse (CRRN), and in 1997 an advanced practice certification for rehabilitation nurses, certified rehabilitation registered nurse-advanced (CRRN-A) was created. In addition to these specialty roles, the Association of Rehabilitation Nurses (ARN) supports a variety of specialized practice roles for rehabilitation nurses including the Home Care Rehabilitation Nurse, Pain Management Rehabilitation Nurse, Pediatric

Rehabilitation Nurse, Rehabilitation Nurse Manager, Rehabilitation Admissions Liaison Nurse, Rehabilitation Case Manager, and Rehabilitation Nurse Educator.

Rehabilitation Settings

Rehabilitation services are offered in freestanding rehabilitation facilities, specialized units in acute care hospitals, long-term care facilities, or in the home. Regardless of the setting, inpatient or outpatient, services should be provided by a team of trained professionals. Rehabilitation services have generally been delivered within a service model that is designed to deliver rehabilitation care to a mixed diagnosis group of clients (Babicki & Miller-McIntyre, 1992). Historically, most facilities have provided a general approach to client with many different types of diagnosis as opposed to specific approaches for specific diagnoses. However, it is becoming more common for rehabilitation facilities to focus their services on specific diagnostic groups of clients, e.g. traumatic brain injury, cerebral palsy, stroke syndromes, spinal cord injuries, cancer, burns, or HIV.

Hospitals and Freestanding Facilities

Some freestanding rehabilitation facilities specialize in one or two conditions, primarily spinal cord injury or traumatic brain injury. Others provide care for all types of clients. Rehabilitation units within hospitals generally have a mixed-diagnosis caseload of clients. These facilities provide comprehensive rehabilitation services, including intensive therapy designed to return the client their pre-injury state or to adapt to their functional limitations as quickly as possible. In general, clients admitted to these facilities and units must be able to tolerate at least three hours of therapy per day, have adequate family or social support, have a goal of discharge to home, and have private insurance or Medicare coverage (Easton, 1999).

Subacute Care Units

Rehabilitation services are frequently provided in subacute care units. These units deliver a lower level of care than traditional acute settings and provide a higher level of care than skilled nursing facilities. These units are considered transition units and bridge care from the acute setting to rehabilitation units, home, or long-term care. Length of stay can range from a few days to several weeks. Clients with rehabilitation needs who are medically complex and unable to tolerate three hours of therapy are frequently admitted to subacute units. Clients with stage III and IV pressure sores, chronic ventilator dependence, or continuous intravenous therapy typically receive care in subacute units or chronic care hospitals.

Long-Term Care Facilities

Skilled nursing facilities may also provide rehabilitation. Although admission to a long-term care facility is often seen as a negative outcome, it may, in fact, be a very appropriate alternative for clients with rehabilitation potential, especially older adults. However, not all skilled nursing facilities provide the same level of rehabilitation services. Some long-term care facilities offer CARF accredited rehabilitation programs and some offer *restorative care* services (Remsburg, Armacost, Radu, & Bennett, 1999; Remsburg, Armacost, Radu, & Bennett, 2001; Resnick & Fleishall, 2002). Consumers of such care need to know the extent of services offered. Skilled nursing settings have some advantages over acute care facilities for the elderly client. The pace is generally slower, lasting months instead of weeks or days, and the focus is on the individual, with less concern as to how fast progress is made (Osterweil, 1990).

At-Home Rehabilitation

A newer approach is providing rehabilitation in the client's home. In general the cost is considerably less than for inpatient services. Some studies comparing outcomes in clients who do and do not receive home care rehabilitation services indicate better outcomes for clients receiving home care rehabilitation services (Robinson, 2000).

Home rehabilitation services may be used to supplement outpatient services. With pressure from Medicare and private insurance, discharge from acute care can occur before the client is sufficiently ready to participate, both physically and emotionally, in an inpatient rehabilitation program, resulting in a need for a modified program. Unfortunately, significant increases in home care services in the 1990s sparked enormous scrutiny by the federal government and led Congress to enact legislation creating a prospective payment system for home care. In 1990, the national average number of home care visits per home health user was 36; by 1997, the average rose to 73 visits (Nusbaum, 2000). The average length of time patients received home care also dropped significantly (McCall & Korb, 2003; Murkofsky, Phillips, McCarthy, Davis, & Hamel, 2003).

Rehabilitation Specialties

Although rehabilitation professionals deal with a number of different chronic diseases, the disabilities produced by these diseases are often very similar. For example, rehabilitation services may be provided for a number of mobility-disabled individuals, but each individual's disability may have originated from a very different impairment. As mentioned previously, some rehabilitation facilities may choose to focus their services on one or more similar conditions. Finally, some rehabilitation programs are targeted as specific age groups, e.g. children or elderly persons. A major advantage of programs that focus on specific conditions is the opportunity for patients with similar conditions to work together toward common goals—encouraging each other and reinforcing rehabilitation training.

Geriatric Rehabilitation

The population over the age of 75 is the fastest growing segment of society (CDC, 2003), and, not surprisingly, their most significant health care problem is chronic disease. Over 80% of elderly persons report having at least one chronic health problem (CDC, 2003). The most common age-related chronic conditions include arthritis, hypertension, hearing and visual disturbances, and heart disease. Elderly clients with chronic disease can live productive, independent lives if given the opportunity to participate in a geriatric rehabilitation program.

Geriatric rehabilitation involves medical care and rehabilitation strategies that are designed to prevent disability, restore function and promote "accommodation to the irreversible effects of normal and pathological aging" (Clark & Siebens, 2005; Felsenthal & Stein, 1996, p.1238). Programs designed specifically for the elderly have different goals, require less intensive rehabilitation, and require different types of care from younger patients (Beers & Berkow, 2004; Lin and Armour, 2004; Routasalo, Arve, & Lauri, 2004; Worsowicz, Stewart, Phillips, & Cifu, 2004). Geriatric rehabilitation is more concerned with a client's abilities, and accentuates residual function, while treating the whole person. The client's disability affects the entire family, and nursing care should include interventions to assist the family as well.

Small gains in independence may enable the older individual to stay at home, with some outside assistance, as compared to living in a long-term care facility. A home health aide assisting the person may be all that is needed so the client can remain in his or her own home. In addition to improving functional capacity and self-care abilities, geriatric rehabilitation can improve coping capacity (Easton, 1999). Finally, geriatric rehabilitation focuses on improving quality of life. Teaching an elderly client to use a transfer board that will enable independent transfers can result in improved self-esteem and self-worth.

Cardiac Rehabilitation

With heart disease the number one cause of mortality in the United States, there are many potential candidates for such rehabilitation (Rash-baum, Walker, & Glassman, 2001). Cardiac rehabilitation programs are longitudinal, preventive in nature, and demand strong client participation. The goals of cardiac rehabilitation are to improve the client's functional capacity and to reduce subsequent morbidity and mortality (Liehr, Leaverton, Yepes, Frazier, & Fuentes, 2003; Singh, Schocken, Williams, & Stamey, 2004). These goals are accomplished through a comprehensive program that includes risk factor reduction, e.g., cessation of smoking, lifestyle alteration, e.g., weight reduction and low fat diet, and exercise training (Glassman, Rashbaum, & Walker, 2001). Cardiac rehabilitation following a myocardial infarction has four phases: Acute Phase, in-hospital; Convalescent Phase, early post-hospitalization; Training Phase, exercise training; and Maintenance Phase, post-training (Shah, 2005; Singh et al., 2004). Cardiac rehabilitation programs focus on physical reconditioning to allow resumption of customary activities, limiting the physiologic and psychological effects of heart disease and decreasing the risk of sudden cardiac arrest or reinfarction. Long-term interventions are aimed at identifying and modifying risk factors; stabilizing or reversing the atherosclerotic process; and enhancing clients' psychological status.

Pulmonary Rehabilitation

The primary goal in pulmonary rehabilitation is to assist clients and their families to adapt to their chronic lung disease (Walker, Glassman, & Rashbaum, 2001). The rehabilitation approach includes medical management, training in coping skills, and exercise reconditioning (Alba, 1996). Managing dyspnea is a major challenge for these clients. As pulmonary disabilities are likely to be permanent and progressive, realistic goals are of utmost importance for the client, family, and interdisciplinary team.

Cancer Rehabilitation

Deaths from cancer have been declining about one percent per year since 1999 (American Cancer

Society, 2005). For all types of cancers diagnosed between 1995 and 2000, the survival rate is 64%, up from 50 percent in 1974–76. Improvements in cancer detection and treatment continue to increase the number of cancer survivors, creating an even greater need for cancer rehabilitation programs. Individuals with cancer may develop a variety of functional deficits that could benefit from rehabilitation. The goals of cancer rehabilitation include both maximizing independence in mobility and ADLs, promoting quality of life and preserving dignity (Beck, 2003; Gillis, Cheville, & Worsowicz, 2001; Vargo & Gerber, 2005). Cancer rehabilitation therapy is guided by the stage of the disease and can be divided into preventative, supportive, and palliative rehabilitative therapy. Preventative therapy focuses on achieving maximal function; supportive therapy focuses on providing adaptive strategies to offset decline associated with progression of the cancer; and palliative therapy focuses on improving or maintaining comfort and function during the end stages of the disease (Gillis et al., 2001; Vargo & Gerber, 2005).

HIV Rehabilitation

It is estimated that the number of persons in the United States with human immunodeficiency virus (HIV) is between 500,000 and 900,000 (Lewinson & Fine, 2005). While current treatments have dramatically increased the life expectancy for many HIV clients, in other clients the infection progresses to acquired immunodeficiency syndrome (AIDS) with the associated neurological, pulmonary, cardiac, and rheumatological manifestations. Rehabilitation programs specifically designed to prevent, and manage impairments associated with these conditions are becoming more common. Rehabilitation therapy is based on the specific manifestation and ranges from compensatory strategies such as memory notebooks and verbal monitoring of tasks for early cognitive decline to the use of assistive devices and strategies that promote independence with ADLs for clients with myelopathy.

Pain Management

Increasingly, health care professionals are recognizing the impact that appropriate pain management has on recovery and function. Both acute and chronic pain can interfere with achievement of rehabilitation goals in any setting; therefore, assessment and management of pain are included in most rehabilitation programs. Additionally, programs that specifically address the management of chronic pain syndromes such as low back pain and headaches are growing. Chronic pain can lead to decreased function, depression, disability, and loss of workdays (Walsh, Dumitru, Schoenfeld, & Ramaurthy, 2005; Harris, 2000; Lipton, Hamelsky, Kolodner, Steiner, & Stewart, 2000). Since chronic pain is a complex problem with medical and psychosocial components, it requires a comprehensive approach and is managed by an interdisciplinary team using a variety of pharmacological and nonpharmacological interventions (see chapter 4, chronic pain).

Assuring Quality in Rehabilitation Facilities

Freestanding and in-hospital rehabilitation facilities can seek accreditation from two organizations, the Joint Commission on the Accreditation of Hospital Organizations (JCAHO) and the Rehabilitation Accreditation Commission (CARF).

Joint Commission on the Accreditation of Hospital Organizations (JCAHO).

The oldest accrediting body is the Joint Commission on the Accreditation of Hospital Organizations (JCAHO), an independent not-for-profit organization. JCAHO's original interest was assessing the quality of rehabilitation programs within hospitals, but its mission has expanded to accrediting freestanding rehabilitation facilities as well. The mission of JCAHO is "to continuously improve the safety and quality of care provided to the public through the provision of health care accreditation and related services that support performance improvement in health care organizations" (JCAHO, 2005). The JCAHO has developed current up-to-date, professionally-based standards and, through the survey process, evaluates the compliance of health care organizations with these standards. The ORYX initiative, a standard set of core performance measures, allows for benchmarking facility performance based on process and actual outcomes of care. JCAHO promotes the implementation of applicable national patient safety standards and establishes provider goals. Examples of these goals include: improving effectiveness of communication among caregivers; improving the safety of using medications; and eliminating wrong site, wrong patient, wrong procedure surgery (JCAHO, 2005).

Rehabilitation Accreditation Commission (CARF)

The Rehabilitation Accreditation Commission (CARF) is a private, not-for-profit organization that accredits both inpatient and outpatient rehabilitation programs and services of a medical, social, or vocational nature (Black & Roberts, 2001). The mission of CARF is " to promote the quality, value, and optimal outcomes of services through a consultative accreditation process that centers on enhancing lives of the persons served" (CARF, 2005). A major focus in the CARF accreditation is involvement of consumers. CARF accredited programs and services actively involve consumers in selecting, planning, and using services while meeting consumer-focused, state-of-the-art national standards of performance. The organization focuses on assisting each consumer in achieving his or her chosen goals and outcomes (CARF, 2005).

Outcomes

An essential component of any rehabilitation program is outcomes assessment. Granger (1998) describes outcomes as "changes and achievements representing the benefits of the rehabilitation program" (p. ix) and suggests that there are four domains of human experience that should be assessed to determine outcomes of the rehabilitation process. These domains include physical functioning, cognitive status, experience with pain, and affective sense of well being.

Several important outcomes in the domain of physical functioning include increased independence in completion of ADLs, whole or partial resumption of family and community role responsibilities, and whole or partial resumption of previous vocational/work responsibilities or successful assumption of new vocational/work responsibilities. The rehabilitation process is primarily focused on improving functional status giving the individual greater independence in activities of daily living and allowing the individual to fulfill life goals to the greatest degree possible. Other related outcomes in this domain include reduction of caregiver burden and caregiver stress and illness associated with being a long-time caregiver of someone with a chronic illness, and reduction of community and societal burden associated with permanent or progressive disability.

Outcomes in the domain of cognitive status include changes in cognitive status that give the individual ability to understand and communicate their needs and prevention or effective management of depression and symptoms of depression.

Client satisfaction with the management of his/her pain is a primary outcome in the domain of pain experience. The reduction or elimination of pain, especially when it interferes with achievement of functional status goals, is a critical outcome for rehabilitation.

While quality of life is a highly subjective and personal concept, maintaining or enhancing the individual's quality of life, e.g., feelings of well-being, self-esteem, dignity, and purpose and meaning of life, is a major goal of rehabilitation and the primary outcome in the domain of affective sense of well-being.

Finally, other outcomes of rehabilitation include reductions in complications associated with disability, e.g. pressure sores, infections, falls, fracture, and reductions in rehabilitation care costs. A major goal for rehabilitation in the future will be to identify strategies to provide cost-effective care, e.g. cost containment or reduction while achieving the outcomes previously described.

1. Describe pathophysiology, impairment, functional limitation, disability, and societal limitation, and relate those terms to chronic illness.
2. Rehabilitation is a philosophy as much as it is a set of techniques. Name five different components of the philosophy and explain each.
3. Identify three problems in the provision of rehabilitation services to the chronically ill.
4. Describe the different settings where rehabilitation services can be provided.

5. HIV rehabilitation is a relatively new concept with special issues of its own. What benefits and problems do you see in this concept?
6. What specific issues in rehabilitation make doing research difficult?
7. Discuss the advantages and disadvantages of the different types of functional assessment tools.

References

Alba, A. (1996). Concepts in Pulmonary Rehabilitation. In R. Braddom (Ed.). *Physical medicine and rehabilitation.* Philadelphia: Saunders.

Allen, P. L. (2004). Children with special health care needs: national survey of prevalence and health care needs. *Pediatric Nursing, 30* (4), 307–14.

American Cancer Society (2005). *Cancer facts and figures 2005.* Atlanta: American Cancer Society.

Anderson, C., Linto, J., & Stewart-Wynne, E. (1995). A population-based assessment of the impact and burden of caregiving for long-term stroke survivors. *Stroke, 26,* 843–849.

Association of Rehabilitation Nurses (ARN). (1995). *Ethical issues.* Available online at www.rehabnurse. org/resources00/position/pethical.htm

Association of Rehabilitation Nurses (1996). *Scope and standards of advanced clinical practice in rehabilitation nursing.* Glenview, IL: Association of Rehabilitation Nurses.

Association of Rehabilitation Nurses (2000). *Standards and scope of rehabilitation nursing practice.* Glenview, IL: Association of Rehabilitation Nurses.

Atchinson, D. (1992). Restorative nursing a concept whose time has come. *Nursing Homes, 4* (1), 9–12.

Athelstan, G. (1982). Vocational assessment and management. In F. Kottke, G. Stillwell, & J. Lehmann (Eds.).

Krusen's handbook of physical medicine and rehabilitation (3rd ed.) (pp. 163–189). Philadelphia: Saunders.

Babicki, C., & Miller-McIntyre, K. (1992). A rehabilitation programmatic model: The clinical nurse specialist perspective. *Rehabilitation Nursing, 17* (2), 145–153.

Balcazar, F. E. (2001). Strategies for reaching out to minority individuals with disabilities. *Research Exchange, 6* (2). Available online at http://www.ncddr. org/du/researchexchange/v06n02/strategies.html

Beck, L. A. (2003). Cancer rehabilitation: Does it make a difference? *Rehabilitation Nursing, 28* (2), 32–7.

Beatty, P. W., Haggland, K. J., Neri, M. T., Dhont, K. R., et al. (2003). Access to health care services among people with chronic or disabling conditions: Patterns and predictors. *Archives of Physical Medicine and Rehabilitation, 84,* 1417-1425.

Beers, M. H., & Berkow, R. (2004). Rehabilitation. *The Merck manual of geriatrics.* Merck & Co., Medical Services, USMEDA, USHH. Available online at http:// www.merck.com/mrkshared/mm_geriatrics/home.jsp

Black, T., & Roberts, P. (2001). Preparing for a successful CARF accreditation. *Rehabilitation Nursing; 26* (6), 208–213.

Blair, C. (1995). Combining behavior management and mutual goal setting to reduce physical dependency in nursing home residents. *Nursing Research, 44,* 160–165.

Brandstater, M. E. (2005). Stroke Rehabilitation. In J. DeLisa and B. Gans (Eds.) *Rehabilitation medicine: Principles and practice* (4th ed.), (pp. 1655–1676). Philadelphia: Lippincott-Raven.

Brandt, E. & Pope, A. (1997). *Enabling America: Assessing the Role of Rehabilitation Science and Engineering.* Committee on Assessing Rehabilitation Science and Engineering. Division of Health Policy. Institute of Medicine. Washington, DC: National Academy Press.

Brouwer, W.B.F., van Exel, N.J.A., van de Berg, B., Dinant, H.J., et al. (2004). Burden of caregiving: evidence of objective burden, subjective burden, and quality of life impacts on informal caregivers of patients with rheumatoid arthritis. *Arthritis and Rheumatism, 51* (4), 570–7.

Brummel-Smith, K. (1990). Introduction. In B. Kemp, K. Brummel-Smith, & J. Ramsdell (Eds.), *Geriatric rehabilitation,* (pp. 3–21). Boston: Little Brown.

Buchanan, L. (1996). Community-based rehabilitation nursing. In S. Hoeman (Ed.), *Rehabilitation nursing: Process and application* (2nd ed.), (pp.114-129). St. Louis: Mosby.

Campinha-Bacote, J. (2001). A model of practice to address cultural competence. *Rehabilitation Nursing, 26* (1), 8–11.

Canam, C., & Acorn, S. (1999). Quality of life for family caregivers of people with chronic health problems. *Rehabilitation Nursing, 24* (5), 192–96.

Center for International Rehabilitation Research Information Exchange (CIRRIE) and the National Institute on Disability and Rehabilitation Research (NIDDR) (2002). *The rehabilitation provider's guide to cultures of the foreign-born.* Available online at http://cirrie.buffalo.edu/mseries.html

Centers for Disease Control and Prevention (CDC) (2002). Fast Stats: Disabilities/Limitations. Available online at http://www.cdc.gov/nchs/fastats/disable.htm

Centers for Disease Control and Prevention (CDC) (2003). Public Health and Aging: Trends in aging in the United States and worldwide. *MMWR, 52* (06), 101–106.

Centers for Medicare and Medicaid Services (2001). Medical review of services for patients with dementia. *Program Memorandum,* CMS Pub.60AB.

Centers for Medicare and Medicaid Services. (2002). RAI Version 2.0 Manual. Available online at http://www.cms.hhs.gov/quality/mds20/

Centers for Medicare and Medicaid Services (2004a). *Welcome to Medicaid.* Available online at http://www.cms.hhs.gov/publications/overview-medicare-medi caid/default4.asp

Centers for Medicare and Medicaid Services (2004b). *Medicare program; changes to the criteria for being classified as an inpatient rehabilitation facility. Final rule.* Available online at http://www.cms.hhs.gov/medicare/

Centers for Medicare and Medicaid Services (2004c). *Medicare program; Changes to the inpatient rehabilitation facility prospective payment system and fiscal year 2004 rates. Final rule.* Available online at http://www.cms.hhs.gov/medicare/

Centers for Medicare and Medicaid Services (2005a). *Medicare Information Resource.* Available online at http://www.cms.hhs.gov/medicare/

Centers for Medicare and Medicaid (2005b). *Medicare inpatient rehabilitation facility classification requirements.* Available online at http://www.cms.hhs.gov/medicare/

Clark G. S., & Siebens H. (2005). Geriatric rehabilitation. In J. DeLisa and B. Gans (Eds.) *Physical Medicine and Rehabilitation: Principles and practice* (4th ed.), (pp. 1531–1560–1676). Philadelphia: Lippincott Williams & Wilkins.

Council of State Administrators of Vocational Rehabilitation (2004–2005). *Investing in America: The gateway to independence public vocational rehabilitation— A program that works.* Available online at http://www.rehabnetwork.org/investing_in_america.htm

Currie, D. M., Atchison, J. W., & Fiedler, I. G. (2002). The challenge of teaching rehabilitative care in medical school. *Academic Medicine, 77* (7), 701–8.

D'Andrea, D. C., & Meyer, J. D. (2004). Workers' compensation reform. *Clinics in Occupational & Environmental Medicine, 4,* 259–71.

das Chagas Medeiros, M., Ferraz, M., & Quaresma, M. (2000). The effect of rheumatoid arthritis on the quality of life of primary caregivers. *Journal of Rheumatology, 27* (1), 76–83.

Dean-Baar, S. (2003). Nursing shortages affect all levels of the profession. *Rehabilitation Nursing, 28* (4), 102.

DeLisa, J., Currie, D. & Martin, G. (1998). Rehabilitation medicine: Past, present and future. In J. DeLisa (Ed.), *Rehabilitation medicine,* (pp. 3–32). Philadelphia: Lippincott.

Department of Veterans Affairs (2004). *Compensation and benefits.* Available online at http://www.vba.va.gov/bln/21/index.htm

Department of Veterans Affairs (2005). *Vocational reha-bilitation and employment services.* Available online at http://www.vba.va.gov/bln/vre/

Dittmar, S. (Ed.) (1989). *Rehabilitation nursing: Practice and application.* St. Louis: Mosby.

Doherty, R. B. (2004). Assessing the new medicare pre-scription drug law. *Annals of Internal Medicine, 141* (5), 391–5.

Doyle, P. J. (2002). Measuring health outcomes in stroke survivors. *Archives of Physical Medicine and Rehabi-litation, 83* (Suppl 2): S39–43.

Druss, B., Marcus, S., Rosenheck, R., Olfson, M., et al. (2000). Understanding disability in mental and gen-eral medical conditions. *American Journal of Psychi-atry, 157* (9), 1485–91.

Easton, K. (1999). *Gerontological rehabilitation nursing.* Philadelphia: Saunders.

Edwards, P. (2000). Rehabilitation nursing: Past, present and future. In P. Edwards (Ed.) *The specialty practice of rehabilitation nursing* (4th ed.). Glenview, IL: As-sociation of Rehabilitation Nurses.

Edwards. P.A. & Reed, R.J. (2000). Ethical, moral, and legal considerations. In P. Edwards (Ed.) *The specialty practice of rehabilitation nursing* (4th ed.). Glenview, IL: Association of Rehabilitation Nurses.

Emmer, S., & Allendorf, L. (2004). The Medicare Pre-scription Drug, Improvement, and Modernization Act of 2003. *Journal of the American Geriatrics So-ciety, 52* (6), 1013–15.

Estores, I. M. (2003). The consumer's perspective and pro-fessional literature: What do persons with spinal cord injury want? *VA Research and Development, 40* (4), S93–98.

Federal Register. (2003). *Medicare program; changes to the inpatient facility prospective payment system and fis-cal year 2004 rates.* Final rule. *68* (148), 45673-728.

Federal Register. (2004). *Changes to the criteria for being classified as an inpatient rehabilitation facility. Final rule. 69* (89), 25751–776.

Felsenthal, G., & Stein, B. (1996). Principles of geriatric re-habilitation. In R. Braddom (Ed.) *Physical medicine and rehabilitation.* Philadelphia: Saunders.

Ferrucci, Guralnik, Bandeen-Roche, Lafferty, et al. (1995). Adaptation to Disability. In J. Guralnik, L. Fried, E. Simonsick, J. Kasper, M. Lafferty (Eds.). *The women's health in aging study: Health and social characteristics of older women with disability.* Bethesda, MD: National Institute on Aging; NIH Pub. No. 95-4009.

Fried, T. R., Bradley, E. H., Williams, C. S. & Tinetti, M. E. (2001). Functional disability and health care expen-ditures for older persons. *Archives of Internal Medi-cine, 161* (21), 2602–7.

Freedman, V. A., Martin, L. G., & Schoeni, R. F. (2002). Recent trends in disability and functioning among older adults in the United States: A systematic review. *Journal of the American Medical Association, 288,* 3137–46.

Fujiura, G. T. (2001). Emerging Trends in Disability. *Pop-ulation Today.* Available online at http://www.prb.org/ Content/NavigationMenu/PT_articles/Jul-Sep01/ Emerging_Trends_in_Disability.htm#webextra.

Fujiura, G. T., & Yamaki, K. (1997). Analysis of ethnic vari-ations in developmental disability prevalence and household economic status. *Mental Retardation, 35* (4), 286–94.

Fujiura, G. T., & Yamaki, K. (2000). Trends in Demography of Childhood Poverty and Disability. *Exceptional Children, 66* (2), 187–199.

Gillis, T. A., Cheville, A. L., & Worsowicz, G. M. (2001). Cardiopulmonary rehabilitation and cancer rehabil-itation: Oncologic rehabilitation. *Archives of Physical Medicine and Rehabilitation, 82* (Suppl 1), 63–8.

Gittler, M. S., McKinley, W. O., Stiens, S. A., Groah, S. L., et al. (2002). Rehabilitation outcomes. *Archives of Physical Medicine and Rehabilitation, 83* (Suppl 1), S65–71.

Glassman, S.J, Rahbaum, I.G., & Walker, W.C. (2001). Cardiopulmonary rehabilitation and cancer reha-bilitation: Cardiac rehabilitation. *Archives of Physi-cal Medicine and Rehabilitiation, 82* (Suppl 1), S47–51.

Granger, C. (1998). Forward. In S. Dittmar & G. Gresham (Eds.) *Functional assessment and outcome measures for the rehabilitation health profession* (p. ix.). Gaith-ersburg, MD: Aspen.

Grant, B.F., Hasin, D.S., Stinson, F.S., Dawson, D.A., et al. (2004). Prevalence, correlates, and disability of per-sonality disorders in the United States: Results from the national epidemiological survey on alcohol and related conditions. Journal of Clinical Psychiatry, 65 (7), 948–58.

Gregg, E., Beckles, G., Williamson, D., Leveille, S., et al. (2000). Diabetes and physical disability among older U.S. adults. *Diabetes Care, 23* (9), 1272–7.

Grimaldi, P. L. (2002). Inpatient rehabilitation facilities are now paid prospective rates. *Journal of Health Care Finance, 28* (3), 32–48.

Grunfeld, E., Coyle, D., Whelan, T., Clinch, J., et al. (2004). Family caregiver burden: results of a longitudinal study of breast cancer patients and their principal caregivers. *Canadian Medical Association Journal, 170* (12), 1795–801.

Hahn, E. A., & Cella, D. (2003). Health outcomes assessment in vulnerable populations: Measurement challenges and recommendations. *Archives of Physical Medicine and Rehabilitation, 84* (Suppl 2), S35–42.

Harris, J. A. (2000). Understanding acute and chronic pain. In P. Edwards (Ed.) *The specialty practice of rehabilitation nursing* (4th ed.). Glenview, IL: Association of Rehabilitation Nurses.

Havercamp, S. M., Scandlin, D., & Roth, M. (2004). Health disparities among adults with developmental disabilities, adults with other disabilities, and adults not reporting disability in North Carolina. *Public Health Reports, 119* (4), 418–26.

Health Insurance of American (2002–2003). *Guide to Insurance.* Available online at http://www.insureusa.org/consumerinfo/guidehi.htm

Hogan, A., McLellan, & Bauman, A. (2000). Health promotion needs of young people with disabilities—a population study. *Disability Research, 22* (8), 352–7.

Hogstel, M. O., Curry, L. C., Walker, C. A., & Burns, P. G. (2004). Ethics committees in long-term care facilities. *Geriatric Nursing, 25* (6), 364–9.

Hubert, H., Bloch, D., Oehlert, J., & Fries, J. (2002). Lifestyle habits and compression of morbidity. *Journal of Gerontology: Medical Sciences, 57A,* 347–51.

Hughes, J.A. (2004). Ethics in the emergency department. *Academy of Emergency Medicine, 11* (9), 995–6.

Hughes, S., Giobbie-Hurder, A., Weaver, F., Kubal, J., et al. (1999). Relationship between caregiver burden and health-related quality of life. *Gerontologist, 39* (5), 534–45.

Jans, L., Stoddard, J. L., & Kraus, L. (2004). *Chartbook on Mental Health Disability. An InfoUse Report.* Washington, DC: Department of Education, National Institute on Disability and Rehabilitation Research. Available online at http://www.infouse.com/disabilitydata/mentalhealth/1prevalence.php

Johnson, J. A. (2004). Withdrawal of medically administered nutrition and hydration: the role benefits and burdens, and of parents and ethics committees. *Journal of Clinical Ethics, 15* (3), 307–11.

Johnston, M. V., Eastwood, E., Wilkerson, D. L., Anderson, L., et al. (2005). Systematically assessing and improving the quality and outcomes of medical rehabilitation programs. In J. DeLisa & B.M. Gans (Eds.), *Rehabilitation medicine: Principles and practice* (3rd ed.), (pp. 1163–1192). Philadelphia: Lippincott-Raven.

Joint Commission on the Accreditation of Hospital Organizations (JCAHO). (2005). *About the Joint Commission.* Available online at http://www.jcaho.org/

Kemp, B. (1986). Psychosocial and mental health issues in rehabilitation of older persons. In S. Brody & G. Ruff (Eds.), *Aging and rehabilitation,* (pp. 122–158). New York: Springer.

Kennedy J. (2001). Unmet and undermet need for activities of daily living and instrumental activities of daily living assistance among adults with disabilities: estimates from the 1994 and 1995 disability follow-back surveys. *Medical Care, 39* (12), 1305–12.

Kielhofner, G., Braveman, B., Finlayson, M., Paul-Ward A., et al. (2004). Outcomes of a Vocational Program for Persons with AIDS. *American Journal of Occupational Therapy, 58* (1), 64–72.

Kingston, R. & Smith, J. (1997). Socioeconomic status and racial differences and ethnic differences in functional status associated with chronic disease. *American Journal of Public Health, 87,* 805-810.

Kirschner, K. L., Stocking, C., Wagner, L. B., Foye, S. J., et al. (2001). Ethical issues identified by rehabilitation clinicians. *Archives of Physical Medicine and Rehabilitation, 82* (12 Suppl 2), S2-8.

Kiselica, D., Sibson, B., & McKenzie-Green, J. (2004). Workers' compensation: A historical review and description of a legal and social insurance system. *Clinics in Occupational and Environmental Medicine, 4,* 237–47.

Klingbeil, H., Baer, H. R., & Wilson, P. E. (2004). Aging with a disability. *Archives of Physical Medicine and Rehabilitation, 85* (7 Suppl 3): S68–73.

Kolanowski, A. M., Fick, D., Waller, J. L., & Shea, D. (2004). Spouses of persons with dementia: Their healthcare problems, utilization, and costs. *Research in Nursing & Health, 27,* 296–306.

Kottke, F., Stillwell, G., & Lehmann, J. (Eds.) (1982). *Krusen's handbook of physical medicine and rehabilitation* (3rd ed.). Philadelphia: Saunders.

Kovacek, P. R., & Kovacek, K. A. (1998). Reimbursement methodologies in physical rehabilitation. In P. R. Kovacek & K. A. Kovacek (Eds.) *Managing physical rehabilitation in a managed care environment,* (pp. 77–97). Harper Woods, MI: Kovacek Management Services, Inc.

Kovner, C. T., Mezey, M., & Harrington, C. (2002). Who cares for older adults? Workforce implications of an aging society. *Health Affairs (Millwood), 21* (5), 78–89.

Kraft, G. H., & Cui, J. Y. (2005). Multiple sclerosis. In J. DeLisa & B. M. Gans (Eds.). *Rehabilitation medicine: Principles and practice* (3rd ed.), (pp. 1753–1770). Philadelphia: Lippincott-Raven.

Krussen, F. Kottke, F., & Ellwood, P. (1971). *Handbook of physical medicine and rehabilitation.* Philadelphia: WB Saunders.

LaPlante, M., & Carlson, D. (1996). *Disability in the United States: Prevalence and causes 1992.* U.S. Department of Education, National Institute on Disability and Rehabilitation Research (NIDRR). Available online at www.ed.gov

LaPlante M., Kaye H. S., Kang T., & Harrington C. (2004). Unmet need for personal assistance services: estimating the shortfall in hours of help and adverse consequences. *The Journal of Gerontology, Series B, Psychological Science and Social Science, 59* (2), S98–S108.

Levinson, S. F., & Fine, S. M. (2005). Rehabilitation of the individual with HIV. In J. DeLisa & B. M. Gans (Eds.). *Rehabilitation medicine: Principles and practice* (3rd ed.), (pp. 1795–1810). Philadelphia: Lippincott-Raven.

Lieberman, M. & Fisher, L. (1995). The impact of chronic illness on the health and well-being of family members. *Gerontologist, 35* (1), 94-102.

Liehr, P., Leaverton, R., Yepes, A., Frazier, L., et al. (2003). Addressing current challenges to cardiac rehabilitation care. *Advanced Practice in Acute Critical Care, 14* (1), 13–24.

Lin, J. L., & Armour, D. (2004). Selected medical management of the older adult rehabilitative patient. *Archives of Physical Medicine and Rehabilitation, 85* (Suppl 3), S76–82.

Lipton, R., Hamelsky, S., Kolodner, K., Steiner, T., et al. (2000). Migraine, quality of life, and depression: A population-based case-control study. *Neurology, 55* (5), 629–35.

Loprest, P., & Davidoff, A. (2004). How children with special health care needs affect employment decisions of low-income parents. *Maternal Child Health Journal, 8* (3), 171–82.

Lutz, B. J., & Bowers, B. J. (2003). Understanding how disability is defined and conceptualized in the literature. *Rehabilitation Nursing, 28* (3), 74–8.

Lysaght, R.M. (2004). Approaches to worker rehabilitation by occupational and physical therapists in the United States: Factors impacting practice. *Work, 23* (2), 139–46.

Manton, K. G., & Gu, X. (2001). Changes in the prevalence of chronic disability in the United States black and nonblack population above age 65 from 1982 to 1999. Proceedings of the National Academy of Sciences of the United States of America (PNAS), May 2001; 10.1073/pnas.111152298. Available online at http:// www.pnas.org/cgi/content/abstract/111152298v1

McCall, N., & Korb, J. (2003). The impact of Medicare home health policy changes on Medicare beneficiaries. *Center for Home Care Policy and Research Policy Briefs, 15,* 1–6.

McNeil, J. (1997). Americans with Disabilities: 1995–1995. *Current Population Reports,* P70-61, Aug., 1997.

Mezey, M., & Fulmer, T. (2002). The future history of gerontological nursing. *Journal of Gerontology A Biological Sciences Medical Sciences, 57* (7), M438-41.

Mills, P., Yu, H., Ziegler, M., Patterson, T., et al. (1999). Vulnerable caregivers of patients with Alzheimer's disease have a deficit in circulating CD62L-T lymphocytes. *Psychosomatic Medicine, 61* (2), 168–74.

Murkofsky, R. L., Phillips, R. S., McCarthy, E. P., Davis, R. B., et al. (2003). Length of stay in home care before and after the 1997 BBA, *Journal of the American Medical Association, 289* (21), 2841–8.

Nadash, P., & Feldman, P.H. (2003). The effectiveness of a "restorative" model of care for home care patients. *Home Healthcare Nurse, 21* (6), 421–3.

National Center for Chronic Disease Prevention and Health Promotion, Centers for Disease Control and Prevention (1999). *Chronic disease notes and reports: Special focus. Healthy Aging, 12,* 3.

National Center for the Dissemination of Disability Research (NCNNR) (1999). Disability, Diversity and Dissemination: A review of the literature on topics related to increasing the utilization of rehabilitation research outcomes among diverse consumer groups Parts 1 & 2. *Research Exchange, 4* (2). Available online at http://www.ncddr.org/du/researchexchange/v04n 02/power.html

National Clearing House of Rehabilitation Training Materials (2003). *Multicultural catalog.* Available online at http://www.nchrtm.okstate.edu

National Council on Rehabilitation (1994). *Symposium on the processes of rehabilitation.* New York.

National Depressive and Manic-Depression Association. (1998). *Overview of depressive illness and its symptoms.* Available online at http://www.ndma.org/depover.htm

National Institute of Mental Health. (1998). *Mental illness.* Auburn University. Available online at www.duc.auburn.edu/~mcquedr/psyinfo/ment_ill.htm

National Organization on Disability (2004). *Executive summary of the 2000 N.O.D./Harris survey of Americans with disabilities.* Available online at www.nod.org

National Therapeutic Recreation Society (1996). *Philosophical position statement.* Online. Internet: www.nrpa.org/branches/ntrs/philos.htm

Neal, I. J. (2001). Using rehabilitation theory to teach medical-surgical nursing to undergraduate students. *Rehabilitation Nursing, 26* (2), 72–5, 77.

Neale, P. (2000). Medical Rehabilitation Case Management Accreditation. *Rehabilitation Nursing, 25* (3), 84–85.

Nelson, W. (2004). Addressing rural ethics issues. The characteristics of rural healthcare settings pose unique ethical challenges. *Healthcare Executive, 19* (4), 36–7.

Newacheck, P. W., Inkelas, M., & Kim, S. E. (2004). Health services use and health care expenditures for children with disabilities. *Pediatrics, 4* (1), 79–85.

Niemeier, J. P., Burnett D. M., & Whitaker D. A. (2003). Cultural competence in the multidisciplinary rehabilitation setting: Are we falling short of meeting needs? *Archives of Physical Medicine and Rehabilitation, 84* (8), 1240–5.

Nusbaum, N. (2000). Issues in home rehabilitation care. *Annals of Long-Term Care, 8* (11), 43–47.

O'Neil, J. H., Zuger, R. R., Fields, A., Fraser, R., et al. (2004). The program without walls: Innovative approach to state agency vocational rehabilitation of persons with traumatic brain injury. *Archives of Physical Medicine and Rehabilitation, 85* (4), S68–72.

Osborn, C., & Marshall, M. (1993). Self-feeding performance in nursing home residents. *Journal of Gerontological Nursing, 19,* 7–14.

Ostchega, Y., Harris, T., Hirsch, R., Parsons, V. et al. (2000). The prevalence of functional limitations and disability in older persons in the U.S.: Data from the National Health and Nutrition Examination Survey III. *Journal of the American Geriatrics Society, 48,* 1132–1135.

Osterweil, D. (1990). Geriatric rehabilitation in the long-term care institutional setting. In B. Kemp, K. Brummel-Smith, & J. Ramsdell (Eds.), *Geriatric rehabilitation,* (pp. 347–456). Boston: Little, Brown.

Pellmar, T. C., Jr. Brandt, E. N., & Baird, M. A. (2002). Health and behavior: The interplay of biological, behavioral, and social influences: Summary of an Institute of Medicine report. *American Journal of Health Promotion, 16* (4), 206–19.

Pope, A., & Tarlov, A. (Eds.). (1991). *Disability in America: Toward a national agenda for prevention.* Washington, DC: National Academy Press.

Power, P. (1989). Working with families: An intervention model for rehabilitation nurses. *Rehabilitation Nursing, 14* (2), 73–76.

Pryor, J. (2002). Rehabilitative nursing: A core nursing function across all settings. *Collegian, 9* (2), 11–15.

Rashbaum, I. G., Walker, W. C., & Glassman, S. J. (2001). Cardiopulmonary rehabilitation and cancer rehabilitation: Cardiac rehabilitation in disabled populations. *Archives of Physical Medicine and Rehabilitation, 82* (Suppl 1): S52–5.

Rehabilitation Accreditation Commission (CARF). (2005). *Mission and purposes.* Available online at http://www.carf.org/consumer.aspx?content=content/About/mission.htm

Reichard A., Sacco T. M., & Turnbull H. R. 3rd. (2004). Access to health care for individuals with developmental disabilities from minority backgrounds. *Ment Retard, 42* (6), 459–70.

Remsburg, R. (2004). Restorative Care Activities. B. Resnick (ed.) *Restorative care nursing for older adults: A guide for all care settings* (pp 74–95). New York: Springer.

Remsburg, R., Armacost, K., Radu, C., & Bennett, R. (1999). Comparison of two models of restorative care in the nursing home. *Geriatric Nursing, 20* (6), 321–326.

Remsburg, R., Armacost, K., Radu, C., & Bennett, R. (2001). Impact of a restorative care program in the nursing home. *Educational Gerontology: An International Journal, 27,* 261–280.

Resnick, B., & Fleishell, A. (2002). Developing a restorative care program: A five-step approach that involves the resident. *American Journal of Nursing, 102* (7), 91–5.

Resnick, B., & Remsburg, R. (2004). Overview of restorative care. In B. Resnick (Ed.). *Restorative care nursing for older adults: A guide for all care settings,* (pp. 1–12). New York: Springer.

Robinson, K. (2000). Efficacy of home care rehabilitation interventions. *Annals of Long-Term Care, 8* (9),69–71.

Rogers, J., Holm, M., Burgio, L., Granieri, E., et al. (1999). Improving morning care routines of nursing home residents with dementia. *Journal of the American Geriatrics Society, 47*, 1049–1057.

Rogers, S. T., Amador, M. J., & Bryan, T. A. (2000). Physical healthcare patterns and nursing interventions. In P. A. Edwards (Ed.) *The specialty of nursing practice of rehabilitation nursing: A core curriculum.* Glenview, IL: Association of Rehabilitation Nurses.

Ross, B. (1992). The impact of reimbursement issues on rehabilitation nursing practice and patient care. *Rehabilitation Nursing, 17* (5), 236–238.

Rothberg, J. (1981). The rehabilitation team: Future direction. *Archives of Physical Medicine and Rehabilitation, 62* (8), 407–10.

Routasalo, P., Arve, S., & Lauri, S. (2004). Geriatric rehabilitation nursing: Developing a model. *International Journal of Nursing Practice, 10* (5), 207–15.

Rusk, H. (1965). Preventive Medicine, curative medicine— The rehabilitation. *New Physician, 59* (4), 156–160.

Santerre, R. E. (2002). The inequity of Medicaid reimbursement in the United States. *Applied Health Economics and Health Policy, 1* (1), 25–32.

Schulz, R., & Beach, S. (1999). Caregiving as a risk factor for mortality: The caregiver health effects study. *Journal of the American Medical Association, 282* (23), 2215–9.

Secrest, J. A. (2000). Rehabilitation and rehabilitation nursing. In P. A. Edwards (Ed.), *The specialty practice of rehabilitation nursing a core curriculum* (4th ed.), (pp. 2–16). Glenview, IL: Association of Rehabilitation Nurses.

Seibert, P. S., Stridh-Igo, P., & Zimmerman, C. G. (2002). A checklist to facilitate cultural awareness and sensitivity. *Journal of Medical Ethics, 28*, 143–146.

Shah, S. K. (2005). Cardiac rehabilitation. In J. DeLisa & B. M. Gans (Eds.). *Rehabilitation medicine: Principles and practice* (3rd ed.), (pp. 1811–1842). Philadelphia: Lippincott-Raven.

Shaw, W., Patterson, T., Ziegler, M., Dimsdale, J., et al. (1999). Accelerated risk of hypertensive blood pressure recordings among Alzheimer caregivers. *Journal of Psychosomatic Medicine, 43* (3), 215–27.

Shirey, L., & Summer, L. (2000). Caregiving: Helping the elderly with activity limitations. *Challenges for the 21st century: Chronic and disabling conditions.* National Academy on An Aging Society, Washington, DC.

Singh, V. N., Williams, K., & Stamey, R. (2004). Cardiac rehabilitation. *EMedicine.* Available online at http://www.emedicine.co/pmr/topic180.htm

Social Security Online (2005). *Social Security handbook.* Available online at http://www.ssa.gov/OP_Home/handbook/ssa-hbk.htm

SoRelle, R. (1999). Global epidemic of cardiovascular disease expected by the year 2050. *Circulation, 100*, 101.

Spillman, B. (2003). *Changes in elderly disability rates and implications for health care utilization and cost.* U.S. Department of Health and Human Services, Office of the Assistant Secretary for Planning and Evaluation. Available online at http://aspe.hhs.gov/daltcp/reports/hcutlcst.htm#execsum

Stineman, M. G. (2002). Prospective payment, prospective challenge. *Archives of Physical Medicine and Rehabilitation, 83* (12), 1802–5.

Stryker, R. (1977). *Rehabilitative aspects of acute and chronic nursing care.* Philadelphia: Saunders.

Stuart, B. (2004). Navigating the new Medicare drug benefit. *American Journal of Geriatric Pharmacotherapy, 2* (1), 75–80.

Taguiam-Hites, S. (1995). The Americans with Disabilities Act of 1990: Implementation and education in rehabilitation nursing. *Rehabilitation Nursing, 20* (1), 42–44.

Tappen, R. (1994). The effect of skill training on functional abilities of nursing home residents with dementia. *Research in Nursing and Health, 17*, 159–165.

Targett, P., Wehman, P., & Young, C. (2004). Return to work for persons with spinal cord injury: Designing work supports. *Neurorehabilitation. 19* (2), 131–9.

Tate, D. G., & Pledger, C. (2003). An integrative conceptual framework of disability. New direction for research. *American Psychologist. 58* (4), 289–95.

Thompson, T. L, Emrich, K., & Moore, G. (2003). The effect of curriculum on the attitudes of nursing students toward disability. *Rehabilitation Nursing, 28* (1), 27–30.

Trupin, L., Sebesta, S., Yelin, E., & LaPlant, M. (1997). Trends in labor force participation among persons with disabilities, 1993–1994. *Disability Statistics Report, 10*, 1–39.

Uniform Data System for Medical Rehabilitation. (1997). FIM™ Instrument. University at Buffalo, Buffalo, NY, 14214.

U.S. Census Bureau. (1999). *Dynamic Diversity: Project changes in U.S. race and ethnicity composition 1995 to 2050.* Available online at http://www.mbda.gov/index.php?section_id=1&bucket_id=16&format_id=19

U.S. Census Bureau, Housing and Household Economic Statistics Division. (2004). *Health insurance coverage: 2003.* Available online at http://www.census.gov/hhes/www/hlthins/hlthin03.html

U.S. Department of Education (2005). Office of Special Education and Rehabilitation Services. Rehabilitation Services Administration. Available online at http://www.ed.gov/about/offices/list/osers/rsa/about.html

U.S. Department of Health and Human Services (DHHS) & The Agency for Health Quality and Research (AHRQ). (2003). *The National Health Disparities Report.* Available online at http://qualitytools.ahrq.gov/disparitiesreport/download_report.aspx

U.S. Equal Opportunity Employment Commission. The Americans with Disabilities Act (ADA): 1990–2002. Available online at http://www.eeoc.gov/ada/

van Dyck, P. C., Kogan, M. D., McPherson, M. G, Weissman, G. R., et al. (2004). Prevalence and characteristics of children with special health care needs. *Archives of Pediatric Adolescent Medicine, 158* (9), 931–2.

Vargo, M. M., & Gerber, L. H. (2005). Rehabilitation for patients with cancer diagnoses. In J. DeLisa and B. Gans (Eds.) *Physical Medicine and Rehabilitation: Principles and practice* (4th ed.), (pp. 1771–1794). Philadelphia: Lippincott Williams & Wilkins.

Verville, R., & DeLisa, J.A. (2001). The evolution of Medicare financing policy for graduate medical education and implications for PM&R: A commentary. *Archives of Physical Medicine and Rehabilitation, 82* (4), 558–62.

Vistnes, J., & Monheit, A. (1997). *Health insurance status of the civilian noninstitutionalized population: 1996.* Agency for Health Care Policy and Research, Rockville, MD. MEPS Research Findings No. 1. AHCPR Publication No. 97-0030.

Waidmann, T., & Liu, K. (2000). Disability trends among elderly persons and implications for the future. *Journal of Gerontology B Psychological Science/Social Science, 55* (5), S298–307.

Walker, W. C., Glassman, S. J., & Rashbaum, I. G. (2001). Cardiopulmonary rehabilitation and cancer rehabilitation: Pulmonary rehabilitation. *Archives of Physical Medicine and Rehabilitation, 82* (Suppl 1): S56–62.

Walsh, N. E., Dumitru, D., Schoenfeld, L. S., & Ramaurthy, S. (2005). Treatment of the patient with chronic pain. In J. DeLisa and B. Gans (Eds.) *Physical Medicine and Rehabilitation: Principles and practice* (4th ed.), (pp. 493–530). Philadelphia: Lippincott Williams & Wilkins.

Watson, P. (1990). The Americans with Disabilities Act: More rights for people with disabilities. *Rehabilitation Nursing 15,* 325–328.

Weitzenkamp, D., Gerhart, K., Charlifue, S., Whiteneck, G., et al. (1997). Spouses of spinal cord injury survivors: The added impact of caregiving. *Archives of Physical Medicine and Rehabilitation, 78* (8), 822–7.

Whyte, J. (1998). Enabling America: A report from the Institute of Medicine on rehabilitation science and engineering. *Archives of Physical Medicine and Rehabilitation, 79,* 1477–1480.

Williams, T. (Ed.) (1984). *Rehabilitation in the Aging.* New York: Raven Press.

Wood, N., Marlow, N., Costeloe, K., Gibson, A., et al. (2000). Neurologic and developmental disability after extremely preterm birth. *New England Journal of Medicine, 343* (6), 378–384.

World Health Organization (WHO). (1980). *International classification of impairments, disabilities and handicaps.* Geneva: WHO.

World Health Organization (WHO). (2002). *Towards a common language for functioning, disability and health ICF.* Available on line at: http://www3.who.int/icf/icftemplate.cfm?myurl=beginners.html&mytitle=Beginner%27s%20Guide

Worsowicz, G. M, Stewart, D. G., Phillips, E.M, & Cifu, D. X. (2004) Geriatric Rehabilitation. Social and economic implications of aging. *Archives of Physical Medicine and Rehabilitation, 85* (Suppl 3), S3–6.

Wu, H., Wang, J., Cacioppo, J., Glaser, R., et al. (1999). Chronic stress associated with spousal caregiving of patients with Alzheimer's dementia is associated with downregulation of B-lymphocyte GH mRNA. *Journal of Gerontology A Biologic Science/Medical Science, 54* (4), M212–5.

CHAPTER 26

Politics and Policy

Betty Smith-Campbell

*Just do it. When you are a frustrated nurse, you are
probably frustrated because of the policy issues that
are going on in your institution or in your state or in
the nation. The only way to deal with that frustration
is to change it.*

Virginia Trotter Betts, RN, JD, MSN, FAAN
(2000, p. 126)

Introduction

Chronic diseases represent a global challenge.
Almost half (47%) of global diseases are considered
chronic noncommunicable diseases and account for
some 60% of global deaths (WHO, 2004). In the
United States, chronic illness and disabling conditions are major public health problems. More than
90 million Americans live with a chronic illness and
seven out of ten die of a chronic illness (CDC,
2004a). Approximately 33 percent or 57 million of
working-aged Americans live with at least one
chronic condition (Tu, 2004). One aspect of providing and improving the care of individuals with
chronic illness is to understand how policy influences the care and life of individuals with chronic
conditions.

Nurses have described caring not only as the
essence of nursing (Benner & Wrubel, 1989; Watson,
1988) but essential if culturally appropriate care is

provided to our clients (Kavanagh & Knowlden,
2004). Most nurses who care for individuals with
chronic illnesses would agree that caring is a part of
their professional practice and perhaps the most important part, yet caring is often viewed only at the
individual level (Smith-Campbell, 1999). Nurses do
not always see the connectedness of an individual's
health to the broader social system and how nursing
practice is influenced by policy and politics (Mason,
Leavitt & Chaffee, 2002). To be involved in the caring process, system factors, including political,
social, cultural, and economic factors, must be
incorporated into the nursing process to impact
clients and nursing practice. It is important that
nurses understand the influence that policies, both
public and private, have on individuals with chronic
conditions. For example, policy affects the availability of health insurance for persons with chronic illness. In the United States, health care is not a right;
therefore, the government is not obligated to provide health insurance to everyone. Some policy initiatives have been very successful; for example, the
elderly and those with the most severe disabilities
have hospitalization coverage. Because of policy
gaps, however, those same individuals who receive
excellent hospital coverage may not be able to receive home care or obtain needed medical equipment or medication. To have an impact on nursing

practice and the types of services available to clients with chronic conditions, nurses must be able to (1) assess and understand current health policies, (2) evaluate the strengths and weaknesses of health care policies, and then (3) act to implement or change health care policy to improve care for clients with chronic illnesses and conditions.

Policy Defined

To better understand how policy influences the care of clients and nursing practice, a definition of *policy* is needed. *Policy* is defined as the "choices society, segments of society, or organizations make regarding its goals and priorities and the ways it will allocate its resources to attain those goals" (Mason et al., 2002, p. 8). *Public policy* is defined "as a guide to government action, whether by legislation, executive order or regulatory mandate" (Milio, 1989, p. 316). Social and health policies are included within the context of public policy. *Social policy* pertains to governmental action that promotes the welfare of the public. For example, the Family Medical Leave Act was passed to promote the welfare of families by allowing parents the right to care for sick children or elderly parents without losing their jobs.

Governmental action that promotes the health of citizens is considered *health policy*. Examples of federal legislation include Medicare and funding to support research into chronic diseases such as Alzheimer's disease, arthritis, and diabetes. Local examples include city or county governments restricting smoking in public buildings. State and local boards of health have policies that monitor water quality and provide minimum safety requirements for nursing homes and day care centers. Regulatory agencies also affect public health policy. State boards of nursing set specific regulations that define who can practice nursing within their state.

Beyond public policy there are also institutional and organization policies that affect individuals with chronic conditions. *Institutional policies* govern the workplace (Mason et al., 2002). Such policies establish the way an institution is operated, its goals and mission, and thus influence how the institution will treat its employees and how employees will work. For example, if a goal of a business is to have a diverse work force, policies may be incorporated to assist employees who have physical or mental disabilities. Rules governing, and positions taken by, organizations are considered to be *organizational policies* (Mason et al., 2002). For example, organizational governing rules may include a nonsmoking rule during all official business meetings or have a policy that requests members not to use strong perfumes to protect members who are sensitive to strong odors.

Policy is never static but is continuously influenced by cultural, political, and financial factors in the environment (Chopoorian, 1986). Policy development and implementation is often not logical, rational, or orderly, and can be influenced during any part of the process. It is important to note that all policies reflect current societal values, beliefs, and attitudes and are shaped by politics (Mason et al., 2002).

Private and governmental policies have developed a multitude of programs that have benefited millions of Americans. The majority of citizens in the United States receive excellent acute care through private insurance paid by their employers. The population with severe disabilities and the very poor receive some health care services. Individuals and their families with present or past military service receive a broad range of health care services, including acute care, home care, and long-term care. Quality standards are being implemented throughout our health care system, and now based on national policy, persons with disabilities have equal access to employment, buildings, and transportation. As a nation, there is much of which to be proud regarding our policies, yet many problems remain.

Problems and Issues

The aging population has been recognized as a "demographic time bomb" set to explode about 25 years from now when the first wave of Baby Boomers turns 80. By the year 2030, nearly 150 million Americans will have some type of chronic illness, and direct medical costs are expected to increase 70 percent (Jones, 2000). However, health care policy makers have taken few decisive steps to restructure health care financing and delivery systems to accommodate the expanding number of vulnerable populations, including individuals with chronic illness and disability (Navarro, 2004).

U.S. Health Care: A System in Trouble

The United States is the only industrialized nation in the world in which health care is not considered a right. This cultural value has directed both past and current public policy decisions regarding health. Historically, the value of individual choice has been predominant. There has been a strong cultural belief that if one works hard enough, one should be able to support oneself and one's family, implying that one should then be able to afford health care (Bellah et al., 1985). Additionally, current health policy is guided by society's value that a competitive market is the best way to provide health care services. Allowing the market to provide the majority of health care services has left policy makers with only the ability to "fix" problems in the health care system. Policy makers, with the approval of society, have agreed that some segments of the population need assistance, such as the elderly, the very poor, and the disabled. This "fixing" of the problem has led to separate programs for the elderly and disabled (Medicare), the poor (Medicaid), and uninsured children (SCHIP—State Children's Health Insurance Program). Policy makers have also agreed to reward, through health care coverage, those who have provided service to the nation, those in the military and veterans, leading to another separate health care system (Veterans Affairs). This mix of private and public health coverage has given us one of the most fragmented and complex health care systems in the world. To better understand this fragmented and complex system, an overview of key policies, health system programs, and their limitations are discussed.

Health Insurance

Although declining, the preponderance of health care in the United States is financed through private insurance (61%), and the majority of U.S. residents under the age of 65 obtains health insurance through their employers (Kaiser, 2004a). It is important to note that the goal, and thus the policy, of private U.S. health insurance companies is to generate revenue. This is accomplished through risk rating—the practice of setting premiums and other terms of the policies, according to age, sex, occupation, health status, and health risks of policyholders. Ideally, insuring large numbers of persons spreads the risk. This philosophy may work in large companies (or governments) with thousands of employees/citizens, but the majority of businesses in the United States are small and their risks of needed health care are not spread over a large group of individuals. For insurance companies to make money, they need to enroll healthy individuals and limit the enrollment of those with high health expenses.

Rising costs have become a major problem for insured people with chronic conditions. The percent of chronically ill people with private insurance who spent more than five percent of their income on out-of-pocket expenses grew from 28 percent in 2001 to 42 percent in just two years (Tu, 2004).

Traditional or Conventional Insurance

In the past the most common type of insurance provided was the traditional fee-for-service plan. The numbers of traditional or conventional plans have declined dramatically from 73% in 1988 to just 5% in 2003 (Kaiser, 2004b). Traditional health insurance plans generally allow the insured to choose the health provider, and the health provider is able to make most health care decisions with little oversight by the insurance company. A majority of covered services are for acute care services, such as hospitalization, medication, and medical equipment, with little to no emphasis on prevention, health maintenance, or supportive health care services. This type of coverage limits the services needed to prevent chronic conditions and provide the long-term care services needed to support individuals with disabilities and chronic illnesses. Another major problem under the traditional fee-for-service plan has been the lack of control on service use and thus cost. Health care providers have little incentive to control cost, and the more services they provide, the more income they generate. Thus, insurance premiums increase to cover rising services. Rising insurance costs have become a major issue for employers, who pay for most of the insurance premiums. As the cost of providing insurance continues to rise above inflation, employers often look for less costly options to provide coverage for their employees. One solution for employers is to look at managed care organizations.

Managed Care Organizations

Originally, managed care organizations (MCOs) were defined as health care delivery systems with a capitated financing mechanism. Currently, MCO generally refers to any non-fee-for-service plan that attempts to contain costs and management of care (Kaiser, 2004b). Types of MCOs include health maintenance organizations (HMOs), preferred provider organizations (PPOs), and point of service (POS) plans. Of those insured through an employer, there has been an inverse relationship in growth with MCOs and traditional health plans. While traditional plans have decreased, the MCOs have risen dramatically from 27% in 1988 to 95% in 2003 (Kaiser, 2004b).

With the resurgence of MCOs in the 1990s, many were hopeful that there would be a system to actually manage care. It was hoped that MCOs would promote health and assist in preventing disease, with a final goal of reducing costs. Managed care organizations could help eliminate inappropriate over utilization of services and also offer advantages in setting standard protocols by providing preventive health care services. Unfortunately, most experts agree that the main system change MCOs, especially HMOs have emphasized is that of controlling costs. This emphasis on controlling costs can

lead to undertreatment of clients who need care, especially individuals with special health needs, such as those with severe mental illness or chronic conditions (Heinrich, 1998).

Medicare

Medicare was implemented in 1965 through the federal act, Title XVIII of the Social Security Act—Health Insurance for the Aged and Disabled (Wakefield, 2001). Medicare is an insurance program that serves over 40 million Americans (CMS, 2004a). This program provides coverage for individuals age 65 years and older, individuals of any age with permanent kidney failure, and individuals under the age of 65 who have long-term disabilities. Medicare covers more than 35 million Americans 65 years or older and six million younger adults with permanent disabilities (Kaiser, 2004c) Before the enactment of Medicare, 50 percent of the elderly did not have health insurance (Vladeck & King, 1997).

Medicare "was designed to primarily support inpatient acute care, 63% of the current Medicare beneficiary population of 40 million people have at least two chronic illnesses that account for 95% of the program spending" (Wakefield, 2001, p. 100). There are two separate programs within Medicare, Part A and Part B. Medicare Part A, covers inpatient hospital services, skilled nursing facility care, hospice care and home health care. Part A is free to most elderly U.S. citizens. To receive Medicare Part B, all beneficiaries must pay a monthly premium. Services provided under Part B include health professional services, including physicians, advanced practice nurses, and other providers; outpatient care; durable medical equipment; and ambulance services. Neither Part A nor Part B of Medicare covers long-term care.

Medicare services seem comprehensive and clearly defined, yet, as with all health insurance programs, when assessing how a policy is implemented either through specific laws or administrative regulatory policy, services are often found to be neither comprehensive nor clearly defined. For example, to receive home health care through Medicare, an individual must meet each of the following requirements: (1) be confined to his or her home; (2) have a physician prescribe treatment; (3) need intermittent skilled nursing care, physical therapy, or speech therapy; and (4) receive services from a certified home health agency participating in Medicare (AAHSA, nd). Therefore, if a nurse practitioner's diabetic client with a history of congestive heart failure needed skilled nursing care for leg ulcers, the client would first have to be referred to a physician. Second, if the client could leave his or her home to obtain groceries from the store across the street but could not physically tolerate the half-hour bus ride to the practitioner's office, the client would technically be ineligible to receive home health services through Medicare. It is important to note that women are more likely to be affected by problems with Medicare. Women are more likely than men to have chronic conditions that lead to illness and disability, and they have fewer social and financial resources with which to cope with these problems (Bierman & Clancy, 2000).

Medicare Prescription Drug, Improvement, and Modernization Act of 2003   Landmark Medicare reform was passed in November 2003, titled the Medicare Prescription Drug, Improvement, and Modernization Act of 2003 (Modernization Act) (Jennings, 2004a). This law creates a subsidized prescription drug benefit for all elderly starting in 2006

(see Table 26-1). In 2004, individuals could purchase a drug discount card, estimated at about $35 a month, that could save them 10%-25% on current drug costs. If an individual's income was not more than $12,569, they qualified for a $600 credit on their discount card to help cover the cost of their prescriptions (CMS, 2004b). The new law does not contain any mechanisms to control the cost of medication. Only time will tell how effective the discount cards will be. A study by *Consumer Reports* found shopping online for prescription medication to be more cost effective than the Medicare drug-discount cards (Medicare cards, 2004).

Prior to the Modernization Act, the Balanced Budget Act (BBA) of 1997 had expanded the role of private plans (traditional fee-for-service and managed care organizations) under Medicare with a new program called Medicare+Choice (M+C) program. The BBA included preferred provider organizations (PPOs), provider-sponsored organizations (PSOs), private fee-for-service plans (PFFS) and medical savings accounts (MSAs). The Medicare+Choice plan was renamed Medicare Advantage (MA) under the Modernization Act and created another optional plan, regional PPOs (CMS, 2004b)

Also, under the new Modernization Act, disease management initiatives must be implemented (Jennings, 2004b). In 2004, the administrator for CMS announced that by the end of the year, ten (10) Medicare chronic care projects would be launched.

TABLE 26-1

Costs of New Medicare Prescription Drug Benefit 2006

In addition to the annual premium of $420.....

If your drug costs are...	you pay	up to...	Cumulative total amount out of your pocket
$0–$250	100%	$250	$250
$251–$2,250	25%	$500	$750
$2,251–$5,100	100%	$2,850	$3,600
Over $5,100	5%	No Limit	$3,600
			plus 5% of costs above $5,100

SOURCE: Families USA (2004b)

It is hoped that increased coordination of care for Medicare beneficiaries will demonstrate health care quality and positive outcomes as well as significant cost savings.

Medicare has greatly improved access to health care for both older Americans and the disabled. Medicare provides coverage for a wide array of essential services and with the enactment of the Modernization Act there is hope that prescription drug coverage will be available and affordable to the elderly and disabled. But many questions and potential problems still need to be addressed. Some of the questions include: How will the government be able to afford the needed medication without cost controls? How will Medicare beneficiaries be able to afford the rising cost of Medicare B premiums? Will Medicare beneficiaries be able to afford the rising cost of medication even with their discount drug card? (Families USA, 2004a; McClellan, 2004). Many questions will be raised during the implementation phase of this Act, and policy makers are sure to make modifications as their constituents bring forward their concerns.

Medicaid

Medicaid was an amendment to the Social Security Act in 1965 and was implemented in 1966. Title XIX of the Social Security Act, Medicaid, was established to provide health insurance to low-income families with dependents. Individual states define the program, and it is jointly funded by federal and state governments (CMS, 2004c). Because coverage by Medicaid is administered at the state level, coverage varies from state to state, and there are vast disparities regarding who is eligible (Rowland & Tallon, 2004). To receive matching federal dollars, the state program must offer certain basic medical services, including inpatient and outpatient hospital care and physician and family nurse practitioner services. Over 50 million people receive essential health care services through Medicaid (Families USA, 2004c). This number includes more than 24 million children, 11 million adults and more than 13 million elderly and disabled peo-

ple (Rowland & Tallon, 2004). Although more than 70 percent of Medicaid beneficiaries are children and parents, they make up only a quarter of Medicaid's spending. The majority of Medicaid dollars are committed to the disabled and elderly (Rowland & Tallon, 2004).

Many individuals are dually eligible for Medicare and Medicaid. Services for persons covered by both programs will first be paid by Medicare, with the difference paid by Medicaid, up to each state's limit (CMS, 2004c). Medicaid will cover additional services such as long-term nursing facility care, prescription drugs, eyeglasses, and hearing aids. Medicaid also covers those with disabilities and the elderly who are enrolled in Medicare but have incomes below a certain level. This limited coverage for low-income Medicare beneficiaries assists with premiums, deductibles, and coinsurance. It is important to note that over 40 percent of nursing home care is financed through Medicaid (CMS, 2004c). One of the problems related to this coverage is the excessive financial burden on the government as the population ages and as the need for LTC increases. These costs, in turn, influence the need for more revenue to be generated to fund the program, typically provided through tax dollars. With society's reluctance to increase taxes, the future of both Medicaid and Medicare is uncertain.

Until major legislative changes in 1996, welfare and Medicaid eligibility were linked (Pulcini, Neary & Mahoney, 2002). Although the new welfare reform law did not change Medicaid directly, determining eligibility has become more complicated now that it is no longer linked with welfare benefits. The advantages of the policy change allowed former welfare recipients and the working poor to obtain health insurance coverage through Medicaid. Thus, it saves many single parent families from making a choice between working and Medicaid coverage for their children. However, the rush to remove individuals from the welfare rolls and save state dollars has also resulted in the denial of assistance to individuals who remain eligible for Medicaid services (Kronebusch, 2004). There had been documentation of states (1) illegally dropping families from Medicaid when they leave the welfare program; (2) providing incorrect counsel to Medicaid applicants; (3) placing applicants on a waiting list, which cannot be imposed under federal law; and (4) not responding to applicants' needs, and often not treating applicants with dignity and respect (Families USA, 2000).

SCHIP: State Children's Health Insurance Program

The Balanced Budget Act (BBA) of 1997 expanded health insurance coverage to children through the new State Child Health Insurance Program (SCHIP). The BBA allocated over $48 billion dollars to enable states to insure children from working families whose incomes have been too high to qualify for Medicaid but too low to afford private insurance (HCFA, 2000a, 2000b). Similar to Medicaid, SCHIP is administered through states, and the type of program offered varies by state. Information and evaluation of individual state programs can be found on the website of the Centers for Medicare and Medicaid Services (http://www.cms.hhs.gov/schip/).

An important benefit of the marketing initiative to enroll children in SCHIP has been increased enrollment of children in Medicaid. Many states initiated statewide campaigns to enroll children in their SCHIP programs and found that many of the children referred to the program were eligible for Medicaid. For example, in one state, for every four children eligible for SCHIP, five children were newly enrolled in Medicaid (Rothschild, 2000). This suggests a previous and, possibly, current problem that many children who met the criteria for Medicaid were not enrolled. This lack of enrollment may occur because families are unaware of their children's eligibility or they do not want to have the stigma of enrolling in a "welfare" program. SCHIP is an important step in decreasing the number of uninsured individuals in the United States. However, many eligible children have still not been enrolled in either the SCHIP or Medicaid programs. In one state, it is believed that greater than 60,000 children could benefit from the SCHIP program, yet only 40,000 children are currently covered by SCHIP or are enrolled in Medicaid (Rothschild, 2000). In other states, children who are no longer eligible for Medicaid have not been informed of their option to enroll in SCHIP, leaving many children exposed to inadequate or no health care. Without health insurance, children often do not receive care to prevent chronic conditions or illnesses such as complications from diseases that could have been prevented by immunizations (i.e., hepatitis) or disabilities created because of lack of treatment (i.e., hearing loss from otitis media).

Federal Initiatives

The Balanced Budget Act (BBA) of 1997 had an enormous impact on federal spending related to Medicare and Medicaid. This law contained the largest reductions in Medicaid spending since 1981 and produced a significant set of structural changes in Medicare (Pulcini et al., 2002). One of the strengths of the new legislation was CHIP, as discussed previously. The Act also restored Medicaid eligibility for legal immigrants who entered the country prior to 1996 and who had since become disabled. Additionally, new block grant funding to states was established to help cover Medicare Part B premiums for certain individuals with low-income Medicare beneficiaries. The BBA also restored Medicaid coverage for some children with disabilities who lost their coverage under a 1996 law that narrowed the definition of childhood disability. The BBA required that coverage be restored to all disabled children who were receiving SSI benefits before the 1996 welfare law (Schneider, 1997).

More recently, the Medicare Prescription Drug, Improvement, and Modernization Act of 2003 is expected to have the greatest impact on the U.S. health care system. As the baby boomers grow in number and add to the number of persons with chronic illness and disabilities, many are concerned that with no cost containment measure in the Modernization Act, there will not be enough funds to assist everyone who is currently eligible. This and other issues related to accessibly and affordability will continue to be debated, and with every new legislative session new policies will be developed and enacted.

Lack of Affordable, Accessible, and Quality Health Care

Affordability

In the early 1990s, when it seemed that health care reform was a possibility, the American Nurses Association (ANA) campaigned for affordable, accessible, and quality health care. The ANA, as well as many other organizations and consumer groups, continue to support change in the health care system, but true reform has never occurred and many Americans continue to lack affordable, accessible, quality health care. The very poor may be eligible for insurance through Medicaid, but obtaining coverage may be cumbersome and demeaning, with coverage varying from state to state. For persons with low to moderate incomes, or persons with a mild disability who may be able to work, affordable health insurance may be not available.

The number of working persons covered by private insurance declined from 68 percent in 1989 to 61 percent in 2004 (NCHS, 1999; Kaiser, 2004a). Due to the strength of the economy, in 1999 the number of insured workers increased for the first time since 1987. In the early 2000s the number of uninsured again began to rise. In 2003, almost 16 percent of the population, or 45 million Americans, did not have health insurance (DeNavas-Walt, Proctor & Mills, 2004). It is estimated that one of every three Americans under the age of 65 was without health insurance for all or part of 2002 and 2003, approximately 81.8 million people (Families USA, 2004d). Of that number, only 15.5% were not in the labor force because "they were disabled, chronically ill, family caregivers or not looking for employment for other reasons" (p. 5).

Persons with low incomes are more often uninsured, and persons who have disabilities live disproportionately in families with low incomes and no insurance. Individuals with disabilities who don't have health insurance face great challenges. Of the disabled without insurance, more than two-thirds (69%) state they have no regular doctor; 67% go without needed equipment such as wheelchairs and hearing aids; 60% skip doses, split pills or do not fill prescriptions due to cost and 66% postpone needed care because of cost (Hanson, Neuman, & Voris, 2003). Uninsured people with chronic illness are not only less likely to receive appropriate care than the insured, but have worse clinical outcomes (IOM, 2002). Similar problems also occurred for the disabled who had only Medicare insurance. Even with broad Medicaid coverage, over 20% said a doctor would not accept their insurance, twice the rate reported by those with insurance (Hanson et al., 2003).

Americans with incomes above the poverty level who lose access to employer-based coverage include the elderly and people with chronic illness. These individuals have difficulty obtaining quality insurance at reasonable rates. Before enactment of the Health Insurance Portability and Accountability Act (HIPAA) of 1997, if an insured person lost her or his insurance for some reason, such as losing a job, new insurance could be denied for preexisting conditions, including chronic illnesses. Today, with HIPAA in effect, if a person has been insured for the past 12 months, a new insurance company cannot refuse to cover the person and cannot impose preexisting conditions or a waiting period before coverage. The law explicitly states that genetic information shall not be considered a preexisting condition (National Partnership, 2002). The limitation of HIPAA is that neither a previous employer nor a new employer has an obligation to cover any part of the new insurance premiums. Often, an individual who loses insurance is no longer included in a group insurance plan, causing the premiums to be very high. Nongroup health insurance rates for families on average cost $277.62 a month to over $1,300 a month, with deductibles up to $5,000, making health insurance unaffordable for the unemployed or low wage worker (eHealthInsurance, 2004).

It has been projected that by 2030 there will be 64 million Americans over 65 years of age. With this growing number of elderly, there will be an increased demand for nursing home services for the aged and the chronically ill. The risk of becoming a resident in a nursing home after age 70 is 42 percent (Knickman & Snell, 2004). The primary insurance for the elderly, Medicare, does not cover long-term use of nursing homes. In 1995, 65 percent of elderly nursing home residents used Medicaid to help pay for their nursing home expenses, while private insurance accounted for just four percent of long-term care costs (Knickman & Snell, 2004).

Accessibility

Health care accessibility continues to be an issue for many. One problem for those who live in a rural community is geographic accessibility. People who live in rural communities often have limited access to health care services, especially to needed specialty services. Individuals with common chronic conditions in rural communities may have access to basic health care services but getting long-term, consistent care for chronic conditions is difficult. Accessibility may also be a problem in urban areas as well. Individuals covered by Medicare or Medicaid may find that there aren't health care providers in their communities that take clients with Medicare or Medicaid, or providers take only a limited number of such clients.

Lack of Access to Health Promotion, Health Maintenance, and Rehabilitation

The United States has one of the best health care systems in the world for individuals with health insurance needing acute care services. With the current focus on acute illness, there has been little emphasis on the prevention of chronic illness, nor are services provided that support persons with chronic conditions. Changing personal health behaviors through preventive screening and counseling have been found to be cost-effective measures and have been noted to reduce morbidity and mortality. Yet, individuals who lack adequate preventive care health coverage are less likely to obtain preventive screen-

ing, and insurance benefits are less likely to include preventative and screening services versus acute care and diagnostic services (IOM, 2002). Beyond preventative services, the current health care system provides little support for supportive long-term care, whether at home or in an alternative housing setting. Often, persons with chronic illnesses do not need medical services but need the supportive service of someone driving them to work, cleaning their house, or helping with their medication set up. Although there are beginning to be some system changes such as the CDC's (2004b) Chronic Disease Center and the New Freedom Initiative (2004), the current health care system offers little assistance for individuals with chronic illnesses who are in need of long-term supportive services.

Quality Issues

Although Florence Nightingale publicized mortality rates of hospitalized patients, it has only been in the past decade that indicators of quality have been developed and disseminated. Health plans that publicly provide performance data are more likely to provide better care than plans that do not (Thompson et al., 2004). The National Committee for Quality Assurance (NCQA), a nonprofit, private organization, is responsible for developing the Health Plan Employer Data and Information Set (HEDIS). HEDIS is a program that sets quality standards for managed care organizations. Programs such as this are beginning to make an impact on client services. Although HEDIS is administered through a private organization, it is heavily influenced by CMS, the largest purchaser of managed care, through Medicare.

Currently, HEDIS is the measurement tool that is used by most health plans in America to measure care and service performance (NCQA, 2003). The status of individual MCOs' accreditation status by NCQA can be found on their website (www.ncqa.org). Employers and consumers can use data from HEDIS to help them choose their health plan. The standards set by HEDIS are considered to be nationally accepted practice protocols and monitor many performance measures related to chronic illness/conditions: cancer, heart disease, smoking, asthma and diabetes (NCQA, 2004). In 2004, a study found that health plans that publicly reported their performance showed gains for the fifth year in a row (NCQA, 2004). But as the President of NCQA stated, "Why don't we have performance data for the other 75% of the U.S. health care system?" (NCQA News, 2004, ¶ 2). This same study found broader gaps in our current health care system with thousands of avoidable deaths (see Table 26-2), and over $1.8 billion in excess medical costs.

Managed care plans have been known to improve the quality of care by organizing care and allocating resources to address the needs of each client. However, there is also the potential for underservice and poor quality of care to maximize profits (Himmelstein & Woolhander, 2004). HEDIS is one of several quality initiatives to measure performance and to hold plans accountable for the quality of their services. In one study, using HEDIS data, it was noted that HMOs "with higher administrative overhead delivered worse-quality care" (Himmelstein & Woolhander, p. 336). In the nursing home industry, there are many documented quality-of-care problems (Consumers Union, 2004).

It has been noted that 97 percent of nursing facilities do not meet recommended staffing levels (Kovner, Mezey & Harrington, 2004).

Quality-of-Life Issues

Social Security Income for the Disabled

Income influences the quality of life for all individuals, including those with chronic illnesses. The United States government, under the Social Security Administration (SSA), has two financial assistance programs for the disabled: the Social Security (SS) disability insurance program and the Supplemental Security Income (SSI) program. The medical requirements are the same for both programs. The SS disability insurance program is based on prior work under Social Security. Disability, as defined by governmental policy, is based on the inability to work. A person can be defined as disabled if unable to do any kind of work, and the disability is expected to last for at least a year or is expected to result in death (SSA, nd). After receiving SS disability insurance for two years, an individual is automatically enrolled in Medicare Part A.

TABLE 26-2

Estimated Deaths Attributable to Failure to Deliver Recommended Care: Selected Measures/Conditions (U.S. Population)

Measure	Avoidable Deaths (range)
Controlling High Blood Pressure	15,000–26,000
Cholesterol Control	6,900–17,000
Diabetes Care–HbA1c Control	4,300–9,600
Smoking Cessation (with medication)	5,400–8,100
Flu Shots	3,500–7,300
Colorectal Cancer Screening	4,200–6,300
Beta-Blocker Treatment	900–1,900
Prenatal Care	600–1,400
Breast Cancer Screening	600–1,000
Cervical Cancer Screening	600–800
Total	42,000–79,400

SOURCE: NCQA News (2004).

The SSI program provides financial assistance to both adults and children with limited incomes who meet the governmental definition of disabled, to persons who have worked in the United States and are age 65 or older, and to individuals who are blind. SSI disability payments are made on the basis of financial need and are not based on prior work. Low-income persons receiving SSI disability payments are frequently eligible for Medicaid and the food stamp program (SSA, nd). Children under 18 years of age may receive income from SSI if they are disabled and come from a home with a limited income or if their parent (or a survivor/spouse of a parent) is collecting retirement or disability benefits. Benefits will continue after the age of 18 only if the child remains classified as disabled.

For a child to be considered disabled, the physical and/or mental condition must result in a severe and marked functional limitation. Under the Persons with Disability and Work Opportunity Reconciliation Act 1996, also known as the welfare reform bill, a child no longer needs an individual assessment to be classified as disabled. Under this law, if a child's disability is included in SSA's listed disability categories, the government will begin making immediate payments.

The Americans with Disabilities Act

The Americans with Disabilities Act (ADA) was passed in 1990. Former U.S. Attorney General Janet Reno, in celebrating ADA's tenth year anniversary in 2000, stated that the ADA was "a landmark civil rights bill that ensures equal opportunity for people with disabilities in employment, public accommodations, transportation, state and local government services, and telecommunications" (USDOJ, 2000, p. 1). To receive protection provided by the ADA, a person must have a disability or have a relationship or association with an individual with a disability. The ADA definition of *disabled* is less restrictive than that of the SS disability insurance or SSI programs. A disabled person, as defined by the ADA, is someone who has a physical or mental impairment that substantially limits one or more major life activities.

The ADA gives individuals with disabilities the right to equal opportunity to employment, restricts questions a potential employer can ask regarding disability, and requires employers to make reasonable accommodations for a person's known physical or mental limitations. This Act is seen as a victory for the disabled, but limits still exist. Provisions of this law restrict its implementation to businesses with 15 or more employees (USDOJ, 2000). The definition of *reasonable accommodations* continues to be argued in the courts. In 1999, the U.S. Supreme Court, in the *Olmstead* decision, found that unnecessary institutionalization is a form of discrimination and prohibited states from unnecessary institutionalization of persons with disabilities (Kannarr, 2002). To assist states in carrying out this law, in 2001 an Executive Order by President Bush announced the *Freedom Initiative,* a nationwide effort to remove barriers to community living for people of all ages with disabilities and long-term illnesses (CMS, 2004d). Controversy continues, and disabled groups continue to disagree with the interpretation of the principles of self-determination and independent living. Additionally there are those who believe that regulations and laws still force many disabled into institutions or to have unmet needs when moved into the community (AAPD, 2004).

The Family and Medical Leave Act

The Family and Medical Leave Act (FMLA), effective in 1993, enables individuals to have time to care for themselves and/or family members who are ill. The Act entitles employees up to 12 work weeks of unpaid leave during any 12-month period for one or more of the following reasons (DOL, 2000):

■ The birth and care of the newborn child of the employee
■ Placement with the employee of a son or daughter for adoption or foster care
■ Care for an immediate family member (spouse, child, or parent) with a serious condition
■ Medical leave when the employee is unable to work because of a serious health condition

Before enactment of FMLA, many U.S. employees were unable to leave work when they or their families had a major health need, for fear of losing their jobs. This law guarantees that people who work for companies with more than 50 employees can take up to 12 weeks of unpaid leave to care for seriously ill family members or to recover from their own serious health conditions. The limitations of this act are that the leave is unpaid and does not affect companies with fewer than 50 employees.

The Older Americans Act

The Older Americans Act (OAA), passed in 1965, established the Administration on Aging (AOA), which was created to organize, coordinate, and provide community-based services and opportunities for older Americans and their families and was amended in 2000 (AOA, 2004). The 2000 amendments included a five-year reauthorization, maintained many of the original objectives of the program and established the National Family Caregiver Support Program (NFCSP). The AOA awards funds to state units on aging, which then distribute funds to Area Agencies on Aging (AAA). The services of AAAs include the following:

- Access services: information and assistance; outreach; transportation; case management
- In-home services: homemaker/home health aides; personal care; visiting and telephone reassurance; chore and supportive services
- Community services: congregate meals; senior center activities; adult day care; ombudsman services; abuse prevention; legal services; employment counseling; health promotion
- Caregiver services: respite; adult day care; counseling and education

Public policy has greatly influenced the U.S. health care system. Basic health services are provided to the majority of U.S. senior citizens and the severely disabled, but, as discussed, the health system is fragmented and complex. Initiating changes in current policies can benefit individuals with chronic illness, but to do so requires political action.

Interventions: Politics, a Caring Action

Each of us is just one personal injustice away from being involved in politics.

(Dodd, 2004, p. 19)

Public and private policies reflect societal values, beliefs, and attitudes and are shaped by politics (Mason et al., 2000). To influence and change policy requires more than a one-time intervention. It requires continued, caring nursing action, which includes being politically active (Smith-Campbell, 1999). Being active in politics allows nurses the ability to shape policy that influences the care individuals with chronic illness receive and gives nurses an opportunity to partner with clients to meet common goals. Helping clients with chronic conditions and their families understand the political process and the power of politics can empower them to work to change the injustices experienced in the health care system.

Politics is often viewed negatively, yet *politics* is a neutral term that has been defined as influencing (Mason et al., 2000). The reason politics is often seen as negative is that *influencing* often means that individuals differ on what policy should or should not be implemented. These differences can arise from conflicting value and belief systems that elicit strong emotional responses, which are often viewed as negative. As a process, politics is neither negative nor positive but aims to influence the decisions of others and wield control over situations and events, usually in attempts to control scarce resources (Mason et al., 2000).

Stages of Influencing Policy

Agenda Setting

Milstead (2004) and Milio (1989) present four stages in which policy can be influenced: (1) agenda setting, (2) legislation/regulation of policy, (3) program implementation, and (4) program evaluation. Identifying a societal problem and bringing it to the attention of government is agenda setting (Milstead). Most national policy agenda setting begins with congressional members or comes from the office of the President. The personal values and beliefs of public officials and the values and desires of their constituents influence governmental officials in determining new agenda items or attempting to change agenda items. Agendas may be pushed to the forefront, at local, state, or national levels, because of a single injustice or tragedy. Before the organization Mothers Against Drunk Driving (MADD) existed, most of the American populace viewed drinking and driving as normal; yet, drunk drivers were causing death and disabling individuals across the nation. Because one mother felt passionate about the injustice of her child being killed by a drunk driver, a new advocacy organization was formed and MADD chapters that fight drinking and driving now exist everywhere. Policies, as well as national values, have changed regarding drinking and driving, all because one woman became passionate about an injustice (Dodd, 2004). MADD was successful because the political climate was ripe for change.

An idea, issue, or problem becomes an agenda when conditions are favorable and society believes that action should be taken (Furlong, 2004). Agenda setting can be influenced by many factors, including publication of research findings. Based on an Institute of Medicine report on errors in the health care system, patients, families, and legislators are asking questions about the quality of health care received (Kohn, Corrigan & Donaldson, 2000). Once an agenda becomes recognized, governmental officials begin to legislate programs and develop and/or change policy to correct problems identified in agenda setting.

Legislation and Regulation

Legislation and regulation are formal responses to problems identified in agenda setting (Milstead,

2004). The key players that influence policy development and exert considerable control throughout the process include Congress, congressional staff, special interest groups and their lobbyists, the executive branch, constituents, and the media (Wakefield, 2004). The process of how a bill becomes law at the national level is outlined in Figure 26-1. The process is similar at the state level, with the endpoint being the governor of the state. The key players not only influence the form of the final bill, but also can have an impact on the bill's continuation or abandonment at any time during the process. Broad language is used to write laws for flexibility and adaptability of their application over time. Regulations interpret the specifics of how a law will be implemented (Loquist, 2004). Once a bill becomes law, it is the responsibility of administrative agencies to write regulations based on the approved law. Examples include the AOA developing regulations for the OAA, and the CMS setting specific fee structures for Medicare based on the Modernization Act of 2003. The development of regulations also can be influenced. At the national level, a draft of specific regulations must be posted in the *Federal Register* (http://www.gpoaccess.gov/fr), and public comment is taken. The administrative agency then reviews the comments and may make changes to the final rules and regulations. Once approved by an executive level agency, the regulations go into effect. After regulations are approved, programs are then established or past programs are modified, based on the new regulations.

Program Implementation

Program implementation occurs when programs are initiated to achieve goals written in either legislation policy or regulation (Milstead, 2004). As in the earlier discussion of policy and the health care system, program implementation can have both positive and negative effects. Positive examples include mandating access to public buildings and transportation for the disabled, and national programs that provide funding to the disabled for

FIGURE 26-1

How a Bill Becomes a Law (Federal Level)

Opportunity to Politically Influence

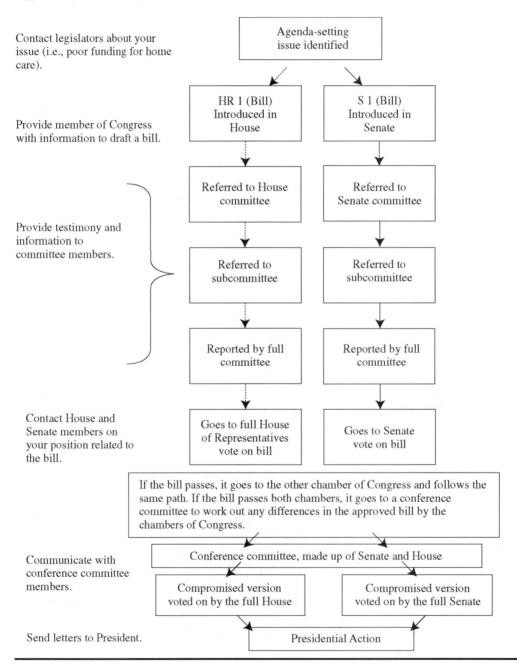

Contact legislators about your issue (i.e., poor funding for home care).

Provide member of Congress with information to draft a bill.

Provide testimony and information to committee members.

Contact House and Senate members on your position related to the bill.

Communicate with conference committee members.

Send letters to President.

Agenda-setting issue identified

HR 1 (Bill) Introduced in House

S 1 (Bill) Introduced in Senate

Referred to House committee

Referred to Senate committee

Referred to subcommittee

Referred to subcommittee

Reported by full committee

Reported by full committee

Goes to full House of Representatives vote on bill

Goes to Senate vote on bill

If the bill passes, it goes to the other chamber of Congress and follows the same path. If the bill passes both chambers, it goes to a conference committee to work out any differences in the approved bill by the chambers of Congress.

Conference committee, made up of Senate and House

Compromised version voted on by the full House

Compromised version voted on by the full Senate

Presidential Action

health insurance and living expenses, as well as nursing home care to those with limited incomes. In turn, other programs have been cut to help balance the budget. It is possible to influence program implementation and encourage the need for program evaluation when problems are seen within the program.

Program Evaluation

Political influence can be used to effect change in a program during the appraisal of the program's performance (Milstead, 2004). For example, when the BBA was enacted it produced major changes within Medicare and Medicaid, which in turn included disastrous effects on home health agencies and reimbursements to hospitals. Because of those effects on the health care institutions and providers, but particularly to those with chronic illness, legislators modified the BBA, including increasing reimbursement rates to hospitals and physicians.

To affect public policy, nurses need to learn the skills necessary to influence policy makers at all stages of policy development. These skills can also be taught to clients with chronic conditions and their families so they, too, can be empowered to change the system on their own behalf.

The Three Cs of Political Influence

Communication

Vance (1985) identified communication, collectivity, and collegiality as the three components of political influence. Skillful communication can be very influential in the political process. Nurses usually are expert one-to-one communicators, but to affect policy, nurses must broaden their communication skills. The first step of communication is listening and learning. It is essential to learn about the political process. Knowing how a bill becomes law is one way of learning about the political process. It is also important to identify the key players at different steps in the process. Knowing when a bill is in

committee and the chairperson and committee membership is important information so that one can then attempt to apply influence. In addition to directly trying to influence public policy makers, indirect influencing is also a strategy. Communicating with congressional/executive staff members, the media, and public policy makers' constituents also can influence policy makers. Knowing who you are trying to influence and how you want to influence their actions are key factors. Once you have determined that, there are several communication strategies that can influence policy makers:

- In-home Send your message and/or position by mail, letter, fax sheet, e-mail, or telegram (Specific tips: see Web sites: Congress.org; UCP) Important to note following the Anthrax attack, email and fax are probably the best way to communicate with legislators.
- In-home Write letters to your newspaper editor; talk on the radio/TV (Specific tips: see Web site: Public Knowledge)
- In-home Visit your legislator and/or this person's staff (Table 26-3).
- In-home Testify at public hearings.
- In-home Vote and get others to vote.

Building relationships with legislators before controversial issues occur can give you an edge in influencing others. There are several ways to build relationships or friendships with legislators prior to critical issues. One way is to assist an individual who is running for office. Help with the campaign, hand out flyers, answer phones, or hold a fund raising event in your home. A nurse activist who holds a national governmental appointment states, "Money is the mother's milk of politics. Give it early and if you don't have it raise it" (Dodd, 2004, p. 19). Campaigns require money, and providing such assistance to the candidate of your choice then opens the door to your influence once the candidate is elected. This does not mean that money buys votes, but it does provide access. If a legislator has limited time and has to choose to see someone who gave him or her money or another who did not, most likely the leg-

Guidelines for Meeting with Policy Makers

1. Make an appointment. Be on time.
2. Always introduce yourself, even if this is your third or fourth meeting. State that you are a registered nurse, or if a client is speaking, have that person share the nature of the chronic condition he or she or the family member has.
3. Begin on a positive note. Thank the legislator for seeing you and then get down to business. Clearly identify the issue you want to discuss; if it is a specific bill, state its number, its title, your position, and what you want the legislator to do.
4. Depending on the time allotted, give examples and facts to illustrate your position. Most importantly, share client stories.
5. Remain positive; keep the atmosphere open and friendly. The purpose of the meeting is to exchange ideas and keep the lines of communication open. Don't engage in threats or ask for the impossible.
6. Be prepared to answer questions. If you don't know the answer, say so, but state that you will get more information, and then follow through.
7. Always leave written literature on the subject (position paper, outline of your key points, etc.) and your business card.
8. Follow up your visit with a thank-you note.
9. Send copies of your written comments or a summary of your meeting to the organization(s) with which you are working.

SOURCE: UCP, 2000; Congress.org (2004).

islator will choose the person who assisted the campaign financially. This access gives the person, the nurse, the client, or family member the opportunity to share their position and influence the legislator. Political activists would probably agree that although money provides access, constituents can also make a difference with their time (i.e., campaigning, writing letters, or calling legislators on issues). Legislators pay attention to those who vote and to those who communicate with them.

Collectivity

Collectivity is crucial to the development of political influence and is built on a foundation of networking, coalition building, and collaboration (Vance, 1985). Building relationships within the profession is key, as it is with representatives of public and private sector organizations who have demonstrated an interest in health care (Wakefield, 2004). Changing legislation requires group action and collaboration. The American Nurses Association (ANA), which speaks for over 2.7 million

nurses, has testified to increase spending for home care services, problems with the Nursing Home Reform Act plus economic and safety issues for nurses. Joining with groups such as ANA, AARP, the National Home Care Association, and the Hospital Association on common issues can be one of the most effective ways to initiate and sustain change.

Personal connections can be an important strategy in moving a critical issue. Consider the nursing student whose mother is a legislator on a health committee discussing reimbursement for health providers. Working with the student nurse, providing education and support to the student to testify in front of the mother's committee, could have a major impact on the direction an issue takes. Networking is key, because sometimes success comes down to having just one important personal connection (Leavitt, Cohen, & Mason, 2002).

Networking with client groups also can be helpful. Having clients communicate with legislators about how they or their families have been or will be affected by legislation is an important strategy to influence policy makers. Working with groups that have been active in advocacy can provide a novice political advocate needed assistance and support. Advocacy groups such as the American Association of People with Disabilities (AAPD) can help professionals or families of the disabled provide testimony at public hearings (AAPD, 2000).

Collegiality

Central to the political process is collegiality, a spirit of cooperation and solidarity with associates (Vance, 1985). To be a political activist and risk taker requires support from colleagues. It is helpful to work with others with an attitude of mutual respect and shared convictions. Sometimes, diverse groups can work together on a mutual issue, even if they are opponents on other issues. Disassociating the emotional context of working with opponents is key. As stated earlier, politics is neither negative nor positive, but each side often has different values and beliefs. Working in solidarity with a group provides support during conflict and can assist in an important factor in political influencing—not taking it personally. As a professional, it is important to address your specific issue and not personally attack those who oppose you. Address only the issue, even if others personally attack you. Eleanor Roosevelt once said, "No one can make you feel inferior without your permission." Often, this is easier said than done. Influencing policy changes requires patience, perseverance, and compromise. Working with those who share similar values, beliefs, and convictions will be of great assistance when working for change.

The strategies discussed in this section emphasize influencing policy at the national level. These same strategies can also be used to influence local and state policy, as well as policy makers in work and community organizations. It is vital that nurses become political, or they risk being excluded from important decisions that affect nursing practice or the care their patients with chronic illnesses receive.

Becoming a political person can be an overwhelming experience as you realize you cannot change a whole system alone. As a beginning political activist, start by voting. Next, choose an issue about which you feel passionate (e.g., the inability of your chronically ill clients to get long-term home care). Educate yourself on the issue, and join others who are interested in the issue. Communicate your position to the key players. Know that your cause is just, and be proud of the political influence you, your clients, and your colleagues can accomplish.

■ Summary and Conclusions

Through public policy, society has made choices to assist many Americans. There are policies to care for the elderly and severely disabled through Medicare, provide health insurance to the poor through Medicaid, and ensure access for the disabled with the ADA. Society's belief in the market system and individual rights has also left many with inadequate or absent health care. Because health care is not a right in the United States, there is no "system" of health care. The system in place is complex, fragmented, and difficult to use, especially for vulnerable populations such as the chronically ill, the disabled, and the elderly. Changes can be made to improve the system. The profession of nursing and clients with chronic illness and their families can influence change through political action. It will take time and perseverance, but as Marian Wright Edema, founder and president of the Children's Defense Fund, states, "We must not, in trying to think about how we can make a big difference, ignore the small daily differences we can make which, over time, add up to big differences that we often cannot see."

Study Questions

1. Describe the trends of chronic illness and how these trends are significant in relation to health policy.

2. Differentiate between Medicare and Medicaid.
3. Identify the major social issues affecting health policy for the individual with chronic illness.

4. How does the current U.S. health care system affect those with chronic illness?

5. Explain how a bill becomes law.

6. Describe HEDIS and its relationship to individuals needing care for chronic illness.

7. What effect will the Modernization Act of 2003 have on the elderly and disabled?

8. Identify the three components of political influence, and explain each.

9. What are the first steps you will engage in to become politically active?

References

AAHSA—American Association of Homes and Services for the Aging. (nd). *Medicare*. Retrieved September 13, 2004 from www.aahsa.org/public/medicbkgd.htm

AAPD—American Association of People with Disabilities. (2000). *AAPD*. Available on-line at http://www.aapd.com/

_____ (2004, March 2). Letter to Tommy Thompson Secretary of the Department of Health and Human Services. Retrieved September 20,2004 from www.familiesusa.org/site/DocServer/Medicaid_Ltr_to_Thompson.doc?docID=3061

AOA—Administration on Aging. (2004, September 9) *Older Americans Act*. Retrieved September 21, 2004 from www.aoa.gov

Bellah, R. N., Madsen, R., Sullivan, W. M., Swidler, A., et al. (1985). *Habits of the heart: Individualism and commitment in American life*. New York: Harper & Row.

Benner, P., & Wrubel, J. (1989). *The primacy of caring*. Menlo Park, CA: Addison-Wesley.

Betts, V. T. (2000). In the health policy spotlight: An interview with Virginia Trotter Betts. *Policy, Politics, and Nursing Practice, 1* (2), 124–127.

Bierman, A. S., & Clancy, C. M. (2000). Making capitated Medicare work for women: Policy and research challenges. *Women's Health Issues, 10*, 59–68.

CDC-Centers for Disease Control and Prevention.(2004a). *The burden of chronic diseases and their risk factors: National and State perspectives 2004. Retrieved September 13, 2004 from http://www.cdc.gov/nccdphp/burdenbook2004/toc.htm*

_____ (2004b) *About CDC's Chronic Disease Center*. Retrieved September 13, 2004 from http://www.cdc.gov/nccdphp/about.htm

Chopoorian, T. J. (1986). Reconceptualizing the environment. In P. Moccia (Ed.), *New approaches to theory development*, (pp. 39–54). New York: National League of Nursing.

CMS-Center for Medicare and Medicaid Services (2004a, August 18*). CMS/HCFA History*. Retrieved September 13, 2004 from http://www.cms.hhs.gov/about/history/

_____ (2004b, February 17*). The facts about upcoming new benefits in Medicare*. Retrieved September 20, 2004 from http://www.medicare.gov/Publications/Pubs/pdf/11054.pdf

_____ (2004c, September 16) *Medicaid: A Brief Summary* Retrieved September 20, 2004 from http://www.cms.hhs.gov/publications/overview-medicare-medicaid/default4.asp

_____ (2004d, September 16). *Fulfilling America's promise to Americans with disabilities New Freedom Initiative*. Retrieved September 21, 2004 from www.cms.hhs.gov/newfreedom

Congress.org. (2004). *Visiting Capitol Hill*. Retrieved September 21, 2004 from http://www.congress.org/congressorg/issues/basics/?style=visit

Consumers Union. (2004, September 21). *Many of the nation's nursing homes continue to have problems and offer questionable care*. Retrieved September 23 from www.Consumerhealthchoices.org

DeNavas-Walt, C., Proctor, B. D., & Mills, R. J. (2004). Income, poverty, and health insurance coverage in the United States. *Current Population Reports, P60-226 [electronic version]*. Washington, DC: U.S. Census Bureau.

Dodd, C. J. (2004). Making the political process work. In C.Harrington & C.L. Estes (Eds.), *Health Policy Crisis and Reform in the U.S. Health Care Delivery System* (4th Ed., pp. 18–28). Boston: Jones & Bartlett.

DOL—Department of Labor. (2000). *Employment standards administration wage and hour division*. Available on-line at http://www.dol/gov/dol/esa/public/regs/compliance/whd/whdfs28.htm

eHealthInsurance (2004, August). *Update on Individual Health Insurance* [#7133-02]. Retrieved September 21, 2004 from www.ehealthinsurance.com

Families USA. (2000, May). *Access denied: Families denied access to Medicaid, food stamps, CHIP, and child care.* Available on-line at www.familiesusa.org/newunin. htm

_____ (2004a, September 14) *Data hidden in 2004 Medicare trustees' report shows huge harm to seniors by new drug law.* Retrieved September 20, 2004 http://www.familiesusa.org/site/PageServer?page name=Media_Statement_Data_Hidden

_____ (2004b, Spring). *Q &A: Understanding the new Medicare prescription drug benefit.* Retrieved September 20, 2004 from http://www.familiesusa.org/ site/DocServer/Q_A_.pdf?docID=2768

_____ (2004c, May). *Medicaid: Good Medicine for State Economies –2004 Update.[Publ. No. 04-102] Retrieved September 20, 2004 from www.familiesusa.org*

_____ (2004d, June). *One in three: Non-Elderly Americans without health insurance, 2002–2003.* Retrieved September 21, 2004 from http://www.familiesusa. org/site/DocServer/82million_uninsured_report.pdf ?docID=3641

Furlong, E. A. (2004). Agenda setting. In J. A. Milstead (Ed.), *Health policy and politics: A nurses' guide* (pp. 37–66). Gaithersburg, MD: Aspen.

Hanson, K., Neuman,T., & Voris, M. (2003, September). *Understanding the health-care needs and experiences of people with disabilities: Findings from a 2003 survey.* Kaiser Family Foundation (Publ. #6106) Retrieved September 21, 2004 from www.kff.org

HCFA (2000a). *Balanced Budget Act of 1997.* Washington, DC: Author. Available on-line at: www.hcfa.gov/init/ bba/bbaintro.htm

——. (2000b, July). *The state children's health insurance program: Preliminary highlights of implementation and expansion.* Washington, DC: Author. Available on-line at: www.hcfa.gov/init/children.htm

Heinrich, J. (1998). Organization and delivery of health care in the United States: The health care system that isn't. In D. J. Mason & J. K. Leavitt (Eds.), *Policy and politics in nursing and health care,* (pp. 59–79). Philadelphia: WB Saunders.

Himmelstein, D. U., & Woolhandler, S. (2004). Taking care of business: HMOs that spend more on administration deliver lower-quality care. In C. Harrington & C. L. Estes (Eds.), *Health PolicyCrisis and Reform in the U.S. Health Care Delivery System* (4th ed.), (pp. 336–338). Boston: Jones & Bartlett.

IOM-Institutes of Medicine (2002). *Care without coverage: Too little, too late.* Washington, DC: National Academy Press.

Jennings, C. P. (2004a) Medicare prescription drug, improvement, modernization act of 2003. *Policy, Politics & Nursing Practice, 5* (1), 57–58.

_____ (2004b). Policy highlight: Medicare's chronic care projects. *Policy, Politics & Nursing Practice, 5* (3), 205–206.

Jones, L. (2000). Rethinking health care to handle an impending chronic care crisis. *Advances—Robert Wood Johnson Foundation Newsletter, 2,* 10,12.

Kaiser Family Foundation. (2004a). *Employer health benefits 2004 summary of findings.* Retrieved September 10, 2004. from www.kff.org/insurance/7148/

_____ (2004b). *Trends and Indicators in the Changing Health Care Marketplace, 2004 Update.* Retrieved September 13, 2004 from www.kff.org/insurance/ 7031/index.cfm

_____ (2004c). Medicare at a glance. In C. Harrington & C. L. Estes (Eds.), *Health Policy Crisis and Reform in the U.S. Health Care Delivery System* (4th Ed.), (pp. 293–307). Boston: Jones & Bartlett.

Kannarr, S. W. (2002, October). *A quick look at the Olmstead decision fro Kansas Policy makers.* Retrieved September 27, 2004 from *http://www.khi.org/trans fers/IssueBrief14.pdf*

Kavanagh, K. H., & Knowlden, V. (2004). *Many voices: Toward caring culture in healthcare and healing.* Madison, WI: University of Wisconsin Press.

Knickman, J. R., & Snell, R. K. (2004). The 2030 problem: caring for aging baby boomers. In C. Harrington & C. L. Estes (Eds.), *Health Policy Crisis and Reform in the U.S. Health Care Delivery System* (4th ed.), (pp. 114–122). Boston: Jones & Bartlett.

Kohn, L. T., Corrigan, J. M., & Donaldson, M. S. (2000). *To err is human: Building a safer health system.* Washington, DC: National Academy Press.

Kovner, C.T., Mezey, M., & Harrington, C. (2004). Whocare for older adults? Workforce implications of an aging society. In C. Harrington & C. L. Estes (Eds.), *Health Policy Crisis and Reform in the U.S. Health Care Delivery System* (4th ed.), (pp. 216–221). Boston: Jones & Bartlett.

Kronebusch, K. (2004). Medicaid for children: Federal mandates, welfare reform, and policy backsliding. In C. Harrington & C. L. Estes (Eds.), *Health Policy Crisis and Reform in the U.S. Health Care Delivery System* (4th ed.), (pp.287–292). Boston: Jones & Bartlett.

Leavitt, J. K., Cohen, S. S. & Mason, D. J. (2002). Political analysis and strategies. In D. J. Mason, J. K. Leavitt, & M. W. Chaffee (Eds.), *Policy and Politics in Nursing and Health Care* (4th ed.), (pp. 71–86). St. Louis, MO: Saunders.

Loquist, R. S. (2004). Government regulation: Parallel and powerful. In J. A. Milstead (Ed.), *Health policy and politics: A nurses' guide* (pp. 89–128). Gaithersburg, MD: Aspen.

Mason, D. J, Leavitt, J. K., & Chaffee, M. W. (2002). *Policy and politics in nursing and health care* (4th ed.). St. Louis, MO: Saunders.

McClellan, M. (2004, September 20). *Questions from Senate Finance Committee to CMS Administrator Transcript.* Retrieved September 20, 2004 from http://www.kaisernetwork.org/health_cast/uploaded_files/092004_cq_transcript.pdf

Medicare cards: No match for online prices. (2004, September). *Consumer Reports,* p. 8.

Milio, N. (1989). Developing nursing leadership in health policy. *Journal of Professional Nursing, 5,* 315–321.

Milstead, J. A. (2004). *Health policy and politics: A nurse's guide* (2nd ed.). Gaithersburg, MD: Aspen.

Navarro, V. (2004). Why congress did not enact health care reform. In C. Harrington & C. L. Estes (Eds.), *Health Policy Crisis and Reform in the U.S. Health Care Delivery System* (4th ed.), (pp. 36–40). Sudbury, MA: Jones & Bartlett.

NCHS–National Center for Health Statistics. (1999). *Health, United States, 1999: With health and aging chartbook.* (PHS 99-1232). Hyattsville, MD: U.S. Department of Health and Human Services.

NCQA–National committee for Quality Assurance. (2003). *The state of health care quality: 2003.* Retrieved September 21 from www.ncqa.org

_____ (2004). *The state of health care quality: 2004.* Retrieved September 23 from www.ncqa.org

NCQA News. (2004, Sepember 23). *NCQA report finds major gains in health care quality, but only for 1/4th of the system.* Retrieved September 24 from www.ncqa.org

New Freedom Initiative. (2004). Centers for Medicare and Medicaid Services. Retrieved Sepember 21, 2004 from http://www.cms.hhs.gov/newfreedom/

Pulcini, J. A., Neary, S. R. & Mahoney, D. F. (2002). Health Care Financing. In D. J. Mason, J. K. Leavitt, & M. W. Chaffee (Eds.), *Policy and Politics in Nursing and Health Care* (4th ed.), (pp. 241–265). St. Louis, MO: Saunders.

Rothschild, S. (2000, August 28). Loss of child health insurance funds has silver lining. *Wichita Eagle,* #9A Wichita, KS.

Rowland, D., & Tallon, J. R. (2004). Medicaid: Lessons from a decade. In C. Harrington & C. L. Estes (Eds.),

Health policy crisis and reform in the U.S. health care delivery system (4th ed.), (pp. 282–286). Sudbury, MA: Jones & Bartlett.

Schneider, A. (1997). *Overview of Medicaid provisions in the Balanced Budget Act of 1997. P.L. 105-33.* Washington, DC: Center on Budget and Policy Priorities. Available on-line at: www.cbpp.org/908mcaid.htm

Smith-Campbell, B. (1999). A case study on expanding the concept of caring from individuals to communities. *Public Health Nursing, 16,* 405–411.

SSA-Social Security Administration (n.d.) *Social Security Online.* Retrieved September 21, 2004 from http://www.ssa.gov/

Thompson, J. W., Pinidiya, S. D., Ryan, K. W., McKinley, E. D., et al. (2004). Health plan quality data: The importance of pubic reporting. In C. Harrington & C. L. Estes (Eds.), *Health policy crisis and reform in the U.S. health care delivery system* (4th ed.), (pp. 233–235). Boston: Jones & Bartlett.

Tu, H.T. (2004, September). *Rising health costs, medical debt and chronic conditions.* Center for Studying Health System Change Retreived September 23, 2004 from http://www.hschange.org/CONTENT/706/706.pdf

UCP. (2000). UCPNet: Understanding disabilities, creating opportunities: Advocacy and public policy. Available on-line at: www.ucp.org.

USDOJ—United States Department of Justice. (2000). *A guide to disability rights laws.* Available on-line at: www.usdoj.gov/crt/ada/adahom.htm.

Vance, C. (1985). Politics: A humanistic process. In D. J. Mason, S. W. Talbott, & J. K. Leavitt (eds.), *Policy and politics for nurses,* (pp. 104–118). Philadelphia: WB Saunders.

Vladeck, B. C., & King, K. M. (1997). Medicare at 30: Preparing for the future. In C. Harrington & C. L. Estes (Eds.), *Health policy and nursing,* (pp. 319–326). Boston: Jones and Bartlett.

Wakefield, M. K. (2001). Medicare at the crossroads. *Policy, Politics & Nursing Practice, 2* (2), 98–102.

Wakefield, M. K. (2004). Government response: Legislation. In J. A. Milstead (Ed.), *Health policy and politics: A nurses' guide ,* (pp. 67–88). Gaithersburg, MD: Aspen.

Watson, J. (1988). *Nursing: Human science and human care a theory of nursing.* New York: National League of Nursing.

WHO-World Health Organization. (2004). World Health Organization: Department of chronic diseases and health promotion. September 13, 2004 retrieved from http://www.who.int/noncommunicable_diseases/about/chp/en/

Internet Resources

AAPD—American Association of People with Disabilities: www.aapd.com

AAHSA—American Association of Homes and Services for the Aging: www.aahsa.org

American Nurse's Association: www.nursingworld.org

Centers for Medicare and Medicaid Services (CMS) http://www.cms.hhs.gov/

Citizens for Long Term Care: www.citizensforltc.org

Congress.org: communication tips: http://www.congress.org/congressorg/issues/basics/?style=comm

Consortium for Citizens with Disabilities: www.c-c-d.org

DVV—Department of Veterans Affairs: www.va.gov

Families USA http://www.familiesusa.org/

Federal Legislative link site: http://thomas.loc.gov/

National Alliance for Caregiving: http://www.caregiving.org/

National Chronic Care Consortium: www.nccconline.org/

National Respite Coalition: http://www.archrespite.org/NRC.htm

National Committee for Quality Assurance (NCQA): http://www.ncqa.org

Preventing Chronic Disease Journal, CDC- http://www.cdc.gov/pcd/

Public Knowledge: http://www.publicknowledge.org/content/policy-papers/grassroots-lobbying-howto

Social Security Administration—Disability benefits: www.ssa.gov

UCPnet, Understanding Disabilities, Creating Opportunities: www.ucp.org

WHO—World Health Organization. www.who.org

CHAPTER 27

Financial Impact

Sonya R. Hardin

Introduction

The continued rise in health care costs is a growing crisis in the United States. These rising costs are linked to several factors, including increased personal income, new technologies, and an increased incidence of defensive medicine costs. However, the most important factor contributing to the rising costs is the demographic change occurring in the United States. The effect of the Baby Boomer generation reaching retirement age in the year 2011 and the effect of the increasing percentage of the population over the age of 65 will significantly impact the provision of health care services and their associated costs.

With the aging of America and the continued advances in acute care technology, the incidence and prevalence of chronic illness will continue to accelerate. Currently, chronic conditions account for 80 percent of all deaths and 90 percent of all morbidity in the United States (Bringewatt, 1998). Nearly 100 million Americans have one or more chronic conditions. Individuals with chronic diseases, such as cancer, diabetes, respiratory disease, Alzheimer's disease, arthritis, and others, are the highest cost, fastest-growing, most complex group of clients in the health care system (Bringewatt, 1998).

According to the National Chronic Care Consortium (Bringewatt, 1998), cost reduction and improved quality of care will not be attained until purchasers, payers, and providers focus on the problems of individuals with chronic disease. To succeed with this task, providers of health care need to move beyond consolidation of services to a transformation of financing, administration, and delivery of care (Bringewatt, 1998).

Services for those with chronic illness are financed by multiple public and private sources. Each of these sources uses a different approach to program administration. Purchasers of benefits under Medicare and Medicaid have seen managed care companies as the primary vehicle to ratchet down costs and ensure customer satisfaction. However, in most cases, managed care companies have functioned as third-party payers, with costs and quality managed through a series of cost- or discounted-based subcontracts, similar to those used in fee-for-service. Problems of chronic illness and disability require that all managed care companies and health system executives shift the focus of financing to whatever combination of care is most cost effective in addressing specific chronic conditions (Bringewatt, 1998).

Currently, the administration, financing, and oversight of government-sponsored programs have produced a fragmented, institutionally-based, reactive, cure-oriented approach to care. Medicare, Medicaid, and a host of other programs available to people at various stages of disability frequently provide incentives to third-party payers and providers to maintain antiquated operations. Rules and regulations provide disincentives for using collaborative, disability prevention methods.

Gauging Health Care Costs

Several economic or financial measures are commonly used to gauge health care expenses. These measures include total costs, a percent of the gross domestic product (GDP), and per capita costs. The continued upward trend in these measures is important to politicians and policy makers in identifying the current crisis in health care and developing solutions.

Total Costs

The National Health Care Expenditure was $1.7 trillion in 2003. In 1970, the National Health Care Expenditure was 7.0% of the Gross Domestic Product (GDP) and in 2003 it was 15.3% (Smith, Cowan, Sensening & Catlin, 2005). However, one must keep in perspective that the population has increased from 210.2 million in 1970 to 285.5 million in 2002 (Centers for Medicare and Medicaid Services, 2003).

Gross Domestic Product

GDP is a measure of the total production and consumption of goods and services in the United States. Most industrialized countries, including the United States, use the GDP instead of the gross national product (GNP) as their chief economic indicator. The GDP measures the values of all goods and services produced within a nation's borders regardless of the nationality of the producer. The share of GDP devoted to health care in 2003 was 15.3 percent, compared with 13.7 percent in 1993 (Smith et al., 2005). Figure 27-1 denotes the rise in health care from 1960 to 2010 (projected).

Per Capita

Per capita expenditures reflect average health care costs per person. This measure is used for group comparisons based on socioeconomic and geographic differences. Per capita data are based on averages and therefore can be misleading. In 2003, $5,670 was spent per capita on health care costs in the United States as compared with $4,094 in 1998 (Smith et al., 2005).

Issues of Rising Health Care Costs

Health care spending had been characterized by unprecedented slow growth during the late 1990s and early 2000s. The most important factor in decelerating public spending was Medicare, with the early impact of the Balanced Budget Act of 1997 (BBA) reducing spending from 6 percent in 1997 to 2.5 percent in 1998 (Levit et al., 2000). Growth in private health insurance premiums picked up its pace in 1998, and it has been suggested that this will continue through 2010. The hospital industry continues to consolidate into regional and national alliances in an attempt to improve operating efficiency. Physician practices continue to increase in size as an attempt to increase their power during negotiation of managed care plans. It is expected that this action will continue as Congress grapples with the budget in an attempt to slow Medicare spending growth.

To more accurately understand the crisis of health care costs in the United States and describe the patterns that caused this crisis, this chapter addresses how health care is paid for, where this money goes, and the amount of money spent.

Paying for Health Care

There are three primary sources of payment: public sources, private insurance, and direct or out-of-pocket expenditures by consumers. During 2003, private expenditures were 55 percent of total national health expenditures, while the government (public sources) spent 45 percent of those expenses.

FIGURE 27-1

National Health Expenditures as a Percentage of Gross Domestic Product, 1960–2010

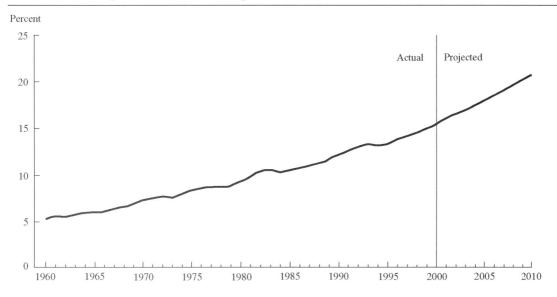

SOURCE: Health Care Financing Administration (2000). Data from the Office of National Health Statistics.

The percentage of private expenditures continues to increase (Smith et al., 2005) (see Table 27-1).

Changes in private funding shares of health spending from 1970 to 2001 came from out-of-pocket payments, which fell from 39.7 percent to 16.6 percent (CMS, 2003). While the out-of-pocket share remained stable in the late 90s, the share coming from private health insurance rose for the first time since 1990, accounting for most of the private share increase. Figure 27-2 depicts the percentages of the different sources of health care spending.

Public Sources

Since the introduction of Medicare and Medicaid in the mid-1960s, the federal government has become the single largest payer for health care.

Medicaid Medicaid spending totaled $258 billion in 2002, an increase of 11.7 percent from 2001. Slow spending rates over the previous four years led to stability in Medicaid's share of overall health spending, at approximately 14.8 percent (CMS, 2003).

Between 2000 and 2002, the number of children and adults eligible for Medicaid grew by 5.6 million. This increase is attributed to an extension of the programs offered under Medicaid and the weak economic environment. This rapid increase in enrollment has caused 45 states to enact measures to control spending such as provider rate freezes or reductions, cuts in benefits and policies to contain growth on prescription drug spending (Levit et al., 2004).

Medicare Medicare is the second largest entitlement program in the United States (after Social Security) and provides 95% of the health insurance coverage to people who are disabled or over the age of 65. In 2001, the federal government spent $241 billion to finance the health care of 78 million

TABLE 27-1

National Health Expenditures by Source of Funds, 1990, 1994, 1998 and 2003

Year	Amount in Billions			
	1990	*1994*	*1998*	*2003*
Total	$697.5	$937.1	$1,149.1	$1,678.9
All private funds	413.1	517.2	626.4	913.2
Consumer				
Total	380.8	478.7	574.4	763.7
Out-of-pocket	148.4	176.0	199.5	230.5
Private health insurance	232.4	302.7	337.0	600.6
Other	32.3	38.6	37.9	82.1
Government				
Total	284.3	419.9	522.7	765.7
Federal	195.8	301.9	376.9	541.7
State and local	88.5	118.0	145.8	224

Source: Smith, C., Cowan, C., Sensening, A., & Catlin, A., (2005) Health spending growth slows in 2003. *Health Affairs, 24* (1), 185–194. Copyright © 2005 by Project Hope. Reproduced with permission of Project Hope in the format Textbook via Copyright Clearance Center.

people (Hoffman et al., 2002). Medicare is divided into two parts: Part A and Part B. Medicare Part A helps pay the cost of inpatient hospital care, skilled nursing facility care, home health care, and hospice care. Medicare Part B provides for various services, such as doctor fees at 80 percent of the approved charge for most reasonable and necessary services, 100 percent of the cost for up to 35 hours per week of skilled nursing and home health aide services, annual immunizations to prevent influenza and pneumonia, annual mammograms for women over the age of 40, annual Pap smears for high-risk women, bone density measurement and colorectal cancer screening for all over the age of 50, diabetes self-management (training for patients, glucose monitors, and test strips), and prostate cancer screening for men age 50 and older. Lastly, Medicare Part B pays 80 percent of durable medical equipment, 50 percent of outpatient hospital services, 80 percent of physical therapy, 100 percent of laboratory tests and x-rays, 80 percent of ambulance service, and 80 percent of blood transfusions after the first three units.

In 2003, Medicare, the largest public payer of health care, spent $246.8 billion for the health care

of 41 million elderly and disabled beneficiaries. This number accounts for 19 percent of the nation's total health care spending (CMS, 2003). Medicare's most recent peak in growth occurred in 2001, as its spending grew 9.5 percent before slowing to 8.4 percent in 2002 (Levit et al., 2004).

Given that the first baby boomers will reach Medicare eligibility in 2011, the Medicare system is expected to be depleted by 2026. The debate on how to structure the Medicare program (including coverage of prescription drugs) and the role of the private sector in providing care is controversial.

Medigap Medigap policies fill some of the gaps in Medicare coverage, such as the 20 percent coinsurance payment for doctors' services. There are ten types of Medigap plans, labeled A through J. Each plan type varies with the number of services offered and the cost. However, none of the plans cover benefits that might be needed for individuals with chronic illness: long-term custodial care at home or in a nursing facility, vision or dental care, hearing aids, private duty nursing, or unlimited prescription drug coverage.

FIGURE 27-2

Distribution of Spending for Personal Health Care by Source of Payment, 1960–2000

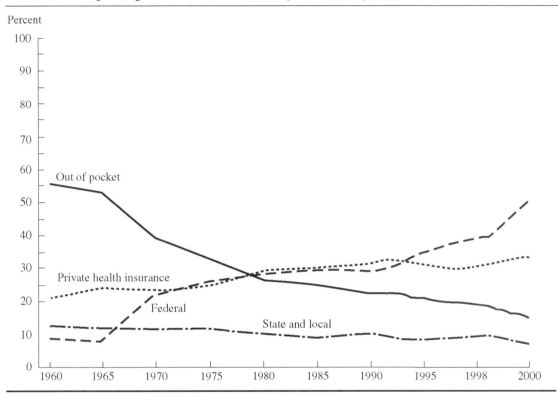

SOURCE: CMS, Office of the Actuary, National Health Statistics Group

Private Health Insurance Private health insurance paid for one-third ($549.6 billion) of the total health care spending in 2002. Premiums increased 10.9 percent in 2002, compared with 10.3 percent in 2001. This represented a reversal when compared with the period 1994 to 1997, when premiums grew more slowly than benefits.

Migration of workers enrolled in employer-sponsored plans from indemnity to managed care plans continues. Consumers are facing higher co-payments and deductibles as well as increases in co-pays for prescription drugs. More than half of the covered workers were enrolled in three-tier plans in 2002, compared with 29 percent in 2000. Covered workers are paying more out-of-pocket expenses for health care than ever before. These out-of-pocket expenses are in the form of drug copayments which often are more costly for the individual than are the premiums (Levit et al., 2004).

Long-term care insurance has been available in the United States since the early 1970s. With most policies, benefits go into effect after a person has demonstrated an inability to perform at least two activities of daily living, such as bathing, dressing, eating, or toileting. However, this coverage is not inexpensive. Policies may cost from $900 to more than $8,000 a year, depending on the age of the buyer and the benefits chosen (Levit et al., 2000). Additionally, roughly one in four people who apply do not qualify because of preexisting health problems, such as multiple sclerosis, Alzheimer's disease, Parkinson's disease, or other chronic conditions, or are already bedridden with a physical or mental disorder. However, most long-term care policies do cover these conditions if the client is diagnosed after enrollment in the plan.

The United Seniors Health Cooperative cautions potential buyers that if paying the premiums is going to cause financial hardship, alternatives should be carefully considered. What is suggested is that no more than seven percent of one's annual income be paid toward the cost of this insurance (Levit et al., 2000).

Out-of-Pocket Expenses Out-of-pocket dollars represent the amount of money individuals pay in deductibles and co-payments to hospitals and nursing homes; for dental, medical care, and other professional services; and for vision care, drugs, and other non-medical durables. For the elderly and clients with chronic illness who use multiple drugs, these expenses may be exorbitant.

The rise in private and public managed care enrollment in the 1990s created an environment in which insured persons gained greater access to drug coverage at lower out-of-pocket costs, thereby increasing demand. Demand increased further as the number of new drugs brought to market soared, which occurred partly as a result of the reduced average time required by the Food and Drug Administration (FDA) to approve a drug for sale (from two years in 1993 to 11.7 months in 1997) (Crippen, 2000).

Most people spend out-of-pocket health care dollars on over-the-counter drugs and insurance costs (premiums, deductibles, and coinsurance). Out-of-pocket expenses as a proportion of income have remained relatively constant (4.6 percent) for Americans in households not headed by an elderly person. For households headed by an elderly person, these costs are a considerably higher percentage (11 percent) of income (CBO, 2000).

Health Care Spending

Health care spending slowed to 7.7% in 2003, much slower than the 9.3 percent growth in 2002 (Smith, Cowan, Sensening & Catlin, 2005). However

for the first time ever, health care spending accounted for over 15% of the gross domestic product (GDP), specifically 15.3 percent of the GDP, up .4% over 2002 data (Smith et al., 2005).

Although aggregate statistics indicate unprecedented slow, stable growth over the past several years, a more detailed examination of these estimates signals important changes taking place in the nation's health care system. Real (inflation-adjusted) health-spending growth, less than 4.5 percent each year from 1995 to 2001, accelerated to 4.9 percent in 2002. More than half of public spending for health care came from private sources. Private health insurance contributed 41 percent and consumers' direct payments accounted for 9 percent of health care costs (Levit et al., 2004).

In 2002, share of spending from Medicaid nearly matched Medicare. The most important factor in decelerating public spending was Medicare. The impact of the BBA of 1997, and continued progress in combating fraud and abuse, combined to reduce Medicare spending. The Medicare provisions of the BBA were Congress' response to projected depletion of the Medicare Hospital Insurance (HI) trust fund and Medicare spending growth that exceeded private insurers' spending growth between 1992 and 2002. BBA provisions that were effective in fiscal year 1998 and additional provisions to be implemented over the subsequent five years have held down Medicare and public spending growth through 2002 (Levit et al., 2004).

Other changes in the health care system affected providers as well. Hospitals' contribution to spending had a growth from 3.7 percent in 2000 to 7.5 percent in 2001, and 9.5 percent in 2002. Hospital spending represented 32 percent of health care expenditures in 2002. Of concern to the public is the poor economic growth which threaten the generosity of health care benefits provided by insurance companies and the ability of health care facilities to write off losses (Levit et al., 2004).

Where Health Care Money Goes

In 2003, national health expenditures topped $1.7 trillion, up 7.7 percent from 2002 (Smith et al.,

2005). This marked the sixth consecutive year in which spending growth increased above 6 percent. On a per capita basis, health care spending increased $5670. Hospitals received 31 percent, physicians 22 percent, drugs 11 percent, nursing homes 7 percent, home care 3 percent, and other professional services 26 percent of the national health expenditure in 2003 (Smith et al., 2005) (Tables 27-2 and 27-3).

Hospitals

Hospital expenditures totaled $515.9 billion in 2003. The growth reflects a demand for services, rising expenses and hospitals asking for higher reimbursement from private payors (Smith et al., 2005).

The largest share of hospital inflation is tied to payroll. Compensation to employees accounts for 62 percent of operating costs. Rising costs associated with the nursing shortage and hospital malpractice insurance have contributed to increased costs. Also influencing hospital costs are the recent increases in inpatient days associated with increased admissions (Levit et al., 2004).

Physicians

Physician services accounted for $369.7 billion in 2003, 22 percent of all health care expenditures (Smith et al., 2005). Public funds paid for 60 percent of physician services, while out-of-pocket payments from the consumer paid for 20 percent (Levit et al., 2004).

TABLE 27-2

Expenditures for Health Services and Supplies, By Type of Service and Source of Funds, Calendar Year 2003

Spending category	Total	Private funds			Public funds			
		Total[a]	Out-of-pocket	Private health insurance	Total	Medicare	Federal and state Medicaid[b]	Other public
Health services and supplies (billions)	$1,614.2	$892.6	$230.5	$600.6	$721.7	$283.1	$268.6	$169.9
Personal health care	1,440.8	809.2	230.5	518.7	631.5	274.9	250.0	106.6
Hospital care	515.9	215.1	16.3	177.4	300.8	156.4	87.5	56.8
Professional services	542.0	356.0	83.8	238.9	186.1	80.7	67.6	37.7
Physician and clinical services	369.7	246.8	37.6	183.6	123.0	73.8	26.4	22.8
Other professional services	48.5	34.9	13.3	18.8	13.6	6.9	2.6	4.2
Dental services	74.3	69.4	32.9	36.5	4.9	0.1	4.2	0.6
Other personal health care	49.5	4.9	—[c]	—[c]	44.6	—[c]	34.4	10.2
Nursing home and home health	150.8	58.6	37.5	15.7	92.2	26.6	61.0	4.6
Home health care[d]	40.0	15.1	6.6	7.3	24.9	12.9	9.9	2.1
Nursing home care[d]	110.8	43.5	30.9	8.5	67.3	13.7	51.0	2.5
Retail outlet sales of medical products	232.1	179.6	92.9	86.7	52.5	11.2	33.9	7.4
Prescription drugs	179.2	136.0	53.2	82.9	43.2	2.8	33.9	6.4
Durable medical equipment	20.4	12.8	9.0	3.8	7.6	6.6	0.0	1.0
Other nondurable medical products	32.5	30.7	30.7	—[c]	1.7	1.7	—[c]	—[c]
Program administration and net cost of private health insurance	119.7	83.3	—[c]	81.9	36.4	8.2	18.6	9.6
Government public health activities	53.8	—[c]	—[c]	—[c]	53.8	—[c]	—[c]	53.8

NOTE: Numbers may not add to totals because of rounding.
[a]Includes other private funds.
[b]Includes Medicaid State Children's Health Insurance Program (SCHIP) expansion (Title XIX).
[c]Not applicable.
[d]Freestanding facilities only. Additional services of this type are provided in hospital-based facilities and counted as hospital care.

SOURCE: Smith C., Cowan C., Senseing A., and Catlin A. (2005). Health spending growth slows in 2003. *Health Affairs*, 24 (1), 185–94.

TABLE 27-3

National Health Expenditures (NHE), Aggregate and Per Capita Amounts, and Share of Gross Domestic Product (GDP), Selected Calendar Years 1970–2003

Spending category	1970	1980	1993	1997	1999	2001	2002	2003
NHE, billions	$73.1	$245.8	$888.1	$1,093.1	$1,222.2	$1,426.4	$1,559.0	$1,678.9
Health services and supplies	67.3	233.5	856.3	1,055.8	1,180.2	1,373.8	1,499.8	1,614.2
Personal health care	63.2	214.6	775.8	959.2	1,065.6	1,235.5	1,342.9	1,440.8
Hospital care	27.6	101.5	320.0	367.6	393.4	446.4	484.2	515.9
Professional services	20.7	67.3	280.7	352.2	397.7	464.4	503.0	542.0
Physician and clinical services	14.0	47.1	201.2	241.0	270.9	315.1	340.8	369.7
Other professional services	0.7	3.6	24.5	33.4	36.7	42.6	46.1	48.5
Dental services	4.7	13.3	38.9	50.2	56.4	65.6	70.9	74.3
Other personal health care	1.3	3.3	16.1	27.7	33.7	41.1	45.3	49.5
Nursing home and home health	4.4	20.1	87.6	119.6	122.9	134.9	143.1	150.8
Home health care[a]	0.2	2.4	21.9	34.5	32.3	33.7	36.5	40.0
Nursing home care[a]	4.2	17.7	65.7	85.1	90.7	101.2	106.6	110.8
Retail outlet sales of medical products	10.5	25.7	87.5	119.8	151.6	189.7	212.6	232.1
Prescription drugs	5.5	12.0	51.3	75.7	104.4	140.8	161.8	179.2
Durable medical equipment	1.6	3.9	12.8	16.2	17.2	18.4	19.6	20.4
Other nondurable medical products	3.3	9.8	23.4	27.9	30.0	30.5	31.1	32.5
Program administration and net cost of private health insurance	2.8	12.1	53.3	61.3	73.3	90.9	105.7	119.7
Government public health activities	1.4	6.7	27.2	35.3	41.2	47.4	51.2	53.8
Investment	5.7	12.3	31.8	37.2	42.0	52.6	59.2	64.6
Research[b]	2.0	5.5	15.6	18.7	23.7	32.9	36.5	40.2
Construction	3.8	6.8	16.2	18.5	18.3	19.7	22.7	24.5
Population (millions)	210.2	230.4	264.8	277.6	284.1	290.3	293.2	296.1
NHG per capita	$348	$1,067	$3,354	$3,938	$4,302	$4,914	$5,317	$5,670
GDP, billions of dollars	$1,039	$2,790	$6,657	$8,304	$9,268	$10,128	$10,487	$11,004
NHE as percent of GDP	7.0%	8.8%	13.3%	13.2%	13.2%	14.1%	14.9%	15.3%
Implicit price deflator for GDP	27.5	54.0	88.4	95.4	97.9	102.4	104.1	106.0
Real GDP, billions of dollars	$3,772	$5,162	$7,533	$8,704	$9,470	$9,891	$10,075	$10,381
Real NHE[c], billions of dollars	$265.3	$454.7	$1,004.8	$1,145.6	$1,248.8	$1,393.0	$1,497.7	$1,583.9
Personal health care deflator[d]	16.0	34.4	81.6	92.2	96.7	103.9	107.9	111.8

[a]Freestanding facilities only. Additional services of this type are provided if hospital-based facilities and counted as hospital care.
[b]Research and development expenditures of drug companies and other manufacturers and providers of medical equipment and supplies are excluded from "research expenditures" but are included in the expenditure class in which the product fails.
[c]Deflated using the implicit price deflator for GDP(2000=100.0).
[d]Personal health care (PHC) implicit price deflator is constructed from the Producer Price Index for hospital care, Nursing Home Input Price Index for nursing home care, and Consumer Price Indices specific to each of the remaining PHC components.

SOURCE: Smith C., Cowan C., Senseing A., and Catlin A. (2005). Health spending growth slows in 2003. *Health Affairs*, 24 (1), 185–94.

The substantial and rapid shift to managed care among employer-sponsored private health insurance and public program enrollment in the early to mid-1990s had a major impact on many aspects of physician services. This is apparent in the stabilization of the share of physician spending covered by private health insurance. The trend toward managed care combined with the phase-in of a Medicare physician payment and volume performance stan- dards helped to restrain growth in spending for physician services (Levit et al., 2000).

Doctors are called "participating providers" if they "accept assignment," indicating they always ac- cept the Medicare-approved amount as payment in full. This means they aren't allowed to charge a client more than Medicare's approved charge for their ser- vices. Medicare pays the physician 80 percent of the approved amount and the individual pays the other

20 percent. Doctors who treat Medicare beneficiaries who are also eligible for Medicaid (dual eligibles) must accept Medicare assignment. Doctors who do not accept assignment can charge no more than 15 percent above Medicare's approved amount. This means the client pays no more than the extra 15 percent, plus any required deductible and coinsurance.

Nursing Homes

Expenditures for care provided by free-standing nursing homes totaled $110.8 billion in 2003. Growth in spending for nursing home care has decreased steadily since 1990. Much of this decrease is the result of slowing growth in medical price increases and expanded use of alternative treatment settings, such as home health care, assisted living facilities, and community-based day care (Levit et al., 2004).

Public sources funded more than 60 percent of nursing home care in 2002, up from 51 percent in 1990. Medicaid's share of nursing home spending remained fairly steady, rising only slightly from 45.5 percent in 1990 to 49 percent in 2002. Meanwhile, states are trying to shifts patients into community-based dwelling such as retirement communities and assisted living. The goal is to maintain independence as long as possible (Levit et al., 2004).

The average cost of nursing home care is nearly $50,000 a year (Crippen, 2000). Medicare covers only short periods of skilled nursing home care after a hospital stay, and few individuals have long-term care insurance. Almost a third of individuals pay all costs out-of-pocket and almost 70 percent receive help from Medicaid. Many nursing home residents are able to pay the full cost of their care when they are admitted, but they deplete their savings and other assets paying for care and eventually qualify for Medicaid. Medicaid covers all of an individuals' nursing home care as well as some basic needs, such as toiletries and over-the-counter medications. Medicaid pays for prescription drugs and some other services not paid for by Medicare.

Home Care

Home health spending, $40 billion in 2003, experienced a wide swing in growth during the 1990s (Smith et al., 2005). There was a 28.2 percent increase from 1990 to 1998. The BBA mandated stringent provisions for home health costs and utilization controls, including restricted access to services and redefined criteria for coverage of visits. The BBA also led to some of the consolidations, mergers, and closures in the industry and to the decline in home health expenditures in 1998 (Levit et al., 1998). Only $6.5 billion of the cost for home care was paid out-of-pocket from consumers while Medicare paid for $11.4 billion in 2002. The majority of the cost for home care is paid by Medicare and Medicaid (see chapter 22, home health care).

Chronic Illness and Costs

The incidence of most chronic diseases increases with age with most individuals over age 65 having one or more such conditions. The leading chronic conditions for individuals 65 and older are: hypertension (51%); arthritis (37%); heart disease (29%) and eye disorders (25%. (Partnership for Solutions, 2004). The medical costs of people with chronic diseases account for more than 75% of the nation's $1.4 trillion medical care costs (CDC, 2004)

Discussing the financial implications of all chronic diseases is outside the scope of this chapter. However, several conditions are discussed to demonstrate the financial impact of having a chronic condition.

Cognitive Disorders

Alzheimer's disease is a progressive, degenerative disease of the brain, and the most common form of dementia. Approximately four million Americans have Alzheimer's disease (Alzheimer's Association, 2001). A national survey conducted in 1993 indicates that approximately 19 million Americans have a family member with Alzheimer's, and 37 million know someone with the disease (Alzheimer's Association, 2001). Fourteen million Americans will have Alzheimer's by 2050 unless a cure or preventative treatment is found (Alzheimer's Association, 2001).

A person with Alzheimer's disease lives an average of eight years and can live as many as 20 years or more from the onset of symptoms. Alzheimer's disease costs the United States at least $100 billion a year (Alzheimer's Association, 2004). Neither Medicare nor private health insurance covers the type of long-term care that most of these individuals need. Alzheimer's disease costs American businesses more than $61 billion annually with $24.6 billion covering health care expenditures and $36.5 billion covering the costs related to caregivers (Alzheimer's Association, 2004).

More than seven of ten people with Alzheimer's disease live at home, with almost 75 percent of home care being provided by family and friends. The remainder is "paid" care costing an average of $12,500 per year, most of which is covered by families as out-of-pocket expenses. Half of all nursing home residents suffer from Alzheimer's or a related disorder. The average per resident cost for nursing home care is $42,000 per year but can exceed $70,000 per year in some areas of the United States. The average lifetime cost per individual with Alzheimer's disease is estimated to be $174,000 (Alzheimer's Association, 2004).

Diabetes Mellitus

Diabetes is thought to affect more than 17 million individuals in the United States. Since 1991 the incidence of diabetes has increased by 61% (CDC, 2004). Diabetes is the leading cause of blindness, end-stage renal failure, and lower extremity amputation (Drass et al., 1998).

The use of health care services by persons with diabetes is high, with a large portion of the cost of diabetes attributed to inpatient hospital care. In 1996, there were 503,000 hospital discharges with diabetes listed as the first diagnosis and 3.8 million discharges listing diabetes as one of seven discharge diagnoses. Diabetes was one of the top three diagnoses for 1.2 million emergency room visits. Approximately 14 percent of persons with diabetes had a diabetes-related emergency room visit in 1996, with the highest rate among individuals over the age of 45 (CDC, 2000).

Spinal Cord and Brain Injuries

There are an estimated 250,000 spinal cord-injured (SCI) individuals living in the United States. On average, 11,000 new injuries are reported every year, with vehicular accidents causing 40 percent of these spinal cord injuries. More than half of the SCI population was injured between the ages of 16 and 30, and the most frequently occurring age at injury is 19. The majority of SCI individuals survive and live a near-normal life span. Initial hospitalization (an average of 100 days), adaptive equipment, and home modification costs following injury average $140,000. Additional lifetime costs average $600,000 and can reach as high as $1.35 million, depending on the severity of injury (Christopher Reeve Paralysis Foundation, 2000) (see http://www.paralysis.org/).

Two million brain injuries occur each year in the United States, resulting in 75,000 to 100,000 deaths each year. The typical brain injury victim is a young male, between the ages of 16 and 24, who is injured in a vehicular accident. A survivor of a severe brain injury incurs costs of between $4.1 million and $9 million in lifetime care (see http://www.paralysis.org/). These individuals typically apply for Medicaid and require significant financial resources for lifetime care.

Chronic Obstructive Pulmonary Disease

Chronic bronchitis and emphysema take a heavy toll on our economy. According to estimates made by the National Heart Lung and Blood Institute, in 1998, the annual cost to the nation for chronic obstructive pulmonary disease was $26 billion. This includes $13.6 billion in direct care expenditures, $6.4 billion in indirect morbidity costs, and $6 billion in direct mortality costs (Asthma and Allergy Foundation, 2000).

Asthma is responsible for 500,000 hospitalizations a year. Direct medical expenditures for asthma amounted to $7.5 billion in 1998, and indirect economic losses accounted for an additional $3.8 billion. Of direct medical care costs, approximately 57 percent was spent on hospitalization, outpatient visits, and emergency department visits (U.S. Department of Health and Human Services, 2000). Asthma accounts for about 1.8 million emergency room visits and 10 million doctor office visits each year (Asthma and Allergy Foundation, 2000).

Osteoporosis

Osteoporosis accounts for approximately 1.5 million new fractures each year, with associated medical charges (including rehabilitation and extended treatment facilities) costing an estimated $17 billion in 2001, according to the National Osteoporosis Foundation. Because osteoporosis affects primarily the elderly, the National Osteoporosis Foundation estimates that these costs will increase to $200 billion by the year 2040 as the number of individuals over the age of 65 increases (National Osteoporosis Foundation, 2004).

Hip fractures are the most serious consequence of osteoporosis. Osteoporosis-related hip fractures result in estimated costs of $12.8 billion to $17.8 billion per year for medical care, extended treatment facilities, and the value of lost wages. Rehabilitation and institutionalization costs, at about $5.1 billion to $7.1 billion, account for 40 percent of the estimated total economic cost of osteoporosis-related hip fractures (Barefield, 1996).

Cardiovascular Disease

The estimated cost of cardiovascular disease and stroke in the United States in 2005 was estimated at $393.5 billion. Of this total, heart disease makes up the largest portion of the expenditure, at $254.8 billion. A majority of these funds are given to hospitals and nursing homes, with nursing homes receiving $39.3 billion and physicians receiving $36 billion (AHA, 2004). Table 27-4 demonstrates estimated direct and indirect costs of cardiovascular diseases.

Cardiovascular medical procedures increased 350 percent from 1979 to 1997. In 1995, 669,000 outpatient cardiovascular surgical procedures were performed. Of these outpatient cardiovascular surgical procedures, 373,000 were done on males and 296,000 on females. Cardiovascular surgical procedures include cardiac catheterization, coronary

TABLE 27-4

Costs of Cardiovascular Disease in Billions of Dollars

	Heart Disease	Coronary Heart Disease	Stroke	Hypertension	Congestive Heart Failure	Total Cardiovascular Disease
Direct costs						
Hospital	$77.7	$39.9	$14.8	$6.0	$14.7	$109.8
Nursing homes	19.1	10.0	13.2	3.9	3.6	39.3
Physician	18.5	10.4	2.9	10.4	1.9	36.0
Drugs/Other medical durables	19.4	9.0	1.2	22.3	2.9	45.9
Home health care	4.8	1.4	2.9	1.6	2.2	10.9
Total expenditure	$139.5	$70.7	$35.0	$44.2	$25.3	$241.9
Indirect costs						
Lost productivity/ morbidity	21.4	9.4	6.3	7.5	NA	34.8
Lost productivity/ mortality	93.9	62.0	25.5	8.0	2.6	116.8
Grand total	$254.8	$142.1	$56.8	$59.7	$27.9	$393.5

SOURCE: American Heart Association, 2004.

artery bypass surgery, heart transplants, and percutaneous transluminal coronary angioplasty (PTCA). The average cost of coronary artery bypass surgery in 1995 was $44,820. The first year following a heart transplant the average cost is $253,200 with yearly follow-up costs of $21,200. The average cost of a PTCA was $20,370 in 1995 (see http://www.americanheart.org).

Children and Chronic Illness

Acute care technology has saved the lives of many infants, but leaves many of them with life-long conditions requiring ongoing health care. Depending on the condition and its severity, children with chronic illness may require any of a wide range of health services and supports. Federal law recognizes this and stipulates that children enrolled in Medicaid are entitled to case management, rehabilitative services, personal care, psychological counseling, recuperative and long-term residential care, and many other services, as long as they are deemed necessary by a physician or other health care providers. Approximately 2.5 million children with chronic conditions are enrolled in the Medicaid program (Newacheck & Hughes, 1994).

Uninsured Children In 1997, there were 11 million uninsured children, and despite changes in Title XXI and Medicaid, only 55 percent of the eligible children were provided some health care coverage. Many of the country's uninsured children live in areas that do not have easy access to health care services, and they may receive less care as parents struggle to find the funds to pay for health care. A majority of uninsured children are Hispanics (30%), followed by Blacks (19.7%) and Whites (14.4%), according to the March 1999 U.S. Census Bureau (Frankenfield et al., 1997).

Impact of Rising Costs

The projected long-range fiscal shortfall in the federal budget is associated with three phenomena: the aging and the eventual retirement of the Baby Boom generation, increased life expectancy, and escalating per capita medical costs. Assumptions of the Social Security trustees are that from 2000 to 2030, the number of elderly people in the United States will nearly double, while the number of people ages 20 to 64 will only increase by 16 percent (CBO, 2000a). With demographic trends such as these, federal programs for the elderly will consume sharply increasing shares of national income and the federal budget. According to Social Security and Medicare trustees, spending for Social Security and Medicare as a percentage of the GDP will rise from 6.5 percent in 2000 to almost 11 percent in 2030. Using similar projections, the CBO expects that in 2030, those programs will constitute more than half of total federal spending, compared with 39 percent in 1999 (CBO, 2000a). In addition, the Medicaid program will experience severe budgetary pressures in meeting the long-term care needs of the low-income elderly population.

Today's children are the taxpayers of the future, and they will be the ones called upon to pay for the increasing portion of the federal budget that will be devoted to caring for the elderly. However, significant wage growth is assumed in most futurist's projections, so today's children will likely be more affluent and may be able and willing to share an increasing portion of their income with the generations that preceded them (CBO, 2000a).

Solutions to Rising Health Care Costs

The resources required to finance the government's obligations are drawn from the overall economy when the obligations are liquidated. Projections are that in 2030, pledges to the elderly as well as other federal priorities—such as national defense, assistance to state and local education agencies, public health services, and transportation projects—will require the government to draw on economic resources available at that time.

One way to prepare for the budgetary pressures expected in the twenty-first century is to save more as a nation. By implementing policies that promote capital accumulation, the nation could boost both its productive capacity and its wealth by essentially helping decrease future consumption. However, adding to the supply of capital requires less current consumption in exchange for more national saving and investment. One approach to increasing national saving is for the federal government to have annual budget surpluses, as long as the policies creating the surpluses do not come at the expense of private saving. Strategies to encourage private saving might also help to pay for future consumption.

Economic growth would expand the capacity to fund Social Security benefits and other federal commitments, and a healthy economy could ease the transfer of additional resources to retirees. Strong growth swells revenues, which, if used for debt reduction, would reduce interest costs and improve the overall outlook for government budgets. Despite those benefits, however, growth will not eliminate the imbalances of the current Social Security program. The reason is that economic growth generally increases real wages, and under the current benefit formula, higher wages subsequently translate into higher Social Security benefits, although with a substantial lag. Therefore, although the nation might be wealthier, it would still face a sharp increase in the budgetary resources necessary to pay for the Social Security and health care costs of the Baby Boom generation during its retirement (CBA, 2000a).

Cycle of Impoverishment

Mr. B. is a 56-year-old truck driver who had to quit work two years ago due to his emphysema. He is currently disabled and on Medicare. He was the sole income for his wife. His children are grown and live in another state. He is on nebulizer treatments four times a day and oxygen prn. After recently being hospitalized with pneumonia, he returns home. He typically has pneumonia two to three times a year and has difficulty recovering from the infections due to his chronic obstructive pulmonary disease. He was evaluated several weeks ago for sleep apnea because of his snoring and wife's persistence that he be evaluated. The results showed that he has sleep apnea lasting 20 seconds. It is recommended that he obtain a cpap machine for sleep at night. He is on eight medications for his chronic illness. He takes Prozac, Singular, and Provental inhaler twice a day; Prevacid each A.M.; a stool softener each P.M.; Lasix twice a day; potassium twice a day; and an Ambien for sleep at night. The cost of his monthly oral medications and the nebulizer medications is approximately $268 a month. His house rent is $600 per month, and the average cost of utilities is $90 month. He receives a disability check each month for $558. His wife now works at a local supermarket, making minimum wage. Her income covers the groceries, gasoline for the car, and the rest of the monthly expenses. The cost of medications, rent, and utilities averages $958. He is $400 short each month in covering his expenses. His wife brings home $800 a month. After paying the $400 toward his expenses, she uses the other $400 to pay for groceries and gasoline. This is a typical scenario of a couple trying to manage from one month to the next with chronic illness.

Questions to ask:

1. What pharmaceutical resources exist for individuals who are at poverty level?
2. Are there less expensive alternatives to Mr. B's current list of medications?
3. What solutions can you see for Mr. B. and his wife? Will it ever be possible to break this "cycle of impoverishment?"

Managing Chronic Conditions

Prevention

The United States cannot effectively address escalating health care costs without addressing the problem of chronic disease. Historically, private and government sources have not funded preventive health care; however, some change in funding is beginning to be realized. Most insurance companies are now willing to pay for some preventive services as well as an annual health physical. Even though Medicare does not pay for routine physical examinations, a number of preventive tests are currently covered under Medicare Part B. These tests include screenings for breast, cervical, vaginal, colorectal, and prostate cancer; testing for loss of bone mass; diabetes monitoring and self-management; and influenza, pneumonia, and hepatitis B vaccinations.

The Centers for Disease Control (2000) reports that prevention of chronic disease has financial implications for health care expenditures. The cost of preventing illness is far less than the expense of treatment of a chronic diseases that may last a lifetime. An example in the literature includes clinical smoking cessation interventions. These interventions would save an estimated $2,587 for each year of life saved, the most cost effective of all clinical preventive services. Another program that is beneficial is mammography screening every two years, at a cost of $8,280 and $9,890 per year of life saved. Increased spending on prevention in this country will occur once research can better demonstrate cost effectiveness.

Expanding Medicare

Medicare is the second largest entitlement program after Social Security. In 2003 this program spent $246.8 billion to finance the health care of 41 million individuals (CMS, 2003). Some political analysts project that the Medicare program will be threatened beginning in 2010, because the demand for services will grow dramatically while the number of people in the labor force will level off. Between 2000 and 2030, the number of individuals covered by Medicare is projected to double (CBO, 2000b).

Medicare's benefit package covers basic services such as hospital stays, postacute care, physicians' services, and other outpatient care. It does not cover outpatient prescription drugs. Spending for out-of-hospital medications accounted for ten percent of the total cost of health care services for the Medicare recipient in 1996 (Levit et al., 1998). Approximately $25 billion was spent on prescriptions, with individuals paying half of this cost out-of-pocket (Levit et al., 1998).

One idea being discussed is to increase the comprehensiveness of Medicare. This would eliminate the need for private insurance supplements and require Medicare to increase spending. Expanding services may decrease fee-for-service care to risk-based Medicare choice plans, such as plans proposed by the Bipartisan Commission on the Future of Medicare. Sample plans include the establishment of multiple plans in each geographic area, allowing recipients to enroll in at least one plan with a modest premium. Expensive plans, with more benefits, would be available for those recipients able to afford them. Competition among plans for enrollment would help to ensure that plans would provide adequate service at the lowest possible costs. Clearly, the long-term benefits of managed competition may or may not slow cost growth, but, certainly, a one-time reduction in cost for enrollees would occur when the individual moves from fee-for-service care to a more efficient managed care plan.

Expanding Health Insurance Coverage

The number of uninsured has risen, from 35 million in 1991 to more than 44 million in 1998 (CBO, 2000a, p. 36). Lack of health insurance coverage is a problem for individuals under the age of 65, because Medicare covers those 65 and over. In 1998, 18.4 percent of individuals under the age of 65 were without insurance coverage. About 15 percent of children do not have health coverage (CBO, 2000b).

Several approaches have been proposed to increase the number of insured in the United States. These include expanding the scope and funding of government insurance programs, providing tax incentives for health insurance, and regulating the private market to expand options for the purchase of lower cost health insurance. Another approach is to expand government funding for public health clinics and free clinics.

In 2000, approximately 60 million people were covered by Medicare, Medicaid, and SCHIP (State Children's Health Insurance Program), at a cost totaling more than $300 billion (Getzen, 2000). Medicare is the only program that is totally federally funded. Medicaid and SCHIP are programs cosponsored by both the federal and state governments. The federal government sets standards for insuring individuals, while the administration of the funds for Medicare and SCHIP is established by the states. Expansion of these programs would be guided by the states.

The number of individuals covered by Medicaid could be increased by expanding the eligibility requirements. Currently, each state defines eligibility and the level of coverage. Eligibility could be more uniform among states by requiring all states to standardize the level of poverty covered. Even if the program were expanded, there are those who would not enroll due to perceived stigma and others who lack the knowledge to enroll.

Expanding SCHIP would increase the number of low-income children covered by health insurance. Currently, federal support ranges from 65 to 85 percent, depending on a state's average per capita income. Federal expenditures for SCHIP were nearly $2 billion for the year 2000 (CBO, 2000a). States decide whether they want to use the SCHIP funds to expand Medicaid, develop or support children's programs, or to pay for specific services. Only 19 states used SCHIP funds in 1998, its first year of operation, and many states spent less than amounts allotted to them by the federal government. The BBA of 1997 gave states three years to spend their allocations. Unspent funds were to be redistributed by the Secretary of Health and Human Services in the fourth year (2001) to states that have spent their allocations. Expanding SCHIP to cover the parents of children covered has been proposed as well.

Providing Tax Incentives for Purchase of Insurance

Currently, the federal government forgoes tax revenues by excluding from income and payroll taxes the contributions that employers make for health benefits and by allowing deductions for certain health expenses. Also, flexible spending accounts are tax-free, and an employee's contribution to long-term care insurance and un-reimbursed medical expenses that exceed 7.5 percent of an individual's adjust gross income are tax-free. These un-reimbursed expenses include health insurance payments made by individuals, out-of-pocket payments, and certain costs for transportation, lodging, and long-term care. These initiatives have benefited more than 150 million people with employment-based insurance. Those who are self-employed may deduct 60 percent of their expenses for health insurance, with new regulations for that deduction to rise to 100 percent in 2003.

The current tax system favors those who are employed and receive employer-based coverage. People in the highest tax brackets benefit the most from this tax incentive. Because the savings depend on the tax rate, those who benefit the most are those who have the highest incomes. Possible expansion of tax benefits proposed by analysts include, the use of broader deductions, exclusions, or tax credits. More likely, a tax credit would be directed toward individuals who do not have access to employment-based coverage. A weakness of this proposal is that it would provide a tax credit only at the time of tax filing. Thus, the individual would still have to have funds available to purchase the health insurance initially, and only be "repaid" with a tax credit much later.

Long-Term Care Services for the Elderly

The demand for long-term care services will double over the next 30 years. In 2000, 7.5 million people over the age of 65, approximately 21 percent of the elderly population, required long-term care assistance (Crippen, 2000). Of these 7.5 million people, 1.5 million will need nursing home care and 2.2

million will be in an assisted-living center, utilizing home care, or living in community rest homes (Crippen, 2000). These statistics demonstrate the continued need to educate nurses in the delivery of long-term care and prepare them to care for the elderly population.

Presently, Medicare and Medicaid finance about half of the nation's nursing home and home care expenses. Medicaid provides catastrophic long-term care coverage for individuals of the middle class who have utilized all personal financial resources to cover the high expenses of long-term care. Private insurance accounted for one percent of spending on nursing home and home care in 1995 (CBO, 2000a, p. 36). It has been estimated that families provide long-term care at a value of $50 billion to $100 billion annually (CBO, 2000b). However, projections are that with smaller family size, the ability of families to provide long-term care will more than likely decrease in the future, leaving long term care costs for Medicaid.

Expanding Medicare and Medicaid for long-term care would require extending eligibility rules. Another possibility is to offer tax subsidies for long-term care services that would benefit low-income individuals. Another proposal is to establish a tax-deferred savings account that could be used for long-term care services. Such an account would be funded with pretax dollars, with interest accruing tax-free. A weakness of this proposal is that the amount of additional savings may be minimal, given the income of some taxpayers.

Expanding long-term insurance may be accomplished through employer-sponsored programs instead of the current individual and group association markets. Tax credits could be established for individuals purchasing long-term insurance; however, this initiative would be more useful to middle- and higher income taxpayers (National Rural Health Association, 2000).

The Future

Health care was a critical issue in the presidential election of 2004. In his first term in office, President George W. Bush had advocated spending taxpayers' money to finance a new government ben-

efit: prescription drug coverage for senior citizens. Enactment of the Medicare Prescription Drug, Improvement and Modernization Act of 2003 will increase costs by $395 billion during the 2004-2013 budget periods. Beginning in 2006, Medicare's new Part D will subsidize prescription drug coverage through managed care plans or employer-sponsored plans. This Act also provides for a drug discount card to cover $600 in prescription drugs per year for certain low-income Medicare recipients. It is estimated that by 2014, Part D will account for 22 percent of all Medicare spending (CBO, 2004). Other provisions of this law include a reduction in fee-for-service to providers of Medicare-insured clients. Medicare payments will be reduced by $28 billion beginning in 2005 (CBO, 2004).

The Republican health care plan has financial implications for the next decade as health care providers attempt to provide care to an aging population with chronic conditions. The National Defense Authorization Act for 2004 expands benefits for disabled retirees of the military with a 50% or greater disability. Under previous law, retired veterans could not receive both full retirement annuities and disability compensation from Veteran Affairs. Beginning in 2014, disabled retirees will be able to receive both their retirement and disability compensation. These provisions increased spending for military retirement by $1 billion in 2004 and $28 billion over the 2004-2013 periods (CBO, 2004).

Summary and Conclusions

To meet today's and tomorrow's challenge of caring for those with chronic illnesses, we must transform our current system of care by establishing person-centered, community-based, system-oriented approaches rooted in the principles of chronic disease management. This means integrated care management, integrated information, integrated financing, and integrated policy.

One must ask whether this nation can continue to devote ever-increasing resources and money to the health care industry. Proponents highlight that we have the finest health care system in the world. Opponents criticize that it is a nonsystem, highly fragmented, lacking coordination, lacking universal coverage, and too focused on acute care. As we come to grips with our inability to afford the current system, we will likely move toward a new and different system.

It is important that nurses expand their knowledge beyond the physical and psychosocial aspects of client care and into new arenas that include health care financing, economics, and insurance. Clients are increasingly faced with serious financial hardships and decisions about their health care. Further, most clients lack a fundamental understanding of health care delivery, costs, financing, and insurance. Nurses serve an important role in supporting and educating clients through their shared concerns, as well as in ex-

amining their own beliefs and practices so they can provide the most cost-effective, quality care possible.

Nurses are increasingly affected by the same economics of health care as their clients. Health care providers' profits and losses influence decisions about acquisitions of equipment used by nurses; budgets for nursing education departments; operational budgets, which include salaries; and allotment of nursing care hours. The future of nursing is in our ability not only to self-examine and change, but also to be leaders and innovators in a changing health care system. Nurses must look beyond the clinical arena and become more involved in the operational, financial, and political decisions of our employers and our governments.

Study Questions

1. Name three key factors that have led to the rise in health care costs over the past 30 years.
2. Identify the three primary sources of payment for health care, and discuss the shifts in payment and their impact on the government in financing health care.
3. Describe out-of-pocket expenses and their implications for the elderly and chronically ill population.
4. If the production of health care is an important part of our national economy, how does the rising cost of health care have a negative impact on business and the economy in general?

5. Describe some of the substantial indirect cost sources associated with chronic illness.
6. Discuss the role of prevention and health promotion in curbing the rise in health care costs.
7. Discuss the process of rationing in health care, and identify nursing's role in shaping this future.
8. Recognizing the importance of science and technology to medicine, nursing, and health care services, discuss current changes and how these will affect health care delivery and future health expenditures.

References

Alzheimer's Association. (2004). Statistics about Alzheimer's Disease. Available on-line at http://www.alz.org/aboutAD/statistics.asp

American Heart Association. (2004). Economic cost of cardiovascular disease. Available on-line at http://www.americanheart.org/statistics/

Asthma and Allergy Foundation. (2000). Facts and statistics. Available on-line at http://www.aafa.org

Barefield, E. (1996). Osteoporosis-related hip fractures cost $13 billion to $18 billion yearly. *Food Review, 1,* 31–36.

Bellandi, D. (1999). A year of more and less: Number of hospital deals drops, but more facilities change hands. *Modern Healthcare, 11,* 48.

Bringewatt, R. J. (1998). Healthcare's next big hurdle. *Healthcare Forum Journal, 41* (5), 14–17.

Casey, M. (1998). Hospital mergers: Where have they gone? *Medical Industry Today.* Available on-line at www.medicaldata.com/MIT

Centers for Disease Control. (2000). *Statistics: Diabetes surveillance, 1999.* Available on-line at http://www.cdc.gov/diabetes/statistics/

Centers for Disease Control (2004). *Chronic Disease Overview.* Available online at: http://www.cdc.gov/ nccd-php/overview.htm

Centers for Medicare and Medicaid (2003). *CMS Statistics.* Baltimore: CMS.

Christopher Reeve Paralysis Foundation (2000). *The facts about spinal cord injury and CNS disorders.* Available on-line at http://paralysis.org/

Congressional Budget Office. (2000a). *The Budget and economic outlook: Fiscal years 2001–2010.* (January) Washington, DC: Government Printing Office.

———. (2000b). *Options to expand federal health, retirement and education activities.* (June). Washington, DC: Government Printing Office.

———. (2004). *The budget and economic outlook: Fiscal years 2005–2014.* Washington, DC: Government Printing Office.

Crippen, D. L. (2000). *Preparing for an aging population.* Congressional Budget Office. Available on-line at http://www.cbo.gov

Drass, J., Kell, S., Osborn, M., Bausell, B., et al. (1998). Diabetes care for Medicare beneficiaries: Attitudes and behaviors of primary care physicians. *Diabetes Care, 21,* (8), 1282–1287.

Enda, J. (2000). Health care is in fashion this year. *Charlotte Observer,* Friday October 20, section 6A.

Frankenfield, D. L., Marciniak, T. A., Drass, J. A., & Jencks, S. (1997). Quality improvement activity directed at the national level: Examples from the Health Care Financing Administration. *Quality Management in Health Care, 5* (4), 12–18.

Getzen, T. E. (2000). Forecasting health expenditure: Short, medium, and long (long) term. *Journal of Health Care Finance, 26* (3), 56–72.

Government Accounting Office. (1999). *Medicare managed care plans: many factors contribute to recent withdrawals; plan interest continues.* Washington, DC: Government Accounting Office.

Groessl, E. J., & Cronan, T. A. (2000). A cost analysis of self-management programs for people with chronic illness. *American Journal of Community Psychology, 28* (4), 455–480.

Hoffman, E. D., McFarland, C. M., & Curtis, C. A. (2002). *Brief Summaries of Medicare and Medicaid.* Office of the Actuary: Centers for Medicare and Medicaid Services.

Levit, K., Cowan, C., Lazenby, H., Sensenig, A., et al. (1999). *Employer health benefits, 1999 annual survey.* Menlo Park, CA: Henry J. Kaiser Family Foundation.

———. (2000). Health spending in 1998: Signals of change. *Health Affairs, 19* (1), 124–132.

Levit, K., Smith, C., Cowan, C., Sensenig, A., et al. (2004). Health spending rebound continues in 2002. *Health Affairs, 23,* 1, 147–159.

National Osteoporosis Foundation. (2004). Statistics. Available on-line at http://www.nof.org/osteoporosis/ diseasefacts.htm

National Rural Health Association. (2000). *Access to health care for the uninsured in rural and frontier America.* Available on-line at http://www.nrharural.org

Newacheck, P., & Hughes, D. (1994). Children with chronic illness and Medicaid managed care. *Pediatrics, 93* (3), 497–451.

Partnership for Solutions (2004). *Chronic conditions: Making the case for ongoing care.* Johns Hopkins University and the Robert Wood Johnson Foundation.

Smith, C., Cowan, C., Sensening, A., & Catlin, A. (2005). Health spending growth slows in 2003. *Health Affairs, 24* (1), 185–94.

U. S. Department of Health and Human Services. (2000). *Healthy People 2010.* (Conference edition, in two volumes). Washington, DC: Government Printing Office.